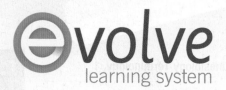

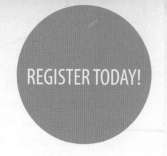
To access your Student Resources, visit:

http://evolve.elsevier.com/Muscolino/muscular

Register today and gain access to:

Student Resources:

* Audio Files
  * Listen to author, Joe Muscolino, read aloud muscle names, attachments, and actions for every muscle covered in the book. Files are downloadable to MP3 devices and CDs for convenient study anywhere you go.
* Practice Test Questions
  * 200 review questions cover all muscle chapters in the book for further study.
* Name That Muscle
  * 169 review exercises help you identify the correct muscle name with its specific muscle image.
* Terminology Crossword Puzzles
  * 22 crossword puzzles help you reinforce muscle names and terminology through fun, interactive activities!
* Drag 'n' Drop Exercises
  * 20 composite muscle illustrations aid in your review of the muscles by dragging the muscle name and dropping it into the correct position on the illustrations.
* Supplementary Appendices
  * 6 appendices posted on the Evolve site provide valuable information for study of muscles on the following topics: soft tissue attachments, palpation guidelines, overview of innervation, overview of arterial supply, additional skeletal muscles, and mnemonics for remembering muscle names.

Instructor Resources:

* TEACH Instructor Resources for The Muscular System Manual: The Skeletal Muscles of the Human Body, ed. 3.
* 1,500 Question ExamView Test Bank
* Image Collection comprised of all images from the third edition textbook
* Image Collection from the second edition textbook

ELSEVIER

THIRD EDITION

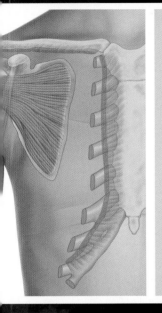

The Muscular System Manual

The Skeletal Muscles of the Human Body

Joseph E. Muscolino, DC

Instructor, Connecticut Center for Massage Therapy
Westport, Connecticut
Owner, The Art and Science of Kinesiology
Redding, Connecticut

ELSEVIER

3251 Riverport Lane
Maryland Heights, Missouri 63043

THE MUSCULAR SYSTEM MANUAL

ISBN: 978-0-323-05723-3

Copyright © 2010 by Mosby, Inc., an affiliate of Elsevier Inc.

Previous editions copyrighted 2003, 2005

Library of Congress Cataloging-in-Publication Data

Muscolino, Joseph E.
 The muscular system manual : the skeletal muscles of the human body / Joseph E. Muscolino.—3rd ed.
  p. ; cm.
 Includes bibliographical references and index.
 ISBN 978-0-323-05723-3 (pbk. : alk. paper)   1. Muscles—Handbooks, manuals, etc.   2. Muscles—Atlases.   3. Manipulation (Therapeutics)—Handbooks, manuals, etc.   4. Manipulation (Therapeutics)—Atlases.   I. Title.
 [DNLM: 1. Musculoskeletal System—anatomy & histology—Atlases.   2. Muscles—physiology—Atlases. WE 17 M9848m 2010]
 QM151.M87 2010
 612.7′4—dc22

                     2009030353

Vice President and Publisher: Linda Duncan
Senior Editor: Kellie White
Senior Developmental Editor: Jennifer Watrous
Publishing Services Manager: Julie Eddy
Senior Project Manager: Celeste Clingan
Design Direction: Amy Buxton

Printed in China

Last digit is the print number: 9 8 7 6 5 4 3 2

This book is dedicated
*to **Simona Cipriani**,*
my wife and angel.

REVIEWERS

David S. Bodoff, DC
Philadelphia, Pennsylvania

Patricia Brady-Lux, DC
Chair of Health Sciences, Department of Education
Connecticut Center for Massage Therapy
Newington, Connecticut

David S. Christian, LMP
Instructor, Department of Kinesiology/Massage Therapy
Everest College
Fife, Washington

Michael Jason Finks, BGS, EMT
Associate Director of Education, Department of Academics
Missouri College
Saint Louis, Missouri

Rebecca S. Fischer, DC, FIACA
Private Practice, Doctors Chiropractic Center, Inc.
Colorado Springs, Colorado
Curriculum Developer/Coordinator
Senior Instructor
Member, Clinical Advisory Board
Activator Methods International
Phoenix, Arizona

David Florkowski, PhD, MEd, ATC, LAT, CEAS, CSCS
Assistant Professor, Department of Kinesiology
Georgia College and State University
Milledgeville, Georgia

Timothy G. Howell, EdD, ATC, CSCS
Athletic Training Education Program Director
Division of Athletic Training
Alfred University
Alfred, New York

Eric W. Mackey, LMT, NCTMB
Lead Instructor, Orthopedic Massage and Sports Massage
Providence Institute of Massage Therapy
Instructor, Neuromuscular Sciences
Arizona School of Acupuncture and Oriental Medicine
Tucson, Arizona

Roger Olbrot
Director of Education, Department of Education
Myotherapy College of Utah
Salt Lake City, Utah
Immediate Past President, American Massage Therapy
    Association
Utah Chapter

Dianne L. Polseno, LPN, LMT
President, Cortiva Institute—Boston
Watertown, Massachusetts

Leigh Simon, LMP, CNA
Instructor, Department of Kinesiology/Massage Therapy
Everest College
Fife, Washington

Karen Stevens, PT, DPT, MS, OCS
Assistant Professor, Department of Physical Therapy
Rosalind Franklin University of Medicine & Science
North Chicago, Illinois

The more than 650 muscles of the human body, when optimally stabilized and integrated, generate an elegant functioning that is truly extraordinary. The static hold of the weightlifter … the leaping twirl of the ballet dancer … the rotational decompression of the pole vaulter at eighteen feet … the stunning accuracy of a left hook … a touchdown pass … or the joyous flip of an exuberant cheerleader. Muscles in motion are the very essence of health, performance, and life itself. Unfortunately, this kinetic symphony sometimes comes to an abrupt halt when pain and injury impact the soft tissues.

As a practicing massage therapist for the past 30 years, I am still often intrigued and amazed by the "stuff" of the athletic injury or the muscular system breakdown: the muscles, tendons, skin, fascia, and ligaments are both promising and puzzling to the dynamics of healing.

This soft tissue "stuff" provides the physiological basis and the therapeutic significance of our hands-on clinical endeavors.

In witnessing the mysterious process of healing, it would seem that the successful hands-on bodyworkers must be adept and comfortable with their right-brain skills. These skills might include postural analysis, revealing global rather than isolated segmental relationships.

Therapeutic compassion and care can jump start the placebo effect. Intuitive hunches often prove more reliable than high tech testing protocols. Clinical reasoning is seldom linear. Skillful palpation includes wandering around in myofascial neighborhoods—and wandering doesn't mean you're lost. Novel explorations and vital discoveries within the soft tissue realm are often guided by literate palpation and three-dimensional visualization.

However, the left-brain skills of anatomical knowledge and objective accuracy are equally vital for successful outcomes. The charismatic extrovert, no matter how reassuring and cheerful, requires a clear understanding of rotator cuff functioning to best serve the client with upper quarter pain. The introverted wisdom of the energy worker is more clinically effective when the attachments and function of the quadratus lumborum are clearly understood. Effective palpation is clearly an art and a science.

Fortunately, compassion and competency are not mutually exclusive skills. Neither are accuracy and artistry. A noted neuromuscular therapist once told me, "To really develop your intuition, know your anatomy!" How true.

So how do we creatively bring the objectivity, the detail and the accuracy of scientific anatomy into the learning process and the ongoing education of the bodywork practitioner?

Some 20 years ago, a groundbreaking event occurred with the publication of Drs. Travell and Simons' *Myofascial Pain and Dysfunction, Volume I.* Physical medicine, manipulative medicine, and bodywork therapies were gifted with a lavishly illustrated and referenced guide to the human muscular system. Massage school curricula began to change. Anatomical competencies were elevated and anatomically-based clinical accuracy was the foundation for many advanced trainings and specialties within the field. "Neutralizing Trigger Points!" became the battle cry for a whole generation of massage therapists. As the therapeutic quest deepened and evolved, it became apparent that trigger points were only one mechanism of pain, dysfunction, and injury … and certainly not the only clinically important aspect of the healing process.

Mystery, nuance, perspective and experimentation, all valid to the therapeutic encounter, seldom develop within rigid formulas. Inquiry, research and dialogue come together to compose a reflective landscape. In recent years, more thoughtful and inclusive bodywork approaches have emerged, encompassing muscle, fascia, function, structure, energetics, mobilization, breathwork, and self-stabilization in forming a new and clinically potent therapeutic philosophy. It became evident that a new foundational textbook, reference and muscular system manifesto was needed … one that would encompass attachments, movement, layers, synergists, palpation skills, an image bank, discussion questions, an instructor's manual, crossword puzzles, and review questions in a four color, user-friendly, and Power Point convertible format.

Such a book has arrived.

The newly revised *The Muscular System Manual,* by Dr. Joseph Muscolino, is a comprehensive, all-in-one resource that scientifically and artfully introduces the student, reinforces the educator, and validates the practitioner in learning and effectively treating the muscular system.

The book's remarkable commitment to precision and detail is underscored by the author's sense of wonder and intellectual curiosity.

The use of color, layout, design, methodology, and muscle group illustration enables the learner to absorb essential information while simultaneously seeing the "big picture" of global and regional relationships. Truly, this is a text that will integratively support the education, clinical practice, and continuing education of the manual therapist.

While conducting a clinical symposium on the iliopsoas complex recently, I used *The Muscular System Manual* as a teaching reference. The drawings, pronunciations, attachments, multiple actions, and learning methodology of this manual greatly facilitated learning outcomes, expertly organized the clinical information, and accurately supported the student learning of palpation and assessment skills. The author's explanation of reverse actions was especially useful, given the multiple action possibilities of this muscle group. The book also documented that psoas minor is absent in 40% of the population, the lumbar plexus is located within the belly of psoas major, and the tenderloin cut of steak is actually the cow's psoas major!

I believe massage therapy education should be informative, interactive and fun. *The Muscular System Manual* not only supports these goals, it stands on its own as a superb teaching reference book.

The author is a practicing chiropractor, massage school anatomy instructor, and an activist for professional standards of competency. He has served as a test specification expert in the fields of anatomy, physiology, and kinesiology for the

National Certification Board of Therapeutic Massage and Bodywork Job Analysis Survey Task Force. He is the author of numerous anatomical and clinical features in *Journal of Bodywork and Movement Therapies* and *Massage Therapy Journal.*

Perhaps equally important, Dr. Muscolino has a twinkle in his eye and a profoundly animated response whenever discussions veer into the realm of muscles and movement. I believe *The Muscular System Manual* reflects his vast knowledge, his creative vision, and the twinkle in his eye. *The Muscular System Manual* is the most current and informative reference for the human muscular system and its potential for function and creative movement.

This book will last you a lifetime.

Robert K. King
August 11, 2004

Although I often wonder why some texts go through second and third editions, such was not the case with Joe Muscolino's *The Muscular System Manual*! This new and spectacularly upgraded edition certainly establishes the author as the leading muscular system expert for manual therapists in this country. Indeed, the upgrades, resources, and knowledge base of this text are nothing short of brilliant.

Initially, Chapters 1 to 3 provide new and innovative material on how the muscular system works with a detailed overview of the roles of bones, joints, and connective tissues. Dr. Muscolino's valuable perspective on the muscular system, the primary user of body energy, provides a perspective and background that would be of value to any manual or movement therapy student, even the individual with a very limited knowledge base. The location terminology, color drawings, bony structure, and movement presentations provide a basic kinesiology foundation that serves as a cornerstone for the rest of the book.

All of the muscles featured (yes, all of them!) are now re-ordered to their respective joints, making the flow and portability of this edition superior to other texts. Furthermore, it coincides with the way that most muscular/myology/kinesiology classes are taught in massage and other bodywork schools. This is an especially useful adjunct for today's student of the healing arts, offering a more systematic portrayal of muscular system and body functioning.

Remarkably enough, this edition is even more thorough than its predecessor in the presentation of muscle function. The author painstakingly presents not only the muscular attachments, but also expands the functional information of each muscle to include the concentric, shortening mover actions, and the reverse mover actions, as well as the eccentric lengthening and isometric stabilization actions. Incredible! These features alone are missing from other bodywork texts, and this material provides a more comprehensive understanding of muscle functioning at all levels.

Reverse mover actions are important because they explain, for instance, why the tensor fasciae latae (TFL) is not only a flexor of the thigh at the hip joint and an abductor and medial rotator of the thigh at the same joint, but also how its reverse actions anteriorly tilt the pelvis and ipsilaterally rotate and depress that side of the pelvis as well. This alone marks TFL as an overlooked source of low back pain, scoliotic compensation, sacroiliac dysfunction and a vitally essential muscle to release in the classic lower crossed syndrome. Useful hands-on and palpatory insights such as this abound throughout this exciting new edition. Simply reviewing this copy generated new clinical insights for me for several clients with whom I currently provide clinical massage. It will be a primary resource in my treatment room for years to come.

Consequently, not only will the student, but also the experienced manual therapist, benefit from this clinically relevant information, presented, once again, in a clear and systematic fashion. Fully expect your knowledge of challenging therapeutic cases to increase with this new edition, which is the most thorough book on muscle functioning currently available. I believe this text will also upgrade, if not revolutionize, the teaching of the muscular system, moving away from useless memorizations and dogma to functionally important information, descriptions, and solid explanations plotted out with careful reasoning.

New and improved color drawings are ubiquitous throughout this edition. Full-color drawings are featured individually, within muscle or function groups and also drawn on real persons, giving learners a vivid presentation of location, palpation, and attachment points. This feature alone will clarify concepts, and stimulate the visual learner to an even deeper awareness of the spectacular movements of the human body and the intricate combination of forces that generate optimal functioning.

An interactive CD is included with the textbook that is a first of its kind! Each of the base illustrations is given showing the body and the skeleton along with a list of all the muscles of that region. The student can then build the muscular system on the illustration, choosing any combination of muscles to show next to each other. Do you want to see the TFL next to the sartorius? Perhaps add in the gluteus medius and/or iliopsoas? You choose. This CD alone will greatly enhance the beginner student's ability to learn the muscles, as well as challenge seasoned therapists to better learn their anatomy. It helps students and therapists alike, not only learn the individual muscles, but also begin the incredibly important and needed clinical task of putting the muscular system back together! This along with audio files of the attachments and actions that allow the student to burn CDs and MP3 files to study on-the-go are alone worth the price of admission to the book.

The newly added Chapter 19 contains functional mover groups of muscles illustrating the concentric, reverse, eccentric, and isometric stabilization functions—once again showcased with excellent new drawings. The second part of this chapter illustrates (with the gracious permission of rolfer and myofascial innovator Tom Myers) the essential myofascial meridians depicting the fascial webbings and relationships of connective tissue that assist with movement and posture. This is yet another feature of *The Muscular System Manual* that underlies its premier status as the most complete book available on this wondrous and vital system of the human body.

The author has truly created a work of science and art masterfully blended for optimal results!

Bob King

August 3, 2009

Bob King, LMT, NCTMB

Bob King has authored manuals, books, videos, curricula, and numerous clinical articles in a massage therapy career spanning more than three decades. He is a Cortiva Educational Consultant and conducts advanced myofascial trainings throughout the country. He is the founder and past president of the Chicago School of Massage Therapy, served two terms as AMTA National President, and is widely regarded as a successful innovator, activist, and educator within the profession. In 2009, Bob was named to the Massage Therapy Hall of Fame. In 2004, he received the Distinguished Service Award for the Massage Therapy Foundation for visionary leadership.

The Muscular System Manual: The Skeletal Muscles of the Human Body, 3rd edition, is meant to be the most thorough atlas of muscle function that is available. Instead of simply listing muscle attachments and actions that are typically taught, The Muscular System Manual comprehensively covers all muscle functions of each muscle. Shortening action functions with their reverse actions are addressed, as well as eccentric and stabilization functions. By offering the student the full picture of muscle function, it actually makes the task of learning the muscles easier, not harder. Students can grasp the information more quickly because they understand it and do not have to memorize it.

■ WHO WILL BENEFIT FROM THIS BOOK?

This book is primarily written for students and practicing therapists of manual and movement therapies, including massage therapy, physical therapy, chiropractic, osteopathy, orthopedists, athletic training, yoga, Pilates, and Feldenkrais. However, anyone who needs to learn the skeletal muscles of the body will find this book invaluable and essential. Unlike many books, you will not outgrow The Muscular System Manual. It will be your guide as you first learn the muscles of the body, and it will remain an invaluable resource on your bookshelf for as long as you are in practice.

■ CONCEPTUAL APPROACH

The approach taken by The Muscular System Manual is unique. Instead of simply listing information, it teaches the information and makes it understandable, allowing for true critical thinking. The beginning chapters set the framework for how muscles work as well as give a five-step approach to learning muscles. Each individual muscle then has notes that explain how the actions can be reasoned out instead of memorized. The goal of this book is to enable the student/therapist/trainer/physician to be able to critically think through muscle functioning when working clinically with clients and patients.

■ ORGANIZATION

The Muscular System Manual is organized into five Parts. Part 1 covers the basic language of kinesiology that the student needs to be able to understand muscle attachments and functions and also communicate with other members of the health care and fitness fields. Parts 2 through 4 systematically cover each of the major muscles of the body, presenting in a clear and organized manner the essential information of every muscle. The beginning of each chapter in these parts opens with large group illustrations of the muscles of the joint region. Each muscle then has an individual layout in which the muscle's attachments, functions, innervation, arterial supply, palpation, relationship to other structures, and other miscellaneous information that is intellectually and clinically relevant are given. Part 5 presents illustrations of all the major functional joint action mover groups of muscles as well as illustrations of the muscles of the pelvic floor and myofascial meridians of the body.

■ DISTINCTIVE FEATURES OF THIS BOOK

There are many features that distinguish this book:
- The most thorough coverage of muscle function available
- Explanations to understand the muscle's actions that promote critical thinking
- Information presented in a layered à la carte approach that allows each student or instructor to determine what content is covered.
- Beautiful illustrations in which the bones and muscles are placed on a photograph of a real person.
- Large group illustrations for every functional group
- Myofascial meridian information for every muscle
- Bulleted clear and easy to follow palpations for each muscle.
- An interactive CD that allows for any combination of muscles to be placed on the skeleton and body.

■ NEW TO THIS EDITION

Although most features of the 2nd edition have been preserved, the 3rd edition of The Muscular System Manual has many new features:
- Updated illustrations that place the muscles and bones on a photograph of a real person for the most accurate understanding of the relationship of the muscles to the client's/patient's body.
- Expanded coverage of muscle function to cover all mover actions and their reverse actions, as well as all antagonist eccentric and isometric stabilization functions.
- Large group illustrations of all the functional mover groups of muscles.
- Myofascial meridian information for every muscle, and myofascial meridian illustrations

- Organization of the muscles by joint action
- An interactive CD that allows the student to learn and study the muscles by placing them in any combination on illustrations.
- An audio feature on the Evolve website in which the author reads aloud the names, attachments, and major actions of all the muscles; ideal for studying and learning while on-the-go.

■ LEARNING AIDS

- The attachment and functions information is presented in a layered à la carte approach that allows the student to decide at what depth to learn the information.
- This book is meant to be used not only as a textbook, but also as an in-class manual. For this reason, checkboxes are provided for each muscle layout as well as each piece of information. This allows the student to check off exactly what content will be learned. Instructors, having students check off content covered allows for extremely clear expectations of what they are responsible for.
- Arrows are placed over the muscle for each individual muscle illustration so that the line of pull of the muscle can be seen and visually understood. This allows for the actions of the muscle to be understood instead of memorized.
- A Miscellaneous section is provided that offers interesting insights to each muscle. Many of these are clinical applications that flesh out and make learning the muscle more interesting.

■ ANCILLARIES

This edition of *The Muscular System Manual* includes an interactive CD that is a first of its kind. A base photograph of the region of the body is presented with the skeleton drawn in. A list of every muscle of that region is given and you can choose any combination of muscles and place them onto the illustration, allowing you to not only see that muscle's attachments, but more importantly, to be able to see the relationship between all the muscles of the region. *Any combination* of muscles can be chosen!

■ EVOLVE ONLINE RESOURCES

This book is backed up by an Evolve website that includes the following student resources:

- An audio feature in which the author reads aloud the names, attachments, and major actions of all the muscles. This allows for studying while commuting or for use with an MP3 device. Ideal for studying and learning while on the go!

- Interactive review exercises such as crossword puzzles, Drag 'n' Drop labelling exercises, and Name That Muscle quizzes for further review of the skeletal muscles of the human body.
- 200 short-answer review questions to reinforce knowledge learned in the book.
- Supplemental appendices featuring valuable information on the following topics: soft tissue attachments, palpation guidelines, overview of innervation, overview of arterial supply, additional skeletal muscles, and mnemonics for remembering muscle names.

■ OTHER RESOURCES

For instructors, the entire book is available in 50-minute PowerPoint lectures, with learning outcomes, discussion topics, and critical thinking questions. There is also an instructor's manual that provides step-by-step approaches to leading the class through learning the muscles, as well as case studies that allow for a critical thinking application of the muscles to common musculoskeletal conditions. Further, a complete image collection that contains every figure in the book, and a test bank in ExamView containing 1,500 questions, are provided.

■ RELATED PUBLICATIONS

The Muscular System Manual is also supported by an excellent coloring book and set of flash cards that can be purchased separately. Look for *Musculoskeletal Anatomy Coloring Book, 2nd Ed.* and *Musculoskeletal Anatomy Flash Cards, 2nd Ed.*, published by Mosby/Elsevier. For more on muscle palpation, look for *The Muscle and Bone Palpation Manual, With Trigger Points, Referral Patterns, and Stretching* (Mosby/Elsevier, 2009).

■ NOTE TO THE STUDENT

This book is thick and packed with information. You can choose exactly how much you want to learn. If you are a beginner to learning muscles, the outstanding illustrations and the simple and clear explanations will make learning muscles easy. If you are an advanced student of the muscular system, the depth of information will help you reach new levels of knowledge and clinical application. You will not outgrow this book. Whether as an in-class manual or a reference text for your bookshelf, you will find this book to be an ideal and essential book now and into the future!

Joseph E. Muscolino, DC

1 Muscle and Group Name (if applicable), covered in a 2–3 page spread.

2 Illustration of individual muscle, with arrows indicating lines of pull. Bony attachments are shaded in brown for easy identification. Muscle is deep to (behind) a bone from this. Figures are full color anatomic illustrations of muscles and bones drawn over photographs to help identify positions of the structures. The positions of muscles and bones in the human body are unmistakable in this overlay artwork.

3 Checkboxes are used throughout the 2–3 page individual muscle spreads so you can mark information to be covered or check it off once you have learned the material.

4 A first look at the name of the muscle to see what free information the name gives us.

5 Derivation and proper pronunciation of the muscle are provided here.

6 Simple attachment (origin) information. (Note: For illustrations of bones, bony landmarks, and muscle attachment sites, see Chapter 2.)

7 More detailed attachment (origin) information.

8 Simple attachment (insertion) information. (Note: If more detailed attachment [insertion] information is present, it will follow directly after this section.)

9 Functions section: This section covers every contraction function of the muscle. This information serves to make The Muscular System Manual more complete, giving a comprehensive presentation of musculoskeletal function. (Note: For an explanation of muscle function, see Chapter 3.)

10 Concentric (Shortening) Mover Actions table: The actions (standard and reverse) that are usually taught at a beginning or intermediate level are in bold print within the table. The remaining actions within the table are for more advanced levels of learning. (Note: For illustrations of joint actions, see Chapter 1.)

11 Standard Mover Action notes: Methodology information that explains the reasoning behind each of the muscle's standard actions.

12 Reverse Mover Action notes: Methodology information that explains the reasoning behind each of the muscle's reverse actions.

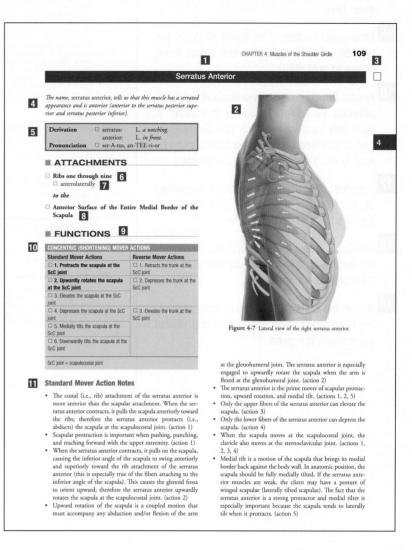

Figure 4-7 Lateral view of the right serratus anterior.

13 Eccentric and Isometric Functions and Notes: The importance of core stabilization (isometric contraction) in exercise and rehabilitation has become increasingly understood in recent years, and negative (eccentric) contractions are used more and more in exercise. Coverage of this information is unique to this book.

14 Additional notes on the muscle's actions are given here.

15 Innervation section: Two levels of detail are provided, with the predominant spinal levels shown in bold print.

16 Arterial Supply section: Two levels of detail are provided. (Note: Arterial supply to muscles is extremely variable. Although specific information is provided here, this variability must be kept in mind when learning this material.)

17 Palpation section: Easy-to-follow numbered steps to palpate the muscle. See the Evolve website for palpation guidelines.

18 Relationship section: Gives information regarding the muscle's anatomic relationship to other musculoskeletal structures.

19 Miscellaneous section: In this section, interesting information about the muscle and clinical applications are given.

---

110   PART 2 The Skeletal Muscles of the Upper Extremity

Serratus Anterior—cont'd

- Downward tilt of the scapula is a motion wherein the inferior angle of the scapula is pulled back against the body wall. In anatomic position, the scapula should be fully downwardly tilted. (action 6)

Reverse Mover Action Notes **12**

- The reverse action of retracting the trunk (i.e., moving it posteriorly) relative to the scapula at the scapulocostal joint is best seen when performing a push-up. At the point in a push-up when the body has been pushed up away from the ground and the elbow joints are fully extended, there is a small additional degree of upward movement of the body. This motion is created by the serratus anterior pulling the trunk up (posteriorly) toward the scapulae, which are now fixed due to the hands being placed on the floor. (reverse action 1)
- The reverse action of depression of the trunk relative to the scapula at the scapulocostal joint might occur if the arms are flexed 180 degrees overhead with the hands fixed to an immovable object when lying down and the body is pulled downward away from the immovable object. (reverse action 2)
- The reverse action of elevation of the trunk relative to the scapula at the scapulocostal joint is not very likely to occur. (reverse action 3)

13 **Eccentric Antagonist Functions**

1. Restrains/slows scapular retraction, downward rotation, depression, elevation, lateral tilt, and upward tilt
2. Restrains/slows protraction, elevation, and depression of the trunk

13 **Isometric Stabilization Functions**

1. Stabilizes the scapula
2. Stabilizes the rib cage

Isometric Stabilization Function Note

1. The stabilization of the scapula function of the serratus anterior is particularly important for maintaining a healthy posture of the scapula. The serratus anterior is the most important muscle for preventing lateral tilt (winging) and upward tilt of the scapula.

14 **Additional Notes on Actions**

1. Some sources state that the uppermost fibers of the serratus anterior can downwardly rotate and laterally tilt the scapula.
2. There is controversy regarding whether or not the serratus anterior is involved with respiration by moving the ribcage. Given its attachments onto the ribs, an accessory respiratory action seems likely.

15 **INNERVATION**
- The Long Thoracic Nerve
  - **C5**, C6, C7

16 **ARTERIAL SUPPLY**
- The Dorsal Scapular Artery (a branch of the Subclavian Artery) and the Lateral Thoracic Artery (a branch of the Axillary Artery)
  - and the Superior Thoracic Artery (a branch of the Axillary Artery)

PALPATION **17**

1. With the client supine and the arm flexed to 90 degrees at the shoulder joint (hand pointed toward the ceiling), place palpating hand on the rib cage on the lateral trunk between the anterior and posterior axillary folds of tissue.
2. Have the client protract the scapula by pushing the hand toward the ceiling and feel for the contraction of the serratus anterior. Resistance may be added.
3. Once located, try to follow the serratus anterior as far anterior as possible (deep to the pectoralis major) and as far posterior as possible (deep to the latissimus dorsi and the scapula).

18 ■ **RELATIONSHIP TO OTHER STRUCTURES**

- From the posterior perspective, the majority of the serratus anterior lies deep to the scapula and the latissimus dorsi. From the anterior perspective, it lies deep to the pectoralis major and minor.
- The serratus anterior is superficial anterolaterally on the trunk where it meets the external abdominal oblique.
- The lowest four to five slips of the costal (i.e., rib) attachments of the serratus anterior interdigitate with the external abdominal oblique.
- The serratus anterior lies next to (anterior to) the subscapularis.
- The serratus anterior is located within the spiral line myofascial meridian.

19 ■ **MISCELLANEOUS**

1. The serrated appearance comes from attaching onto separate ribs, which creates the notched look of a serrated knife.
2. In very well-developed individuals, the serratus anterior looks like ribs standing out in the anterolateral trunk.
3. The serratus anterior can be considered to have three parts: the first part attaching from ribs one and two to the superior angle of the scapula, the second part from ribs two and three to the length of the medial border of the scapula, and the third part from ribs four through nine to the inferior angle of the scapula. The third part (most inferior part) of the serratus anterior is the strongest.
4. The serratus anterior usually blends into the rhomboids on the anterior side of the scapula.

No book of this magnitude can be achieved without help. I would like to express my gratitude to so many people who aided and supported me in the production of this book. This book would not exist today if it were not for the help and support that all of you have given me.

Much of the beauty and success of this book rests in the beautiful illustrations of muscles and bones drawn over photographs of models. Photography was done by Yanik Chauvin and the principle model is Audrey Van Herck, both of Montreal, Canada. The artists are Frank Forney and Dave Carlson of Colorado and Giovanni Rimasti of Canada. A big thank you is also due to Jodie Bernard of Laserwords in Canada. Many of the illustrations from Chapters 1–3 were artfully done by Jean Luciano of Connecticut and Jeanne Robertson of St. Louis and borrowed from my Kinesiology textbook.

The art direction and layout set the tone of this book. Thank you to Julia Dummitt for making a muscle book so attractive to look at and so easy to negotiate. Putting together a book of this size is no small feat. Thank you to the Production people at Elsevier, especially Celeste Clingan and Linda McKinley. And a special thank you to the Editorial team at Elsevier, who worked hand in hand with me throughout this entire project. Thank you to Kellie White for shepherding this project along. And unending appreciation to Jennifer Watrous, my Developmental Editor. Jennifer has worked with me on every step of this project, large and small, along the way.

A continuing thank you to Dr. Sharon Sawitzke, Ph.D., Associate Professor, Division of Anatomical Sciences at the University of Bridgeport, College of Chiropractic, who lent her expertise to provide the information regarding the arterial supply to the muscles. I could not have simplified and organized this material without her. And continuing thanks to David Elliot, Ph.D. of the Touro University College of Osteopathic Medicine, my content editor, who combed through the original edition of this book, ensuring that the informational content was correct. He also fielded countless questions from me, helping me organize the content and provided needed information when the boundaries of my knowledge had been reached.

Thank you also to Tom Myers of Maine who graciously lent of his knowledge and was generous with illustrations from the second edition of his book, *Anatomy Trains*.

I would like to thank Dr. Michael Carnes, my first anatomy instructor, of Western States Chiropractic College in Portland, Oregon. He first whetted my appetite for learning, understanding, and appreciating the beauty of anatomy and physiology.

I believe that textbook writing is essentially "teaching on pages." I am so lucky to have had the best field training that anyone could ask for. Teaching at the Connecticut Center for Massage Therapy (CCMT) over the past 23 years has shaped me as a writer. I don't think my students realize just how much I was, and am still, learning along with them. Thank you to the many teaching assistants I was lucky enough to have through the years. So many of them not only assisted in the classroom, but also improved my teaching by showing me ways of more clearly explaining and demonstrating the material to our students. Thank you also to the staff and faculty at CCMT. They change teaching at CCMT from being simply a job, to feeling as if I am part of an extended family away from home. And I always reserve a special acknowledgement to one student (and now a fellow instructor), William Courtland, who one day uttered the simple words, "You should write a book." Those words began my writing career.

Lastly, I must express my love and appreciation to my entire family for their unending love, support, and understanding as I sat at my computer hour after hour after hour working on this book.

Dr. Joe Muscolino has been teaching musculoskeletal and visceral anatomy and physiology, kinesiology, neurology, and pathology courses at the Connecticut Center for Massage Therapy (CCMT) for over 23 years. He has also been instrumental in course manual development and assisted with curriculum development at CCMT.

Dr. Muscolino has also published:
- Musculoskeletal Anatomy Coloring Book
- Kinesiology: The Skeletal System and Muscle Function
- The Muscle and Bone Palpation Manual, with Trigger Points, Referral Patterns, and Stretching
- Musculoskeletal Anatomy Flashcards
- Flashcards for Bones, Joints, and Actions of the Human Body
- Flashcards for Palpation, Trigger Points, and Referral Patterns
- Mosby's Trigger Point Flip Chart with Referral Patterns and Stretching.

Dr. Muscolino writes the column article, Body Mechanics, in The **Massage Therapy Journal** (MTJ) and has written for the Journal of Bodywork and Movement Therapies (JBMT).

Dr. Muscolino teaches continuing education workshops on such topics as body mechanics, deep tissue massage, stretching and advanced stretching, joint mobilization, palpation, orthopedic assessment, musculoskeletal pathologic conditions, anatomy and physiology, kinesiology, and cadaver workshops.

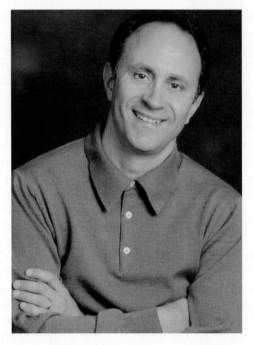

He also runs instructor in-services for kinesiology instructors. He is an approved provider of continuing education (CE); and CE credit is available through the NCBTMB for Massage Therapists and Bodyworkers toward certification renewal. He is also a member of the NCBTMB Exam Committee.

Dr. Joe Muscolino holds a Bachelor of Arts degree in Biology from the State University of New York at Binghamton, Harpur College. He attained his Doctor of Chiropractic Degree from Western States Chiropractic College in Portland, Oregon and is licensed in Connecticut, New York, and California. Dr. Muscolino has been in private practice in Connecticut for more than 24 years and incorporates soft tissue work into his chiropractic practice for all of his patients.

If you would like further information regarding *The Muscular System Manual: The Skeletal Muscles of the Human Body* or any of Dr. Muscolino's other publications, or if you are an instructor and would like information regarding the many supportive materials such as *PowerPoint* slides, test banks of questions, or TEACH instructor's manuals, please visit http://www.us.elsevierhealth.com. If you would like information regarding Dr. Muscolino's workshops, or if you would like to contact Dr. Muscolino directly, please visit his website: www.learnmuscles.com.

xvii

Basic Kinesiology Terminology

It is not possible to discuss muscle function without fluency in the language of kinesiology (Box 1-1). The reason why specific kinesiology terms exist is that they help us to avoid the ambiguities of lay language. Therefore embracing and using these terms is extremely important in the health care field, where someone's health depends on clear communication. The purpose of this chapter is to provide an overview of the basic terms of kinesiology that are needed. ⓔvolve Further explanation of kinesiology terminology is provided on the Evolve website that accompanies this book. For an indepth and thorough discussion of the terminology of kinesiology, see *Kinesiology: The Skeletal System and Muscle Function* (Elsevier, 2007).

■ MAJOR BODY PARTS

Motions of the body involve movement of body parts. To be able to describe the body part's motion, we must be able to accurately name it. Figure 1-1 illustrates the major divisions and body parts of the human body. The two major divisions are the axial body and the appendicular body. The appendicular body can be divided into the upper extremities and the lower extremities.

The names of most body parts are identical to the lay English names for them. However, there are a few cases where kinesiology terms are very specific and need to be observed. For example, the term *arm* is used to refer to the region of the upper extremity that is located between the shoulder and elbow joints. The term *forearm* refers to the body part that is located between the elbow and wrist joints; the forearm is a separate body part and not considered to be part of the arm. Similarly, the term *leg* describes the region of the lower extremity that is located between the knee and ankle joints, whereas the term *thigh* is used to describe an entirely separate body part that is located between the hip and knee joints; the thigh is not part of the leg. The precise use of these terms is essential so that movements of the leg and thigh are not confused with each other, and movements of the arm and forearm are not confused with each other. Another term that should be noted is *pelvis*. The pelvis is a separate body part from the trunk and is located between the trunk and thighs.

BOX 1-1

The term *kinesiology* literally means the study of motion. Given that motion of our body occurs when bones move at joints, and that muscles are the primary creator of the forces that move the bones, kinesiology is the study of the musculoskeletal system. Because the muscles are controlled and directed by the nervous system, it might be more accurate to expand kinesiology to be the study of the neuromusculoskeletal system.

■ ANATOMIC POSITION

Anatomic position is a standard reference position that is used to define terms that describe the physical location of structures of the body and points on the body. In anatomic position, the person is standing erect, facing forward, with the arms at the sides, the palms facing forward, and the fingers and toes extended (Figure 1-2). Note: Given that movement terminology is based on location terminology, anatomic position is ultimately the foundation for movement terminology as well.

■ LOCATION TERMINOLOGY

Now that anatomic position has been defined, it can be used as the reference position for location terms that describe the relative locations of body parts, structures, and points on the body to each other. Location terminology is composed of directional terms that come in pairs, each member of the pair being the opposite of the other.

Pairs of Terms

Anterior/Posterior
Anterior means farther to the front; *posterior* means farther to the back. These terms can be used for the entire body, axial and appendicular.

Note: The term *ventral* is sometimes used for anterior, and the term *dorsal* is sometimes used for posterior. The true defini-

1

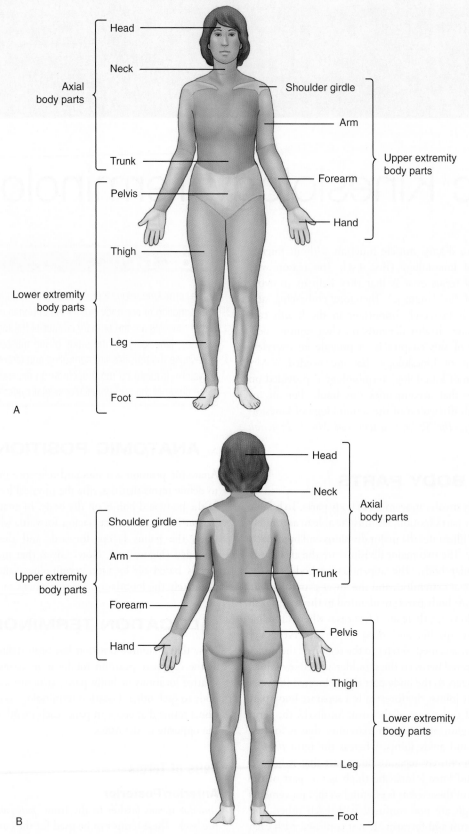

Figure 1-1 The three major divisions of the body are the axial body and the two divisions of the appendicular body. The appendicular body is composed of the upper extremities and lower extremities. Furthermore, the body parts within these major divisions are shown. **A,** Anterior view. **B,** Posterior view.

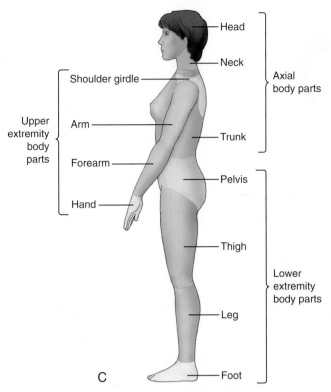

Figure 1-1, cont'd C, Lateral view.

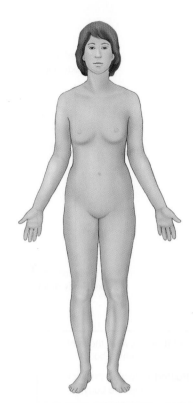

Figure 1-2 Anatomic position is a reference position of the body in which the person is standing erect, facing forward, with the arms at the sides, the palms facing forward, and the fingers and toes extended.

tion of ventral is the soft belly surface of a body part; dorsal refers to the harder surface on the other side of the body part. In the lower extremity, anterior/ventral and posterior/dorsal are not synonymous. The ventral surface of the thigh is the medial surface, of the leg is the posterior surface, and of the foot is the plantar surface.

Medial/Lateral

Medial means closer to an imaginary midline that divides the body into left and right halves; *lateral* means farther from this imaginary midline. These terms can be used for the entire body, axial and appendicular.

Superior/Inferior

Superior means above (toward the head); *inferior* means below (away from the head). These terms are usually used for the axial body only.

Proximal/Distal

Proximal means closer (i.e., more proximity) to the axial body; *distal* means farther (i.e., more distant) from the axial body. These terms are used for the appendicular body only.

Superficial/Deep

Superficial means closer to the surface of the body; *deep* means farther from the surface of the body (i.e., more internal). These terms can be used for the entire body, axial and appendicular. Note: When employing the terms *superficial* and *deep,* it is recommended to always state from which perspective you are viewing the body.

Radial/Ulnar

The terms *radial* and *ulnar* can be used for the forearm and hand in place of the terms *lateral* and *medial,* respectively. The radius is the lateral bone of the forearm; the ulna is the medial bone.

Tibial/Fibular

The terms *tibial* and *fibular* can be used for the leg and sometimes the foot in place of the terms *medial* and *lateral,* respectively. The tibia is the medial bone of the leg; the fibula is the lateral bone.

Palmar/Dorsal

The terms *palmar* and *dorsal* can be used for the hand in place of the terms *anterior* and *posterior,* respectively.

Plantar/Dorsal

The terms *plantar* and *dorsal* can be used for the foot. The plantar surface of the foot is the undersurface that is planted on the ground. The dorsal surface is the top or dorsum of the foot.

Cranial/Caudal

Cranial means toward the head; *caudal* means toward the "tail" of the body. These terms are used for the axial body only.

Combining Terms of Location

These terms that describe location can be combined together. Similar to combining terms such as *north* and *west* to create

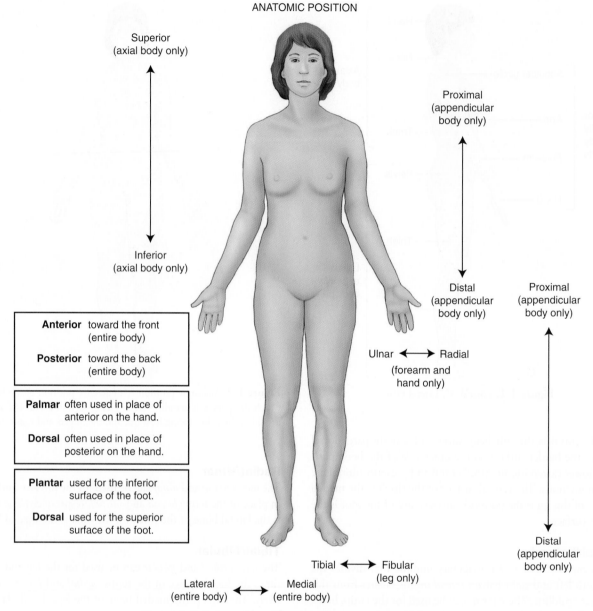

ANATOMIC POSITION

Superior
(axial body only)

Proximal
(appendicular
body only)

Inferior
(axial body only)

Distal
(appendicular
body only)

Proximal
(appendicular
body only)

Anterior toward the front
(entire body)

Posterior toward the back
(entire body)

Palmar often used in place of
anterior on the hand.

Dorsal often used in place of
posterior on the hand.

Plantar used for the inferior
surface of the foot.

Dorsal used for the superior
surface of the foot.

Ulnar ←→ Radial
(forearm and
hand only)

Distal
(appendicular
body only)

Tibial ←→ Fibular
(leg only)

Lateral
(entire body)

Medial
(entire body)

Figure 1-3 Various terms of location relative to anatomic position.

northwest, location terms can be combined. When doing this, the end of the first word is usually dropped and the letter *o* is placed to connect the two words. For example, anterior and lateral combine to become anterolateral. Although there is no hard and fast rule, anterior and posterior are usually placed first when combined with other terms.

Figure 1-3 is an anterior view of a person, illustrating the terms of relative location as they pertain to the body.

■ PLANES

Planes are flat surfaces that cut through and can be used to map three-dimensional space. Because space is three-dimensional, there are three major planes, known as cardinal planes. The three cardinal planes are the sagittal plane, frontal plane, and transverse plane (Box 1-2). A sagittal plane divides the body into left

BOX 1-2

The frontal plane is also known as the coronal plane. The transverse plane is also known as the horizontal plane.

and right portions. A frontal plane divides the body into front and back (anterior and posterior) portions. A transverse plane divides the body into upper and lower (superior and inferior or proximal and distal) portions. Each of the three cardinal planes is perpendicular to the other two cardinal planes. Any plane that is not perfectly sagittal, frontal, or transverse is described as an oblique plane. Therefore an oblique plane has components of two or three cardinal planes. Figure 1-4 illustrates two examples each of the three cardinal planes and an oblique plane.

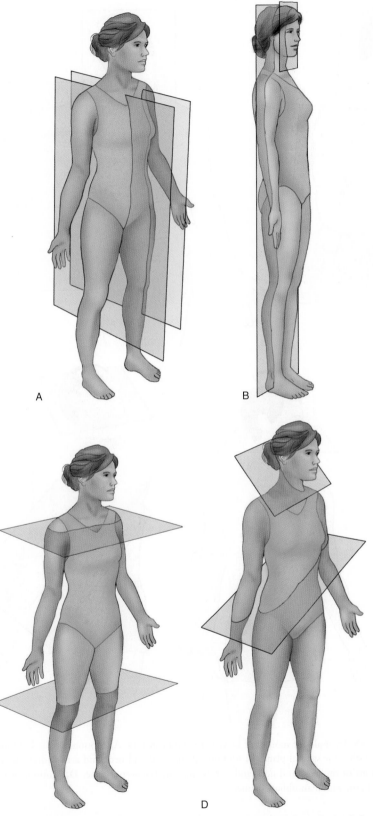

Figure 1-4 Anterolateral views of the body, illustrating the three cardinal planes (sagittal, frontal, and transverse) and oblique planes. **A,** Two examples of sagittal planes; a sagittal plane divides the body into left and right portions. **B,** Two examples of frontal planes; a frontal plane divides the body into anterior and posterior portions. **C,** Two examples of transverse planes; a transverse plane divides the body into upper (superior and/or proximal) and lower (inferior and/or distal) portions. **D,** Two examples of oblique planes; an oblique plane is a plane that is not exactly sagittal, frontal or transverse (i.e., it has components of two or three cardinal planes). The upper oblique plane has frontal and transverse components to it; the lower oblique plane has sagittal and transverse components to it.

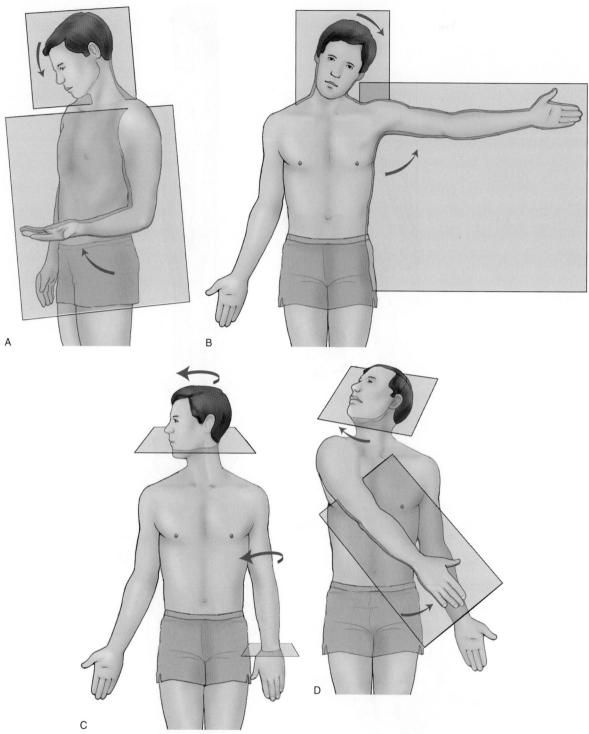

Figure 1-5 Examples of motion of body parts within planes. **A,** Motions of the head and neck and forearm within the sagittal plane. **B,** Motions of the head and neck and arm within the frontal plane. **C,** Motions of the head and neck and arm within the transverse plane. **D,** Motions of the head and neck and arm within an oblique plane.

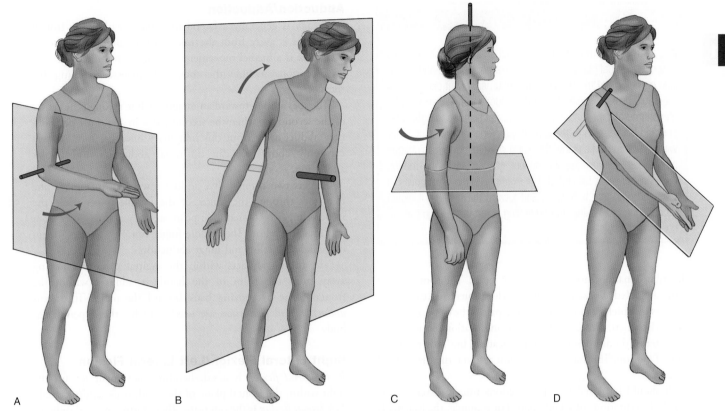

Figure 1-6 A to D, Anterolateral views that illustrate the corresponding axes for the three cardinal planes and an oblique plane; the axes are shown as red tubes. Note that an axis always runs perpendicular to the plane in which the motion is occurring. **A,** Motion occurring in the sagittal plane; because this motion is occurring around an axis that is running horizontally in a medial to lateral orientation, it is called the mediolateral axis. **B,** Motion occurring in the frontal plane; because this motion is occurring around an axis that is running horizontally in an anterior to posterior orientation, it is called the antero-posterior axis. **C,** Motion occurring in the transverse plane; because this motion is occurring around an axis that is running vertically in a superior to inferior orientation, it is called the superoinferior axis, or more simply, the vertical axis. **D,** Motion occurring in an oblique plane; this motion is occurring around an axis that is running perpendicular to that plane (i.e., it is the oblique axis for this oblique plane).

Motion of the Body within Planes

Planes become extremely important when we describe the motion of a body part through space, because the body part moves within a plane. Hence, by defining the planes of space, we can describe the path of motion of a body part when it moves. Note that the sagittal and frontal planes are vertical and the transverse plane is horizontal. Therefore motions within the sagittal and frontal planes move vertically up and down and motions within the transverse plane move horizontally. Figure 1-5 illustrates examples of motion within the three cardinal planes and an oblique plane.

■ AXES

An *axis* (plural: *axes*) is an imaginary line around which a body part moves. If a body part moves in a circular path around an axis, it is described as an axial motion. If the body part moves in a straight line, it is described as a nonaxial motion. Both axial and nonaxial motions of a body part move within a plane.

However, an axial motion moves within a plane and moves around an axis. The orientation of an axis for movement is always perpendicular to the plane within which the movement is occurring.

Each plane has its own corresponding axis; therefore there are three cardinal axes. The axis for sagittal plane movements is oriented side to side and described as the mediolateral axis, the axis for frontal plane movements is oriented front to back and described as anteroposterior, and the axis for transverse plane movements is oriented up and down and described as superoinferior or simply vertical. Each oblique plane also has its own corresponding axis, which is perpendicular to it. Figure 1-6 illustrates axial motions that occur within planes and around their corresponding axes.

■ MOVEMENT TERMINOLOGY

Using anatomic position, we are able to define terms that describe static locations on the body. We now need to define terms that

1

BOX 1-3

It is extremely important to point out that joint action terms describe cardinal plane motions. For example, flexion and extension of the arm at the shoulder (glenohumeral) joint occur within the sagittal plane, abduction and adduction of the arm at the glenohumeral joint occur within the frontal plane, and right rotation and left rotation of the arm at the glenohumeral joint occur within the transverse plane. If the arm were to move in an oblique plane, then to describe its motion, its cardinal plane motion components must be stated. For example, if the arm moves in a straight line that is forward and toward the midline, it would be described as flexing and adducting, even though it moves in only one direction.

describe dynamic movements of the body. These movement terms are called *joint actions.* Similar to location terms, they come in pairs in which each member of the pair is the opposite of the other (Box 1-3). However, different from location terms, movement terms do not describe a static location, but rather a direction of motion. The major pairs of joint action terms are defined here.

It should be noted that joint actions usually describe cardinal plane motions of a body part. For example, the brachialis muscle brings the forearm anteriorly in the sagittal plane at the elbow joint, so its action is described as flexion of the forearm at the elbow joint. If a muscle creates an oblique plane motion, then this motion is described by breaking it into its component cardinal plane joint action motions. An example is the coracobrachialis muscle, which moves the arm anteriorly (in the sagittal plane) and medially (in the frontal plane). When describing this motion, it is said that the coracobrachialis flexes and adducts the arm at the shoulder (glenohumeral) joint. It actually causes one motion, but this one motion is described as having two cardinal (sagittal and frontal) plane components. For more information on this, please go to the Evolve website that accompanies this book or see *Kinesiology: The Skeletal System and Muscle Function* (Elsevier, 2007).

Following the definitions of joint action terms is a joint action atlas that contains illustrations that demonstrate all the joint actions of the body.

Pairs of Terms

Flexion/Extension

Flexion is generally an anterior movement of a body part within the sagittal plane; *extension* is generally a posterior movement within the sagittal plane.

Exceptions include movements of the legs, feet, toes, and thumbs. From the knee joint and further distally, flexion of a body part moves posteriorly (extension is therefore an anterior movement). The thumb moves medially within the frontal plane when it flexes, and laterally within the frontal plane when it extends. The terms *flexion* and *extension* can be used for the entire body, axial and appendicular.

Abduction/Adduction

Abduction is generally a lateral movement within the frontal plane that is away from the imaginary midline of the body; *adduction* is a medial movement toward the midline.

Exceptions include the toes and fingers, including the thumbs.

The toes adduct toward an imaginary line through the center of the second toe when the second toe is in anatomic position; they abduct away from this imaginary line. Toe number two can only abduct; it can do tibial abduction and fibular abduction.

Fingers two through five adduct toward an imaginary line that goes through the center of the middle finger when the middle finger is in anatomic position; they abduct away from this imaginary line. The middle finger can only abduct; it can do radial abduction and ulnar abduction.

The thumb abducts within the sagittal plane by moving away from the palm of the hand; it adducts within the frontal plane by moving back toward the palm. The terms *abduction* and *adduction* are used only for the appendicular body.

Right Lateral Flexion/Left Lateral Flexion

Right lateral flexion is a side-bending movement toward the right within the frontal plane of the head, neck, and/or trunk. *Left lateral flexion* is the opposite. These terms are used only for the axial body.

Lateral Rotation/Medial Rotation

Lateral rotation is a movement within the transverse plane in which the anterior surface of the body part moves to face more laterally (away from the midline); *medial rotation* moves the anterior surface to face more medially (toward the midline).

Lateral rotation is also known as external rotation; medial rotation is also known as internal rotation. These terms are used only for the appendicular body.

Right Rotation/Left Rotation

Right rotation is a movement within the transverse plane in which the anterior surface of the body part moves to face more to the right; *left rotation* moves the anterior surface to face more to the left. These terms are used for the axial body only.

Note: The terms *ipsilateral rotator* and *contralateral rotator* are often used to describe muscles that produce right or left rotation. Ipsilateral and contralateral rotation are not joint action terms. Rather they are ways to describe that a muscle on one side of the body either produces rotation to that same (ipsilateral) side, or to the opposite (contralateral) side.

Elevation/Depression

Elevation is a movement wherein the body part moves superiorly; *depression* occurs when the body part moves inferiorly.

Protraction/Retraction

Protraction is a movement wherein the body part moves anteriorly; *retraction* is a posterior movement of the body part.

Right Lateral Deviation/Left Lateral Deviation

Lateral deviation is a linear movement that occurs in the lateral direction.

Pronation/Supination

The terms *pronation* and *supination* can be applied to motion of the forearm at the radioulnar joints and motion of the foot at the subtalar (tarsal) joint.

Pronation of the forearm results in the posterior surface of the radius facing anteriorly (when in anatomic position); supination is the opposite. Note: It is easy to confuse forearm pronation with medial rotation of the arm at the glenohumeral joint, and forearm supination with lateral rotation of the arm.

Pronation of the foot at the subtalar joint is a triaxial motion that is made up primarily of eversion; it also includes dorsiflexion and lateral rotation (also known as abduction) of the foot at the subtalar joint. Supination of the foot is primarily made up of inversion; it also includes foot plantarflexion and medial rotation (also known as adduction) at the subtalar joint.

Inversion/Eversion

The foot inverts at the subtalar (tarsal) joint when it turns its plantar surface toward the midline of the body; it everts when its plantar surface is turned outward away from the midline. *Inversion* is the principal component of supination of the foot; *eversion* is the principal component of pronation of the foot.

Dorsiflexion/Plantarflexion

The foot dorsiflexes when it moves superiorly (in the direction of its dorsal surface); it plantarflexes when it moves inferiorly (in the direction of its plantar surface). Technically, dorsiflexion is extension and plantarflexion is flexion.

Opposition/Reposition

The thumb opposes at the saddle (carpometacarpal) joint when its pad meets the pad of another finger; it repositions when it returns back toward anatomic position. Opposition is actually a composite of abduction, flexion, and medial rotation of the thumb; reposition is a composite of adduction, extension, and lateral rotation of the thumb.

The little finger can also oppose and reposition at its carpometacarpal joint. Little finger opposition is composed of flexion, adduction, and lateral rotation of the little finger; little finger reposition is composed of extension, abduction, and medial rotation.

Upward Rotation/Downward Rotation

The scapula upwardly rotates when its glenoid fossa is moved to face more superiorly; downward rotation is the opposite motion.

The clavicle upwardly rotates when its inferior surface moves to face anteriorly; downward rotation is the opposite motion.

Note: These actions of the scapula and clavicle cannot be isolated. Rather, they must couple with motions of the arm at the glenohumeral joint.

Lateral Tilt/Medial Tilt and Upward Tilt/Downward Tilt

The scapula laterally tilts when its medial border lifts away from the body wall; medial tilt is the opposite motion wherein the medial border moves back toward the body wall.

The scapula upwardly tilts when its inferior angle lifts away from the body wall; downward tilt is the opposite motion wherein the inferior angle moves back toward the body wall.

Horizontal Flexion/Horizontal Extension

Horizontal flexion is a movement of the arm or thigh in which it begins in a horizontal position (i.e., abducted to 90 degrees) and then moves anteriorly toward the midline of the body. Horizontal extension is the movement in the opposite direction.

Note: Horizontal flexion is also known as horizontal adduction; horizontal extension is also known as horizontal abduction.

Hyperextension and Circumduction

Hyperextension

The term *hyperextension* is often used to describe extension beyond anatomic position. This text does not use hyperextension in this manner. Extension beyond anatomic position is called extension, just as flexion and abduction beyond anatomic position are called flexion and abduction. The prefix *hyper* denotes excessive, therefore the term *hyperextension* would be better and more consistently defined as a range of extension motion that occurs beyond what is normal or beyond what is healthy.

Circumduction

Circumduction is not a joint action. Rather, circumduction is a sequence of four joint actions performed one after the other. For example, if a person moves his or her arm at the glenohumeral joint into flexion, then abduction, then extension, and then adduction, and does this by rounding the corners of the four motions, it creates a circular motion pattern that is called circumduction. It should also be noted that circumduction does not contain any rotation motion. Any joint that allows motion within two or more planes (biaxial or triaxial joints) can allow circumduction to occur.

■ JOINT ACTION ATLAS

Upper Extremity

Scapula at the Scapulocostal Joint

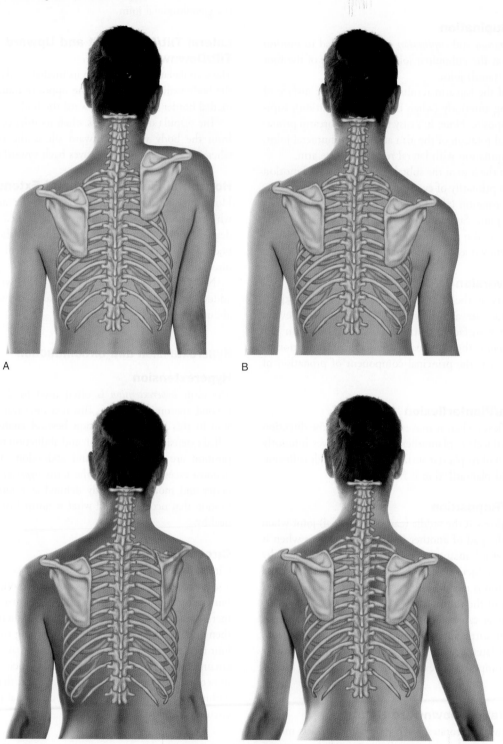

Figure 1-7 Nonaxial actions of elevation/depression and protraction/retraction of the scapula at the scapulocostal (ScC) joint. **A,** Elevation of the right scapula. **B,** Depression of the right scapula. **C,** Protraction of the right scapula. **D,** Retraction of the right scapula. The left scapula is in anatomic position in all figures. (Note: All views are posterior.)

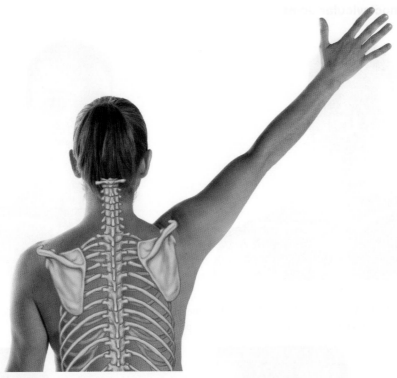

Figure 1-8 Upward rotation of the right scapula at the scapulocostal (ScC) joint. The left scapula is in anatomic position, which is full downward rotation. (Note: The scapular action of upward rotation cannot be isolated. It must accompany humeral motion. In this case, the humerus is abducted at the glenohumeral joint.) (Note: This is a posterior view.)

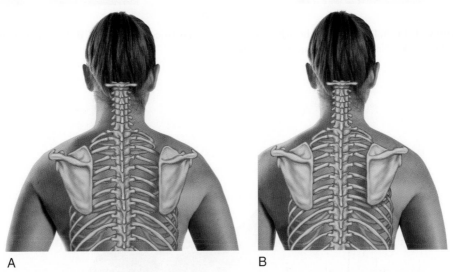

A   B

Figure 1-9 Tilt actions of the scapula at the scapulocostal (ScC) joint. **A,** Upward tilt of the right scapula; the left scapula is in anatomic position of downward tilt. **B,** Lateral tilt of the right scapula; the left scapula is in anatomic position of medial tilt. (Note: Both views are posterior.)

Clavicle at the Sternoclavicular Joint

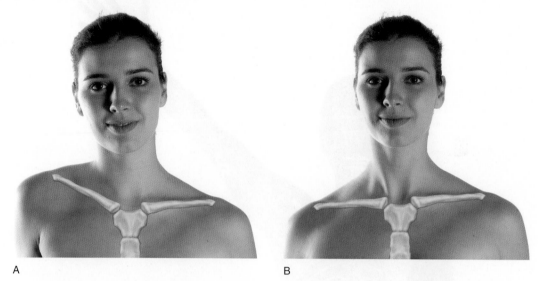

A   B

Figure 1-10 A, Elevation of the right clavicle at the sternoclavicular (SC) joint. **B,** Depression of the right clavicle. (Note: The left clavicle is in anatomic position. Both views are anterior.)

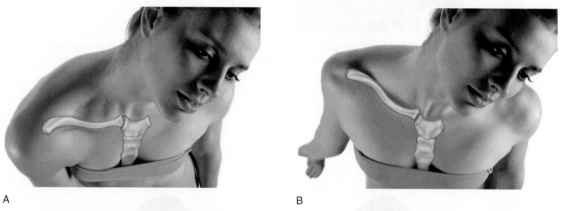

A   B

Figure 1-11 A, Protraction of the right clavicle at the sternoclavicular (SC) joint. **B,** Retraction of the right clavicle. (Note: Both views are anteroinferior.)

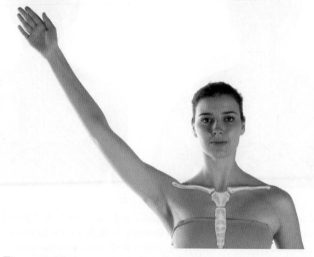

Figure 1-12 Anterior view that illustrates upward rotation of the right clavicle at the sternoclavicular (SC) joint; the left clavicle is in anatomic position, which is full downward rotation. (Note: Upward rotation of the clavicle cannot be isolated. In this figure the arm is abducted at the glenohumeral joint, resulting in the scapula upwardly rotating, which results in upward rotation of the clavicle.)

Arm at the Glenohumeral Joint

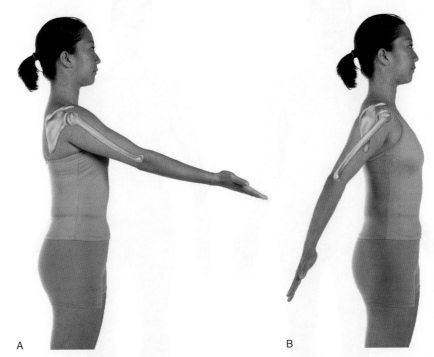

A   B

Figure 1-13 Sagittal plane actions of the arm at the glenohumeral (GH) joint. **A,** Flexion. **B,** Extension. (Note: Both views are lateral.)

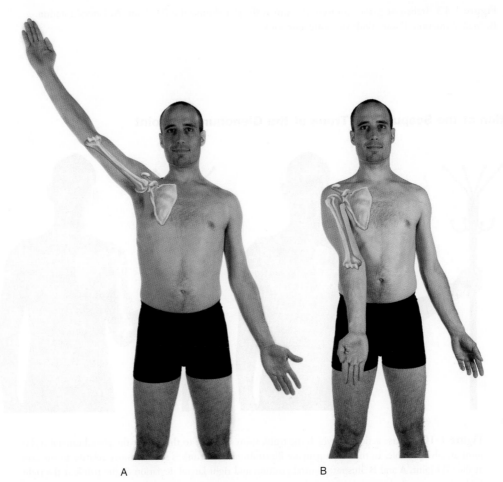

A   B

Figure 1-14 Frontal plane actions of the arm at the glenohumeral (GH) joint. **A,** Abduction. **B,** Adduction. (Note: Both views are anterior.)

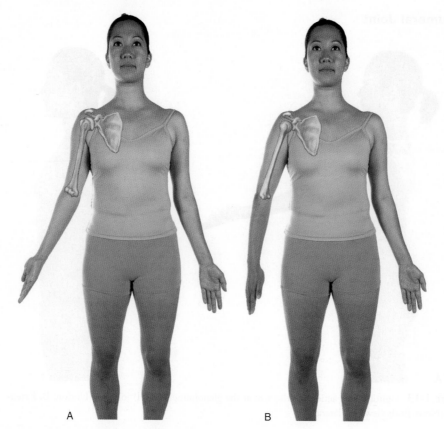

Figure 1-15 Transverse plane actions of the arm at the glenohumeral (GH) joint. **A,** Lateral rotation. **B,** Medial rotation. (Note: Both views are anterior.)

Reverse Action of the Scapula and Trunk at the Glenohumeral Joint

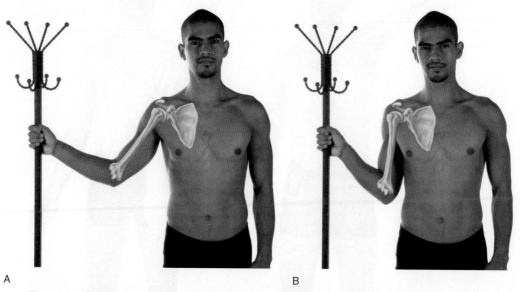

Figure 1-16 Reverse actions in which the trunk moves relative to the arm at the glenohumeral (GH) joint are also possible. In the accompanying illustrations, the trunk is seen to move relative to the arm at the GH joint. **A** and **B** illustrate neutral position and right lateral deviation of the trunk at the right GH joint, respectively.

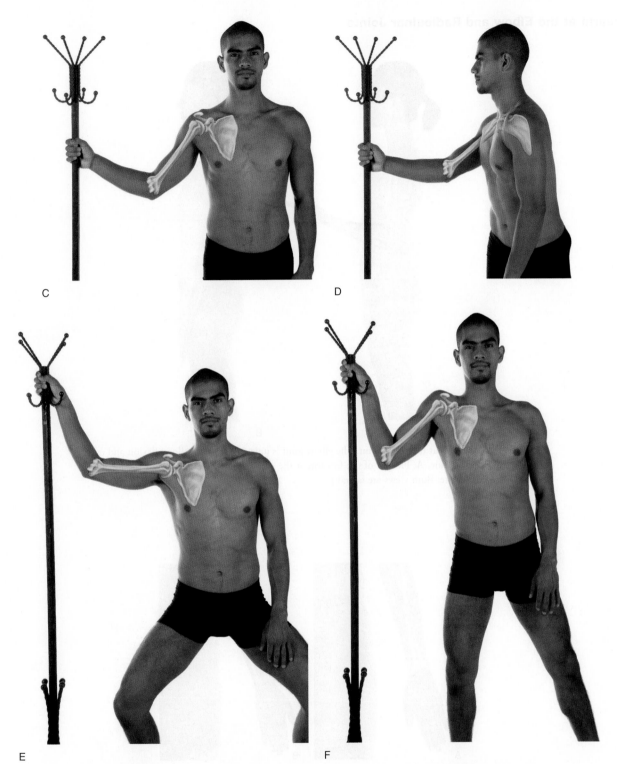

Figure 1-16, cont'd C and **D** illustrate neutral position and right rotation of the trunk at the right GH joint, respectively; and **E** and **F** illustrate neutral position and elevation of the trunk at the right GH joint, respectively. In all three cases, note the change in angulation between the arm and trunk at the GH joint (for lateral deviation **B** and elevation **F**, the elbow joint has also flexed). (Note: All views are anterior.)

Forearm at the Elbow and Radioulnar Joints

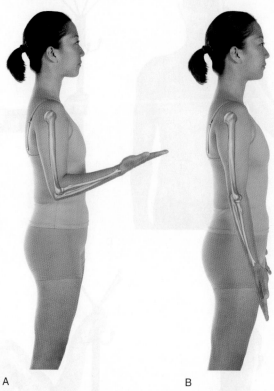

A   B

Figure 1-17 Motion at the elbow joint. The elbow joint is uniaxial and only allows flexion and extension in the sagittal plane. **A,** Flexion of the forearm at the elbow joint. **B,** Extension of the forearm at the elbow joint. (Note: Both views are lateral.)

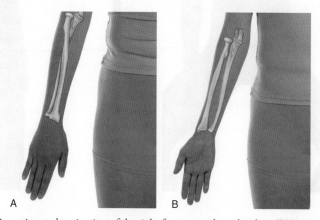

A   B

Figure 1-18 Pronation and supination of the right forearm at the radioulnar (RU) joints. **A,** Pronation. **B,** Supination, which is anatomic position for the forearm. Pronation and supination are joint actions created by a combination of motions at the proximal, middle, and distal RU joints. (Note: Both figures are an anterior view of the forearm.)

Hand at the Wrist Joint

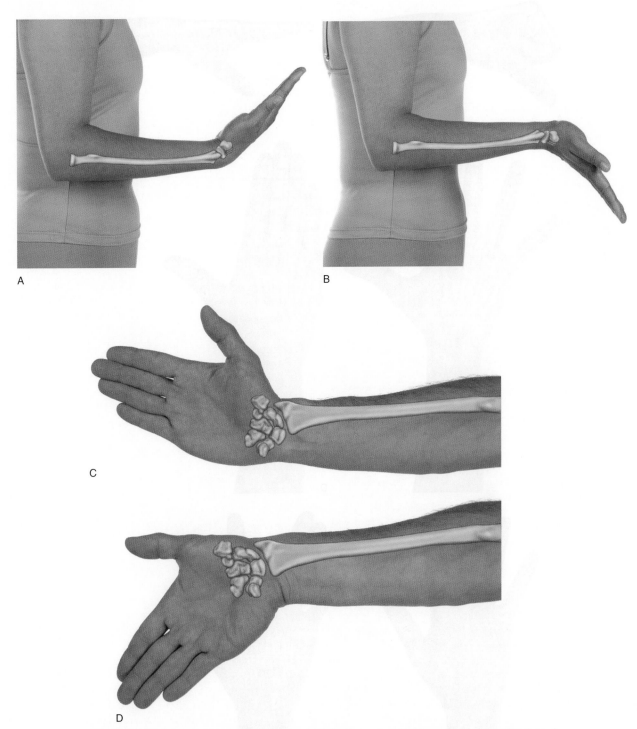

A

B

C

D

Figure 1-19 Motions of the hand at the wrist joint (radiocarpal and midcarpal joints). **A** and **B,** Lateral views illustrating flexion and extension of the hand, respectively. **C** and **D,** Anterior views illustrating radial deviation and ulnar deviation, respectively. Radial deviation of the hand is also known as *abduction*; ulnar deviation is also known as *adduction*.

Fingers 2 through 5 at the Metacarpophalangeal and Interphalangeal Joints

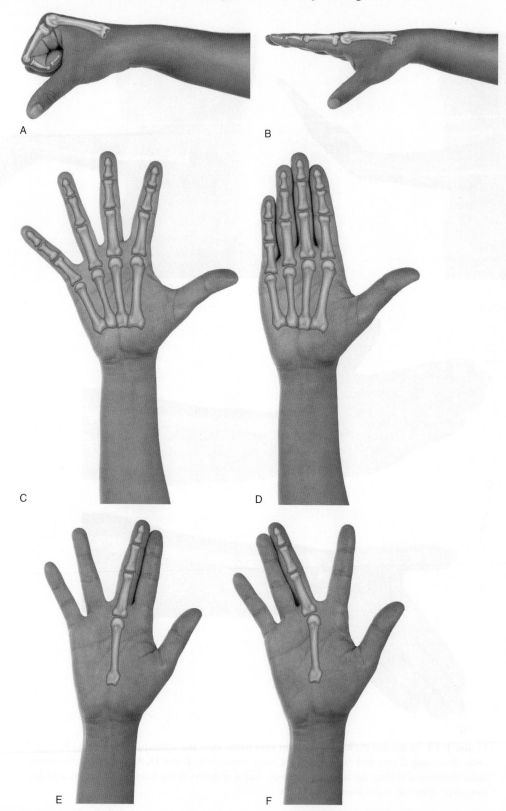

A

B

C

D

E

F

Figure 1-20 Actions of the fingers at the metacarpophalangeal (MCP) joints of the hand. An MCP joint is biaxial, allowing flexion and extension in the sagittal plane and abduction and adduction in the frontal plane. **A** and **B,** Radial (i.e., lateral) views illustrating flexion and extension, respectively, of fingers two through five at the MCP joints. Flexion of the fingers at the interphalangeal joints is also seen. **C** and **D,** Anterior views illustrating abduction and adduction of fingers two through five at the MCP joints, respectively. (Note: The reference line for abduction/adduction of the fingers is an imaginary line through the center of the middle finger when it is in anatomic position.) **E** and **F,** Anterior views illustrating radial abduction and ulnar abduction of the middle finger at the third MCP joint, respectively.

Thumb at the Carpometacarpal Joint

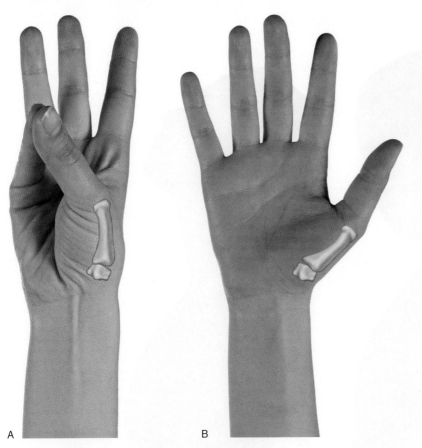

Figure 1-21 Actions of the thumb at the first carpometacarpal (CMC) joint (also known as the *saddle joint of the thumb*). **A** and **B,** Anterior views that illustrate opposition and reposition of the thumb, respectively. Opposition and reposition are actually combinations of actions; the component actions of opposition and reposition are shown in **C** to **F. C** and **D,** Anterior views that illustrate flexion and extension, respectively; these actions occur within the frontal plane. **E** and **F,** Lateral views that illustrate abduction and adduction, respectively; these actions occur within the sagittal plane. Medial rotation and lateral rotation in the transverse plane are not shown separately, because these actions cannot occur in isolation; they must occur in conjunction with flexion and extension, respectively. (Note: Flexion of the phalanges of the thumb and/or little finger at metacarpophalangeal joint is also seen in **A** and **C;** flexion of the thumb at the interphalangeal joint is also seen in **C**).

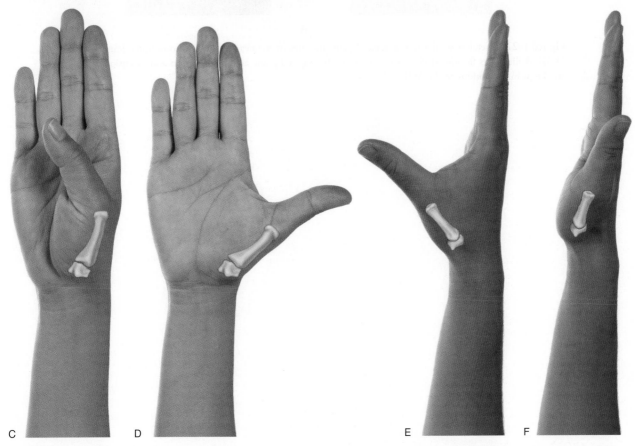

Axial Body

Head at the Atlanto-Occipital Joint

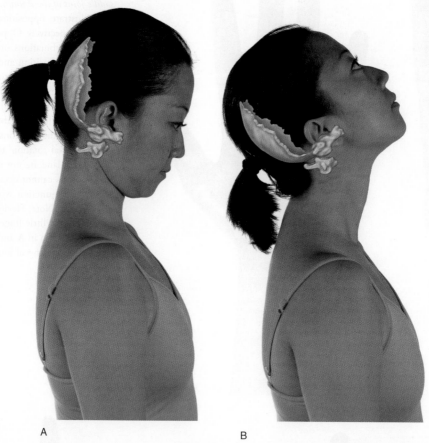

A   B

Figure 1-22 Lateral views illustrating sagittal plane motions of the head at the atlanto-occipital joint (AOJ). **A** illustrates flexion; **B** illustrates extension. The sagittal plane actions of flexion and extension are the primary motions of the AOJ.

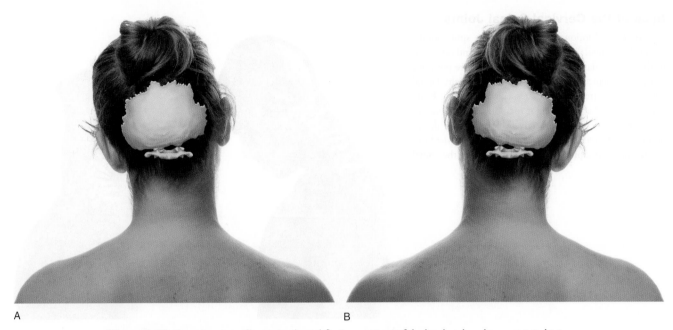

Figure 1-23 Posterior views illustrating lateral flexion motions of the head at the atlanto-occipital joint (AOJ). **A** illustrates left lateral flexion; **B** illustrates right lateral flexion. These actions occur in the frontal plane.

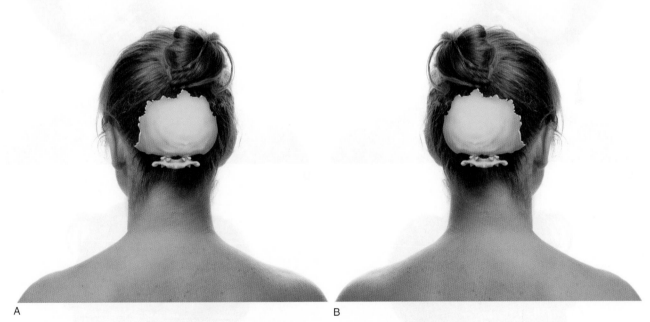

Figure 1-24 Posterior views that illustrates rotation motions of the head at the atlanto-occipital joint (AOJ). **A** illustrates left rotation; **B** illustrates right rotation. These actions occur in the transverse plane.

Neck at the Cervical Spinal Joints

Figure 1-25 Motions of the neck at the spinal joints. **A** and **B** are lateral views that depict flexion and extension in the sagittal plane, respectively. **C** and **D** are posterior views that depict left lateral flexion and right lateral flexion in the frontal plane, respectively. **E** and **F** are anterior views that depict right rotation and left rotation in the transverse plane, respectively. Note: **A** to **F** depict motions of the entire craniocervical region (i.e., the head at the atlanto-occipital joint and the neck at the spinal joints).

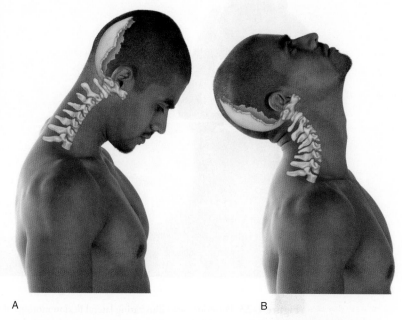

A   B

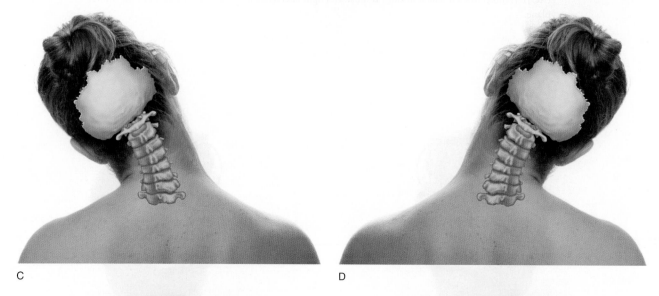

C   D

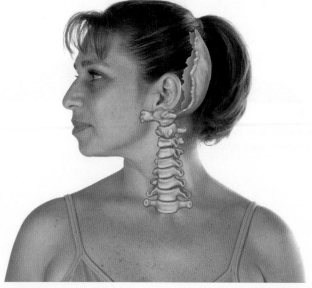
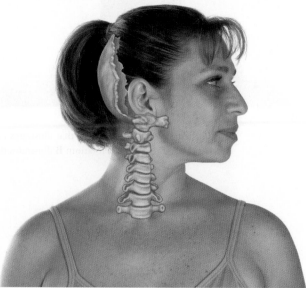

E   F

Trunk at the Thoracolumbar Spinal Joints

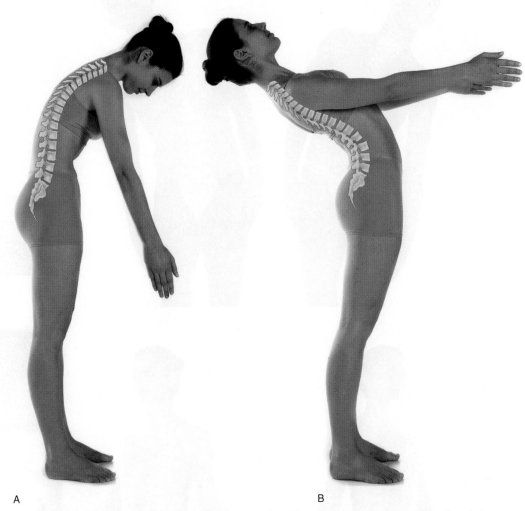

A   B

Figure 1-26 Motions of the thoracolumbar spine (trunk) at the spinal joints. **A** and **B** are lateral views that illustrate flexion and extension of the trunk, respectively, in the sagittal plane.

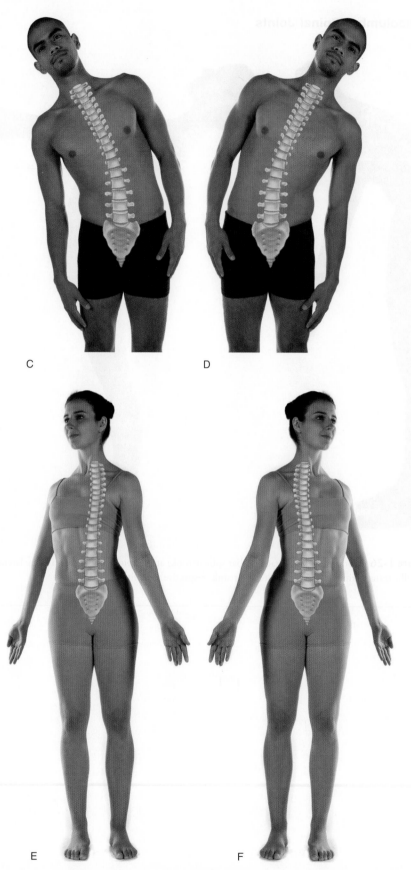

C   D

E   F

Figure 1-26, cont'd **C** and **D** are anterior views that illustrate right lateral flexion and left lateral flexion of the trunk, respectively, in the frontal plane. **E** and **F** are anterior views that illustrate right rotation and left rotation of the trunk, respectively, in the transverse plane.

Pelvis at the Lumbosacral Joint

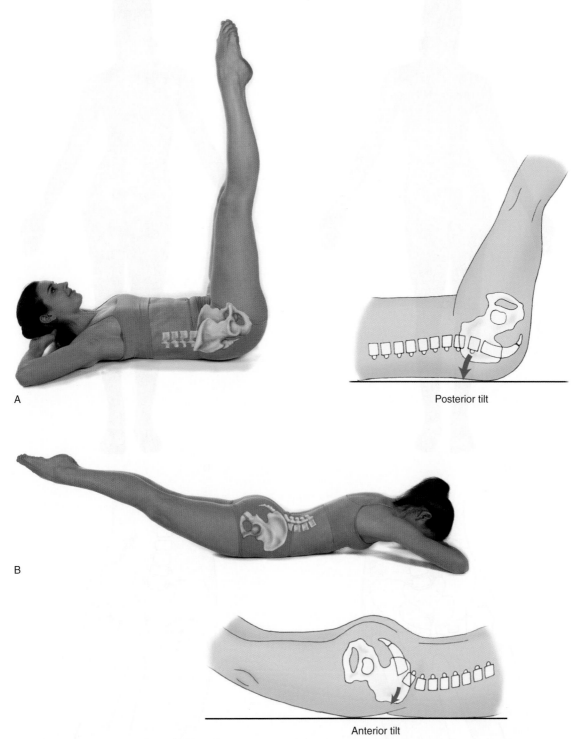

Posterior tilt

A

B

Anterior tilt

Figure 1-27 Motion of the pelvis at the lumbosacral (LS) joint. **A** and **B,** Lateral views illustrating posterior tilt and anterior tilt, respectively, of the pelvis at the LS joint. (Note: In **A** and **B** no motion is occurring at the hip joints; therefore the thighs are seen to "go along for the ride," resulting in the lower extremities changing their orientation.)

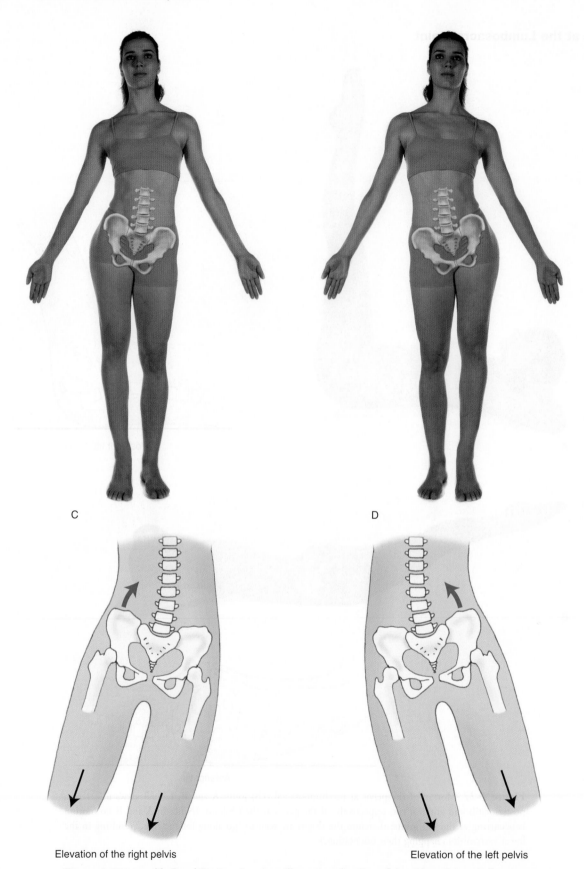

C   D

Elevation of the right pelvis   Elevation of the left pelvis

Figure 1-27, cont'd C and **D,** Anterior views illustrating elevation of the right pelvis and elevation of the left pelvis, respectively, at the LS joint. (Note: In the drawn illustrations of **C** and **D,** no motion is occurring at the hip joints; therefore the thighs are seen to "go along for the ride," resulting in the lower extremities changing their orientation.)

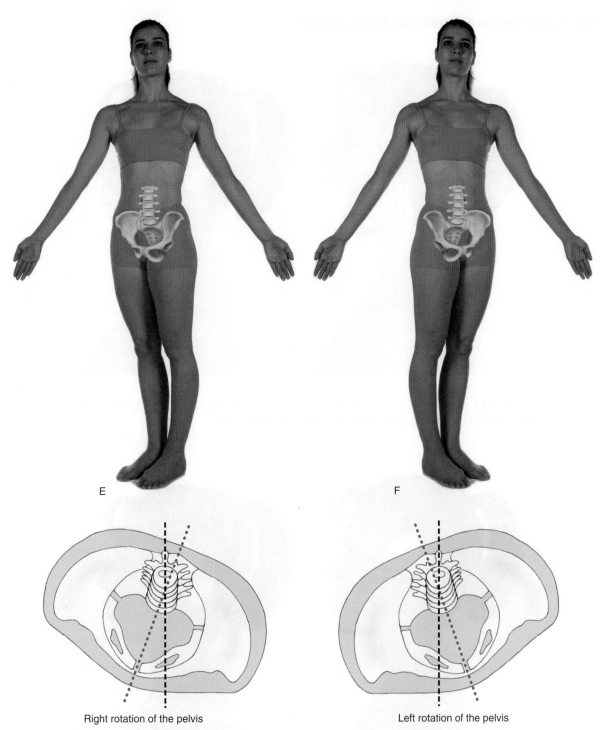

E

F

Right rotation of the pelvis

Left rotation of the pelvis

Figure 1-27, cont'd E and **F,** Anterior and superior views illustrating rotation of the pelvis to the right and rotation to the left, respectively, at the LS joint. (Note: In **E** and **F** the dashed black line represents the orientation of the spine and the red dotted line represents the orientation of the pelvis. Given the different directions of these two lines, it is clear that the pelvis has rotated relative to the spine; this motion has occurred at the LS joint.)

Mandible at the Temporomandibular Joints (TMJs)

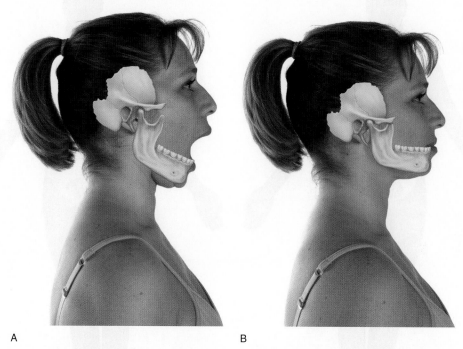

A   B

Figure 1-28 A and **B,** Lateral views that illustrate depression and elevation, respectively, of the mandible at the temporomandibular joints (TMJs). These are axial motions.

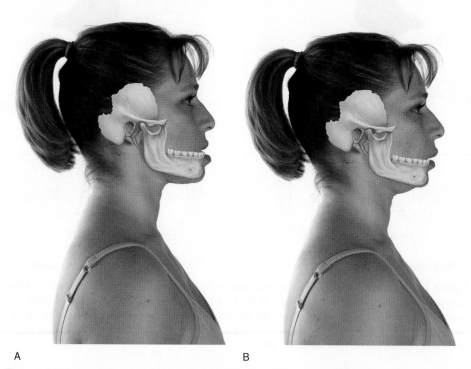

A   B

Figure 1-29 A and **B,** Lateral views that illustrate protraction and retraction, respectively, of the mandible at the temporomandibular joints (TMJs). These are nonaxial glide motions.

1

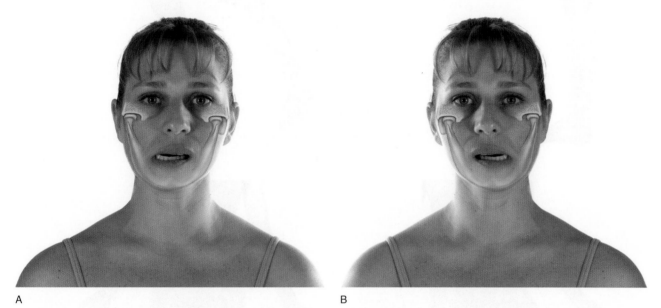

A   B

Figure 1-30 A and **B,** Anterior views that illustrate right lateral deviation and left lateral deviation, respectively, of the mandible at the temporomandibular joints (TMJs). These are nonaxial glide motions.

Lower Extremity

Thigh at the Hip Joint

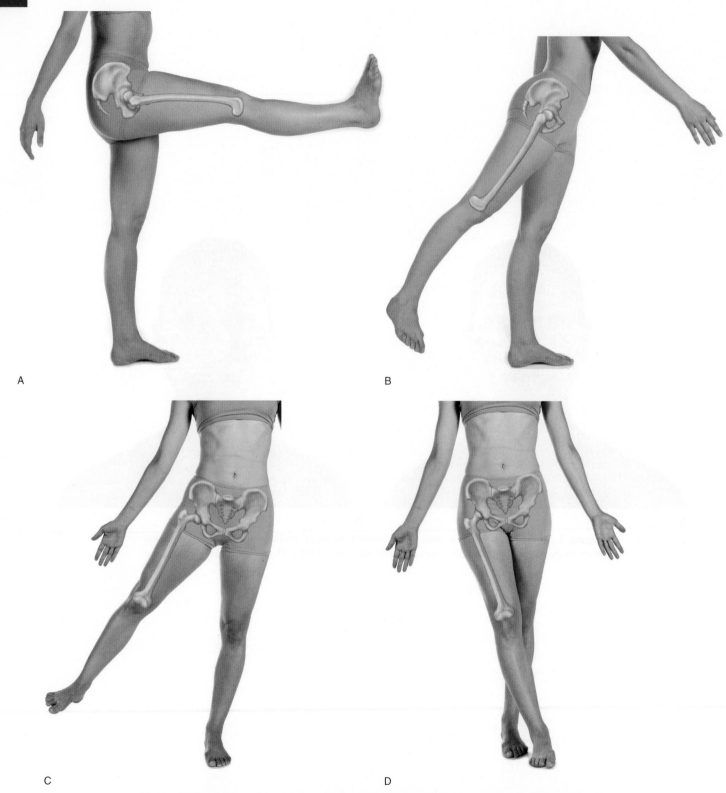

A

B

C

D

Figure 1-31 Motions of the thigh at the hip joint. **A** and **B,** Lateral views illustrating flexion and extension, respectively. **C** and **D,** Anterior views illustrating abduction and adduction, respectively.

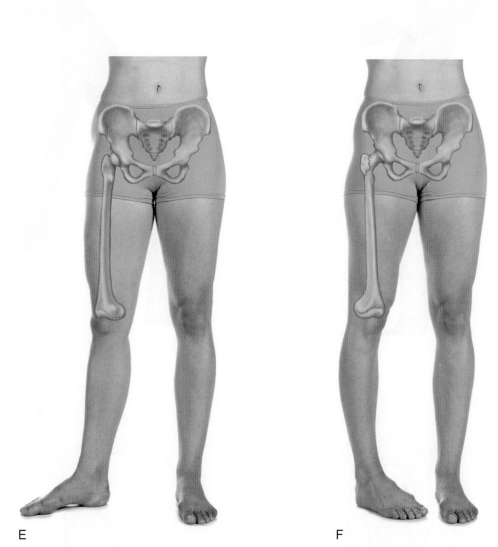

E

F

Figure 1-31, cont'd **E** and **F,** Anterior views illustrating lateral rotation and medial rotation, respectively.

Pelvis at the Hip Joint

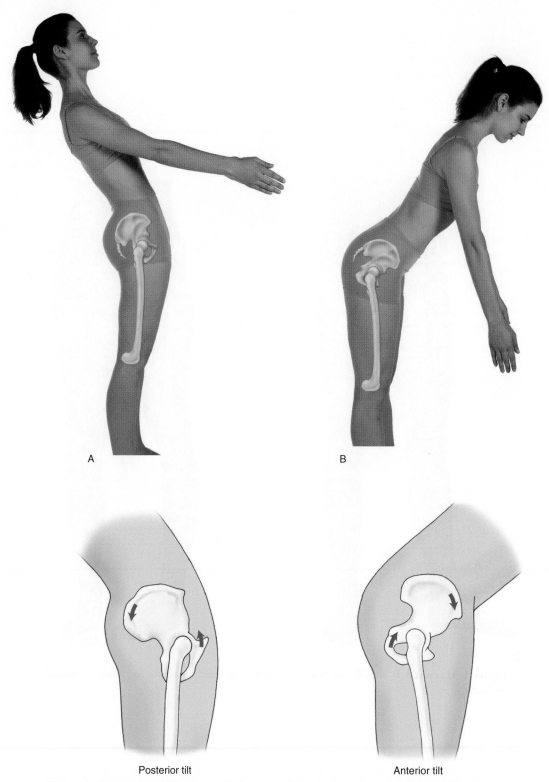

Posterior tilt

Anterior tilt

Figure 1-32 Motion of the pelvis at the hip joint. (Note: In **A** to **D** no motion is occurring at the lumbosacral joint; therefore the trunk is seen to "go along for the ride," resulting in the upper body changing its orientation.) **A** and **B,** Lateral views illustrating posterior tilt and anterior tilt, respectively, of the pelvis at the hip joint.

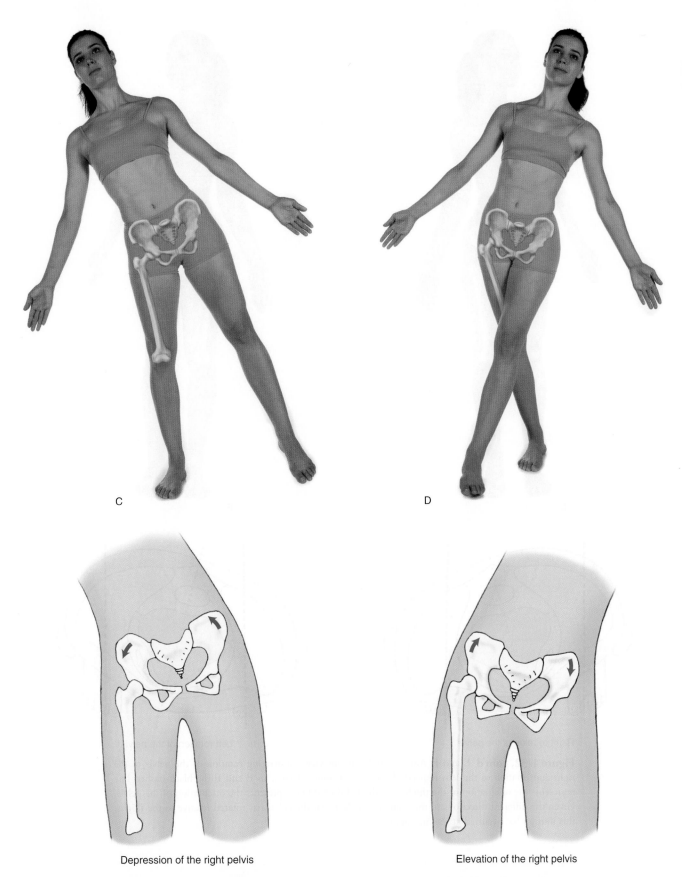

C

D

Depression of the right pelvis

Elevation of the right pelvis

Figure 1-32, cont'd **C** and **D,** Anterior views illustrating depression of the right pelvis and elevation of the right pelvis, respectively, at the right hip joint. (Note: When the pelvis elevates on one side, it depresses on the other, and vice versa.)

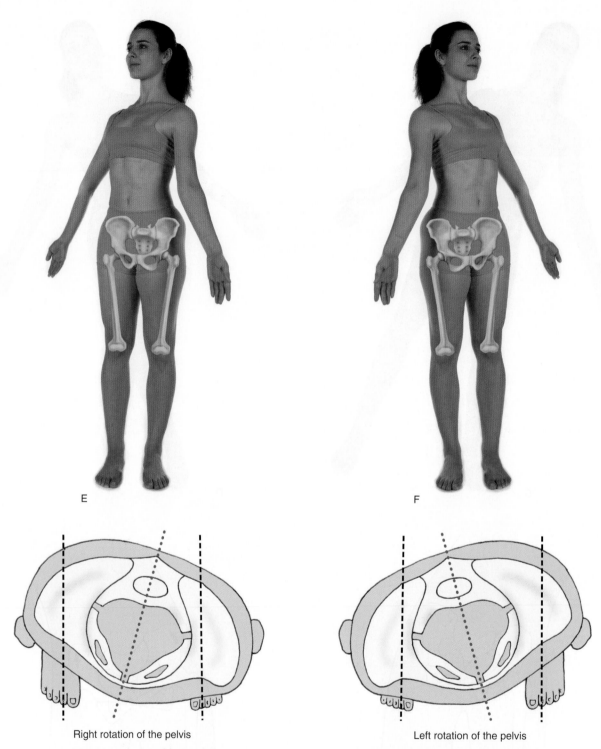

E

F

Right rotation of the pelvis

Left rotation of the pelvis

Figure 1-32, cont'd **E** and **F,** Anterior and superior views illustrating rotation of the pelvis to the right and rotation to the left, respectively, at the hip joints. (Note: In **E** and **F** the black dashed line represents the orientation of the thighs and the red dotted line represents the orientation of the pelvis. Given the different directions of these lines, it is clear that the pelvis has rotated relative to the thighs; this motion has occurred at the hip joints.)

Leg at the Knee Joint

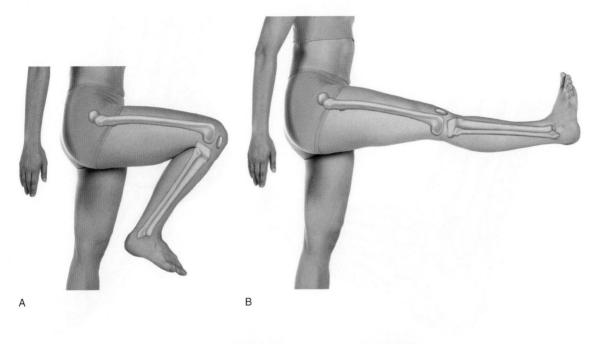

A   B

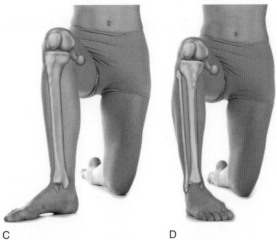

C   D

Figure 1-33 Motions possible at the tibiofemoral (i.e., knee) joint. **A** and **B,** Lateral views illustrating flexion and extension of the leg at the knee joint, respectively. **C** and **D,** Anterior views illustrating lateral and medial rotation of the leg at the knee joint, respectively. (Note: The knee joint can only rotate if it is first flexed.)

Foot at the Ankle Joint

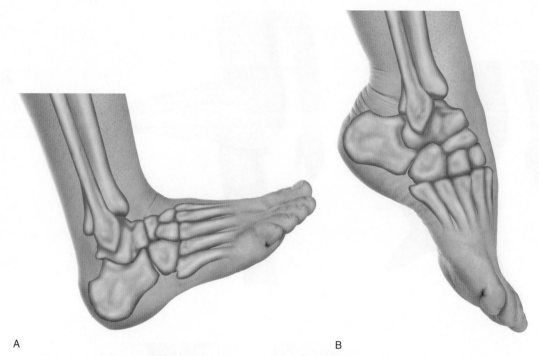

A   B

Figure 1-34 A and **B,** Lateral views illustrating dorsiflexion and plantarflexion of the foot at the talocrural (i.e., ankle) joint, respectively.

Foot at the Subtalar (Tarsal) Joint

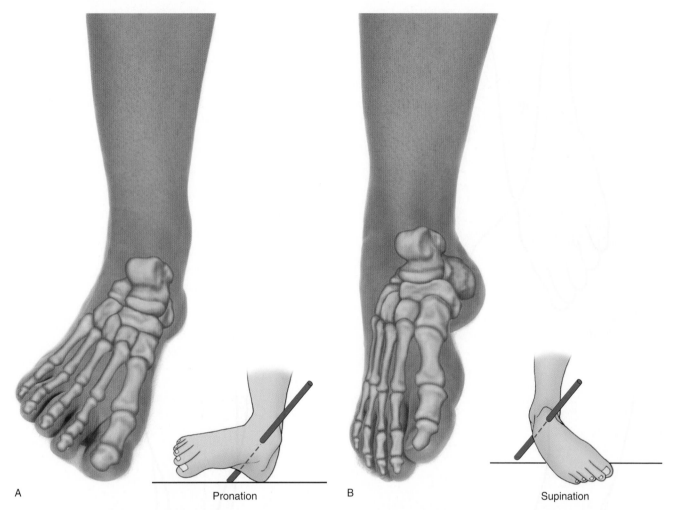

A   Pronation

B   Supination

Figure 1-35 Motions of the foot at the subtalar (tarsal) joint. **A,** Pronation of the foot. Pronation is an oblique plane movement composed of three cardinal plane components: (1) eversion, (2) dorsiflexion, and (3) lateral rotation (also known as abduction) of the foot. The principle component of pronation is eversion. **B,** Supination of the foot. Supination is an oblique plane movement composed of three cardinal plane components: (1) inversion, (2) plantarflexion, and (3) medial rotation (also known as adduction) of the foot. The principle component of supination is inversion.

Foot at the Subtalar and Ankle Joints

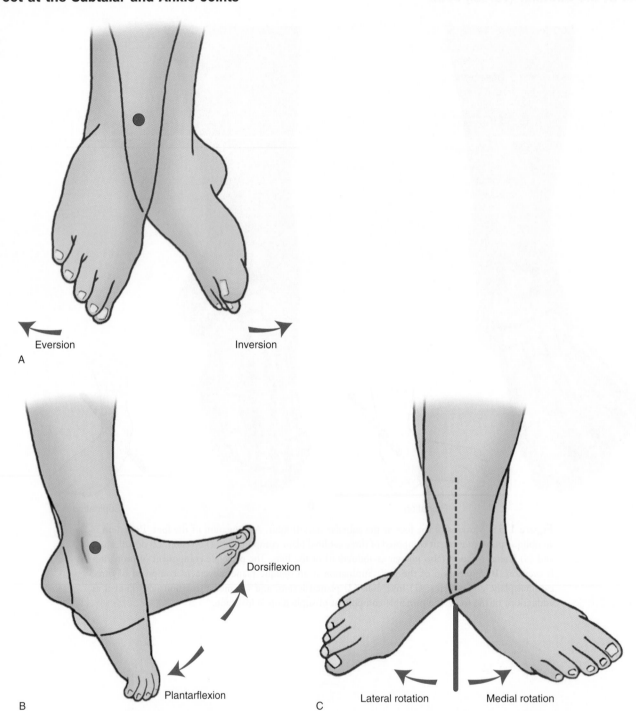

Figure 1-36 Cardinal plane components of foot motion at the subtalar and ankle joints. **A,** Frontal plane components of eversion/inversion. **B,** Sagittal plane components of dorsiflexion/plantarflexion. **C,** Transverse plane components of lateral rotation/medial rotation (abduction/adduction). (Note: In **A** and **B,** the axis is represented by the red dot.)

Toes at the Metatarsophalangeal and Interphalangeal Joints

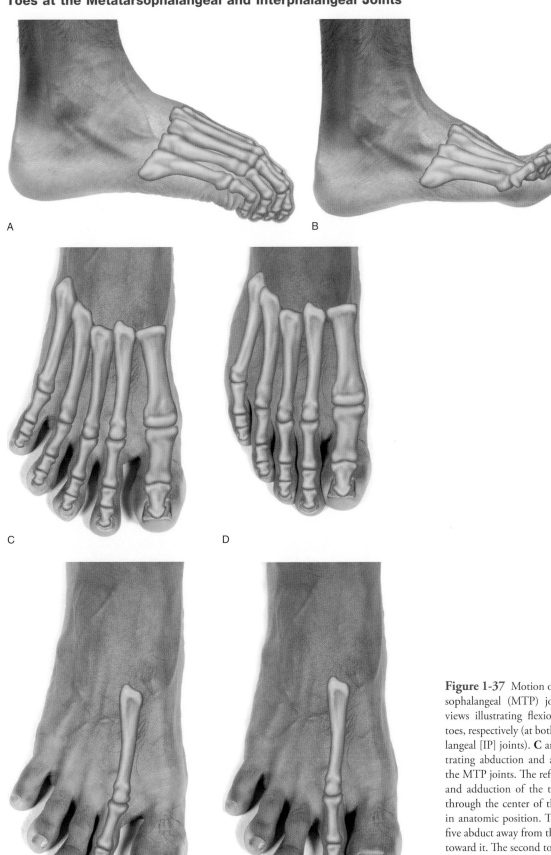

Figure 1-37 Motion of the toes at the metatarsophalangeal (MTP) joints. **A** and **B,** Lateral views illustrating flexion and extension of the toes, respectively (at both the MTP and interphalangeal [IP] joints). **C** and **D,** Dorsal views illustrating abduction and adduction of the toes at the MTP joints. The reference line for abduction and adduction of the toes is an imaginary line through the center of the second toe when it is in anatomic position. Toes one, three, four, and five abduct away from the second toe and adduct toward it. The second toe abducts in either direction it moves. **E,** Fibular abduction of the second toe at the MTP joint. **F,** Tibial abduction of the second toe at the MTP joint.

The Skeletal System

■ THE SKELETON

The skeletal system is composed of approximately 206 bones and can be divided into bones of the axial body and bones of the appendicular body. Figure 2-1 is an anterior view of the full skeleton. Figure 2-2 is a posterior view.

■ JOINTS

Wherever two or more bones come together, in other words join, a joint is formed.

Structural Classification of Joints

Structurally, the definition of a joint is having the two (or more) bones united by a soft tissue. There are three structural classifications of joints: fibrous, cartilaginous, and synovial. Fibrous joints are united by dense fibrous fascial tissue, cartilaginous joints are united by fibrocartilage, and synovial joints are united by a thin fibrous capsule that is lined internally by a synovial membrane, enclosing a joint cavity that contains synovial fluid. Only synovial joints possess a joint cavity and have articular cartilage that covers the joint surfaces of the bones. Figure 2-3 illustrates the three types of structural joints.

Functional Classification of Joints

Functionally, a joint is defined by its ability to allow motion between two (or more) bones. There are three functional classifications of joints: synarthrotic, amphiarthrotic, and diarthrotic. Synarthrotic joints permit very little motion; amphiarthrotic joints allow limited to moderate motion; and diarthrotic joints allow a great deal of motion.

Generally, there is a correlation between the structural and functional classifications of joints. Fibrous joints are usually classified as synarthrotic because they allow very little motion; cartilaginous joints are usually classified as amphiarthrotic because they allow a limited to moderate amount of motion;

and synovial joints are usually classified as diarthrotic because they allow a great deal of motion.

Types of Synovial Joints

Diarthrotic synovial joints can be subdivided based on the number of axes around which they permit motion to occur. The four categories are uniaxial, biaxial, triaxial, and nonaxial. These categories can be further subdivided based on the shape of the joint.

Uniaxial Joints

There are two types of synovial uniaxial joints: hinge and pivot. Hinge joints act similar to the hinge of a door. One surface is concave and the other is spool-like in shape. Flexion and extension are allowed in the sagittal plane around a mediolateral axis. The humeroulnar (elbow) joint is a classic example of a hinge joint (Figure 2-4).

The other type of synovial uniaxial joint is the pivot joint. A pivot joint allows only rotation (pivot) motions in the transverse plane around a vertical axis. The atlantoaxial joint of the spine is a classic example of a uniaxial pivot joint (Figure 2-5).

Biaxial Joints

There are two types of synovial biaxial joints: condyloid and saddle. A condyloid joint has one bone whose surface is concave and the other bone's surface is convex. The convex surface of one bone fits into the concave surface of the other. Flexion and extension are allowed within the sagittal plane around a mediolateral axis, and abduction and adduction are allowed within the frontal plane around an anteroposterior axis. The metacarpophalangeal joint of the hand is an example of a condyloid joint (Figure 2-6).

The other type of synovial biaxial joint is the saddle joint. Both bones of a saddle joint have a convex and concave shape. The convexity of one bone fits into the concavity of the other and vice versa. Flexion and extension are allowed in one plane and abduction and adduction are allowed in a second plane. Interestingly, a saddle joint also allows medial rotation and

2

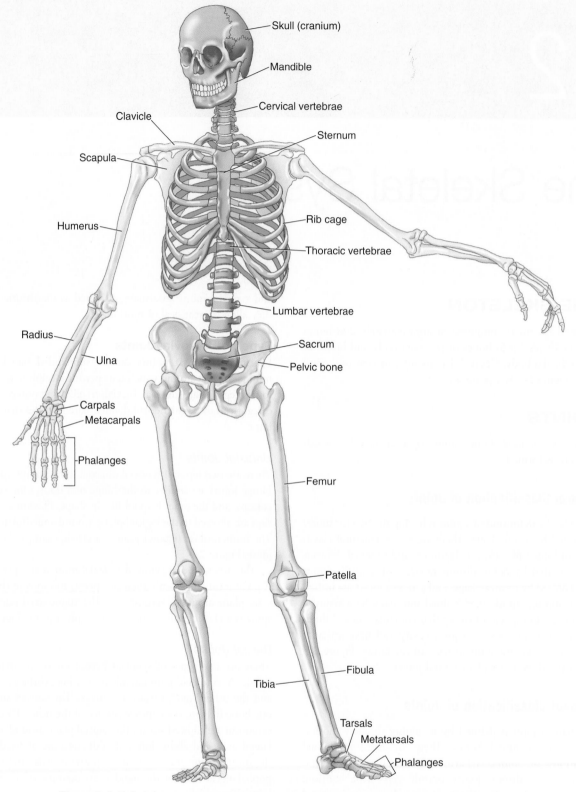

Figure 2-1 Full skeleton—anterior view. Green, axial skeleton; cream, appendicular skeleton. (From Muscolino JE: *Kinesiology: the skeletal system and muscle function,* enhanced edition, St Louis, 2007, Mosby.)

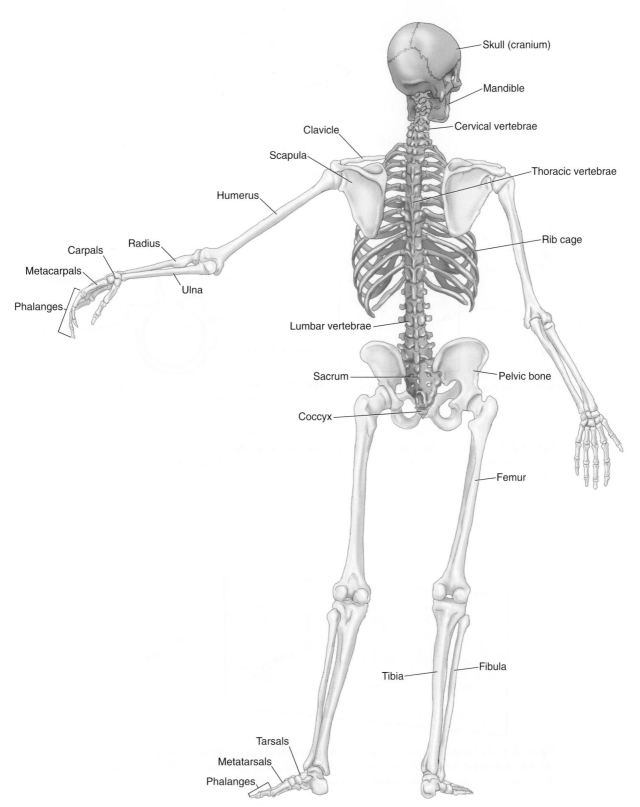

Figure 2-2 Full skeleton—posterior view. Green, axial skeleton; cream, appendicular skeleton. (From Muscolino JE: *Kinesiology: the skeletal system and muscle function,* enhanced edition, St Louis, 2007, Mosby.)

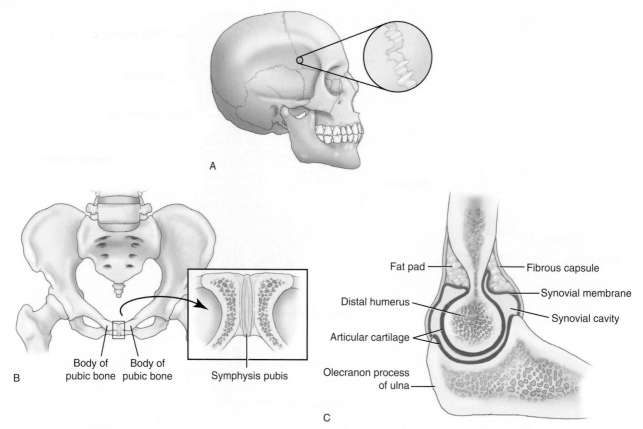

Figure 2-3 Structurally, there are three types of joints: **A,** fibrous; **B,** cartilaginous; and **C,** synovial. (From Muscolino JE: *Kinesiology: the skeletal system and muscle function,* enhanced edition, St Louis, 2007, Mosby.)

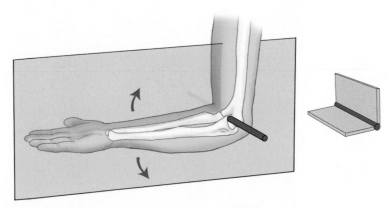

Figure 2-4 The humeroulnar joint of the elbow is an example of a uniaxial hinge joint. It allows flexion and extension within the sagittal plane around a mediolateral axis. (From Muscolino JE: *Kinesiology: the skeletal system and muscle function,* enhanced edition, St Louis, 2007, Mosby.)

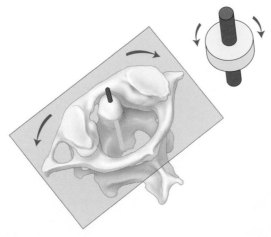

Figure 2-5 The atlantoaxial (C1–C2) joint of the spine between the atlas and axis is an example of a uniaxial pivot joint. It allows right and left rotations within the transverse plane around a vertical axis. (From Muscolino JE: *Kinesiology: the skeletal system and muscle function,* enhanced edition, St Louis, 2007, Mosby.)

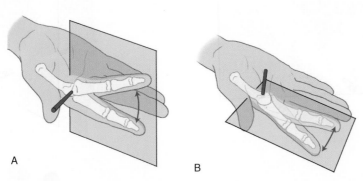

A   B

Figure 2-6 The metacarpophalangeal joint of the hand is an example of a biaxial condyloid joint. It allows flexion and extension in the sagittal joint around a mediolateral axis **(A),** and abduction and adduction in the frontal plane around an anteroposterior axis **(B).** (From Muscolino JE: *Kinesiology: the skeletal system and muscle function,* enhanced edition, St Louis, 2007, Mosby.)

lateral rotation to occur in the third plane, so some might consider a saddle joint to be triaxial. However, because these rotation actions cannot be actively isolated, a saddle joint is still considered to be biaxial. The carpometacarpal joint of the thumb is a classic example of a saddle joint (Figure 2-7).

Box 2-1

The saddle (carpometacarpal) joint of the thumb does allow rotation motions within the transverse plane around a vertical axis. However, medial rotation can only occur as the thumb flexes, and lateral rotation can only occur as the thumb extends. Because rotation actions cannot be actively isolated—that is, they cannot be actively performed by themselves—the saddle joint of the thumb is considered to be biaxial.

Triaxial Joints

There is only one major type of synovial triaxial joint: the ball-and-socket joint. As its name implies, one bone is shaped like a ball and fits into the socket shape of the other bone. A ball-and-socket joint allows the following motions: flexion and extension in the sagittal plane around a mediolateral axis; abduction and adduction in the frontal plane around an antero-posterior axis; and medial rotation and lateral rotation in the transverse plane around a vertical axis. The hip joint is a classic example of a ball-and-socket joint (Figure 2-8).

Nonaxial Joints

Synovial nonaxial joints permit motion within a plane, but the motion is a linear gliding motion and not a circular (axial) motion around an axis. The surfaces of nonaxial joints are usually flat or curved. Intercarpal joints between individual carpal bones of the wrist are examples of nonaxial joints (Figure 2-9).

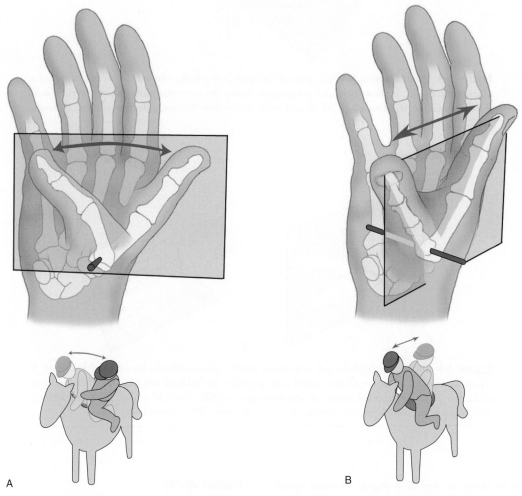

Figure 2-7 The carpometacarpal joint of the thumb is an example of a biaxial saddle joint. It allows flexion and extension as shown in **A**; and abduction and adduction as shown in **B**. It also allows medial and lateral rotation around a third axis; however these motions cannot be actively isolated. They must be coupled with flexion and extension respectively, so the saddle joint is considered to be biaxial. (Modified from Neumann DA: *Kinesiology of the musculoskeletal system: foundations for physical rehabilitation*, St Louis, 2002, Mosby.)

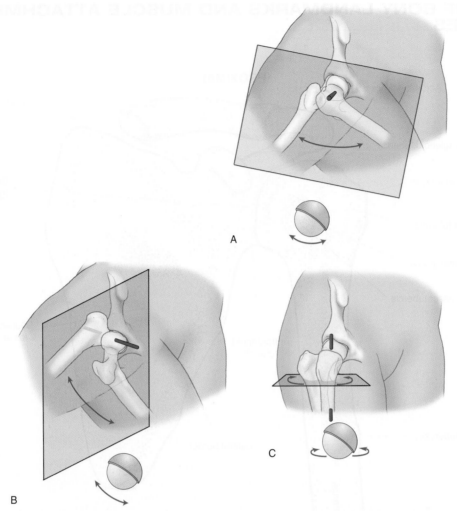

Figure 2-8 The hip joint between the head of the femur and the acetabulum of the pelvic bone is an example of a triaxial ball-and-socket joint. It allows flexion and extension in the sagittal plane around a mediolateral axis **(A)**, abduction and adduction in the frontal plane around an anteroposterior axis **(B)**, and medial rotation and lateral rotation in the transverse plane around a vertical axis **(C).** (From Muscolino JE: *Kinesiology: the skeletal system and muscle function,* enhanced edition, St Louis, 2007, Mosby.)

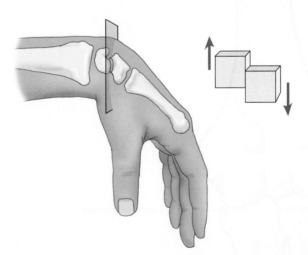

Figure 2-9 An intercarpal joint of the wrist is an example of a nonaxial joint. Linear gliding motion is allowed within a plane, but this motion does not occur around an axis, hence it is nonaxial. (From Muscolino JE: *Kinesiology: the skeletal system and muscle function,* enhanced edition, St Louis, 2007, Mosby.)

■ ATLAS OF BONY LANDMARKS AND MUSCLE ATTACHMENT SITES ON BONES

Upper Extremity

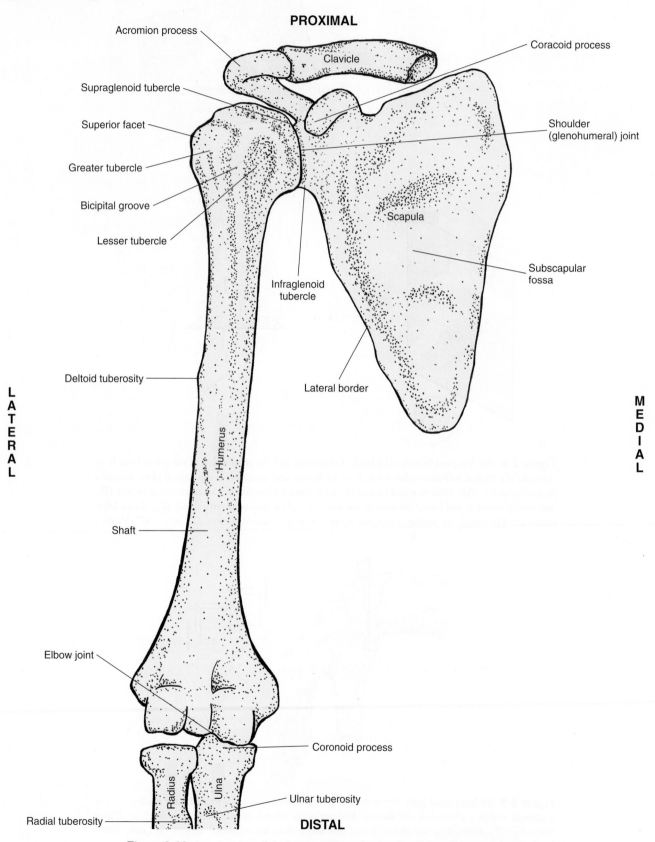

Figure 2-10 Anterior view of the bones and bony landmarks of the right scapula/arm.

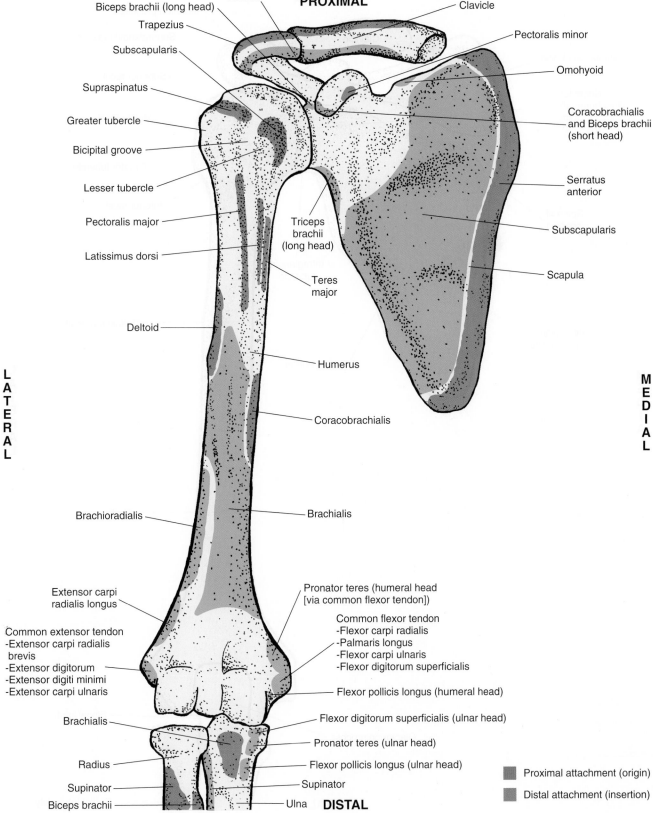

Figure 2-11 Anterior view of muscle attachment sites on the right scapula/arm.

2

PROXIMAL

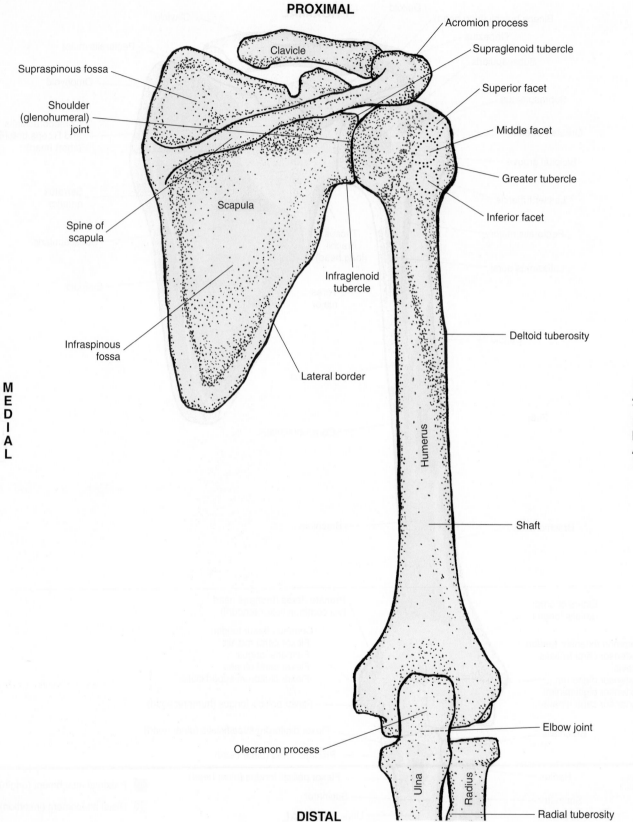

Supraspinous fossa

Shoulder
(glenohumeral)
joint

Spine of
scapula

Infraspinous
fossa

Clavicle

Scapula

Infraglenoid
tubercle

Lateral border

Acromion process

Supraglenoid tubercle

Superior facet

Middle facet

Greater tubercle

Inferior facet

Deltoid tuberosity

Shaft

Humerus

Olecranon process

Elbow joint

Ulna

Radius

Radial tuberosity

MEDIAL

LATERAL

DISTAL

Figure 2-12 Posterior view of bones and bony landmarks of the right scapula/arm.

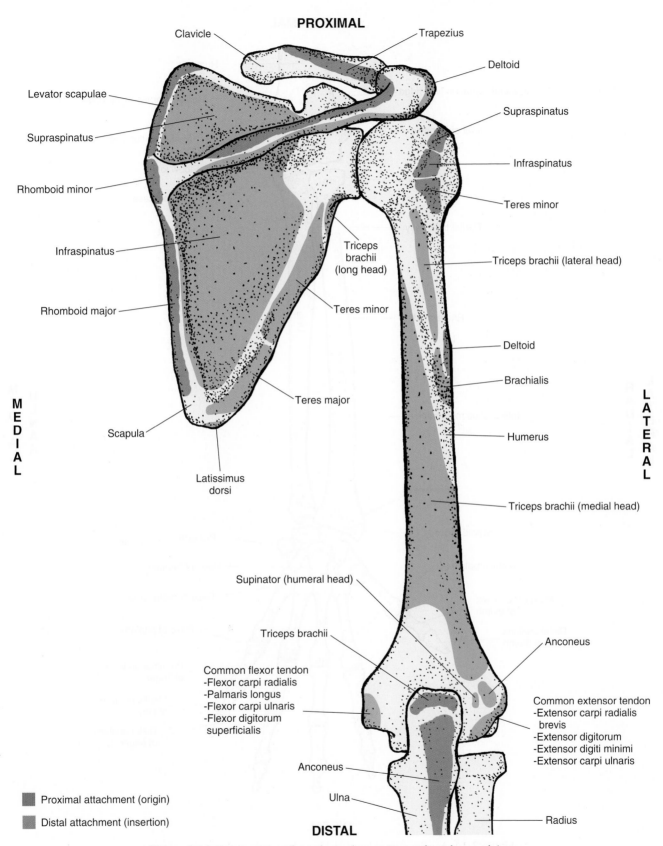

Figure 2-13 Posterior view of muscle attachment sites on the right scapula/arm.

2

PROXIMAL

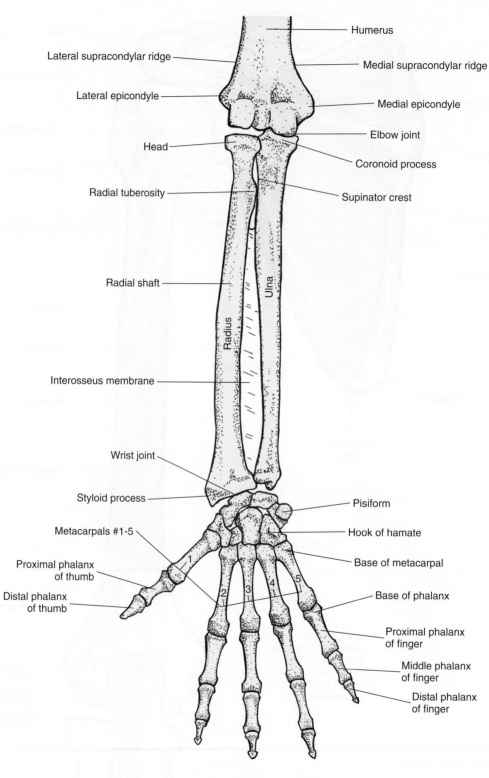

Humerus

Lateral supracondylar ridge — Medial supracondylar ridge

Lateral epicondyle — Medial epicondyle

Elbow joint

Head — Coronoid process

Radial tuberosity — Supinator crest

Radial shaft

Radius

Ulna

Interosseus membrane

Wrist joint

Styloid process

Pisiform

Metacarpals #1-5 — Hook of hamate

Proximal phalanx of thumb — Base of metacarpal

Distal phalanx of thumb — Base of phalanx

Proximal phalanx of finger

Middle phalanx of finger

Distal phalanx of finger

LATERAL RADIAL

ULNAR MEDIAL

DISTAL

Figure 2-14 Anterior view of bones and bony landmarks of the right forearm.

PROXIMAL

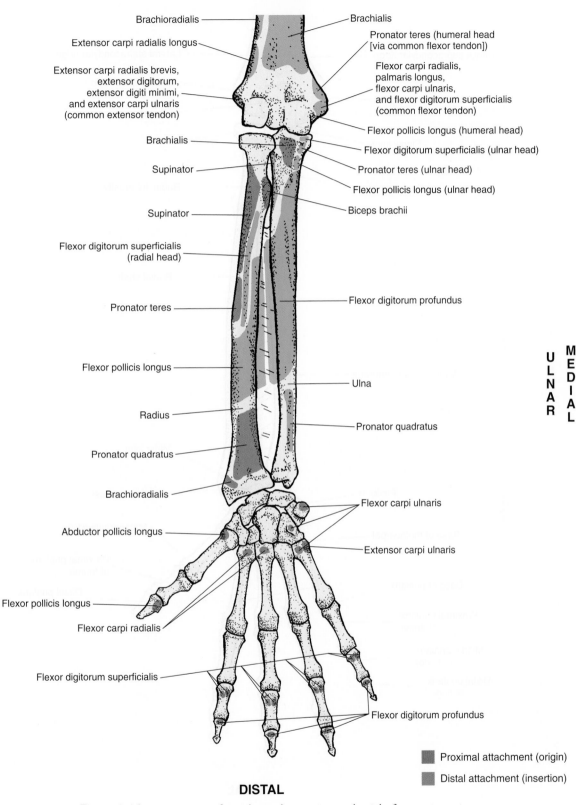

Figure 2-15 Anterior view of muscle attachment sites on the right forearm.

PROXIMAL

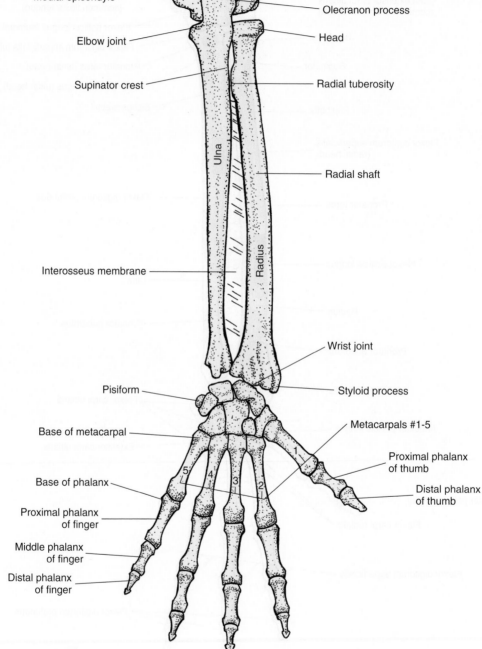

Humerus

Medial supracondylar ridge

Lateral supracondylar ridge

Lateral epicondyle

Medial epicondyle

Olecranon process

Elbow joint

Head

Supinator crest

Radial tuberosity

Ulna

Radius

Radial shaft

Interosseus membrane

MEDIAL ULNAR

RADIAL LATERAL

Wrist joint

Pisiform

Styloid process

Base of metacarpal

Metacarpals #1-5

Proximal phalanx of thumb

Base of phalanx

Distal phalanx of thumb

Proximal phalanx of finger

Middle phalanx of finger

Distal phalanx of finger

DISTAL

Figure 2-16 Posterior view of bones and bony landmarks of the right forearm.

PROXIMAL

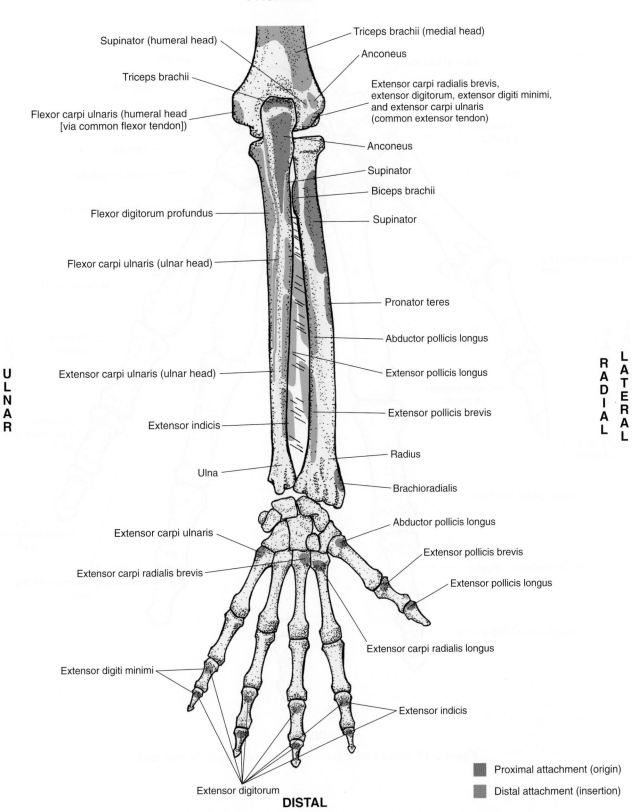

Supinator (humeral head)

Triceps brachii

Flexor carpi ulnaris (humeral head [via common flexor tendon])

Flexor digitorum profundus

Flexor carpi ulnaris (ulnar head)

Extensor carpi ulnaris (ulnar head)

Extensor indicis

Ulna

Triceps brachii (medial head)

Anconeus

Extensor carpi radialis brevis, extensor digitorum, extensor digiti minimi, and extensor carpi ulnaris (common extensor tendon)

Anconeus

Supinator

Biceps brachii

Supinator

Pronator teres

Abductor pollicis longus

Extensor pollicis longus

Extensor pollicis brevis

Radius

Brachioradialis

MEDIAL ULNAR

RADIAL LATERAL

Extensor carpi ulnaris

Extensor carpi radialis brevis

Extensor digiti minimi

Abductor pollicis longus

Extensor pollicis brevis

Extensor pollicis longus

Extensor carpi radialis longus

Extensor indicis

Extensor digitorum

Proximal attachment (origin)

Distal attachment (insertion)

DISTAL

Figure 2-17 Posterior view of muscle attachment sites on the right forearm.

PROXIMAL

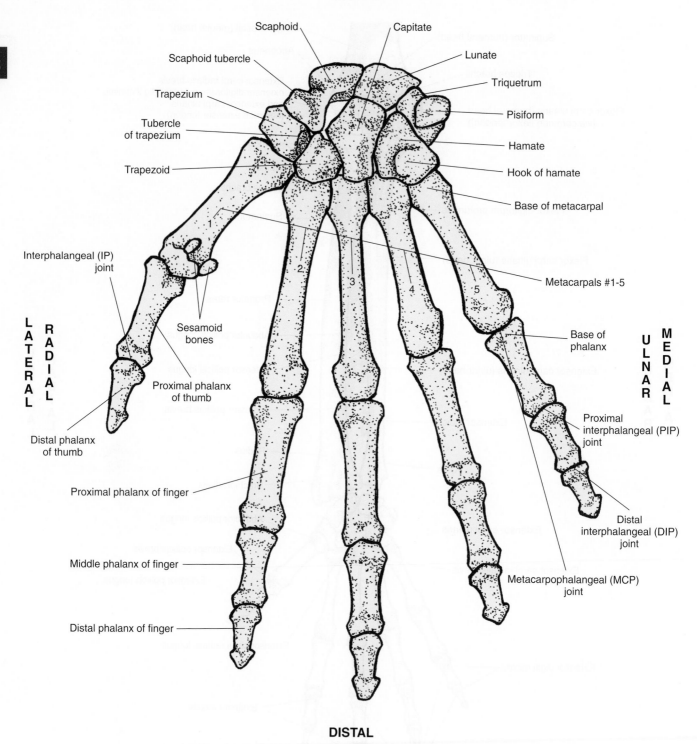

DISTAL

Figure 2-18 Palmar view of bones and bony landmarks of the right hand.

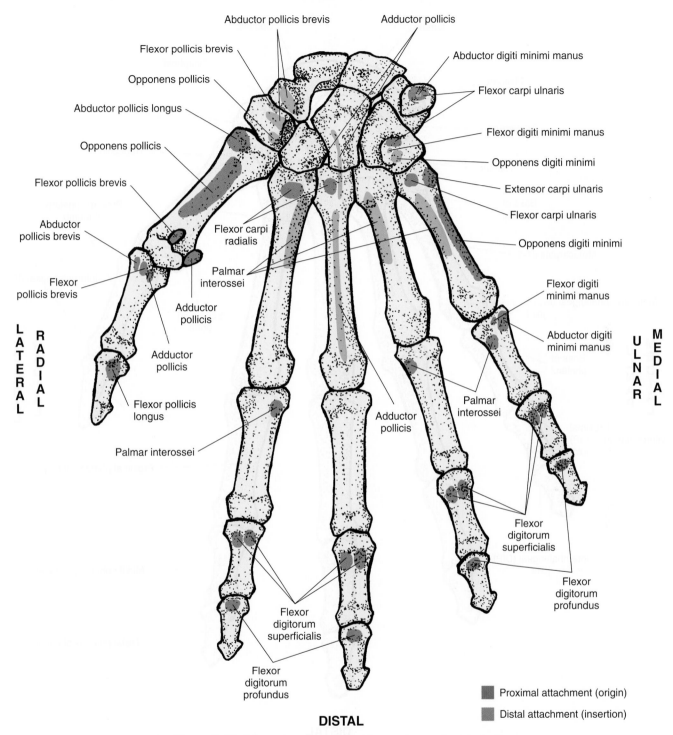

Figure 2-19 Palmar view of muscle attachment sites on the right hand.

2

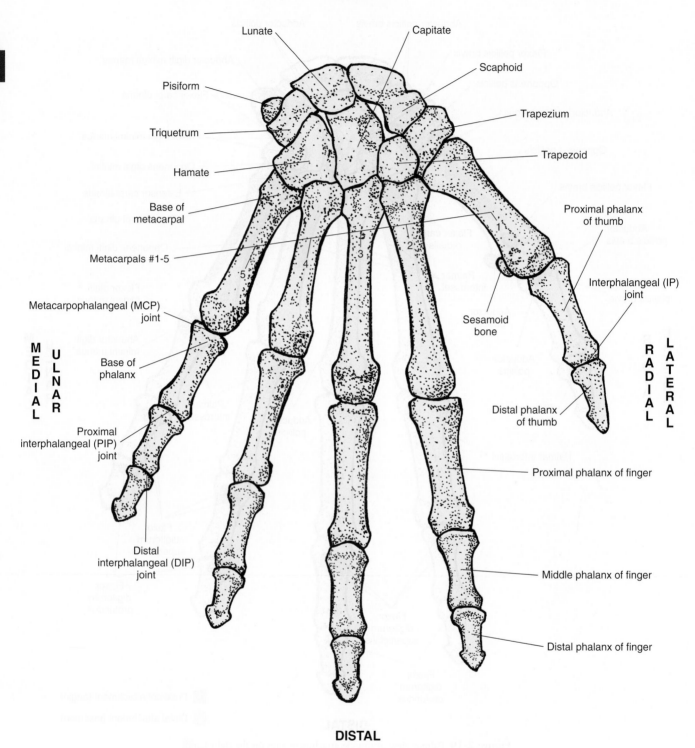

Figure 2-20 Dorsal view of bones and bony landmarks of the right hand.

PROXIMAL

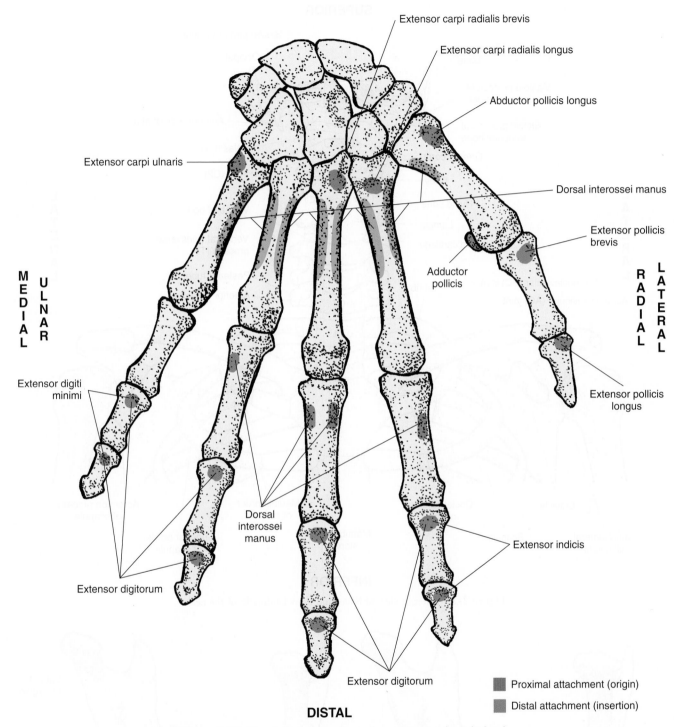

Extensor carpi radialis brevis

Extensor carpi radialis longus

Abductor pollicis longus

Extensor carpi ulnaris

Dorsal interossei manus

Extensor pollicis brevis

Adductor pollicis

Extensor pollicis longus

M E D I A L   U L N A R

R A D I A L   L A T E R A L

Extensor digiti minimi

Dorsal interossei manus

Extensor indicis

Extensor digitorum

Extensor digitorum

■ Proximal attachment (origin)

■ Distal attachment (insertion)

DISTAL

Figure 2-21 Dorsal view of muscle attachment sites on the right hand.

Axial Body

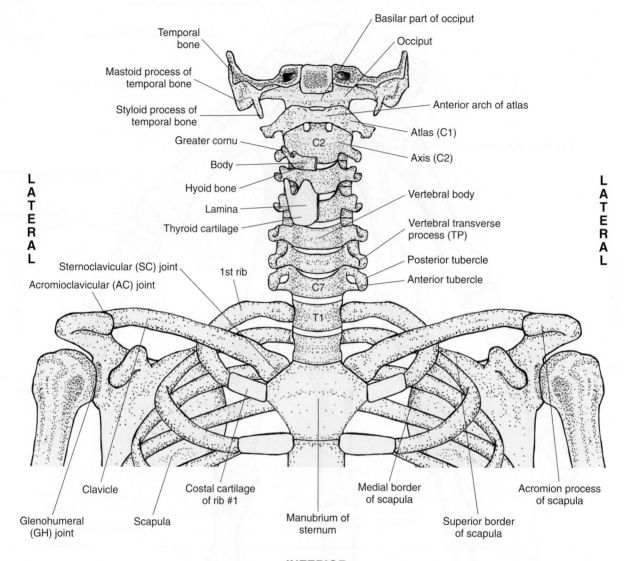

SUPERIOR

Temporal bone

Basilar part of occiput

Occiput

Mastoid process of temporal bone

Styloid process of temporal bone

Anterior arch of atlas

Atlas (C1)

Greater cornu

Axis (C2)

Body

Hyoid bone

Vertebral body

Lamina

Vertebral transverse process (TP)

Thyroid cartilage

Posterior tubercle

Anterior tubercle

Sternoclavicular (SC) joint

Acromioclavicular (AC) joint

1st rib

Clavicle

Costal cartilage of rib #1

Medial border of scapula

Acromion process of scapula

Glenohumeral (GH) joint

Scapula

Manubrium of sternum

Superior border of scapula

L A T E R A L

L A T E R A L

C2

C7

T1

INFERIOR

Figure 2-22 Anterior view of bones and bony landmarks of the neck.

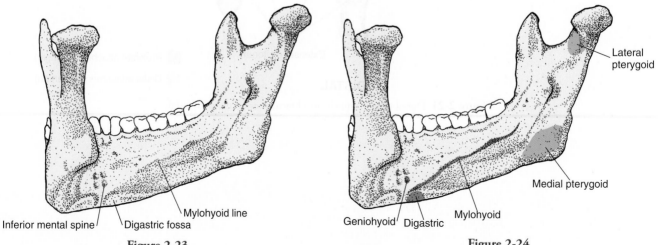

Inferior mental spine

Digastric fossa

Mylohyoid line

Figure 2-23

Lateral pterygoid

Medial pterygoid

Mylohyoid

Geniohyoid

Digastric

Figure 2-24

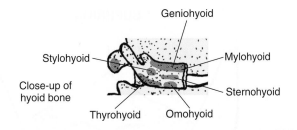

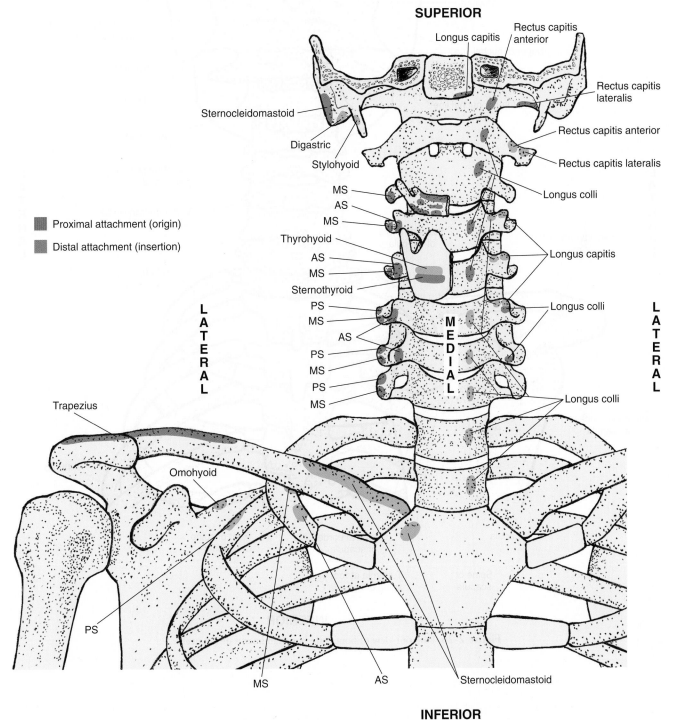

Figure 2-25 Anterior view of muscle attachment sites on the neck. AS, anterior scalene; MS, middle scalene; PS, posterior scalene.

SUPERIOR

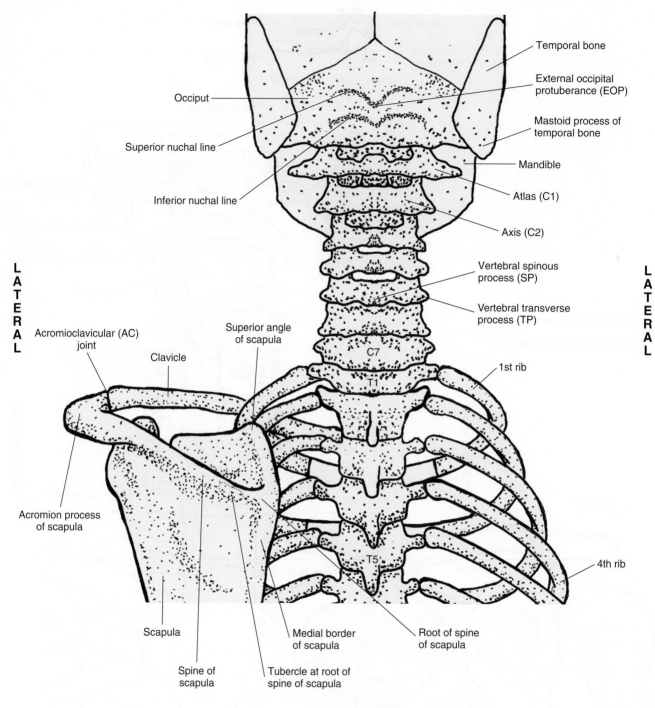

Temporal bone

External occipital protuberance (EOP)

Occiput

Superior nuchal line

Mastoid process of temporal bone

Mandible

Inferior nuchal line

Atlas (C1)

Axis (C2)

Vertebral spinous process (SP)

LATERAL

Acromioclavicular (AC) joint

Clavicle

Superior angle of scapula

Vertebral transverse process (TP)

C7

T1

1st rib

LATERAL

Acromion process of scapula

T5

4th rib

Scapula

Medial border of scapula

Root of spine of scapula

Spine of scapula

Tubercle at root of spine of scapula

INFERIOR

Figure 2-26 Posterior view of bones and bony landmarks of the neck.

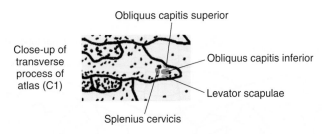

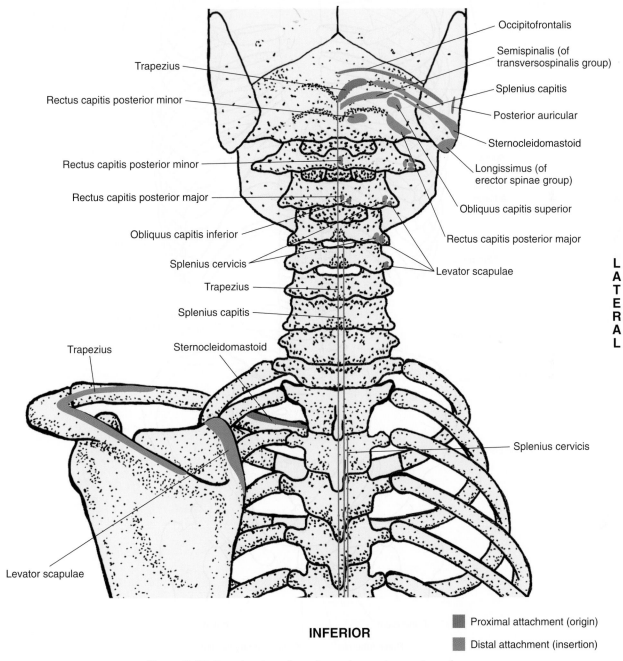

Figure 2-27 Posterior view of muscle attachment sites on the neck.

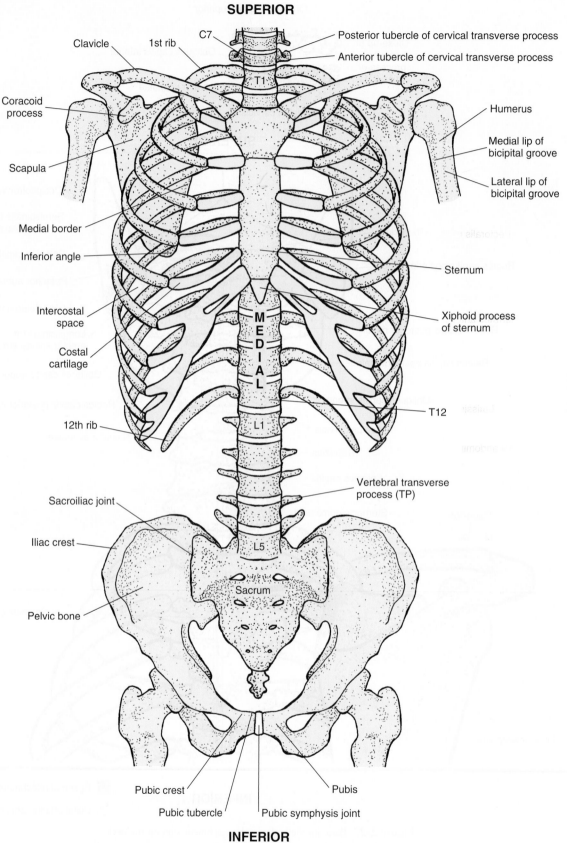

SUPERIOR

Clavicle

1st rib

C7

Posterior tubercle of cervical transverse process

Anterior tubercle of cervical transverse process

T1

Coracoid process

Humerus

Medial lip of bicipital groove

Scapula

Lateral lip of bicipital groove

Medial border

Inferior angle

Sternum

Intercostal space

Xiphoid process of sternum

Costal cartilage

MEDIAL

T12

12th rib

L1

Vertebral transverse process (TP)

Sacroiliac joint

Iliac crest

L5

Pelvic bone

Sacrum

Pubic crest

Pubis

Pubic tubercle

Pubic symphysis joint

LATERAL

LATERAL

INFERIOR

Figure 2-28 Anterior view of bones and bony landmarks of the trunk.

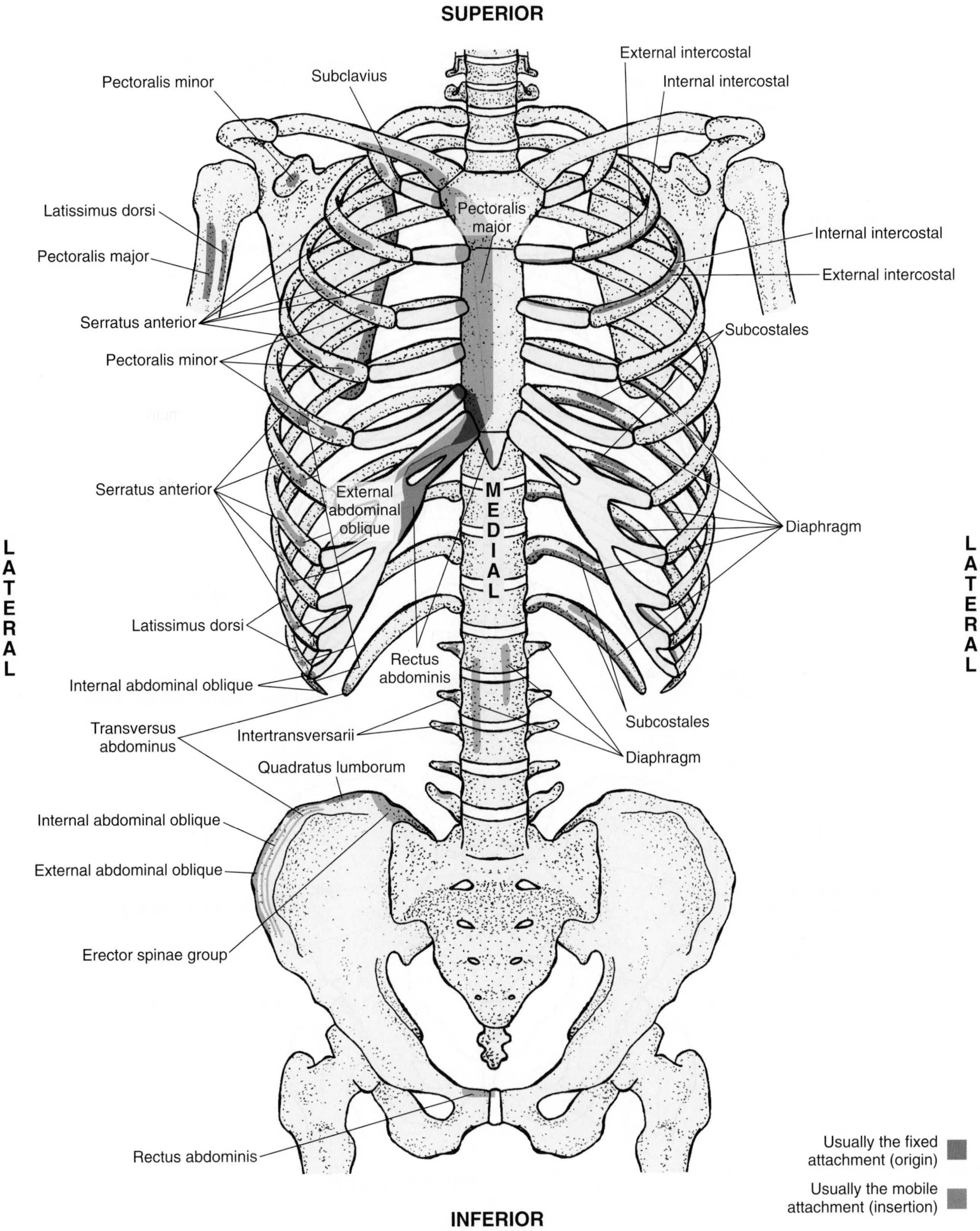

SUPERIOR

Pectoralis minor

Subclavius

External intercostal

Internal intercostal

Latissimus dorsi

Pectoralis major

Pectoralis major

Internal intercostal

External intercostal

Serratus anterior

Subcostales

Pectoralis minor

Serratus anterior

External abdominal oblique

MEDIAL

Diaphragm

Latissimus dorsi

Rectus abdominis

Internal abdominal oblique

Subcostales

Diaphragm

Transversus abdominus

Intertransversarii

Quadratus lumborum

Internal abdominal oblique

External abdominal oblique

Erector spinae group

Usually the fixed attachment (origin)

Usually the mobile attachment (insertion)

Rectus abdominis

L A T E R A L

L A T E R A L

INFERIOR

Figure 2-29 Anterior view of muscle attachment sites on the trunk.

SUPERIOR

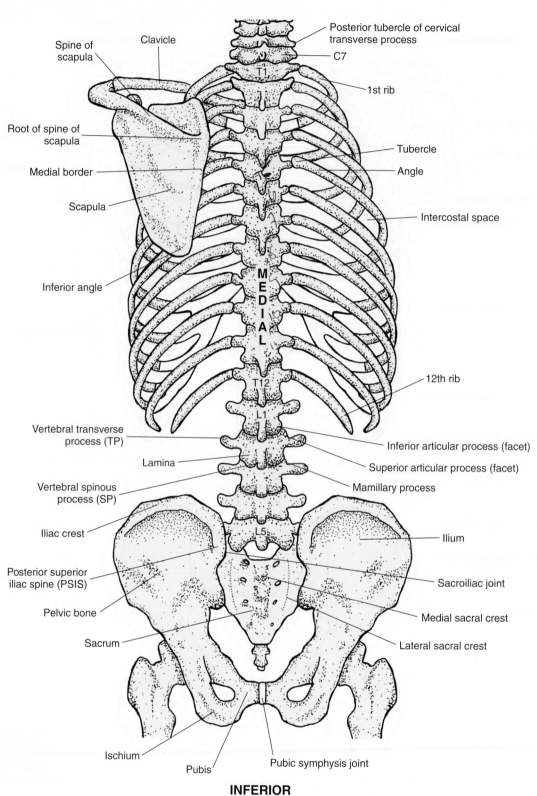

Clavicle

Spine of scapula

Posterior tubercle of cervical transverse process

C7

1st rib

Root of spine of scapula

Medial border

Scapula

Inferior angle

Tubercle

Angle

Intercostal space

LATERAL

MEDIAL

LATERAL

12th rib

Vertebral transverse process (TP)

Lamina

Vertebral spinous process (SP)

Iliac crest

Posterior superior iliac spine (PSIS)

Pelvic bone

Sacrum

Inferior articular process (facet)

Superior articular process (facet)

Mamillary process

Ilium

Sacroiliac joint

Medial sacral crest

Lateral sacral crest

Ischium

Pubis

Pubic symphysis joint

INFERIOR

Figure 2-30 Posterior view of bones and bony landmarks of the trunk.

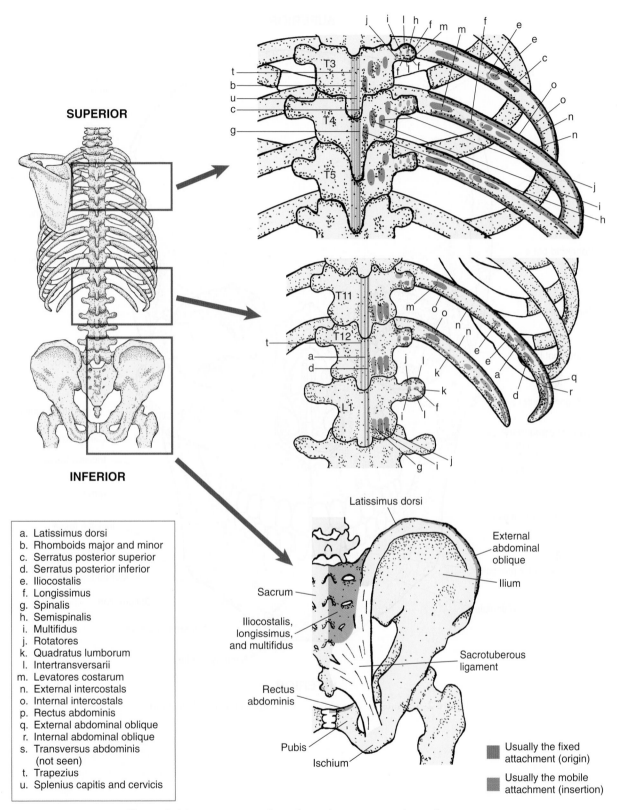

a. Latissimus dorsi
b. Rhomboids major and minor
c. Serratus posterior superior
d. Serratus posterior inferior
e. Iliocostalis
f. Longissimus
g. Spinalis
h. Semispinalis
i. Multifidus
j. Rotatores
k. Quadratus lumborum
l. Intertransversarii
m. Levatores costarum
n. External intercostals
o. Internal intercostals
p. Rectus abdominis
q. External abdominal oblique
r. Internal abdominal oblique
s. Transversus abdominis
   (not seen)
t. Trapezius
u. Splenius capitis and cervicis

Figure 2-31 Posterior view of muscle attachment sites on the trunk.

SUPERIOR

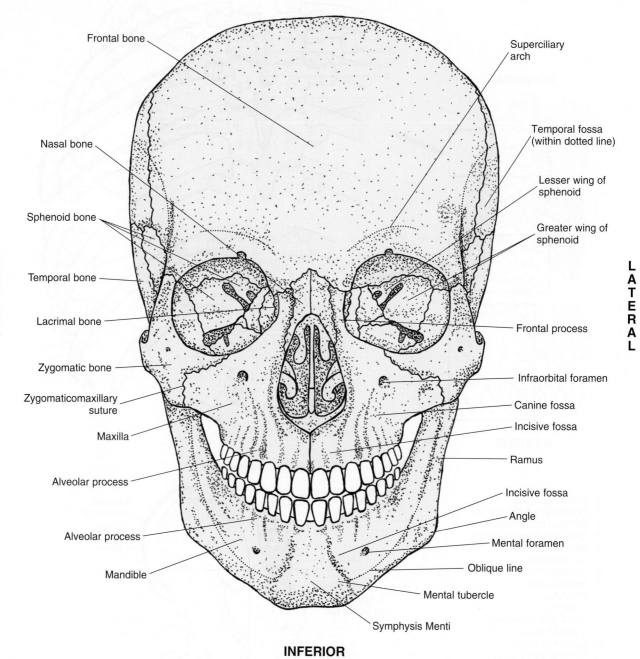

Frontal bone

Nasal bone

Sphenoid bone

Temporal bone

Lacrimal bone

Zygomatic bone

Zygomaticomaxillary
suture

Maxilla

Alveolar process

Alveolar process

Mandible

Superciliary
arch

Temporal fossa
(within dotted line)

Lesser wing of
sphenoid

Greater wing of
sphenoid

Frontal process

Infraorbital foramen

Canine fossa

Incisive fossa

Ramus

Incisive fossa

Angle

Mental foramen

Oblique line

Mental tubercle

Symphysis Menti

LATERAL

LATERAL

INFERIOR

Figure 2-32 Anterior view of bones and bony landmarks of the head.

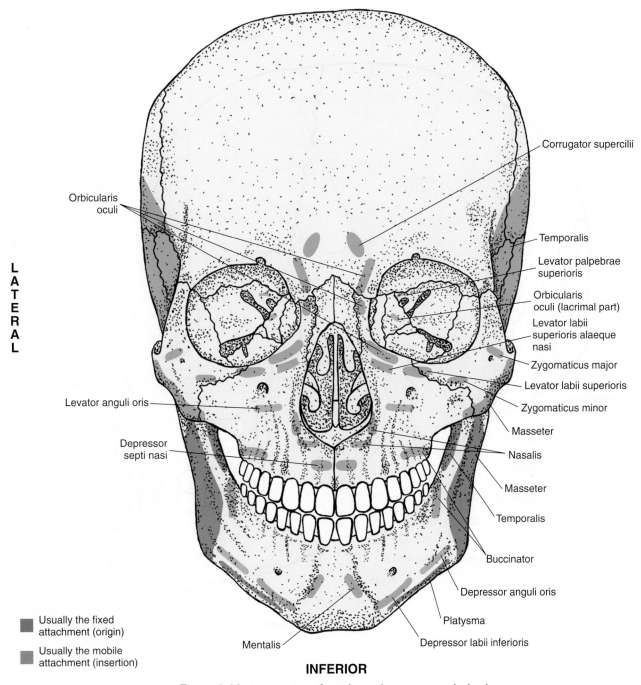

SUPERIOR

Corrugator supercilii

Orbicularis
oculi

Temporalis

Levator palpebrae
superioris

Orbicularis
oculi (lacrimal part)

Levator labii
superioris alaeque
nasi

Zygomaticus major

Levator labii superioris

Levator anguli oris

Zygomaticus minor

Masseter

Depressor
septi nasi

Nasalis

Masseter

Temporalis

Buccinator

Depressor anguli oris

Platysma

Mentalis

Depressor labii inferioris

LATERAL

LATERAL

Usually the fixed
attachment (origin)

Usually the mobile
attachment (insertion)

INFERIOR

Figure 2-33 Anterior view of muscle attachment sites on the head.

2

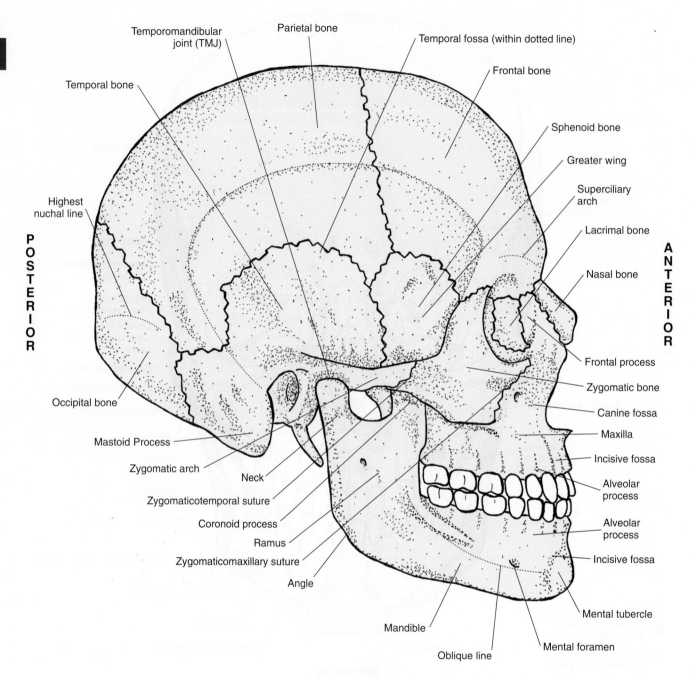

SUPERIOR

Temporomandibular joint (TMJ)

Parietal bone

Temporal fossa (within dotted line)

Temporal bone

Frontal bone

Sphenoid bone

Greater wing

Superciliary arch

Highest nuchal line

Lacrimal bone

Nasal bone

P O S T E R I O R

A N T E R I O R

Occipital bone

Frontal process

Zygomatic bone

Canine fossa

Maxilla

Mastoid Process

Incisive fossa

Zygomatic arch

Alveolar process

Neck

Zygomaticotemporal suture

Coronoid process

Alveolar process

Ramus

Incisive fossa

Zygomaticomaxillary suture

Angle

Mental tubercle

Mandible

Mental foramen

Oblique line

INFERIOR

Figure 2-34 Lateral view of bones and bony landmarks of the head.

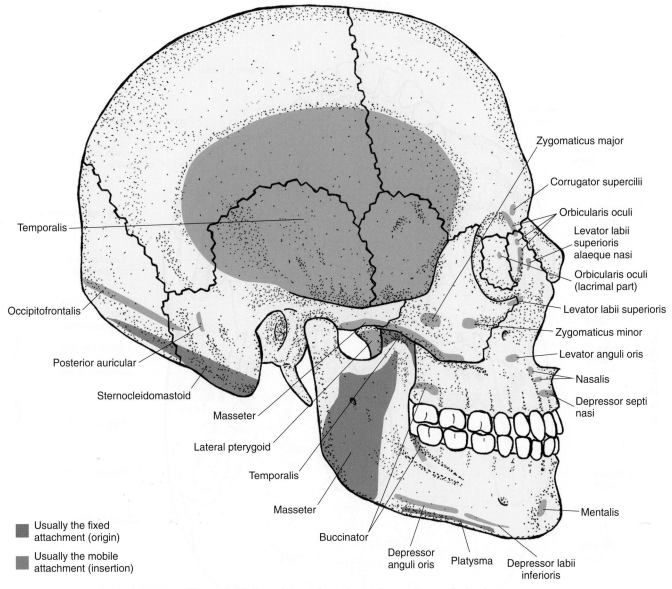

Figure 2-35 Lateral view of muscle attachment sites on the head.

Zygomaticus major

Corrugator supercilii

Orbicularis oculi

Levator labii superioris alaeque nasi

Orbicularis oculi (lacrimal part)

Levator labii superioris

Zygomaticus minor

Levator anguli oris

Nasalis

Depressor septi nasi

Mentalis

Temporalis

Occipitofrontalis

Posterior auricular

Sternocleidomastoid

Masseter

Lateral pterygoid

Temporalis

Masseter

Buccinator

Depressor anguli oris

Platysma

Depressor labii inferioris

■ Usually the fixed attachment (origin)

■ Usually the mobile attachment (insertion)

ANTERIOR

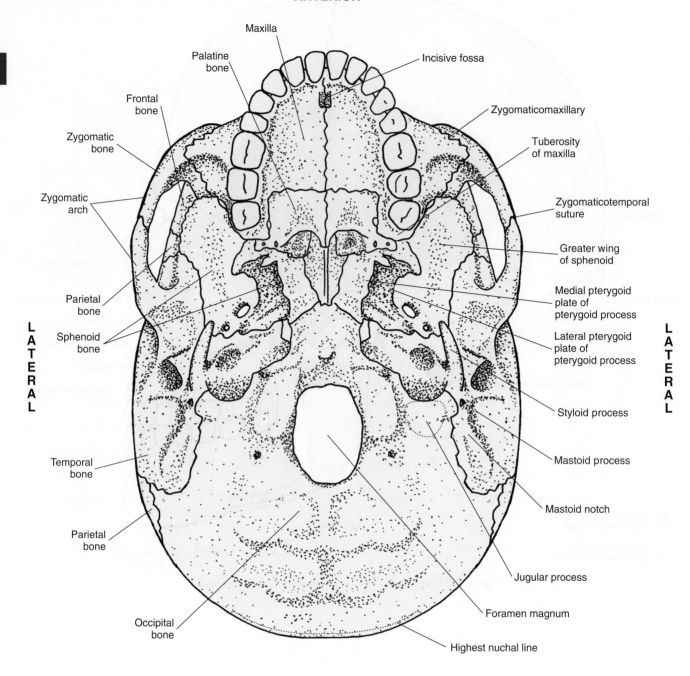

POSTERIOR

Figure 2-36 Inferior view of bones and bony landmarks of the head.

2

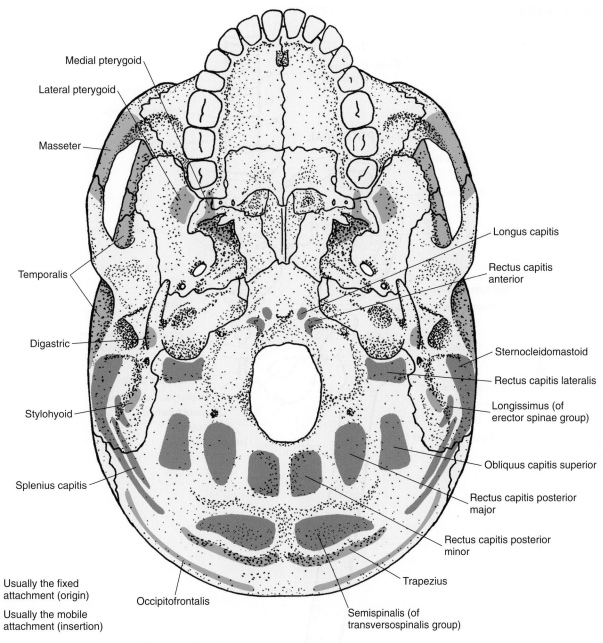

Medial pterygoid

Lateral pterygoid

Masseter

Temporalis

Digastric

Stylohyoid

Splenius capitis

Longus capitis

Rectus capitis anterior

Sternocleidomastoid

Rectus capitis lateralis

Longissimus (of erector spinae group)

Obliquus capitis superior

Rectus capitis posterior major

Rectus capitis posterior minor

Trapezius

Semispinalis (of transversospinalis group)

Occipitofrontalis

Usually the fixed attachment (origin)

Usually the mobile attachment (insertion)

Figure 2-37 Inferior view of muscle attachment sites on the head.

Lower Extremity

2

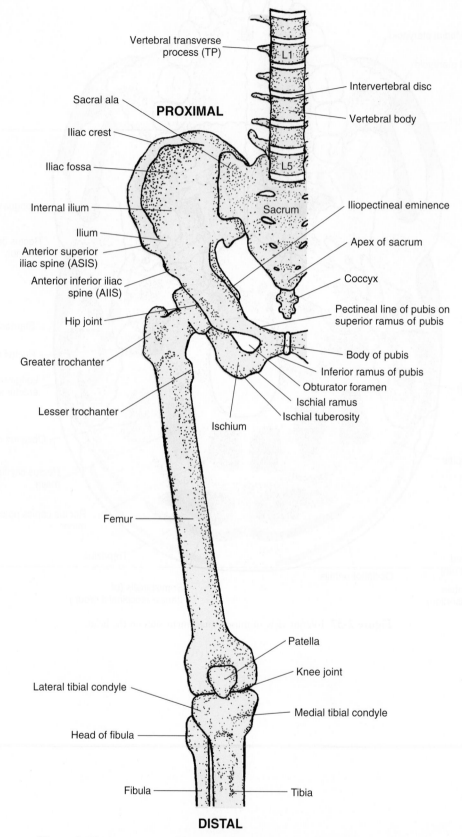

Figure 2-38 Anterior view of bones and bony landmarks of the right pelvis and thigh.

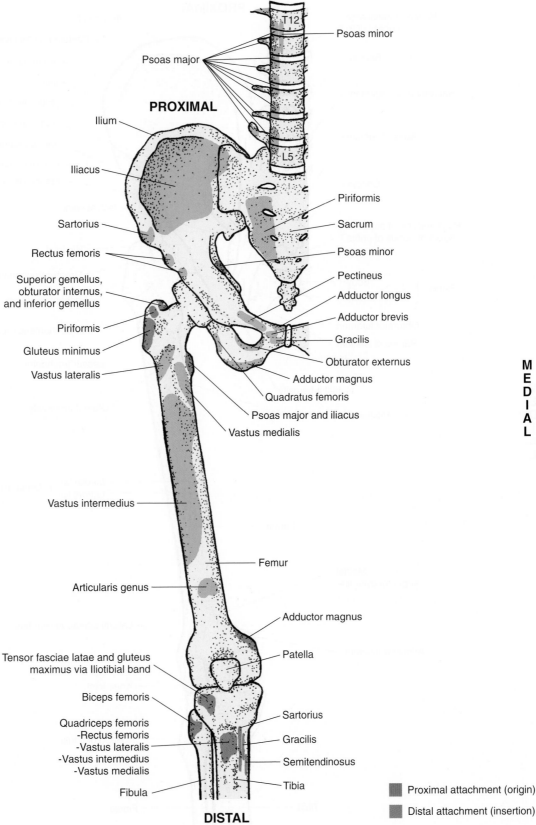

Figure 2-39 Anterior view of muscle attachment sites on the right pelvis and thigh.

2

PROXIMAL

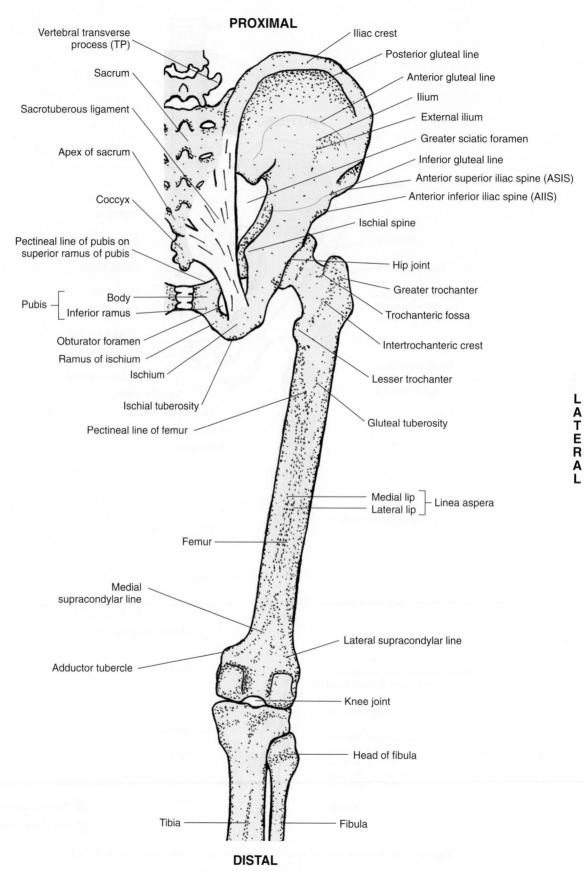

Vertebral transverse process (TP)

Sacrum

Sacrotuberous ligament

Apex of sacrum

Coccyx

Pectineal line of pubis on superior ramus of pubis

Pubis {
Body
Inferior ramus
}

Obturator foramen

Ramus of ischium

Ischium

Ischial tuberosity

Pectineal line of femur

Iliac crest

Posterior gluteal line

Anterior gluteal line

Ilium

External ilium

Greater sciatic foramen

Inferior gluteal line

Anterior superior iliac spine (ASIS)

Anterior inferior iliac spine (AIIS)

Ischial spine

Hip joint

Greater trochanter

Trochanteric fossa

Intertrochanteric crest

Lesser trochanter

Gluteal tuberosity

M E D I A L

L A T E R A L

Medial lip
Lateral lip
} Linea aspera

Femur

Medial supracondylar line

Adductor tubercle

Lateral supracondylar line

Knee joint

Head of fibula

Tibia

Fibula

DISTAL

Figure 2-40 Posterior view of bones and bony landmarks of the right pelvis and thigh.

PROXIMAL

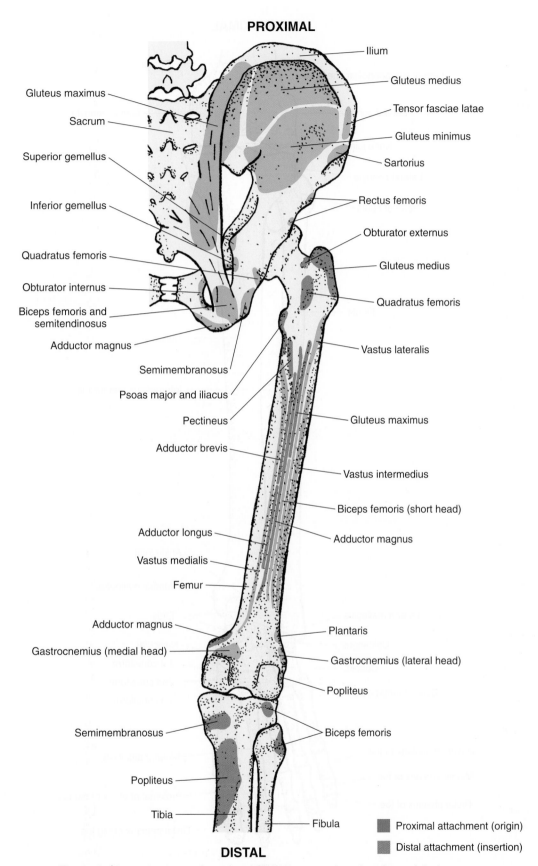

Ilium

Gluteus medius

Tensor fasciae latae

Gluteus minimus

Sartorius

Rectus femoris

Obturator externus

Gluteus medius

Quadratus femoris

Vastus lateralis

Gluteus maximus

Vastus intermedius

Biceps femoris (short head)

Adductor magnus

Plantaris

Gastrocnemius (lateral head)

Popliteus

Biceps femoris

Fibula

Gluteus maximus

Sacrum

Superior gemellus

Inferior gemellus

Quadratus femoris

Obturator internus

Biceps femoris and semitendinosus

Adductor magnus

Semimembranosus

Psoas major and iliacus

Pectineus

Adductor brevis

Adductor longus

Vastus medialis

Femur

Adductor magnus

Gastrocnemius (medial head)

Semimembranosus

Popliteus

Tibia

M E D I A L

L A T E R A L

Proximal attachment (origin)

Distal attachment (insertion)

DISTAL

Figure 2-41 posterior view of muscle attachment sites on the right pelvis and thigh.

2

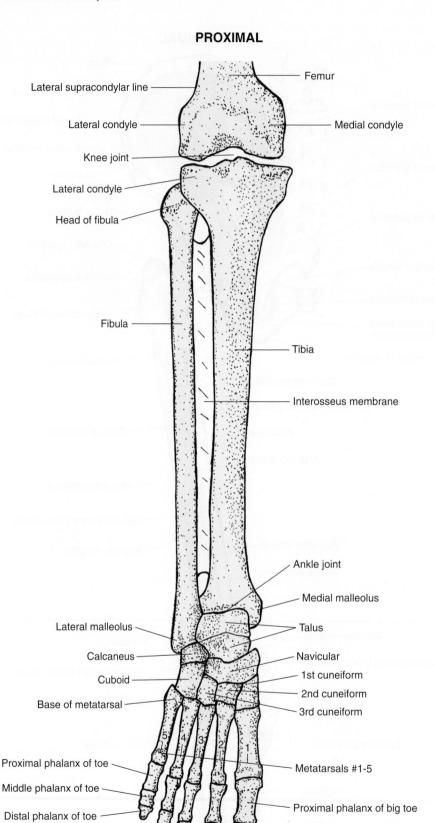

PROXIMAL

Lateral supracondylar line — ——— Femur

Lateral condyle — ——— Medial condyle

Knee joint —

Lateral condyle —

Head of fibula —

Fibula — ——— Tibia

——— Interosseus membrane

——— Ankle joint

——— Medial malleolus

Lateral malleolus — ——— Talus

Calcaneus — ——— Navicular

Cuboid — ——— 1st cuneiform

Base of metatarsal — ——— 2nd cuneiform

——— 3rd cuneiform

5 4 3 2 1

Proximal phalanx of toe — ——— Metatarsals #1-5

Middle phalanx of toe —

Distal phalanx of toe — ——— Proximal phalanx of big toe

——— Distal phalanx of big toe

DISTAL

L A T E R A L

M E D I A L

Figure 2-42 Anterior view of bones and bony landmarks of the right leg.

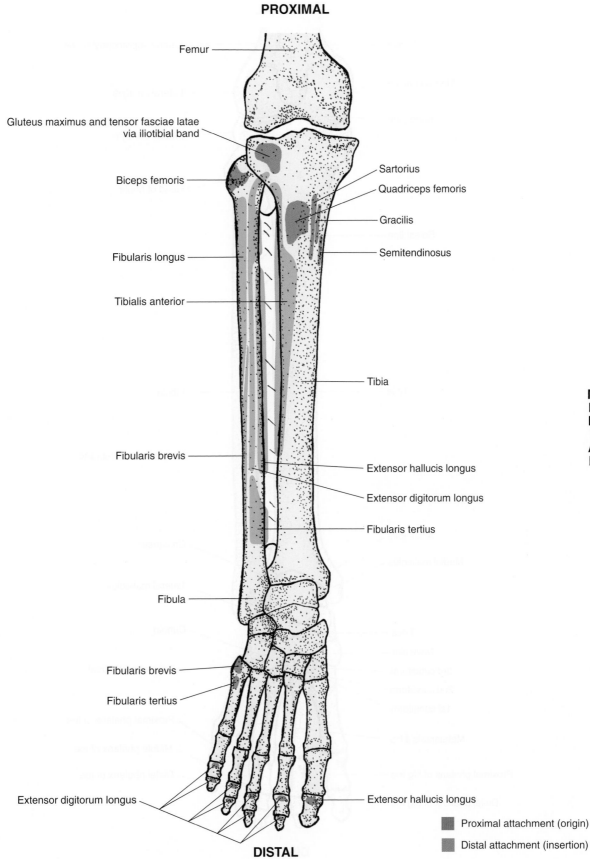

PROXIMAL

Femur

Gluteus maximus and tensor fasciae latae
via iliotibial band

Biceps femoris

Sartorius

Quadriceps femoris

Gracilis

Fibularis longus

Semitendinosus

Tibialis anterior

Tibia

Fibularis brevis

Extensor hallucis longus

Extensor digitorum longus

Fibularis tertius

Fibula

Fibularis brevis

Fibularis tertius

Extensor digitorum longus

Extensor hallucis longus

LATERAL

MEDIAL

Proximal attachment (origin)

Distal attachment (insertion)

DISTAL

Figure 2-43 Anterior view of muscle attachment sites on the right leg.

2

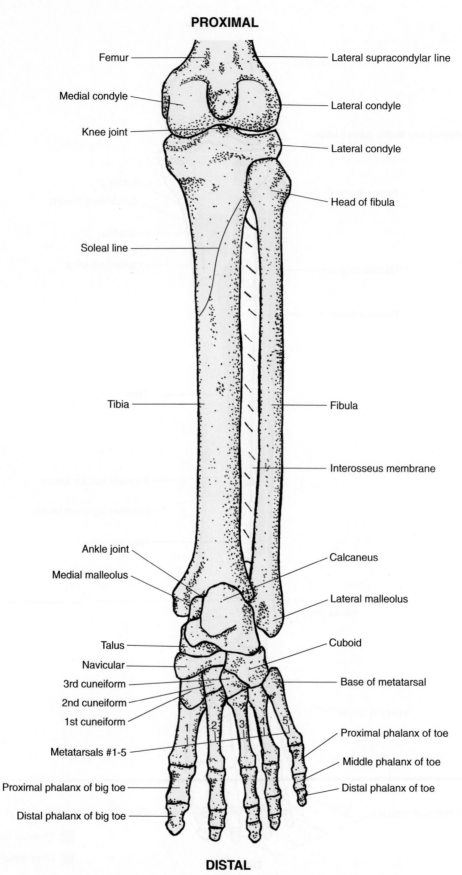

PROXIMAL

Femur — Lateral supracondylar line

Medial condyle — Lateral condyle

Knee joint — Lateral condyle

Head of fibula

Soleal line

M E D I A L

Tibia — Fibula

Interosseus membrane

L A T E R A L

Ankle joint — Calcaneus

Medial malleolus — Lateral malleolus

Talus — Cuboid

Navicular —

3rd cuneiform — Base of metatarsal

2nd cuneiform

1st cuneiform

1 2 3 4 5

Metatarsals #1-5 — Proximal phalanx of toe

Middle phalanx of toe

Proximal phalanx of big toe — Distal phalanx of toe

Distal phalanx of big toe

DISTAL

Figure 2-44 Posterior view of bones and bony landmarks of the right leg.

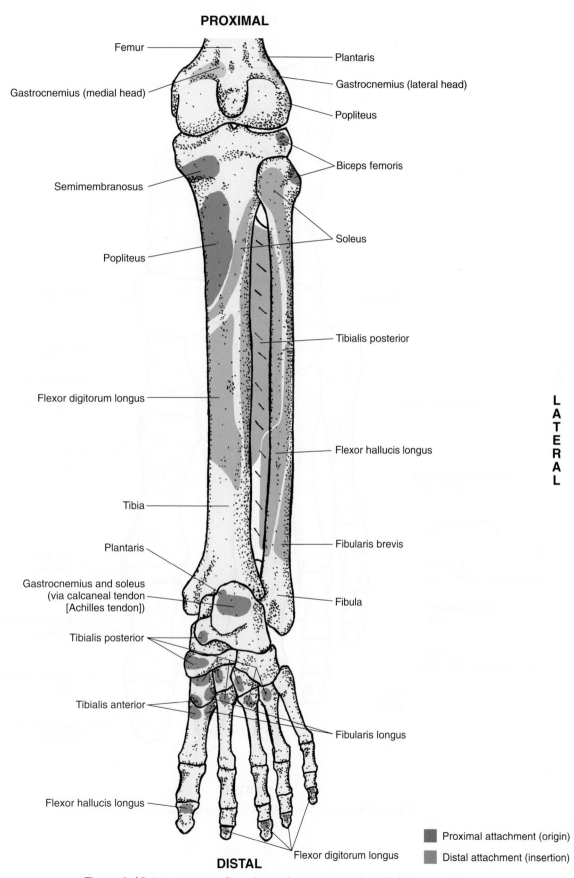

Figure 2-45 Posterior view of muscle attachment sites on the right leg.

PROXIMAL

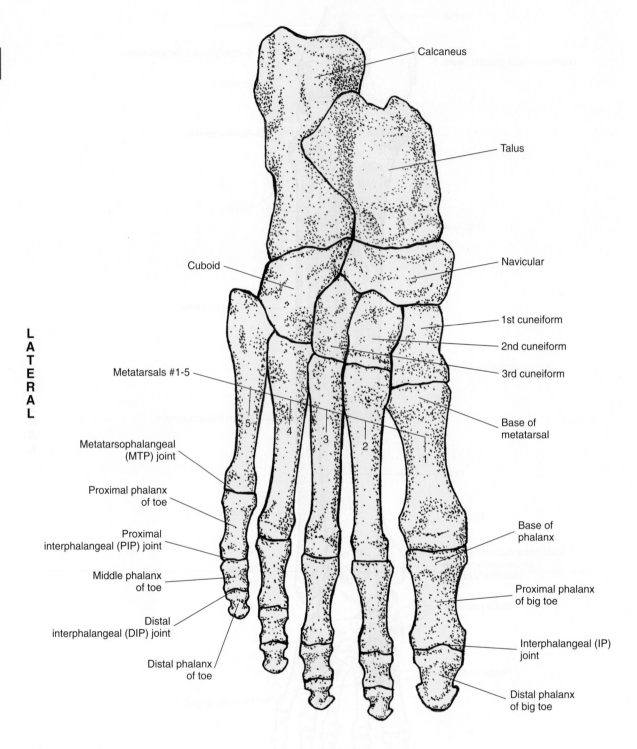

LATERAL

MEDIAL

Calcaneus

Talus

Cuboid

Navicular

1st cuneiform

2nd cuneiform

3rd cuneiform

Metatarsals #1-5

Base of
metatarsal

Metatarsophalangeal
(MTP) joint

Proximal phalanx
of toe

Proximal
interphalangeal (PIP) joint

Middle phalanx
of toe

Distal
interphalangeal (DIP) joint

Distal phalanx
of toe

Base of
phalanx

Proximal phalanx
of big toe

Interphalangeal (IP)
joint

Distal phalanx
of big toe

DISTAL

Figure 2-46 Dorsal view of bones and bony landmarks of the right foot.

PROXIMAL

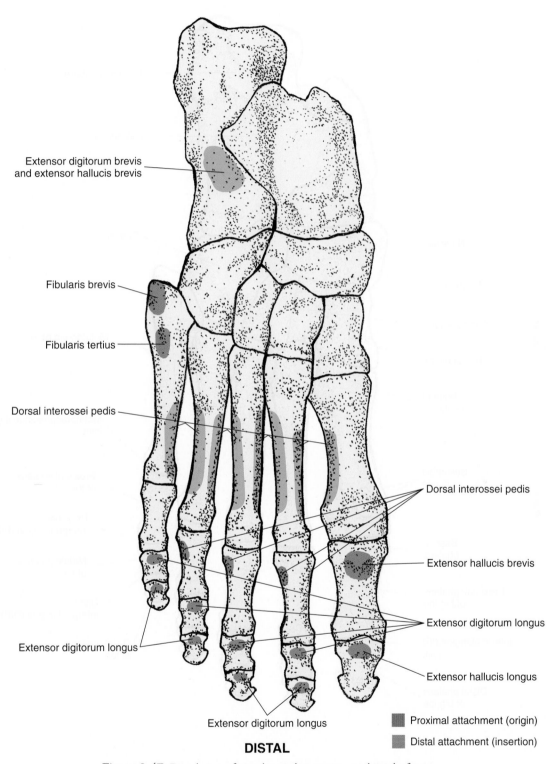

Extensor digitorum brevis
and extensor hallucis brevis

Fibularis brevis

Fibularis tertius

Dorsal interossei pedis

LATERAL

MEDIAL

Dorsal interossei pedis

Extensor hallucis brevis

Extensor digitorum longus

Extensor digitorum longus

Extensor hallucis longus

Extensor digitorum longus

Proximal attachment (origin)

Distal attachment (insertion)

DISTAL

Figure 2-47 Dorsal view of muscle attachment sites on the right foot.

2

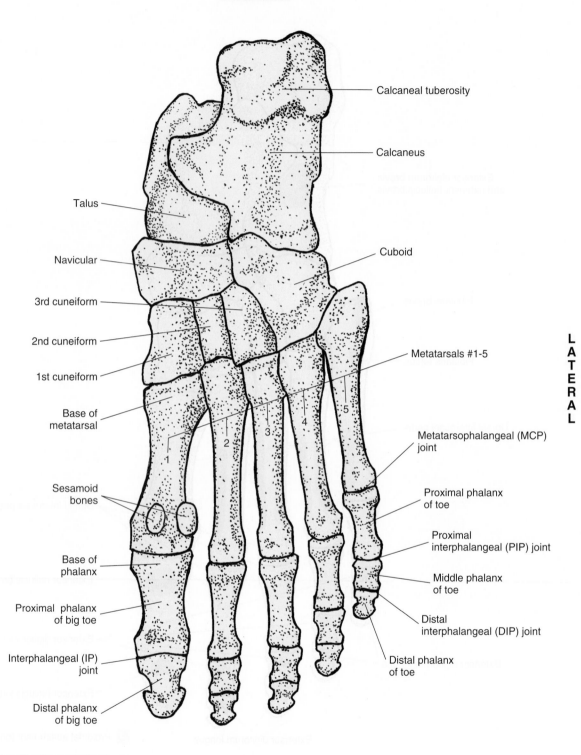

PROXIMAL

M E D I A L

L A T E R A L

Calcaneal tuberosity

Calcaneus

Talus

Navicular

Cuboid

3rd cuneiform

2nd cuneiform

1st cuneiform

Metatarsals #1-5

Base of
metatarsal

Metatarsophalangeal (MCP)
joint

Proximal phalanx
of toe

Sesamoid
bones

Proximal
interphalangeal (PIP) joint

Middle phalanx
of toe

Base of
phalanx

Proximal phalanx
of big toe

Distal
interphalangeal (DIP) joint

Interphalangeal (IP)
joint

Distal phalanx
of toe

Distal phalanx
of big toe

DISTAL

Figure 2-48 Plantar view of bones and bony landmarks of the right foot.

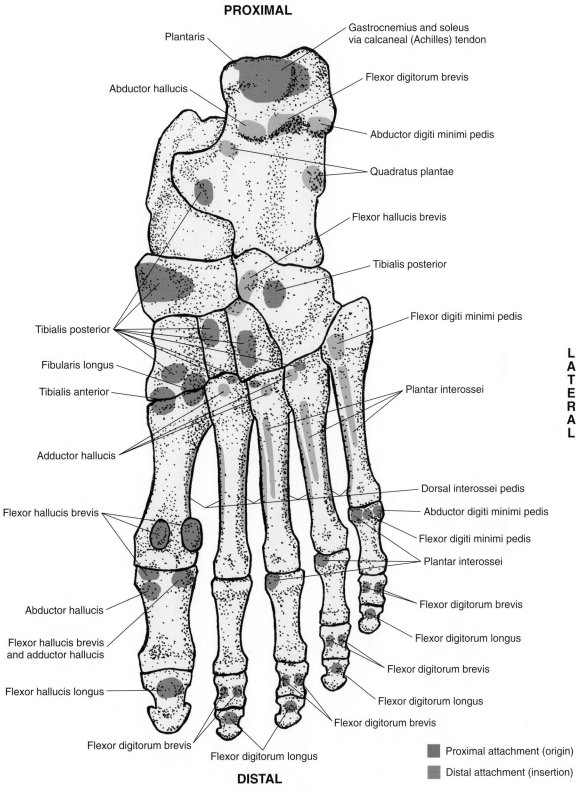

PROXIMAL

Plantaris

Gastrocnemius and soleus
via calcaneal (Achilles) tendon

Abductor hallucis

Flexor digitorum brevis

Abductor digiti minimi pedis

Quadratus plantae

Flexor hallucis brevis

Tibialis posterior

Flexor digiti minimi pedis

Tibialis posterior

Fibularis longus

Plantar interossei

Tibialis anterior

Adductor hallucis

Dorsal interossei pedis

Abductor digiti minimi pedis

Flexor digiti minimi pedis

Plantar interossei

Flexor hallucis brevis

Flexor digitorum brevis

Flexor digitorum longus

Abductor hallucis

Flexor digitorum brevis

Flexor hallucis brevis
and adductor hallucis

Flexor digitorum longus

Flexor hallucis longus

Flexor digitorum brevis

Flexor digitorum brevis

Flexor digitorum longus

MEDIAL

LATERAL

■ Proximal attachment (origin)

■ Distal attachment (insertion)

DISTAL

Figure 2-49 Plantar view of muscle attachment sites on the right foot.

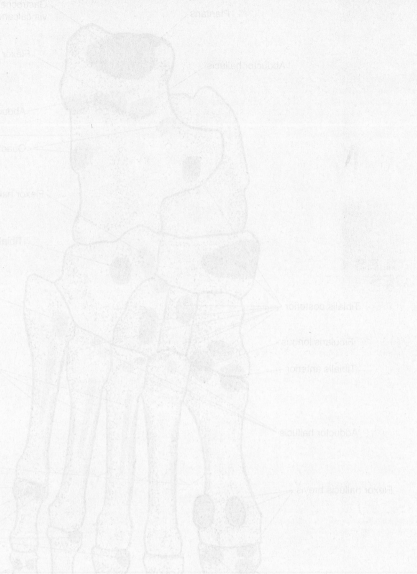

How Muscles Function

■ MUSCLES CREATE PULLING FORCES

The essence of muscle function is that muscles create pulling forces. It is as simple as that. When a muscle contracts, it *attempts* to pull in toward its center. This results in a pulling force being placed on its attachments. If this pulling force is sufficiently strong, the muscle will succeed in shortening and it will move one or both of the body parts to which it is attached. It is also important to realize that this pulling force is equal on both of its attachments. A muscle does not and cannot choose to pull on one of its attachments and not the other. In effect, a muscle is nothing more that a simple "pulling machine." When ordered to contract by the nervous system, it pulls on its attachments; when not ordered to contract, it relaxes and does not pull (Box 3-1).

Box 3-1

To call a muscle nothing more than a simple "pulling machine" does not lessen the amazing and awe-inspiring complexity of movement patterns that the muscular system produces. Any one muscle is a simple machine that pulls. But when different aspects of various muscles are co-ordered to contract in concert with each other and in temporal sequence with each other, the sum of many "simple" pulling forces results in an amazingly fluid and complex array of movement patterns. The director of this symphony who coordinates these pulling forces is the nervous system.

It is usually extremely helpful when confronted with a new kinesiology term to see if there is a cognate, in other words, a similar term in lay English. This helps us to intuitively understand the new kinesiology term instead of having to memorize its meaning. When it comes to the study of muscle function, the operative word is *contract* because that is what muscles do. However, in this case, it can be counterproductive to try to understand muscle contraction by relating it to how the term *contract* is defined in English. In English, the word "contract" means "to shorten." This leads many students to assume that when a muscle contracts, it shortens. This is not necessarily true, and making this assumption can limit our ability to truly grasp how the muscular system functions. In fact, most muscle contractions do not result in the muscle shortening, and to look at the muscular system this way is to overlook much of how the muscular system functions.

■ WHAT IS A MUSCLE CONTRACTION?

When a muscle contracts, it *attempts* to shorten. Whether or not it does succeed in shortening is based on the strength of its contraction compared to the resistance force it encounters that is opposed to its shortening. For a muscle to shorten, it must move one or both of its attachments. Therefore the resistance to shortening is usually the weight of the body parts to which the muscle is attached. Let's look at the brachialis muscle that attaches from the humerus in the arm to the ulna in the forearm (Figure 3-1).

For the brachialis to contract and shorten, it must move the forearm toward the arm and/or move the arm toward the forearm. The resistance to moving the forearm is the weight of the forearm, plus the weight of the hand that must move (*go along for the ride*) with the forearm. The resistance to moving the arm is the weight of the arm, plus the weight of much of the upper part of the body that must move (*go along for the ride*) when the arm moves toward the forearm. Therefore, for the brachialis to contract and shorten, it must generate a force that is greater than the weight of the forearm (and hand) or the arm (and upper body). Because the forearm and hand weigh less than the arm and upper body, when the brachialis contracts and shortens, the forearm usually moves, not the arm. Thus the minimum force necessary that the brachialis must generate if it is to contract and shorten is the weight of its lighter attachment, the forearm.

However, even if the brachialis contracts with insufficient strength to shorten, it is important to understand that it is still exerting a pulling force on its attachments. This pulling force

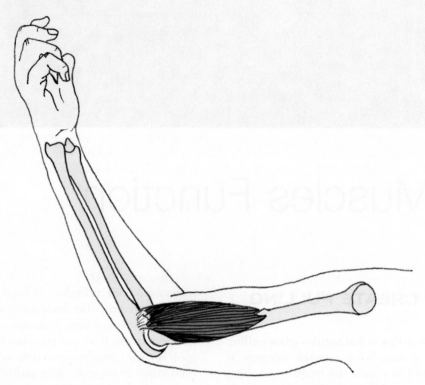

Figure 3-1 The brachialis muscle attaches from the humerus in the arm to the ulna in the forearm. For the brachialis to contract and shorten, it must move the forearm toward the arm and/or move the arm toward the forearm.

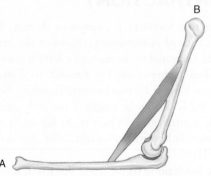

Figure 3-2 A "typical" muscle is shown. It attaches to bone *A* and bone *B* and crosses the joint that is located between them.

can play an important role in musculoskeletal function. When a muscle's function is described, it is usually stated in terms of its joint actions, which are its shortening contractions. For this reason, there is a tendency to overly focus on the shortening contraction of a muscle and overlook the importance of its contraction when it does not shorten.

Concentric Contraction

Let's first look at what happens when a muscle contracts and does shorten. A shortening contraction of a muscle is called a *concentric contraction*. The word "concentric" literally means "with center." In other words, when a concentric contraction occurs, the muscle moves toward its center. As we have said, for

a muscle to contract and shorten, it must move at least one of its attachments. Let's explore the idea of concentric contraction by looking at a "typical" muscle (Figure 3-2).

A muscle attaches to two bones and in doing so, it crosses the joint that is located between them (Box 3-2). Let's call one of the attachments *A* and the other attachment *B*. When the muscle contracts, it creates a pulling force on both bones. If this pulling force is strong enough, a concentric contraction can occur in three possible ways: the muscle can either succeed in pulling bone *A* toward bone *B*, or it can pull bone *B* toward bone *A*, or it can pull both bones *A* and *B* toward each other (Figure 3-3). The bone that moves is described as the *mobile attachment* and the bone that does not move is described as the *fixed attachment*. For a concentric contraction to occur, at least one of the attachments must be mobile and move. Regardless of which attachment moves, when a muscle contracts and does generate sufficient force to move one or both of its attachments, it is the mover of the joint action that is occurring and called

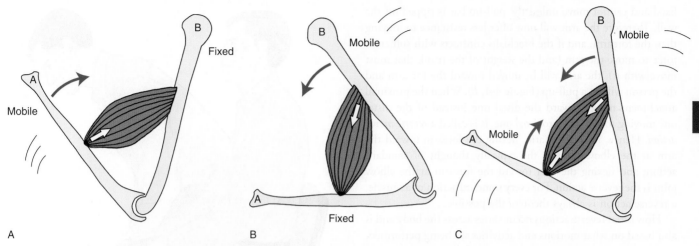

Figure 3-3 A muscle can concentrically contract and cause motion in one of three ways. By naming the muscle's attachments *A* and *B*, we can describe these three scenarios. In **A,** bone *A* moves toward bone *B*. In **B,** bone *B* moves toward bone *A*. And in **C,** both bones *A* and *B* move toward each other.

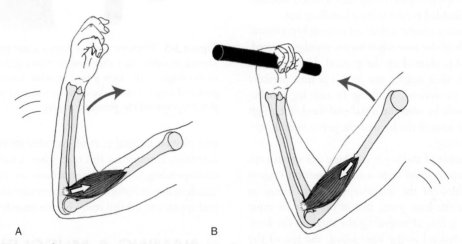

Figure 3-4 A, The standard mover action of the brachialis muscle in which the distal forearm moves toward the proximal arm. **B,** When the hand is fixed, the reverse mover action occurs; the proximal arm moves toward the distal forearm.

the *mover* or *agonist*. By definition, when a mover muscle contracts, it contracts concentrically.

If we now explore concentric contraction a little further and ask which attachment will be the mobile one that does the moving, the answer will be the one that offers the least resistance to moving. That will usually be the lighter attachment. When we are looking at muscles on the extremities of the body, the lighter attachment is usually the distal one. In the upper extremity, the hand is lighter than the forearm, the forearm is lighter than the arm, and the arm is lighter than the shoulder girdle/trunk. In the lower extremity, the foot is lighter than the leg, the leg is lighter than the thigh, and the thigh is lighter than the pelvis. Furthermore, as we have stated, for the more proximal attachment to move, the core of the body usually must move with it, which adds even more weight and resistance to moving. Therefore, when a muscle concentrically contracts, it usually moves its distal attachment. For this reason, when a

muscle's joint actions are learned, they are usually presented and demonstrated with the proximal attachment fixed and the distal attachment mobile. These are what can be termed the *standard mover actions* of the muscle.

Reverse Actions

Although the more common and typically thought of muscle action (the standard action) is one in which the proximal attachment stays fixed and the distal attachment moves, this is not always the case. In fact, it often is not. Let's look at a concentric contraction of the brachialis muscle across the elbow joint. When the brachialis contracts, it would most likely move the distal attachment toward the proximal attachment, moving the forearm and hand toward the arm as in Figure 3-4, *A.* However, if the hand holds onto an immovable object such as a pull-up bar, then because the hand is fixed, the forearm is also

3

fixed and cannot move unless the pull-up bar is ripped off the wall. Therefore the arm will now offer less resistance to moving than the forearm, and if the brachialis contracts with sufficient force to move the arm (and the weight of the trunk that must move with it), the arm will be moved toward the forearm and the person will do a pull-up (Figure 3-4, *B*). When the proximal attachment moves toward the distal one instead of the distal one moving toward the proximal one, it is called a *reverse mover action*. Hence, in this scenario, flexing the forearm toward the arm at the elbow joint is the typically thought of standard action; and flexing the arm toward the forearm at the elbow joint is the reverse action. For every standard action of a muscle, a reverse action is always theoretically possible.

How often reverse actions occur varies across the body and is also based on what motions and activities are being performed. In the upper extremity, reverse actions usually occur whenever the hand is gripping an immovable object. A pull-up bar as illustrated in Figure 3-4 is one example of this. Many other examples in everyday life exist, such as using a banister when walking up the stairs, someone helping to pull you up from a seated to standing position, and a disabled person using a handicap bar.

In the lower extremity, reverse actions are extremely common. This is because much of the time when we are standing, seated, or walking, our foot is planted on the ground. Unless we are on ice or some other slick surface, our foot is at least partially fixed and resistant to moving, resulting in our leg moving toward the foot. Similarly, with the distal end fixed, the thigh would have to move toward the leg and the pelvis would have to move toward the thigh.

An excellent example of this is when we use our quadriceps femoris muscle group to stand from a seated position (Figure 3-5). We usually think of the quadriceps femoris group as extending the leg at the knee joint. But in this case, it must perform the reverse action of extending the thigh at the knee joint. As the thighs extend at the knee joints, the rest of the body must also be lifted. If you palpate the quadriceps femoris in your anterior thighs as you stand up from a seated position, you will easily feel their contraction. In fact, it is because of this frequent activity of daily life that our quadriceps femoris group needs to be so large and powerful.

In the axial body, we do not use the terms *proximal* and *distal*. Here, the usually thought of regular muscle action moves the superior attachment toward the inferior one. This is because the upper axial body (head, neck, and upper trunk) is both lighter than the lower axial body (lower trunk) and because when we are sitting or standing, our lower body is more fixed and consequently more resistant to moving. Therefore, when a muscle of the axial body moves the lower trunk toward the upper trunk, neck, and head, it is a reverse mover action. These reverse actions happen quite often when we are lying down, for example, when moving in bed or doing floor exercises.

When students first study muscle system function and the specific actions of muscles, it is extremely important to not develop too rigid a mindset and only look at a muscle as moving its distal (or superior) attachment when it concentrically contracts. Remember that a reverse mover action is always theoretically possible. Although some rarely occur, others occur frequently

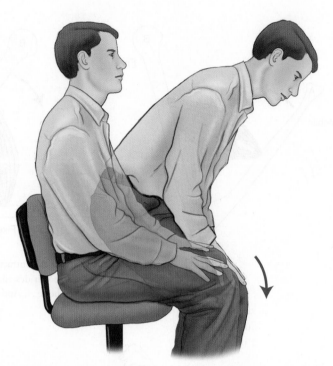

Figure 3-5 When we stand up from a seated position, the quadriceps femoris muscles create their reverse mover action, which is extension of the thighs at the knee joints; in other words, extending the more proximal thighs toward the distal legs instead of extending the more distal legs toward the proximal thighs.

and play an integral part of everyday movement patterns and activities. Throughout this text, when a muscle is discussed, its corresponding reverse mover actions are presented next to its standard mover actions so that the reader can better understand and appreciate the full realm of that muscle's function.

■ NAMING A MUSCLE'S ATTACHMENTS: ORIGIN AND INSERTION VS. ATTACHMENTS

The classic method to name a muscle's attachments is to describe one attachment as the *origin* and the other as the *insertion*. Although the exact definitions have varied, the origin is usually defined as the more fixed attachment and the insertion as the more mobile attachment. Because the proximal attachment usually is the more fixed attachment and the distal attachment usually is the more mobile attachment, some medical dictionaries even define the origin as the more proximal attachment and the insertion as the more distal attachment.

In recent years, use of the terms *origin* and *insertion* has been decreasing in favor. Perhaps the reason is that teaching students who are first learning muscles that one attachment of the muscle is usually fixed tends to promote the idea that it is always fixed. This can lead to less flexibility in how the students view muscular function because they tend to ignore the reverse actions of muscles wherein the insertion stays fixed and the origin moves. Given how often these reverse actions actually occur can handicap the student as he or she begins to use and apply muscle knowledge clinically with clients. Furthermore, asking students who are first learning muscles, and are already overwhelmed trying to remember the names, attachment sites, and actions of the muscles, to now also learn which attachment is designated as the origin and which one is designated as the insertion can be more of a burden.

For these reasons, naming a muscle's attachments by simply describing their location is gaining favor. After all, if the origin can also be defined as the proximal attachment and the insertion can also be defined as the distal attachment, why not skip use of the terms *origin* and *insertion* entirely and simply learn the names of the attachments as proximal and distal? Or, if the muscle is running superiorly and inferiorly or medially and laterally, simply name the attachments using these locational terms. This approach is not only simpler, it also has the advantage of pointing out to the student what the fiber direction of the muscle is. This helps the student to see the muscle's line of pull, which is the most crucial step in figuring out its actions.

This text does not use origin/insertion terminology. For those who would like to use these terms, the first attachment given for each muscle is the attachment usually defined as the origin, and the second attachment given is the attachment usually defined as the insertion. What is most important is that the student learns that a muscle has two attachments, that either one can potentially move, and that what determines which one actually does move in any particular scenario depends on its relative resistance to being moved.

Eccentric Contractions

We have already discussed concentric contractions. They occur when a muscle contracts with a force that is greater than an attachment's resistance force to moving. Therefore the muscle moves the attachment and succeeds in shortening. As we have stated, a muscle does not always succeed in shortening when it contracts.

If a muscle contracts, attempting to pull in toward its center, but the resistance force is greater than the muscle's contraction force, not only will the muscle not succeed in shortening, the muscle's attachment will actually be pulled farther away from the center of the muscle. This will result in a lengthening of the muscle as it contracts. A lengthening contraction is defined as an *eccentric contraction*.

Eccentric contractions happen most often when a muscle is working against gravity. For example, if I am holding an object and want to lower it down to a tabletop, I can let gravity bring my forearm and hand down. However, if the object is fragile, I need to lower it slowly so that it does not crash down onto the table and break. This requires me to contract musculature that opposes gravity so that the object can be lowered slowly and safely (Figure 3-6). In this instance, the muscle contraction's purpose is not to beat gravity and raise the object; rather its purpose is to lose to gravity, but do so slowly so that the effect of the force of gravity is slowed and the object is lowered slowly. Therefore the purpose of an eccentric contraction is to slow or restrain a joint action that is caused by another force, usually gravity. Because the muscle that eccentrically contracts

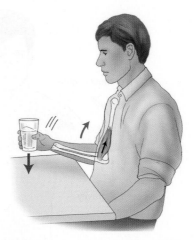

Figure 3-6 While the force of gravity causes extension of the forearm at the elbow joint to lower the person's forearm and hand down toward the table, the person's musculature (brachialis muscle) contracts with an upward pull toward flexion of the forearm at the elbow joint to slow the descent of the glass of water. In this scenario, the person's muscle lengthens as it contracts. Even though it does not succeed in shortening, its lengthening contraction is critically important to slow and restrain the force of gravity so that gravity does not cause the glass to come crashing down and break. In this scenario, this muscle is eccentrically contracting as an antagonist to the joint action that is occurring.

Box 3-3

By definition, when a mover muscle contracts and shortens, it contracts concentrically; and when an antagonist muscle contracts and lengthens, it contracts eccentrically. This does not mean that every muscle that is shortening is concentrically contracting or that every muscle that is lengthening is eccentrically contracting. A muscle can be relaxed as it shortens or lengthens.

opposes the joint action movement that is occurring, it is called the *antagonist*. By definition, when an antagonist muscle contracts, it contracts eccentrically (Box 3-3).

Isometric Contractions

A concentric contraction occurs when the force of the muscle's contraction is greater than the resistance force; an eccentric contraction occurs when the force of the muscle's contraction is less than the resistance force. An isometric contraction occurs when the force of the muscle's contraction is equal to the resistance force. Because the two forces are equal, the muscle is neither able to win and shorten nor lose and lengthen. Instead, it stays the same length as it contracts. This is defined as an *isometric contraction*. In fact, the term *isometric* literally means *same length*. If the muscle stays the same length, its attachments do not move. The function of an isometrically contracting muscle can be critically important because it fixes, in other words, stabilizes its bony attachment (Figure 3-7).

3

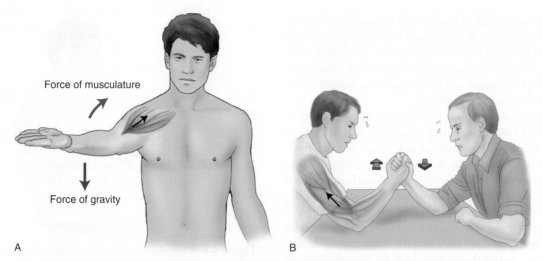

Force of musculature

Force of gravity

A

B

Figure 3-7 A, The person's deltoid muscle isometrically contracts with a force that is equal to the force of gravity so that the person's arm does not move. In this scenario, the deltoid acts as a fixator, in other words, a stabilizer muscle. **B,** The musculature of the person arm wrestling is isometrically contracting because the resistance force from the opponent is exactly equal to the muscle's contraction force. Therefore, no movement occurs.

■ ROLES OF MUSCLES

As we have seen, muscle function can be viewed very simply: muscles contract and create pulling forces. However, muscles can contract concentrically and shorten as movers, contract eccentrically and lengthen as antagonists, or contract isometrically and stay the same length as stabilizers. All too often, students who first learn muscle function focus only on the muscle's standard mover concentric contractions. For a deeper understanding of muscle function, we need to understand and appreciate all types of contractions and all roles that a muscle can play in our movement patterns. Only this deeper understanding will allow for the critical thinking necessary for clinical application when it comes to assessment and treatment of clients.

■ SLIDING FILAMENT MECHANISM

To truly understand the bigger picture of concentric, eccentric, and isometric contractions, it is helpful to examine the actual mechanism that defines muscle contraction. This mechanism occurs on a microscopic level and is known as the *sliding filament mechanism.*

A muscle is made up of thousands of *muscle cells,* also known as *muscle fibers.* Within a muscle, these fibers are bundled together into groups called *fascicles.* A muscle also contains numerous layers of fibrous fascia that are identical to each other in structure but are given different names based on their location. *Endomysium* (plural: endomysia) surrounds each individual muscle fiber; *perimysium* (plural: perimysia) surrounds each fascicle; and *epimysium* surrounds the entire muscle (Figure 3-8). The endomysia, perimysia, and epimysium continue beyond each end of the muscle to create the fibrous tissue attachment of the muscle onto the bone. If this attachment is

Box 3-4

There are also additional layers of fibrous fascia that envelop and surround groups of muscles within a region of the body. These layers are often called *intermuscular septa.*

cordlike in shape, it is called a *tendon.* If it is broad and flat, it is called an *aponeurosis.* The major purpose of the tendon/ aponeurosis is to transmit the pulling force of the muscle belly to its bony attachment (Box 3-4).

If we look more closely at an individual muscle fiber, we see that it is filled with structures called *myofibrils.* Myofibrils run longitudinally within the muscle fiber and are composed of filaments (see Figure 3-8). These filaments are arranged into structures called *sarcomeres.* The term *sarcomere* literally means "unit of muscle." To truly understand how a muscle functions, it is necessary to understand how a sarcomere functions.

Sarcomeres are composed of thin and thick filaments. The thin filaments are *actin* and are arranged on both sides of the sarcomere and attach to the *Z-lines,* which are the borders of the sarcomere. The thick filament is a *myosin* filament and is located in the center and contains projections called heads. When a stimulus from the nervous system is sent to the muscle, binding sites on the actin filaments become exposed and the myosin heads attach onto them, creating *cross-bridges.* The myosin heads then attempt to bend in toward the center of the sarcomere, creating a pulling force on the actin filaments. If the pulling force is sufficiently strong, the actin filaments will be pulled in toward the center of the sarcomere, sliding along the myosin filament, hence the name *sliding filament mechanism.* This will cause the Z-lines to be pulled in toward the center and the sarcomere will shorten (Figure 3-9).

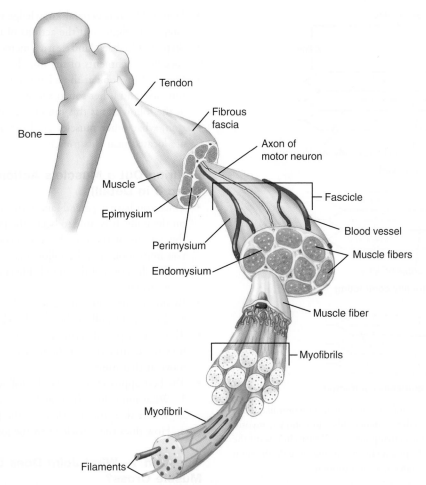

Figure 3-8 Cross sections of a muscle. A muscle is composed of fascicles, which are bundles of fibers. The fibers themselves are filled with myofibrils, which are composed of filaments. Fibrous fascial sheaths called endomysia, perimysia, and epimysium surround the fibers, fascicles, and entire muscle, respectively.

Whatever happens to one sarcomere happens to all the sarcomeres of all the myofibrils of the muscle fiber. If we extrapolate this concept, we see that if all the sarcomeres of a myofibril shorten, the myofibril itself will shorten. If all the myofibrils of a muscle fiber shorten, the muscle fiber will shorten. If enough muscle fibers shorten, the muscle itself will shorten, pulling one or both of its attachments in toward the center, causing motion of the body. This is how a concentric contraction occurs.

When a muscle's contraction was said to create a pulling force toward its center, that pulling force is the sum of the bending forces of all the myosin heads. If the sum of these forces is greater than the resistance to shortening, the actin filaments will be pulled in toward the center of the sarcomere and a concentric contraction occurs. If the sum of these forces is less than the resistance to shortening, the actin filaments will be pulled away from the center of the sarcomere and an eccentric contraction occurs. If the sum of the forces of the myosin heads is equal to the resistance force, the actin filaments will not move and an isometric contraction occurs. Therefore the definition of muscle contraction is having myosin heads creating cross-bridges and pulling on actin filaments.

■ MUSCLE FIBER ARCHITECTURE

Not all muscles have their fibers arranged in the same manner. There are two major architectural types of muscle fiber arrangement. They are longitudinal and pennate. A longitudinal muscle has its fibers running along the length of the muscle. A pennate muscle has its fibers running obliquely to the length of the muscle. The major types of longitudinal muscles are demonstrated in Figure 3-10. The major types of pennate muscles are demonstrated in Figure 3-11.

■ LEARNING MUSCLES

- Essentially, when learning about muscles, two major aspects must be learned: (1) the attachments of the muscle and (2) the actions of the muscle.
- Generally speaking, the attachments of a muscle must be memorized. However, times exist when clues are given about the attachments of a muscle by the muscle's name.

3

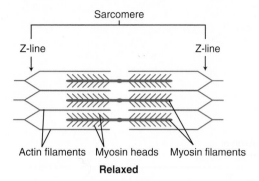

Relaxed

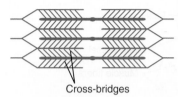

Cross-bridges

Concentrically contracting

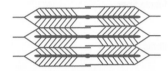

Fully concentrically contracted

Figure 3-9 A sarcomere is composed of actin and myosin filaments. When the nervous system orders a muscle fiber to contract, myosin heads attach to actin filaments, attempting to pull them in toward the center of the sarcomere. If the pulling force is strong enough, the actin filaments will move and the sarcomere will shorten.

- For example, the name *coracobrachialis* tells us that the cora-cobrachialis muscle has one attachment on the coracoid process of the scapula and that its other attachment is on the brachium (i.e., the humerus).
- Similarly, the name *zygomaticus major* tells us that this muscle attaches onto the zygomatic bone (and that it is bigger than another muscle called the *zygomaticus minor*).
- Unlike muscle attachments, muscle actions do not have to be memorized. Instead, by understanding the simple concept that a muscle pulls at its attachments to move a body part, the action or actions of a muscle can be reasoned out.

Five-Step Approach to Learning Muscles

When first confronted with having to study and learn about a muscle, the following five-step approach is recommended:

- Step 1: Look at the name of the muscle to see if it gives you any "free information" that saves you from having to memo-rize attachments or actions of the muscle.
- Step 2: Learn the general location of the muscle well enough to be able to visualize the muscle on your body. At this point, you need only know it well enough to know the following:
  - What joint it crosses
  - Where it crosses the joint (e.g., anteriorly, medially, etc.)
  - How it crosses the joint (i.e., the direction in which its fibers are running, i.e., vertically or horizontally)

- Step 3: Use this general knowledge of the muscle's location (step 2) to figure out the actions of the muscle.
- Step 4: Go back and learn (memorize, if necessary) the specific attachments of the muscle.
- Step 5: Now look at the relationship of this muscle to other muscles (and other soft tissue structures) of the body. Look at the following: Is this muscle superficial or deep? In addi-tion, what other muscles (and other soft tissue structures) are located near this muscle?

Figuring Out a Muscle's Actions (Step 3 in Detail)

- Once you have a general familiarity with a muscle's location on the body, it is time to begin the process of reasoning out the actions of the muscle. The most important thing that you must look at is the following:
  - The direction of the muscle fibers relative to the joint that it crosses
- By doing this, you can see the following:
  - The line of pull of the muscle relative to the joint
- This line of pull determines the actions of the muscle (i.e., how the contraction of the muscle causes the body parts to move at that joint).
- The best approach is to ask the following three questions:
  1. What joint does the muscle cross?
  2. Where does the muscle cross the joint?
  3. How does the muscle cross the joint?

Question 1—What Joint Does the Muscle Cross?

- The first question to ask and answer in figuring out the action(s) of a muscle is to simply know what joint it crosses.
- The following rule applies: If a muscle crosses a joint, it can have an action at that joint. (Note: *This, of course, assumes that the joint is healthy and allows movement to occur.*)
- For example, if we look at the coracobrachialis (see Figure 5-7), knowing that it crosses the shoulder (glenohumeral [GH]) joint tells us that it must have an action at the GH joint.
- We may not know what the exact action of the coracobra-chialis is yet, but at least we now know at what joint it has its actions.
- To figure out exactly what these actions are, we need to look at questions 2 and 3.
- Note: It is worth pointing out that the converse of the rule about a muscle having the ability to create movement (i.e., an action) at a joint that it crosses is also generally true. In other words, if a muscle does not cross a joint, it cannot have an action at that joint. (There are exceptions to this rule.)

Questions 2 and 3—Where Does the Muscle Cross the Joint? How Does the Muscle Cross the Joint?

- These two questions must be looked at together.
- The *where* of a muscle crossing a joint is whether it crosses the joint anteriorly, posteriorly, medially, or laterally.

3

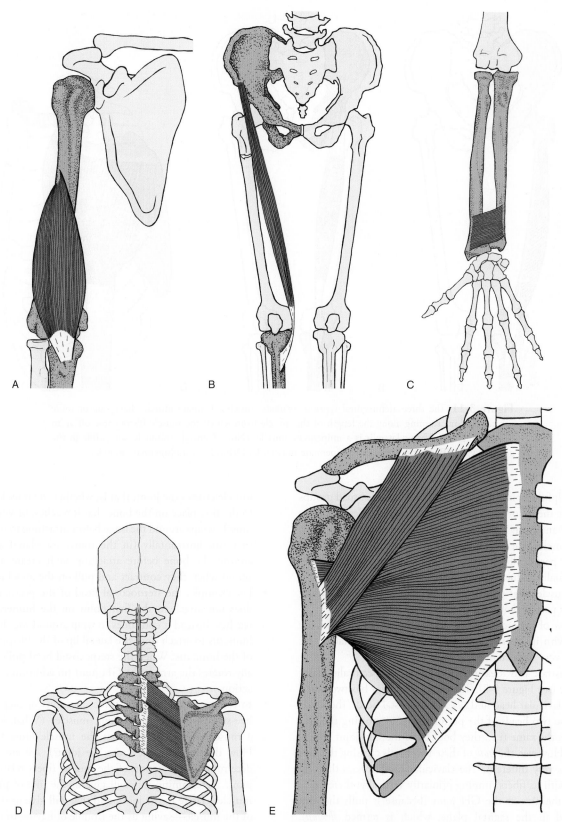

Figure 3-10 Various architectural types of longitudinal muscles. **A,** Brachialis demonstrates a fusiform-shaped (also known as spindle-shaped) muscle. **B,** Sartorius demonstrates a strap muscle. **C,** Pronator quadratus demonstrates a rectangular-shaped muscle. **D,** Rhomboid muscles demonstrate rhomboidal-shaped muscles. **E,** Pectoralis major demonstrates a triangular-shaped (also known as fan-shaped) muscle.

3

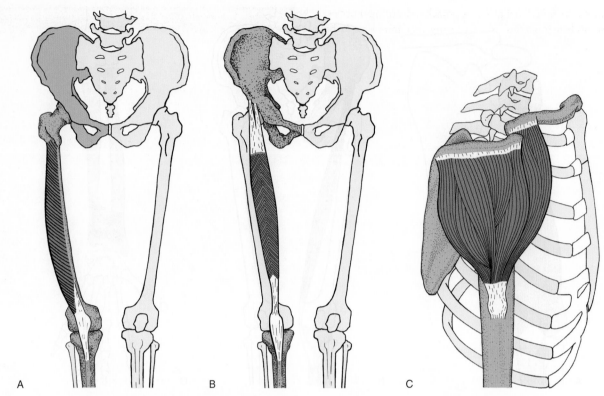

Figure 3-11 The three architectural types of pennate muscles. Pennate muscles have one or more central tendons running along the length of the muscle from which the muscle fibers come off at an oblique angle. **A,** Vastus lateralis is a unipennate muscle. (Note: Central tendon is not visible in the anterior view.) **B,** Rectus femoris is a bipennate muscle. **C,** Deltoid is a multipennate muscle.

- It is helpful to place a muscle into one of these broad groups because the following general rules apply: muscles that cross a joint anteriorly will usually flex a body part at that joint, and muscles that cross a joint posteriorly will usually extend a body part at that joint; muscles that cross a joint laterally will usually abduct or laterally flex a body part at that joint, and muscles that cross a joint medially will usually adduct a body part at that joint.

- The *how* of a muscle crossing a joint is whether it crosses the joint with its fibers running vertically or horizontally. This is also very important.

- To illustrate this idea we will look at the pectoralis major muscle (see Figure 5-8). The pectoralis major has two parts: (1) a clavicular head and (2) a sternocostal head. The *where* of these two heads of the pectoralis major crossing the GH joint is the same (i.e., they both cross the GH joint anteriorly). However, the *how* of these two heads crossing the GH joint is very different. The clavicular head crosses the GH joint with its fibers running primarily vertically; therefore it flexes the arm at the GH joint (because it pulls the arm upward in the sagittal plane, which is termed *flexion*). However, the sternocostal head crosses the GH joint with its fibers running horizontally, therefore it adducts the arm at the GH joint (because it pulls the arm from lateral to medial in the frontal plane, which is termed *adduction*).

- With a muscle that has a horizontal direction to its fibers, another factor must be considered when looking at *how* this muscle crosses the joint; that is, whether the muscle attaches to the first place on the bone that it reaches, or whether the muscle wraps around the bone before attaching to it. Muscles that run horizontally (in the transverse plane) and wrap around the bone before attaching to it create a rotation action when they contract and pull on the attachment.

- For example, the sternocostal head of the pectoralis major does not attach to the first point on the humerus that it reaches. Instead it continues to wrap around the shaft of the humerus to attach onto the lateral lip of the bicipital groove of the humerus. When the sternocostal head pulls, it medially rotates the arm at the GH joint (in addition to its other actions).

- In essence, by asking the three questions of Step 3 of the five-step approach to learning muscles (What joint does a muscle cross? Where does the muscle cross the joint? How does the muscle cross the joint?), we are trying to determine the direction of the muscle fibers relative to the joint. Determining this will give us the line of pull of the muscle relative to the joint, and that will give us the actions of the muscle—saving us the trouble of having to memorize this information!

Functional Group Approach to Learning Muscles

Once the five-step approach to learning muscles has been used a few times and learned, it is extremely helpful to begin to transition to the functional group approach to learning muscles. This approach places emphasis on seeing that muscles can be placed into a functional group, based on their common joint action. For example, if the biceps brachii has been studied and it is seen that it crosses the elbow joint anteriorly and flexes it, then it is easier to see and learn that the brachialis also flexes the elbow joint because it also crosses it anteriorly. In fact, all muscles that cross the elbow joint anteriorly belong to the functional group of elbow joint flexors. Similarly, all muscles that cross the elbow joint posteriorly belong to the functional group of elbow joint extensors. Applying the functional group approach to the GH joint, it is seen that all muscles that cross it anteriorly with a vertical fiber direction (or at least a vertical component to their fiber direction) flex it. All muscles that cross it posteriorly with a vertical fiber direction extend it. All muscles that cross it laterally, abduct it; and all muscles that cross it medially adduct it. Functional groups of medial and lateral rotators are not as segregated location-wise, but with closer inspection, it is seen that all medial rotators of the GH joint wrap in the same direction, and all lateral rotators wrap in the other direction. Chapter 19 contains illustrations of all the major functional groups of muscles.

Visual and Kinesthetic Exercise for Learning a Muscle's Actions

Rubber Band Exercise

- An excellent method for learning the actions of a muscle is to place a large, colorful rubber band (or large, colorful shoelace or string) on your body, or the body of a partner, in the same location that the muscle you are studying is located.
- Hold one end of the rubber band at one of the attachment sites of the muscle, and hold the other end of the rubber band at the other attachment site of the muscle.
- Make sure that you have the rubber band running/oriented in the same direction as the direction of the fibers of the muscle. If it is not uncomfortable, you may even loop or tie the rubber band (or shoelace) around the body parts that are the attachments of the muscle.
- Once you have the rubber band in place, pull one of the ends of the rubber band toward the other attachment of the rubber band to see the action that the rubber band/muscle has on that body part's attachment. Once done, return the attachment of the rubber band to where it began and repeat this exercise for the other end of the rubber band to see the action that the rubber band/muscle has on the other attachment of the muscle (Box 3-5).
- By placing the rubber band on your body or your partner's body, you are simulating the direction of the muscle's fibers relative to the joint that it crosses.
- By pulling either end of the rubber band toward the center, you are simulating the line of pull of the muscle relative to the joint that it crosses. The resultant movements that occur are the mover actions that the muscle would have. This is an excellent exercise both to visually see the actions of a

Box 3-5

When doing the rubber band exercise it is extremely important that the attachment of the rubber band that you are pulling on is pulled exactly toward the other attachment and in no other direction. In other words, your line of pull should be *exactly* the same as the line of pull of the muscle (which is essentially determined by the direction of the fibers of the muscle).

When doing the rubber band exercise, the attachment of the muscle that you are pulling on would be the mobile attachment in that scenario; the end that you do not move is the fixed attachment in that scenario. Further, by doing this exercise twice (i.e., by then repeating it by reversing which attachment you hold fixed and which one you pull on and move), you are simulating the standard mover action and the reverse mover action of the muscle.

muscle and to kinesthetically experience the actions of a muscle.

- This exercise can be used to learn all muscle actions, and can be especially helpful for determining actions that may be a little more difficult to visualize, such as rotation actions.
- Note: The use of a large, colorful rubber band is more helpful than a shoelace or string, because when you stretch out a rubber band and place it in the location where a muscle would be, the natural elasticity of a rubber band creates a pull on the attachment sites that nicely simulates the pull of a muscle on its attachments when it contracts.
- If you can, you should work with a partner to do this exercise. Have your partner hold one of the "attachments" of the rubber band while you hold the other "attachment." This leaves one of your hands free to pull the rubber band attachment sites toward the center.
- A further note of caution: If you are using a rubber band, be careful that you do not accidentally let go and have the rubber band hit you or your partner. For this reason, it would be preferable to use a shoelace or string instead of a rubber band when working near the face.

■ PALPATION GUIDELINES

Learning to palpate muscles is both a science and an art. The science is based on knowing the attachments and actions of the target muscle that you want to palpate. By knowing its attachments, you know where to place your palpating fingers. By knowing its actions, you know what action to ask the client to perform so that the target muscle contracts and hardens, thereby standing out among the adjacent soft tissues. The art of muscle palpation involves many other guidelines. For more on muscle palpation, see the Evolve website. ⓔvolve For a much fuller discussion of muscle and bone palpation, see *The Muscle and Bone Palpation Manual, with Triggers Points, Referral Patterns, and Stretching* (Elsevier, 2009).

CHAPTER

4

Muscles of the Shoulder Girdle Joints

CHAPTER OUTLINE

CHAPTER OVERVIEW

The muscles addressed in this chapter are the muscles whose principal function is usually considered to be movement of the shoulder girdle (scapula and clavicle at the scapulocostal and sternoclavicular joints). Other muscles in the body can also move the shoulder girdle, but they are placed in different chapters because their primary function is usually considered to be at another joint. These muscles cross and move the glenohumeral joint and are covered in Chapter 5.

Overview of Structure

Structurally, muscles that move the shoulder girdle attach from the trunk to the scapula and/or clavicle. The bellies of these muscles may be located posteriorly, such as the trapezius, rhomboids, and levator scapulae; or they may be located anteriorly, such as the serratus anterior, pectoralis minor, and subclavius.

Overview of Function

The following general rules regarding actions can be stated for the functional groups of muscles of the shoulder girdle:
☐ If a muscle attaches to the scapula and its other attachment is superior to the scapula, it can elevate the scapula at the scapulocostal joint.

☐ If a muscle attaches to the scapula and its other attachment is inferior to the scapula, it can depress the scapula at the scapulocostal joint.
☐ If a muscle attaches to the scapula and its other attachment is medial to the scapula on the posterior side (i.e., closer to the spine), it can retract (adduct) the scapula at the scapulocostal joint.
☐ If a muscle attaches to the scapula and its other attachment is lateral to the scapula (i.e., closer to the anterior surface of the body), it can protract (abduct) the scapula at the scapulocostal joint.
☐ If a muscle attaches to the scapula away from the axis of scapular rotation (off-axis), it can either upwardly rotate or downwardly rotate the scapula at the scapulocostal joint. Which rotation it performs depends on where it attaches.
☐ Any muscle that moves the scapula at the scapulocostal joint can do the same motion of the clavicle at the sternoclavicular joint (and vice versa).
☐ Reverse actions of these standard mover actions involve the scapula being fixed and the other attachment moving toward the scapula at the scapulocostal joint.

Review the muscles and bones from this chapter on the enclosed CD!

Posterior View of the Muscles of the Shoulder Girdle Region

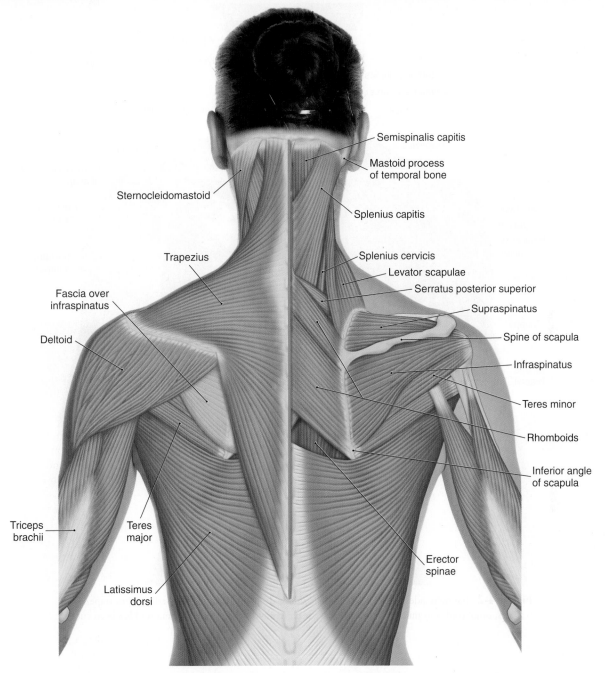

Semispinalis capitis

Mastoid process
of temporal bone

Sternocleidomastoid

Splenius capitis

Trapezius

Splenius cervicis

Levator scapulae

Serratus posterior superior

Fascia over
infraspinatus

Supraspinatus

Deltoid

Spine of scapula

Infraspinatus

Teres minor

Rhomboids

Inferior angle
of scapula

Triceps
brachii

Teres
major

Erector
spinae

Latissimus
dorsi

Figure 4-1 The left side is superficial. The right side is deep (the deltoid, trapezius, sternocleidomastoid, and infraspinatus fascia have been removed).

Anterior View of the Muscles of the Shoulder Girdle Region

4

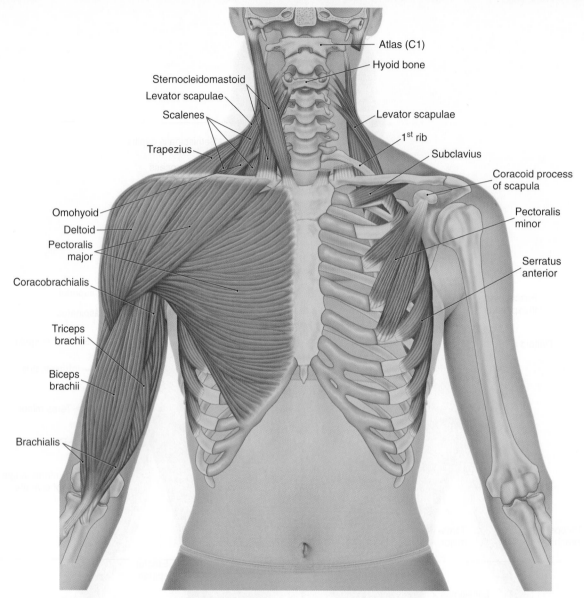

Atlas (C1)
Hyoid bone
Sternocleidomastoid
Levator scapulae
Scalenes
Levator scapulae
1st rib
Trapezius
Subclavius
Coracoid process of scapula
Omohyoid
Deltoid
Pectoralis minor
Pectoralis major
Coracobrachialis
Serratus anterior
Triceps brachii
Biceps brachii
Brachialis

Figure 4-2 The right side is superficial. The left side is deep (the deltoid, pectoralis major, trapezius, scalenes, omohyoid, and muscles of the arm have been removed; the sternocleidomastoid has been cut).

Right Lateral View of the Muscles of the Shoulder Girdle and Neck Region

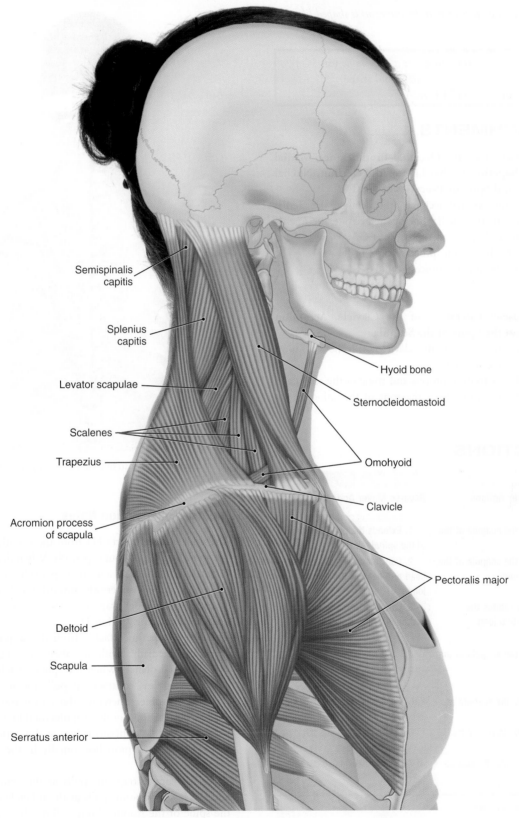

Semispinalis capitis

Splenius capitis

Levator scapulae

Scalenes

Trapezius

Acromion process of scapula

Deltoid

Scapula

Serratus anterior

Hyoid bone

Sternocleidomastoid

Omohyoid

Clavicle

Pectoralis major

Figure 4-3

4

Trapezius ("Trap")

The name, trapezius, *tells us that the trapezius is shaped like a trapezoid (▷).*

| **Derivation** | ☐ trapezius: Gr: *a little table* (or trapezoid shape). |
| **Pronunciation** | ☐ tra-PEE-zee-us |

■ ATTACHMENTS

☐ **Entire Muscle: External Occipital Protuberance, Medial ⅓ of the Superior Nuchal Line of the Occiput, Nuchal Ligament, and Spinous Processes of C7-T12**
  ☐ UPPER: the external occipital protuberance, the medial ⅓ of the superior nuchal line of the occiput, the nuchal ligament, and the spinous process of C7
  ☐ MIDDLE: the spinous processes of T1-T5
  ☐ LOWER: the spinous processes of T6-T12

to the

☐ **Entire Muscle: Lateral ⅓ of the Clavicle, Acromion Process, and the Spine of the Scapula**
  ☐ UPPER: lateral ⅓ of the clavicle and the acromion process of the scapula
  ☐ MIDDLE: acromion process and spine of the scapula
  ☐ LOWER: the tubercle at the root of the spine of the scapula

■ FUNCTIONS

CONCENTRIC (SHORTENING) MOVER ACTIONS	
Standard Mover Actions	**Reverse Mover Actions**
UPPER	
☐ **1. Elevates the scapula at the ScC joint**	☐ **1. Extends the head and neck at the spinal joints**
☐ **2. Retracts the scapula at the scapulocostal joint**	☐ **2. Contralaterally rotates the head and neck at the spinal joints**
☐ **3. Upwardly rotates the scapula at the ScC joint**	☐ **3. Laterally flexes the head and neck at the spinal joints**
MIDDLE	
☐ **4. Retracts the scapula at the ScC joint**	☐ 4. Contralaterally rotates the trunk at the spinal joints
LOWER	
☐ **5. Depresses the scapula at the ScC joint**	☐ 5. Extends the trunk at the spinal joints
☐ 6. Retracts the scapula at ScC joint	☐ 6. Contralaterally rotates the trunk at the spinal joints
☐ 7. Upwardly rotates the scapula at the ScC joint	☐ 7. Laterally flexes the trunk at the spinal joints

ScC joint = scapulocostal joint

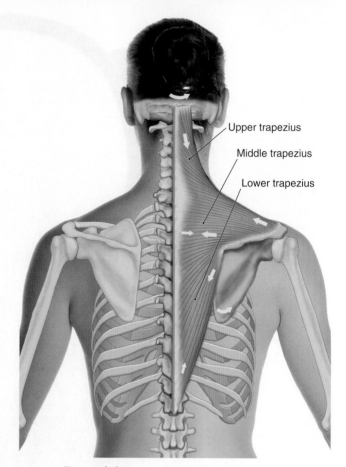

Upper trapezius
Middle trapezius
Lower trapezius

Figure 4-4 Posterior view of the right trapezius.

Standard Mover Action Notes

- The upper trapezius attaches from the scapula inferiorly, to the spine and the occiput superiorly. When the spinal/occipital attachment is fixed and the upper trapezius contracts, it pulls the scapula superiorly toward the head and neck. Therefore the upper trapezius elevates the scapula at the scapulocostal joint. (action 1)
- The entire trapezius attaches from the scapula laterally to the spine medially (with its fibers running horizontally in the frontal plane). When the spinal attachment is fixed and the trapezius contracts, it pulls the scapula medially toward the spine. Therefore the entire trapezius retracts (adducts) the scapula at the scapulocostal joint. Of the three parts, the middle trapezius is best at this action because its fibers are oriented most horizontally in the frontal plane. (actions 2, 4, 6)
- When the upper trapezius pulls at the acromion process and the lower trapezius pulls at the tubercle of the root of the spine of the scapula, both pull on the scapula in such a manner that the scapula rotates, orienting the glenoid fossa superiorly (both upper and lower trapezius rotate the right scapula counter-clockwise in Figure 4-4 above). There-

Trapezius ("Trap")—cont'd

fore the upper and lower trapezius upwardly rotate the scapula at the scapulocostal joint. (actions 3, 7)

- The lower trapezius attaches from the scapula superiorly to the spine inferiorly. When the spinal attachment is fixed and the lower trapezius contracts, it pulls the scapula inferiorly toward the spine. Therefore the lower trapezius depresses the scapula at the scapulocostal joint. (action 5)

- Via the direct pull of the upper trapezius on the clavicle, and the indirect pull of the entire trapezius via its attachment to the scapula, the trapezius can create the same actions of the clavicle (at the sternoclavicular joint) as its actions of the scapula (at the scapulocostal joint). (actions 1, 2 , 3, 4, 5, 6, 7)

- If the lower trapezius pulls the scapula inferiorly toward the spine and the scapula is fixed to the trunk, the upper trunk (with the scapula fixed to it) will extend in the sagittal plane toward the lower spinal attachment. (action 5)

Reverse Mover Action Notes

- The upper trapezius crosses the joints of the cervical spine and the atlanto-occipital joint posteriorly (with fibers running vertically in the sagittal plane). Therefore the upper trapezius extends the neck at the cervical spinal joints and the head at the atlanto-occipital joint. (reverse action 1)

- The upper trapezius crosses the joints of the cervical spine and the atlanto-occipital joint posteriorly (with fibers running somewhat horizontally in the transverse plane). When the upper trapezius contracts, it pulls the more medial attachment (the spinal/occipital attachment) toward the lateral attachment (the scapula/clavicle), causing the anterior surface of the neck and/or head to face the opposite side of the body from the side of the body to which the trapezius is attached. Therefore the upper trapezius contralaterally rotates the neck at the cervical spinal joints and the head at the atlanto-occipital joint. (reverse action 2)

- The upper trapezius crosses the joints of the cervical spine and the atlanto-occipital joint laterally (with fibers running vertically in the frontal plane). Therefore the upper trapezius laterally flexes the neck at the cervical spinal joints and the head at the atlanto-occipital joint. (reverse action 3)

- If the scapula is fixed and the middle and lower trapezius pull on their spinal attachments, the spinous processes will be pulled toward the scapula. This causes the anterior bodies of the vertebrae to come to face the opposite side of the body. Therefore the middle and lower trapezius contralaterally rotate the trunk at the spinal joints. (reverse actions 4, 6)

- The lower trapezius crosses the joints of the thoracic spine posteriorly (with its fibers running vertically in the sagittal plane). If the scapula is fixed and the inferior spinal attachment is pulled superiorly toward the scapula, the trunk will extend at the thoracic spinal joints. (reverse action 5)

Eccentric Antagonist Functions

Upper

1. Restrains/slows depression, protraction, and downward rotation of the scapula at the scapulocostal joint
2. Restrains/slows flexion, opposite-side lateral flexion, and ipsilateral rotation of the head and neck at the spinal joints

Middle

1. Restrains/slows protraction of the scapula at the scapulocostal joint
2. Restrains/slows ipsilateral rotation of the trunk at the spinal joints

Lower

1. Restrains/slows elevation, protraction, and downward rotation of the scapula at the scapulocostal joint
2. Restrains/slows flexion, ipsilateral rotation, and opposite-side lateral flexion of the trunk at the spinal joints

Isometric Stabilization Functions

1. Stabilizes the scapula and clavicle
2. Stabilizes the head, neck, and trunk at the spinal joints

Additional Notes on Actions

1. In addition to its other actions, the scapula can also tilt. If the medial border of the scapula were to move away from the body wall, contraction of the middle and lower trapezius would pull it back to its position against the body wall. The medial border of the scapula moving toward the body wall is called *medial tilt;* therefore the middle trapezius and lower trapezius medially tilt the scapula. The action of medial tilt of the scapula is particularly important when the scapula is protracted because the scapula tends to laterally tilt (i.e., wing out) when it protracts. Muscles that medially tilt the scapula prevent the scapula from laterally tilting (winging out).

2. The muscle actions of the upper trapezius are often written stating that bilateral contraction of the upper trapezius creates extension of the head and neck at the spinal joints. This is certainly true. However, this should not be interpreted to mean that unilateral contraction of the upper trapezius does not cause extension; it does (because of its line of pull being posterior to the spinal joints in the sagittal plane). In fact, unilateral contraction of the upper trapezius will cause extension, same-side (ipsilateral) lateral flexion, and contralateral rotation of the head and neck because its line of pull is across all three planes. So, even though bilateral contraction of the upper trapezius causes pure extension of the head and neck (the opposite lateral flexions cancel each other out and the opposite rotations cancel each other out), unilateral contraction can cause extension too. Note: This concept is true for extension and flexion for all spinal muscles.

4

INNERVATION
☐ Spinal Accessory Nerve (CN XI)
   ☐ and C3, **C4**

ARTERIAL SUPPLY
☐ The Transverse Cervical Artery (a branch of the Thyrocervical Trunk) and the Dorsal Scapular Artery (a branch of the Subclavian Artery)

✋ PALPATION

1. With the client prone, place palpating hand over the trapezius.
2. Ask the client to actively abduct the arm at the glenohumeral joint and slightly retract the scapula at the scapulocostal joint.
3. Palpate all three parts of the trapezius, lower, middle, and upper, by strumming perpendicular to the fibers.
4. To further bring out the upper trapezius, have the client perform slight extension of the head and neck at the spinal joints.

■ RELATIONSHIP TO OTHER STRUCTURES

☐ The entire trapezius is superficial in the neck and the back (except for the most anterior portion, which is deep to the platysma).
☐ Directly deep to the trapezius in the neck are the semispinalis capitis, the splenius capitis, and the levator scapulae. Directly deep to the trapezius in the trunk are the supraspinatus, the rhomboids, and the most superior part of the latissimus dorsi.
☐ Directly anterior to the anterior border of the trapezius are the splenius capitis, the levator scapulae, and the scalenes (in the *posterior triangle of the neck*).
☐ The trapezius is located within the superficial back arm line myofascial meridian.

■ MISCELLANEOUS

1. The trapezius is usually considered to have three functional parts: upper, middle, and lower.
2. The trapezius' lateral attachments are the same as the proximal attachments of the deltoid, namely, the lateral clavicle, the acromion process, and the spine of the scapula.
3. When a person has his or her head inclined anteriorly, the center of gravity of the head is such that it would fall into flexion if it were not for the isometric contraction of head and neck extensor musculature. Because this type of posture is so often assumed, posterior cervical muscles, including the upper trapezius, are probably the most commonly found tight muscles in the human body.

4. Whenever a purse or any type of bag is carried on the shoulder (regardless of the weight), the bag should slide off given the downward slope of the shoulder. However, people usually prevent this by subconsciously elevating the scapula on the side on which the bag is being carried. This posture causes elevators of the scapula (including the upper trapezius) to isometrically contract for long periods of time and therefore become tight and painful. This is a common posture that may cause tightness of the upper trapezius.
5. Whenever a phone is crimped between the head and the shoulder instead of being held by the hand, lateral flexors of the neck and/or elevators of the scapula (including the upper trapezius) on that side of the body must isometrically contract to hold the phone in place. This posture, if held for prolonged periods of time, will cause tension and pain in the muscles involved. This is a common posture that may cause tightness of the upper trapezius.
6. *Rounded shoulders* is a common postural condition in which the scapulae are protracted (abducted) and depressed (at the scapulocostal joints) and the humeri are medially rotated (at the glenohumeral joints). Given the trapezius' action of retraction of the scapulae (especially the middle trapezius), when the trapezius muscles are weak, they can contribute to this condition because they are unable to efficiently oppose protraction of the scapulae. This is especially true if the protractors of the scapulae (often the pectoralis minor and major muscles) are tight.
7. The greater occipital nerve, which innervates the posterior half of the scalp, pierces through the upper trapezius (and the semispinalis capitis of the transversospinalis group). When the upper trapezius is tight, the greater occipital nerve can be compressed, causing a *tension headache* that is felt in the posterior head. (This condition is also known as *greater occipital neuralgia.*)
8. Whenever a heavy weight is held in the hand, a downward force is exerted on the scapula and clavicle. Another important function of the trapezius is to isometrically contract to support the distal clavicle and the scapula from being pulled inferiorly by this downward force. Therefore long periods of carrying a heavy weight in the hand can result in tension and soreness in the upper trapezius.
9. Whenever the arm is abducted at the glenohumeral joint, the abductor musculature (most likely the deltoid) will create a downward rotation force on the scapula (at the glenohumeral and scapulocostal joints). Upward rotator muscles such as the upper trapezius must contract to fix (stabilize) the scapula from downwardly rotating. Therefore holding the arm in a position of abduction is another common posture that may cause tightness of the upper trapezius. If the arm is abducted approximately 30 degrees or more, the upward rotator muscles must contract to create upward rotation of the scapula as a coupled action to accompany the arm abduction.

Rhomboids Major and Minor

The name, rhomboids, *tells us that these muscles have the geometric shape of a rhombus (a parallelogram or diamond shape).* Major *tells us that the rhomboid major is the larger muscle of the two;* minor *tells us that the rhomboid minor is smaller.*

Derivation	□ rhomb:	Gr. *rhombos* (the geometric shape).
	oid:	Gr. *shape, resemblance.*
	major:	L. *larger.*
	minor:	L. *smaller.*
Pronunciation	□ ROM-boyd, MAY-jor, MY-nor	

■ ATTACHMENTS

- □ **THE RHOMBOIDS: Spinous Processes of C7-T5**
  - □ MINOR: spinous processes of C7-T1 and the inferior nuchal ligament
  - □ MAJOR: spinous processes of T2-T5

to the

- □ **THE RHOMBOIDS: Medial Border of the Scapula From the Root of the Spine to the Inferior Angle of the Scapula**
  - □ MINOR: at the root of the spine of the scapula
  - □ MAJOR: between the root of the spine and the inferior angle of the scapula

■ FUNCTIONS

CONCENTRIC (SHORTENING) MOVER ACTIONS	
Standard Mover Actions	**Reverse Mover Actions**
□ **1. Retracts the scapula at the ScC joint**	□ 1. Contralaterally rotates the trunk at the spinal joints
□ **2. Elevates the scapula at the ScC joint**	□ 2. Extends the trunk at the spinal joints
□ **3. Downwardly rotates the scapula at the ScC joint**	
□ 4. Medially tilts the scapula at the ScC joint	□ 3. Contralaterally rotates the trunk at the spinal joints

ScC joint = scapulocostal joint

Standard Mover Action Notes

- The rhomboids attach from the spine medially, to the scapula laterally (with their fibers running somewhat horizontally). When the rhomboids contract, they pull the scapula medially toward the spine; therefore the rhomboids retract (adduct) the scapula at the scapulocostal joint. (action 1)
- The rhomboids attach from the spine superiorly, to the scapula inferiorly (with their fibers running somewhat vertically). When the rhomboids contract, they pull the scapula superiorly toward the spine; therefore the rhomboids elevate the scapula at the scapulocostal joint. (action 2)

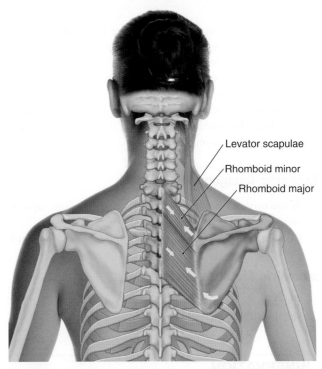

Figure 4-5 Posterior view of the right rhomboids major and minor. The levator scapulae has been ghosted in.

- When the rhomboids contract, they pull on the scapula, causing the inferior angle of the scapula to swing up toward the spine. This will cause the glenoid fossa to orient downward; therefore the rhomboids downwardly rotate the scapula at the scapulocostal joint. The rhomboid major is more powerful than the rhomboid minor at downward rotation because its attachment on the scapula is more inferior. From there it has better leverage to rotate the scapula because it attaches farther from the axis of scapular rotation. (action 3)
- Downward rotation of the scapula at the scapulocostal joint is the best joint action to engage and palpate the rhomboids. (action 3)
- Medial tilt is a motion of the scapula that brings its medial border back against the body wall. In anatomic position, the scapula should be fully medially tilted. The action of medial tilt of the scapula is particularly important when the scapula is protracted because the scapula tends to laterally tilt (i.e., wing out) when it protracts. Therefore muscles that medially tilt the scapula keep the scapula from laterally tilting, or winging out. (action 4)

Reverse Mover Action Notes

- When the scapula is fixed and the rhomboids contract, they pull the spinous processes of the vertebrae toward the scapula. This will cause the anterior bodies of these vertebrae

4

Rhomboids Major and Minor—*cont'd*

to rotate to the opposite side of the body. Therefore the rhomboids can contralaterally rotate the trunk at the spinal joints. (reverse actions 1, 3)

- The rhomboids cross the spinal joints posteriorly with a vertical direction to their fibers. If the scapula is fixed, the spinal attachment is pulled inferiorly toward the scapula. Therefore, the rhomboids can extend the trunk at the spinal joints. (reverse action 2)

Eccentric Antagonist Functions

1. Restrains/slows scapular protraction, depression, upward rotation, and lateral tilt
2. Restrains/slows flexion and ipsilateral rotation of the trunk

Isometric Stabilization Functions

1. Stabilizes the scapula
2. Stabilizes C7-T5 vertebrae

INNERVATION
- ☐ The Dorsal Scapular Nerve
  - ☐ C4, C5

ARTERIAL SUPPLY
- ☐ The Dorsal Scapular Artery (a branch of the Subclavian Artery)

✋ PALPATION

1. With the client seated or prone and the hand placed in the small of the back, place palpating hand between the scapula (at a level that is between the inferior angle and the root of the spine of the scapula) and the spine.
2. Ask the client to move the hand away from the back and feel for the contraction of the rhomboids.
3. Palpate the entirety of the rhomboids.

■ RELATIONSHIP TO OTHER STRUCTURES

- ☐ The rhomboids are deep to the trapezius.
- ☐ The rhomboid minor is directly superior to the rhomboid major.
- ☐ The rhomboid minor attaches onto the scapula, inferior to the levator scapulae's attachment onto the scapula.
- ☐ Deep to the rhomboids are the splenius capitis, the splenius cervicis, the serratus posterior superior, and the erector spinae and transversospinalis groups.
- ☐ The rhomboids are located within the spiral line and deep back arm line myofascial meridians.

■ MISCELLANEOUS

1. The rhomboids major and minor are considered together because they have identical fiber direction and therefore identical lines of pull and identical actions (except for the greater downward rotation force of the rhomboid major).
2. Sometimes there is a small interval of space between the two rhomboids, but often there is not. These two muscles may even blend together.
3. The rhomboids often blend into the serratus anterior on the anterior side of the scapula.
4. The rhomboid muscles are sometimes called the *Christmas tree* muscles. When you look at the rhomboids bilaterally with the spinal column between them, they look like a Christmas tree in shape.
5. *Rounded shoulders* is a common postural condition in which the scapulae are protracted (abducted) and depressed at the scapulocostal joints and the humeri are medially rotated at the shoulder joints. Given the rhomboids' actions of both retraction and elevation of the scapulae, when the rhomboid muscles are weak, they can contribute to this condition because they are unable to efficiently oppose protraction and depression of the scapulae. This is especially true if the protractors and/or depressors of the scapulae (often the pectoralis minor and major muscles) are tight.

Levator Scapulae

The name, levator scapulae, *tells us that this muscle elevates the scapula.*

Derivation	☐ levator:	L. *lifter.*
	scapulae:	L. *of the scapula.*
Pronunciation	☐ le-VAY-tor, SKAP-you-lee	

■ ATTACHMENTS

☐ **Transverse Processes of C1-C4**
  ☐ the Posterior Tubercles of the Transverse Processes of C3 and C4

to the

☐ **Medial Border of the Scapula, from the Superior Angle to the Root of the Spine of the Scapula**

■ FUNCTIONS

CONCENTRIC (SHORTENING) MOVER ACTIONS	
Standard Mover Actions	**Reverse Mover Actions**
☐ **1. Elevates the scapula at the ScC joint**	☐ **1. Extends the neck at the spinal joints**
☐ 2. Downwardly rotates the scapula at the ScC joint	☐ **2. Laterally flexes the neck at the spinal joints**
☐ 3. Retracts the scapula at the ScC joint	☐ 3. Ipsilaterally rotates the neck at the spinal joints

ScC joint = scapulocostal joint

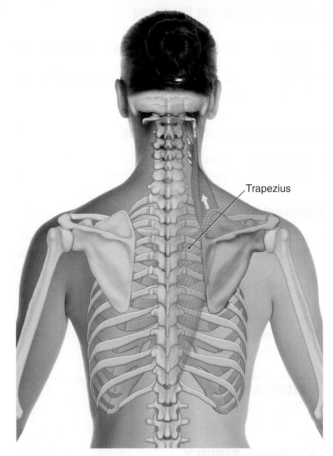

Figure 4-6 Posterior view of the right levator scapulae. The trapezius has been ghosted in.

Standard Mover Action Notes

• The levator scapulae attaches from the scapula inferiorly, to the cervical spine superiorly (with its fibers running vertically). When the cervical spine is fixed and the levator scapulae contracts, it pulls the scapula superiorly toward the cervical spine. Therefore the levator scapulae elevates the scapula at the scapulocostal joint. (action 1)

• When the cervical spine is fixed and the levator scapulae contracts, it pulls the superior angle of the scapula superiorly and the inferior angle moves superiorly and medially. This causes the glenoid fossa to orient inferiorly. Therefore the levator scapulae downwardly rotates the scapula at the scapulocostal joint. (action 2)

• The levator scapulae attaches from the spine medially to the scapula laterally (with its fibers running somewhat horizontally). When the levator scapulae contracts, it pulls the scapula medially toward the spine. Therefore the levator scapulae retracts (adducts) the scapula at the scapulocostal joint. (action 3)

Reverse Mover Action Notes

• The levator scapulae crosses the cervical spine posteriorly (with its fibers running vertically in the sagittal plane). When the scapula is fixed and the levator scapulae contracts, it pulls the cervical spine posteriorly and inferiorly toward the scapula. Therefore it extends the neck at the cervical spinal joints. (reverse action 1)

• The levator scapulae crosses the cervical spine laterally (with its fibers running vertically in the frontal plane). When the scapula is fixed and the levator scapulae contracts, it pulls the cervical spine laterally and inferiorly toward the scapula. Therefore the levator scapulae laterally flexes the neck at the cervical spinal joints. (reverse action 2)

• The levator scapulae's fibers wrap around the cervical spine to attach onto the transverse processes (with its fibers oriented somewhat horizontally, from posterior to anterior, in the transverse plane). When the levator scapulae contracts, it pulls the transverse processes posteromedially, causing the anterior surface of the neck to face the same side of the body to which the levator scapulae is attached. Therefore the levator scapulae ipsilaterally rotates the neck at the cervical spinal joints. Note the similar line of pull to the adjacent splenius capitis and cervicis muscles, which are also ipsilateral rotators. (reverse action 3)

Levator Scapulae—*cont'd*

4

Eccentric Antagonist Functions

1. Restrains/slows scapular depression, upward rotation, and protraction
2. Restrains flexion, opposite-side lateral flexion, and contra-lateral rotation of the neck

Isometric Stabilization Functions

1. Stabilizes the scapula
2. Stabilizes the upper cervical spinal joints

Additional Note on Actions

1. In addition to its other actions, the scapula can also tilt. When the levator scapulae pulls on the scapula, it can pull the scapula in such a manner that the scapula is pulled superiorly and the inferior angle moves superiorly and away from the posterior body wall. The inferior angle of the scapula coming away from the body wall is called *upward tilt;* therefore the levator scapulae upwardly tilts the scapula at the scapulocostal joint.

INNERVATION
☐ Dorsal Scapular Nerve
  ☐ C3, C4, C5

ARTERIAL SUPPLY
☐ The Dorsal Scapular Artery (a branch of the Subclavian Artery)

✋ PALPATION

1. With the client seated and the hand in the small of the back (to relax the trapezius), place palpating hand just superior to the superior angle of the scapula.
2. Ask the client to perform a short, gentle range of motion of elevation of the scapula and feel for the contraction of the levator scapulae.
3. Continue palpating the levator scapulae superiorly into the posterior triangle of the neck (the area between the sternocleidomastoid and the upper trapezius). When palpating in the posterior triangle of the neck, the client's hand does not need to be in the small of the back and the client can contract more forcefully, and against resistance if desired.

■ RELATIONSHIP TO OTHER STRUCTURES

☐ Inferiorly, the levator scapulae is deep to the trapezius. Superiorly, the levator scapulae is deep to the sternocleidomastoid.
☐ There is a part of the middle to upper levator scapulae that is superficial between the trapezius and splenius capitis posteriorly, and the sternocleidomastoid and scalenes anteriorly, in the *posterior triangle of the neck.*
☐ The scapular attachment of the levator scapulae is superior to the attachment of the rhomboids.
☐ The transverse process attachment of the levator scapulae is directly deep (anterior) to the transverse process attachment of the splenius cervicis and directly superficial (posterior) to the transverse process attachment of the scalenes.
☐ The levator scapulae is located within the deep back arm line myofascial meridian.

■ MISCELLANEOUS

1. At approximately the midpoint of the levator scapulae, there is a twist in the fibers that creates an increased density in the middle of the muscle. This increased density may be mistaken for a trigger point. (Of course, it is possible that a trigger point may be present at this location.)
2. Because the cervical transverse process attachment of the levator scapulae is more anterior than the scapular attachment, some sources state that the levator scapulae has the ability to pull the scapula anteriorly. Therefore the levator scapulae is able to protract (abduct) the scapula at the scapulocostal joint. Whether the levator scapulae retracts or protracts the scapula is due to the posture of the individual. The more posturally protracted the client is—in other words, the more rounded the client's shoulders are—the more likely that the levator scapulae can protract the scapula.
3. Many students/therapists have a hard time palpating the superior aspect of the levator scapulae because they do not have a good sense of where the transverse process of the atlas (C1) is located. The transverse process of the atlas is easily palpable just posterior to the posterior border of the ramus of the mandible, directly inferior to the ear, and directly anterior to the mastoid process of the temporal bone.

Serratus Anterior

The name, serratus anterior, *tells us that this muscle has a serrated appearance and is anterior (anterior to the serratus posterior superior and serratus posterior inferior).*

Derivation	☐ serratus:	L. *a notching.*
	anterior:	L. *in front.*
Pronunciation	☐ ser-A-tus, an-TEE-ri-or	

■ ATTACHMENTS

☐ **Ribs one through nine**
   ☐ anterolaterally

to the

☐ **Anterior Surface of the Entire Medial Border of the Scapula**

■ FUNCTIONS

CONCENTRIC (SHORTENING) MOVER ACTIONS	
Standard Mover Actions	**Reverse Mover Actions**
☐ **1. Protracts the scapula at the ScC joint**	☐ 1. Retracts the trunk at the ScC joint
☐ **2. Upwardly rotates the scapula at the ScC joint**	☐ 2. Depresses the trunk at the ScC joint
☐ 3. Elevates the scapula at the ScC joint	
☐ 4. Depresses the scapula at the ScC joint	☐ 3. Elevates the trunk at the ScC joint
☐ 5. Medially tilts the scapula at the ScC joint	
☐ 6. Downwardly tilts the scapula at the ScC joint	

ScC joint = scapulocostal joint

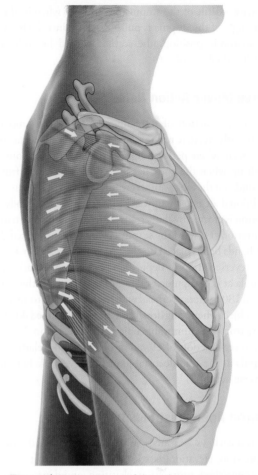

Figure 4-7 Lateral view of the right serratus anterior.

Standard Mover Action Notes

- The costal (i.e., rib) attachment of the serratus anterior is more anterior than the scapular attachment. When the serratus anterior contracts, it pulls the scapula anteriorly toward the ribs; therefore the serratus anterior protracts (i.e., abducts) the scapula at the scapulocostal joint. (action 1)
- Scapular protraction is important when pushing, punching, and reaching forward with the upper extremity. (action 1)
- When the serratus anterior contracts, it pulls on the scapula, causing the inferior angle of the scapula to swing anteriorly and superiorly toward the rib attachment of the serratus anterior (this is especially true of the fibers attaching to the inferior angle of the scapula). This causes the glenoid fossa to orient upward; therefore the serratus anterior upwardly rotates the scapula at the scapulocostal joint. (action 2)
- Upward rotation of the scapula is a coupled motion that must accompany any abduction and/or flexion of the arm

at the glenohumeral joint. The serratus anterior is especially engaged to upwardly rotate the scapula when the arm is flexed at the glenohumeral joint. (action 2)
- The serratus anterior is the prime mover of scapular protraction, upward rotation, and medial tilt. (actions 1, 2, 5)
- Only the upper fibers of the serratus anterior can elevate the scapula. (action 3)
- Only the lower fibers of the serratus anterior can depress the scapula. (action 4)
- When the scapula moves at the scapulocostal joint, the clavicle also moves at the sternoclavicular joint. (actions 1, 2, 3, 4)
- Medial tilt is a motion of the scapula that brings its medial border back against the body wall. In anatomic position, the scapula should be fully medially tilted. If the serratus anterior muscles are weak, the client may have a posture of winged scapulae (laterally tilted scapulae). The fact that the serratus anterior is a strong protractor and medial tilter is especially important because the scapula tends to laterally tilt when it protracts. (action 5)

4

- Downward tilt of the scapula is a motion wherein the inferior angle of the scapula is pulled back against the body wall. In anatomic position, the scapula should be fully downwardly tilted. (action 6)

Reverse Mover Action Notes

- The reverse action of retracting the trunk (i.e., moving it posteriorly) relative to the scapula at the scapulocostal joint is best seen when performing a push-up. At the point in a push-up when the body has been pushed up away from the ground and the elbow joints are fully extended, there is a small additional degree of upward movement of the body. This motion is created by the serratus anterior pulling the trunk up (posteriorly) toward the scapulae, which are now fixed due to the hands being placed on the floor. (reverse action 1)
- The reverse action of depression of the trunk relative to the scapula at the scapulocostal joint might occur if the arms are flexed 180 degrees overhead with the hands fixed to an immovable object when lying down and the body is pulled downward away from the immovable object. (reverse action 2)
- The reverse action of elevation of the trunk relative to the scapula at the scapulocostal joint is not very likely to occur. (reverse action 3)

Eccentric Antagonist Functions

1. Restrains/slows scapular retraction, downward rotation, depression, elevation, lateral tilt, and upward tilt
2. Restrains/slows protraction, elevation, and depression of the trunk

Isometric Stabilization Functions

1. Stabilizes the scapula
2. Stabilizes the rib cage

Isometric Stabilization Function Note

1. The stabilization of the scapula function of the serratus anterior is particularly important for maintaining a healthy posture of the scapula. The serratus anterior is the most important muscle for preventing lateral tilt (winging) and upward tilt of the scapula.

Additional Notes on Actions

1. Some sources state that the uppermost fibers of the serratus anterior can downwardly rotate and laterally tilt the scapula.
2. There is controversy regarding whether or not the serratus anterior is involved with respiration by moving the ribcage. Given its attachments onto the ribs, an accessory respiratory action seems likely.

INNERVATION
- The Long Thoracic Nerve
  - **C5**, C6, C7

ARTERIAL SUPPLY
- The Dorsal Scapular Artery (a branch of the Subclavian Artery) and the Lateral Thoracic Artery (a branch of the Axillary Artery)
  - and the Superior Thoracic Artery (a branch of the Axillary Artery)

✋ PALPATION

1. With the client supine and the arm flexed to 90 degrees at the shoulder joint (hand pointed toward the ceiling), place palpating hand on the rib cage on the lateral trunk between the anterior and posterior axillary folds of tissue.
2. Have the client protract the scapula by pushing the hand toward the ceiling and feel for the contraction of the serratus anterior. Resistance may be added.
3. Once located, try to follow the serratus anterior as far anterior as possible (deep to the pectoralis major) and as far posterior as possible (deep to the latissimus dorsi and the scapula).

■ RELATIONSHIP TO OTHER STRUCTURES

- From the posterior perspective, the majority of the serratus anterior lies deep to the scapula and the latissimus dorsi. From the anterior perspective, it lies deep to the pectoralis major and minor.
- The serratus anterior is superficial anterolaterally on the trunk where it meets the external abdominal oblique.
- The lowest four to five slips of the costal (i.e., rib) attachments of the serratus anterior interdigitate with the external abdominal oblique.
- The serratus anterior lies next to (anterior to) the subscapularis.
- The serratus anterior is located within the spiral line myofascial meridian.

■ MISCELLANEOUS

1. The serrated appearance comes from attaching onto separate ribs, which creates the notched look of a serrated knife.
2. In very well-developed individuals, the serratus anterior looks like ribs standing out in the anterolateral trunk.
3. The serratus anterior can be considered to have three parts: the first part attaching from ribs one and two to the superior angle of the scapula, the second part from ribs two and three to the length of the medial border of the scapula, and the third part from ribs four through nine to the inferior angle of the scapula. The third part (most inferior part) of the serratus anterior is the strongest.
4. The serratus anterior usually blends into the rhomboids on the anterior side of the scapula.

Pectoralis Minor

The name, pectoralis minor, *tells us that this muscle is located in the pectoral (chest) region and is small (smaller than the pectoralis major).*

Derivation	☐ pectoralis:	L. *refers to the chest.*
	minor:	L. *smaller.*
Pronunciation	☐ PEK-to-ra-lis, MY-nor	

■ ATTACHMENTS

☐ **Ribs three through five**

to the

☐ **Coracoid Process of the Scapula**
   ☐ the medial aspect

■ FUNCTIONS

CONCENTRIC (SHORTENING) MOVER ACTIONS	
Standard Mover Actions	**Reverse Mover Actions**
☐ 1. Protracts the scapula at the ScC joint	☐ 1. Elevates ribs three through five at the sternocostal and costospinal joints
☐ 2. Depresses the scapula at the ScC joint	
☐ 3. Downwardly rotates the scapula at the ScC joint	
☐ 4. Laterally tilts the scapula at the ScC joint	
☐ 5. Upwardly tilts the scapula at the ScC joint	

ScC joint = scapulocostal joint

Standard Mover Action Notes

• The pectoralis minor attaches from the scapula posteriorly, to the ribs anteriorly (with its fibers running horizontally). When the pectoralis minor contracts, it pulls the scapula anteriorly toward the rib cage attachment. Therefore the pectoralis minor protracts (abducts) the scapula at the scapulocostal joint. (action 1)

• The pectoralis minor attaches from the scapula superiorly, to the ribs inferiorly (with its fibers running vertically). When the pectoralis minor contracts, it pulls the scapula inferiorly toward the rib cage attachment. Therefore the pectoralis minor depresses the scapula at the scapulocostal joint. (action 2)

• When the pectoralis minor contracts and pulls on the coracoid process of the scapula, it rotates the scapula in such a manner that the coracoid process (anteriorly) is pulled inferiorly and laterally, and the inferior angle of the scapula (posteriorly) elevates and moves medially. This rotation

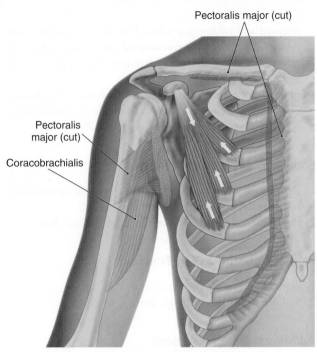

Figure 4-8 Anterior view of the right pectoralis minor. The coracobrachialis and cut pectoralis major have been ghosted in.

causes the glenoid fossa of the scapula to orient downward; therefore the pectoralis minor downwardly rotates the scapula at the scapulocostal joint. (action 3)

• Downward rotation of the scapula at the scapulocostal joint is the best joint action to engage and palpate the pectoralis minor. (action 3)

• Lateral tilt is a motion of the scapula that brings its medial border away from the body wall. In anatomic position, the scapula should be fully medially tilted. When the pectoralis minor contracts and pulls on the scapula, it pulls the coracoid process medially in front, which pulls the medial border of the scapula away from the posterior body wall. A tight pectoralis minor can result in a laterally tilted scapula, known in lay terms as a *winged scapula.* (action 4)

• Upward tilt is a motion of the scapula that brings its inferior angle away from the body wall. In anatomic position, the scapula should be fully downwardly tilted. When the pectoralis minor contracts and pulls on the scapula, it pulls the coracoid process down in front, which lifts the inferior angle of the scapula up and away from the posterior body wall. (action 5)

Reverse Mover Action Notes

• The pectoralis minor attaches from the scapula superiorly, to the ribs inferiorly (with its fibers running vertically). When the scapula is fixed and the pectoralis minor contracts, it pulls the ribs superiorly toward the scapula. Therefore the pectoralis minor elevates ribs three through five at the ster-

4

nocostal and costospinal joints. Even though the pectoralis minor can perform five actions of the scapula, only one reverse action of the ribs (elevation) is possible. (reverse action 1)

- Elevation of ribs helps to increase the volume of the thoracic cavity and therefore the lungs. Hence, the pectoralis minor is a muscle of inspiration. (reverse action 1)

Eccentric Antagonist Functions

1. Restrains/slows scapular retraction, elevation, upward rotation, medial tilt, and downward tilt
2. Restrains/slows depression of ribs three through five

Isometric Stabilization Functions

1. Stabilizes the scapula
2. Stabilizes ribs three through five

Additional Note on Actions

1. When the scapula is moved at the scapulocostal joint, the clavicle is also moved at the sternoclavicular joint.

INNERVATION
- The Medial and Lateral Pectoral Nerves
  - C5, C6, **C7**, **C8**, T1

ARTERIAL SUPPLY
- The Pectoral Branches of the Thoracoacromial Trunk (a branch of the Axillary Artery)
  - and the Posterior Intercostal Arteries (branches of the Aorta) and the Lateral Thoracic Artery (a branch of the Axillary Artery)

✋ **PALPATION**

1. With the client seated and the hand relaxed in the small of the back, place palpating fingers just inferior to the coracoid process of the scapula.
2. Have the client lift the hand away from the back and feel for the contraction of the pectoralis minor.
3. Palpate the entirety of the muscle.

■ RELATIONSHIP TO OTHER STRUCTURES

- The pectoralis minor is deep to the pectoralis major.
- Deep to the pectoralis minor are the serratus anterior and the rib cage.
- The superior attachment of the pectoralis minor is the coracoid process. The short head of the biceps brachii and the coracobrachialis also attach onto the coracoid process of the scapula.
- The pectoral minor is located within the deep front arm line myofascial meridian.

■ MISCELLANEOUS

1. The brachial plexus of nerves and the subclavian artery and vein are sandwiched between the pectoralis minor and the rib cage. Therefore this is a common entrapment site for these nerves and blood vessels. If the pectoralis minor is tight, these vessels and nerves may be compressed and the condition is called *pectoralis minor syndrome* (one of three types of *thoracic outlet syndrome*).
2. *Rounded shoulders* is a common postural condition in which the scapulae are protracted (abducted) and depressed (at the scapulocostal joints) and the humeri are medially rotated (at the glenohumeral joints). Given the pectoralis minor's actions of both protraction and depression of the scapula, when the pectoralis minor muscles are tight, they can significantly contribute to this condition.
3. A tight pectoralis minor, by rounding the shoulders, can also contribute to the clavicle dropping toward the first rib, decreasing the space between these two bones (costoclavicular space). Given that the brachial plexus of nerves and subclavian artery and vein travel in this space, they may be impinged. When this occurs, it is called *costoclavicular syndrome* (one of the three types of *thoracic outlet syndrome*).

Subclavius

The name, subclavius, *tells us that this muscle is "under" (i.e., inferior to) the clavicle.*

Derivation	☐ sub:	L. *under.*
	clavius:	L. *key.*
Pronunciation	☐ sub-KLAY-vee-us	

■ ATTACHMENTS

☐ **First Rib**
  ☐ at the junction with its costal cartilage

to the

☐ **Clavicle**
  ☐ the middle ⅓ of the inferior surface

■ FUNCTIONS

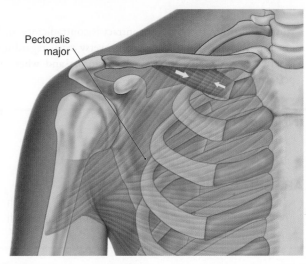

Figure 4-9 Anterior view of the right subclavius. The pectoralis major has been ghosted in.

CONCENTRIC (SHORTENING) MOVER ACTIONS	
Standard Mover Actions	**Reverse Mover Actions**
☐ 1. Depresses the clavicle at the SC joint	☐ 1. Elevates the first rib at the sternocostal and costospinal joints
☐ 2. Protracts the clavicle at the SC joint	
☐ 3. Downwardly rotates the clavicle at the SC joint	
SC joint = sternoclavicular joint	

Standard Mover Action Notes

- The subclavius attaches from the first rib inferiorly to the clavicle superiorly, (with its fibers running somewhat vertically). When the first rib is fixed and the subclavius contracts, it pulls the clavicle inferiorly toward the first rib. Therefore the subclavius depresses the clavicle at the SC joint. (action 1)
- The clavicular attachment is also slightly posterior to the first rib attachment, so when the subclavius contracts, it pulls the clavicle anteriorly toward the first rib attachment. Therefore the subclavius protracts the clavicle at the SC joint.
- When the subclavius contracts, it pulls the clavicle in an anteroinferior direction, causing the anterior surface of the clavicle to face inferiorly (because its pull is anterior to the axis about which the clavicle rotates). Therefore the subclavius downwardly rotates the clavicle at the SC joint. Note: The clavicle is fully downwardly rotated in anatomic position, so the subclavius must downwardly rotate a clavicle that is first upwardly rotated. (action 3)
- Given that the clavicle and scapula often move as a unit, when the subclavius moves the clavicle at the SC joint, it can also create the same movement of the scapula at the scapulocostal joint. (actions 1, 2, 3)

Reverse Mover Action Notes

- The subclavius attaches to the first rib inferiorly, from the clavicle superiorly. When the clavicle is fixed and the subclavius contracts, it pulls the first rib superiorly toward the clavicle. Therefore the subclavius elevates the first rib at the sternocostal and costospinal joints. (reverse action 1)
- Elevation of ribs helps to increase the volume of the thoracic cavity and therefore the lungs. Hence, the subclavius can assist with inspiration. (reverse action 1)

Eccentric Antagonist Functions

1. Restrains/slows clavicular elevation, retraction, and upward rotation
2. Restrains/slows depression of the first rib

Isometric Stabilization Functions

1. Stabilizes the clavicle and first rib

Isometric Stabilization Function Note

- Many sources state that the major function of the subclavius is to stabilize the clavicle during motions of the arm at the glenohumeral joint. Its medial to lateral horizontal line of pull helps to hold the medial end of the clavicle into the manubrium of the sternum.

Additional Note on Actions

1. The actions listed here for the subclavius are posited based on the lines of pull of this muscle on the bones to which it attaches. Electromyographic evidence as to when the subcla-

4

Subclavius—*cont'd*

vius is and is not recruited to contract is contradictory and unclear. Therefore considerable controversy exists regarding exactly which actions this muscle performs and when it performs them.

INNERVATION
□ A Nerve from the Brachial Plexus
  □ C5, C6

ARTERIAL SUPPLY
□ The Clavicular Branch of the Thoracoacromial Trunk (a branch of the Axillary Artery) and the Suprascapular Artery (a branch of the Thyrocervical Trunk)

👋 PALPATION

1. With the client supine and the arm medially rotated and resting at the side of the body, place palpating fingers slightly inferior to the middle ⅓ of the clavicle.
2. Now curl your fingers under the clavicle and feel for the subclavius against the inferior surface of the clavicle.
3. To engage the subclavius, have the client depress the shoulder girdle and feel for its contraction.

■ RELATIONSHIP TO OTHER STRUCTURES

□ The subclavius is located between the clavicle and the first rib.
□ The subclavius is deep to the pectoralis major.
□ Deep to the subclavius are the brachial plexus of nerves and the subclavian artery and vein.
□ The subclavius is located within the deep front arm line myofascial meridian.

■ MISCELLANEOUS

1. A somewhat common anomaly is for the subclavius to attach to the coracoid process of the scapula in addition to or instead of attaching to the clavicle.
2. The brachial plexus of nerves and the subclavian artery and vein are located deep to the subclavius, between the clavicle and the first rib. If the subclavius is tight, it can pull the clavicle and first rib toward each other, lessening the space between these two bones (costoclavicular space) and possibly compressing these neurovascular structures. When entrapment of these nerves and/or vessels occurs in this location, it is called *costoclavicular syndrome* (one of three types of *thoracic outlet syndrome*).

Muscles of the Glenohumeral Joint

CHAPTER **OUTLINE**

CHAPTER **OVERVIEW**

The muscles addressed in this chapter are the muscles whose principal function is usually considered to be movement of the glenohumeral joint. Other muscles in the body can also move the glenohumeral joint, but they are placed in different chapters because their primary function is usually considered to be at another joint. These muscles are the biceps brachii and triceps brachii covered in Chapter 6.

Overview of Structure
☐ Structurally, muscles of the glenohumeral joint are varied. Two of them are large, expansive muscles that arise proximally on the trunk and make their way to attach onto the humerus, crossing the glenohumeral joint along the way. One of these two is the pectoralis major, which is anterior; the other is the latissimus dorsi, which is posterior. The rest of the glenohumeral joint muscles travel from the scapula (and perhaps the clavicle) to attach to the humerus. These muscles include the deltoid, the coracobrachialis, the teres major, and the rotator cuff group.
☐ The larger, more superficial muscles are primarily important for creating motion. The deeper, smaller ones, especially the rotator cuff group muscles, function primarily to stabilize the head of the humerus at the glenohumeral joint.

Overview of Function
The following general rules regarding actions can be stated for the functional groups of muscles of the glenohumeral joint:

☐ If a muscle crosses the glenohumeral joint anteriorly with a vertical direction to its fibers, it can flex the arm at the glenohumeral joint by moving the anterior surface of the arm toward the scapula.
☐ If a muscle crosses the glenohumeral joint posteriorly with a vertical direction to its fibers, it can extend the arm at the glenohumeral joint by moving the posterior surface of the arm toward the scapula.
☐ If a muscle crosses the glenohumeral joint laterally (superiorly, over the top of the joint), it can abduct the arm at the glenohumeral joint by moving the lateral surface of the arm toward the scapula.
☐ If a muscle crosses the glenohumeral joint medially (inferiorly, below the center of the joint), it can adduct the arm at the glenohumeral joint by moving the medial surface of the arm toward the scapula.
☐ Medial rotators of the arm wrap around the humerus from medial to lateral, anterior to the glenohumeral joint.
☐ Lateral rotators of the arm wrap around the humerus from medial to lateral, posterior to the glenohumeral joint.
☐ Reverse actions of these standard mover actions involve the scapula being moved relative to the humerus at the glenohumeral joint (the scapula will also be moved relative to the ribcage at the scapulocostal joint). These reverse actions are usually either rotation or tilt actions of the scapula.

Posterior View of the Muscles of the Glenohumeral Joint and Shoulder Girdle Region

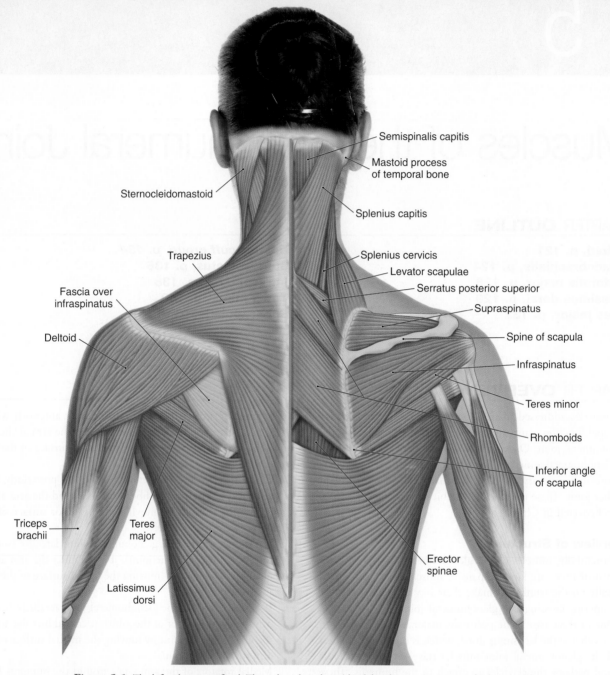

Figure 5-1 The left side is superficial. The right side is deep (the deltoid, trapezius, sternocleidomastoid, and infraspinatus fascia have been removed).

Anterior View of the Muscles of the Glenohumeral Joint and Shoulder Girdle Region

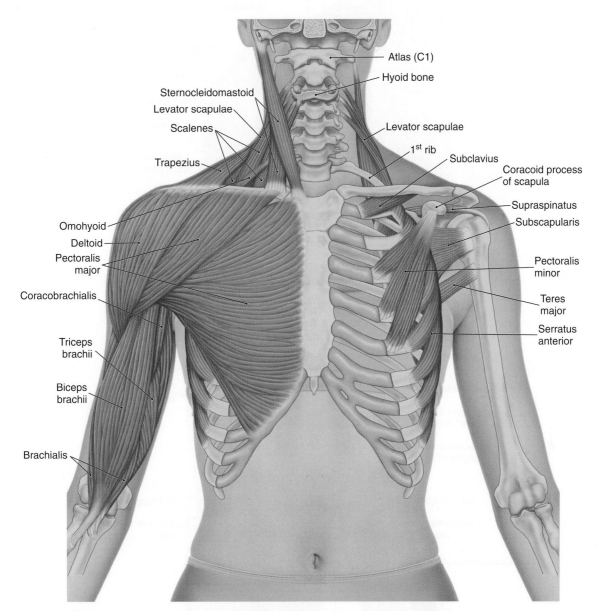

Figure 5-2 The right side is superficial. The left side is deep (the deltoid, pectoralis major, trapezius, scalenes, omohyoid, and muscles of the arm have been removed; the sternocleidomastoid has been cut).

Posterior and Anterior Views of the Muscles of the Glenohumeral Joint

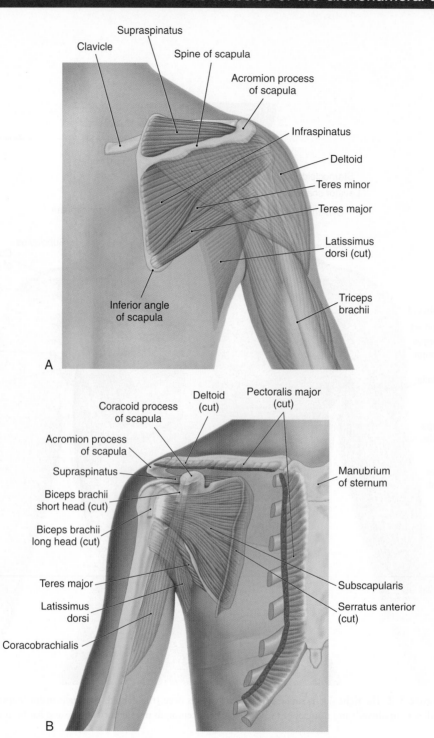

Figure 5-3 **A,** Posterior view. The deltoid, triceps brachii, and latissimus dorsi have been ghosted in. **B,** Anterior view. The rib cage has been cut. The coracobrachialis has been ghosted in.

Anterior View of a Frontal Plane Section through the Right Glenohumeral Joint

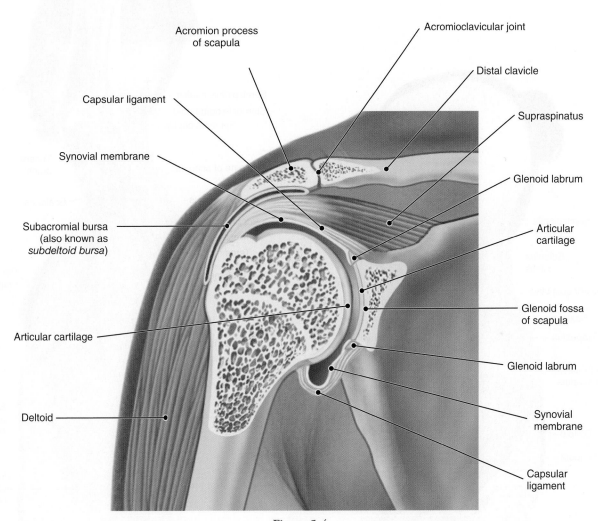

Acromion process
of scapula

Acromioclavicular joint

Distal clavicle

Capsular ligament

Supraspinatus

Synovial membrane

Glenoid labrum

Subacromial bursa
(also known as
subdeltoid bursa)

Articular
cartilage

Articular cartilage

Glenoid fossa
of scapula

Glenoid labrum

Deltoid

Synovial
membrane

Capsular
ligament

Figure 5-4

5

Right Lateral Views of the Muscles of the Neck, Shoulder Girdle, and Trunk Regions

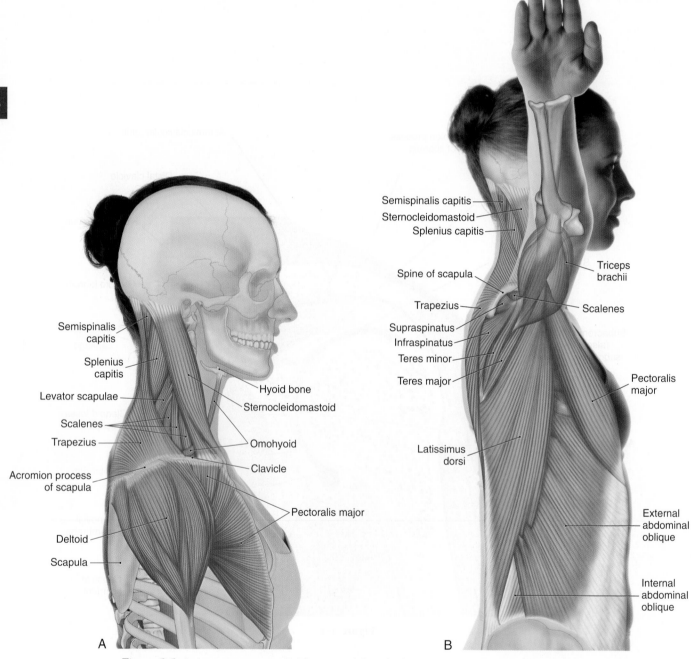

Semispinalis capitis

Splenius capitis

Levator scapulae

Scalenes

Trapezius

Acromion process of scapula

Deltoid

Scapula

Hyoid bone

Sternocleidomastoid

Omohyoid

Clavicle

Pectoralis major

A

Semispinalis capitis

Sternocleidomastoid

Splenius capitis

Spine of scapula

Trapezius

Supraspinatus

Infraspinatus

Teres minor

Teres major

Latissimus dorsi

Triceps brachii

Scalenes

Pectoralis major

External abdominal oblique

Internal abdominal oblique

B

Figure 5-5 A, Anatomic position. **B,** The arm is abducted. The triceps brachii has been ghosted in.

Deltoid

The name, deltoid, *tells us that this muscle has a triangular shape similar to the Greek letter delta (Δ).*

Derivation	☐ delta: Gr. *the letter delta (Δ).* oid: Gr. *resemblance.*
Pronunciation	☐ DEL-toid

■ ATTACHMENTS

☐ **Lateral Clavicle, Acromion Process, and the Spine of the Scapula**
    ☐ the lateral ⅓ of the clavicle

to the

☐ **Deltoid Tuberosity of the Humerus**

■ FUNCTIONS

CONCENTRIC (SHORTENING) MOVER ACTIONS	
Standard Mover Actions	**Reverse Mover Actions**
☐ 1. Abducts the arm at the GH joint (entire muscle)	☐ 1. Downwardly rotates the scapula at the GH and scapulocostal joints
☐ 2. Flexes the arm at the GH joint (anterior deltoid)	☐ 2. Ipsilaterally rotates the trunk
☐ 3. Medially rotates the arm at the GH joint (anterior deltoid)	
☐ 4. Horizontally flexes the arm at the GH joint (anterior deltoid)	
☐ 5. Extends the arm at the GH joint (posterior deltoid)	☐ 3. Contralaterally rotates the trunk
☐ 6. Laterally rotates the arm at the GH joint (posterior deltoid)	
☐ 7. Horizontally extends the arm at the GH joint (posterior deltoid)	

GH joint = glenohumeral joint

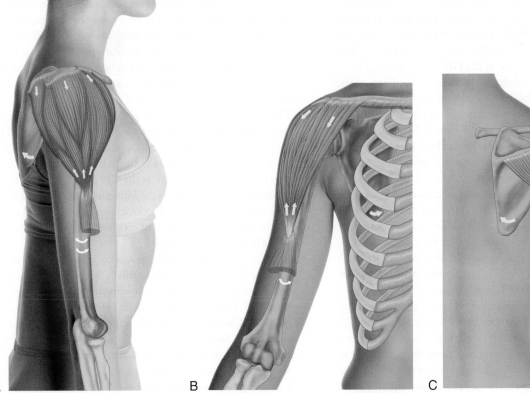
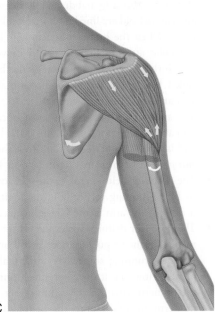

Figure 5-6 The right deltoid. **A,** Lateral view. The proximal end of the brachialis has been ghosted in. **B,** Anterior view. The proximal ends of the pectoralis major and brachialis have been ghosted in. **C,** Posterior view. The proximal end of the triceps brachii has been ghosted in.

5

Standard Mover Action Notes

- The deltoid crosses over the top of the GH joint on the lateral side (with its fibers running vertically in the frontal plane); therefore it abducts the arm at the GH joint. The anterior and posterior parts of the deltoid can abduct the arm at the GH joint, but the fibers of the middle deltoid have the best line of pull for this action. (action 1)
- Although the deltoid can abduct the arm at the GH joint throughout its entire range of motion, the deltoid's activity is strongest between 90 degrees and 120 degrees. (action 1)
- The lowest fibers of the anterior deltoid and posterior deltoid can adduct the arm at the GH joint because they pass inferior to the axis of motion of the GH joint. (action 1)
- The anterior deltoid crosses the GH joint anteriorly (with its fibers running vertically in the sagittal plane); therefore it flexes the arm at the GH joint. The anterior deltoid is considered to be the prime mover of flexion of the arm at the GH joint. (action 2)
- The middle deltoid also has a component of flexion of the arm because the scapula is oriented approximately 35 degrees off the frontal plane toward the sagittal plane. (action 2)
- The anterior deltoid crosses the GH joint anteriorly from medial on the clavicle to more lateral on the humerus (with its fibers running somewhat horizontally in the transverse plane). However, it does not attach onto the first aspect of the humerus that it reaches, but rather it wraps around the humerus to attach onto the deltoid tuberosity. Therefore when the anterior deltoid contracts, the anterior surface of the humerus rotates medially. This movement is called medial rotation of the arm at the GH joint. (action 3)
- When the arm is first abducted 90 degrees, the fibers of the anterior deltoid are lined up horizontally in front of the GH joint. When the humeral attachment is pulled toward the clavicular attachment, the arm is moved horizontally and anteriorly, toward the midline of the body; this motion is called horizontal flexion (or horizontal adduction) of the arm at the GH joint. (action 4)
- The anterior deltoid is a powerful horizontal flexor of the arm at the GH joint. In fact, this is the best action to engage and isolate the anterior deltoid from the middle and posterior deltoid when palpating it. (action 4)
- The posterior deltoid crosses the GH joint posteriorly (with its fibers running vertically in the sagittal plane); therefore it extends the arm at the GH joint. (action 5)
- The posterior deltoid crosses the GH joint posteriorly from medial on the scapula to more lateral on the humerus (with its fibers running somewhat horizontally in the transverse plane). However, it does not attach onto the first aspect of the humerus that it reaches, but rather it wraps around the humerus to attach onto the deltoid tuberosity. Therefore when the posterior deltoid contracts, the anterior surface of the humerus rotates laterally. This movement is called lateral rotation of the arm at the GH joint. (action 6)
- When the arm is first abducted 90 degrees, the fibers of the posterior deltoid are lined up horizontally in back of the GH joint. When the humeral attachment is pulled toward the attachment on the spine of the scapula, the arm is moved horizontally and posteriorly, away from the midline of the body; this motion is called horizontal extension (or horizontal abduction) of the arm at the GH joint. (action 7)
- The posterior deltoid is a powerful horizontal extensor of the arm at the GH joint. In fact, this is the best action to engage and isolate the posterior deltoid from the middle and anterior deltoid when palpating it. (action 7)

Reverse Mover Action Notes

- When the arm is fixed and the deltoid contracts, the deltoid pulls directly on the scapula (and indirectly on the scapula by pulling on the lateral clavicle), pulling the acromion process inferiorly toward the humerus. This causes the inferior angle of the scapula to swing up toward the vertebral column and causes the glenoid fossa to orient downward. Therefore the deltoid downwardly rotates the scapula relative to the humerus at the GH joint and relative to the rib cage at the scapulocostal joint. (reverse action 1)
- The reverse action of downward rotation of the scapula by the deltoid is extremely important. If this action is not opposed by an upward rotator muscle (usually the upper trapezius) when the deltoid contracts to abduct the humerus, the humeral head and acromion process of the scapula will approximate each other, pinching the rotator cuff tendon and subacromial bursa between them. (reverse action 1)
- If the arm is fixed and the anterior deltoid pulls on the clavicle, the clavicle would normally be moved at the sternoclavicular joint (into depression, downward rotation, and protraction). However, if the clavicle and scapula are fixed to the trunk, the trunk will be pulled with the clavicle and scapula and will be rotated such that it faces the same side of the body on which the anterior deltoid is located. This action may be called ipsilateral rotation of the trunk at the GH joint (in reality, it is a scapular motion relative to the humerus at the GH joint and the trunk, being fixed to the clavicle and scapula, goes along for the ride, rotating such that it comes to face the same side of the body). (reverse action 2)
- If the arm is fixed and the posterior deltoid pulls on the scapula, the scapula would normally be moved at the GH and scapulocostal joints (into downward rotation and downward tilt). However, if the scapula is fixed to the trunk, the trunk will be pulled with the scapula and will be rotated such that it faces the opposite side of the body from where the posterior deltoid is located. This action may be called contralateral rotation of the trunk at the GH joint (in reality, it is a scapular motion relative to the humerus at the GH joint; and the trunk, being fixed to the scapula, goes along for the ride, rotating such that it comes to face the other side of the body). (reverse action 3)

Deltoid—*cont'd*

Eccentric Antagonist Functions

1. Restrains/slows arm adduction, extension, horizontal extension, flexion, horizontal flexion, lateral rotation, and medial rotation
2. Restrains/slows contralateral rotation and ipsilateral rotation of the trunk
3. Restrains/slows clavicular elevation, upward rotation, and retraction
4. Restrains/slows scapular upward rotation and upward tilt

Eccentric Antagonist Function Note

• Upward tilt of the scapula is a motion in which the inferior angle of the scapula lifts away from the rib cage wall.

Isometric Stabilization Functions

1. Stabilizes the GH joint
2. Stabilizes the scapula and clavicle

INNERVATION
☐ The Axillary Nerve
  ☐ **C5**, C6

ARTERIAL SUPPLY
☐ The Anterior and Posterior Circumflex Humeral Arteries (branches of the Axillary Artery)
  ☐ and the Pectoral and Deltoid branches of the Thoracoacromial Trunk (a branch of the Axillary Artery)

✋ PALPATION

1. With the client seated, place palpating hand just distal to the acromion process of the scapula.
2. Have the client abduct the arm at the glenohumeral joint and feel for the contraction of the deltoid. Resistance can be added.
3. Continue palpating the deltoid anteriorly for the anterior fibers and posteriorly for the posterior fibers. Palpate all fibers distally to the deltoid tuberosity of the humerus.
4. Note: Horizontal flexion can be used for the anterior fibers; horizontal extension can be used for the posterior fibers.

■ RELATIONSHIP TO OTHER STRUCTURES

☐ The deltoid is superficial and found at the anterior, lateral, and posterior shoulder. It gives the shoulder its characteristic shape.
☐ The anterior deltoid lies next to the clavicular head of the pectoralis major.
☐ Inferior to the posterior deltoid are the infraspinatus, the teres minor, the teres major, and the triceps brachii.
☐ The following muscles all have tendons that are deep to the deltoid: the pectoralis minor, the coracobrachialis, and the short head of the biceps brachii (all attaching to the coracoid process of the scapula); the supraspinatus, the infraspinatus, the teres minor, and the subscapularis (rotator cuff muscles attaching to the greater and lesser tubercles of the humerus); and the pectoralis major, the long head of the biceps brachii, and the long and lateral heads of the triceps brachii.
☐ The deltoid is located within the superficial back arm line myofascial meridian.

■ MISCELLANEOUS

1. The deltoid is considered to have three parts: anterior, middle, and posterior.
2. The anterior deltoid crosses the glenohumeral joint anteriorly and attaches to the lateral clavicle proximally. The middle deltoid crosses the glenohumeral joint laterally and attaches to the acromion process of the scapula proximally. The posterior deltoid crosses the glenohumeral joint posteriorly and attaches to the spine of the scapula proximally.
3. The proximal attachments of the deltoid are the same as the lateral attachments of the trapezius, namely, the lateral clavicle, the acromion process, and the spine of the scapula.
4. Note how the deltoid fans around the glenohumeral joint. It crosses the glenohumeral joint anteriorly, laterally, and posteriorly. This orientation is similar to the orientation of the gluteus medius to the hip joint. Therefore both of these muscles can do the same actions at their respective joints. The deltoid abducts, flexes, extends, medially rotates, and laterally rotates the arm at the glenohumeral joint. The gluteus medius abducts, flexes, extends, medially rotates, and laterally rotates the thigh at the hip joint.
5. The anterior and posterior fibers of the deltoid are longitudinal (nonpennate). The middle fibers are multipennate.
6. Because it is pennate, the middle deltoid functions more for stabilization (in the frontal plane). The anterior and posterior fibers, being longitudinal (nonpennate), function more for movement (in the sagittal plane).

Coracobrachialis

The name, coracobrachialis, *tells us that this muscle is related to the coracoid process and the brachium (the arm), hence its attachments onto the coracoid process of the scapula and the humerus.*

Derivation	☐ coraco:	Gr. *refers to the coracoid process of the scapula.*
		brachialis: L. *refers to the arm.*
Pronunciation	☐ KOR-a-ko-BRA-key-AL-is

■ ATTACHMENTS

☐ **Coracoid Process of the Scapula**
  ☐ the apex

to the

☐ **Medial Shaft of the Humerus**
  ☐ the middle ⅓

■ FUNCTIONS

CONCENTRIC (SHORTENING) MOVER ACTIONS	
Standard Mover Actions	**Reverse Mover Actions**
☐ **1. Flexes the arm at the GH joint**	☐ 1. Upwardly tilts the scapula at the GH and ScC joints
☐ **2. Adducts the arm at the GH joint**	☐ 2. Downwardly rotates the scapula at the GH and ScC joints
☐ 3. Horizontally flexes the arm at the GH joint	☐ 3. Protracts the scapula at the GH and ScC joints

GH joint = glenohumeral joint; ScC joint = scapulocostal joint

Standard Mover Action Notes

- The coracobrachialis crosses the GH joint anteriorly (with its fibers running vertically in the sagittal plane); therefore it flexes the arm at the GH joint. (action 1)
- The coracobrachialis crosses the GH joint medially (with its fibers running vertically in the frontal plane); therefore it adducts the arm at the GH joint. (action 2)
- The coracobrachialis is a strong horizontal flexor of the arm at the GH joint. In fact, horizontally flexing the arm against resistance is probably the most effective way to engage and palpate the coracobrachialis. (action 3)

Reverse Mover Action Notes

- When the scapula moves relative to the arm at the GH joint, it also moves relative to the rib cage at the scapulocostal joint. (reverse actions 1, 2, 3)
- Pulling the coracoid process in front anteriorly and down causes the inferior angle in back to lift up and posteriorly away from the rib cage wall. Lifting the inferior angle of the scapula away from the rib cage is called upward tilt. (reverse action 1)
- Pulling the coracoid process in front down and laterally causes the inferior angle in back to lift up and medially. This causes the glenoid fossa to orient downward. Therefore, the

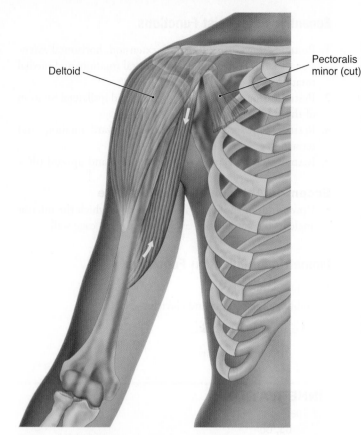

Figure 5-7 Anterior view of the right coracobrachialis. The deltoid and proximal end of the pectoralis minor have been ghosted in.

coracobrachialis downwardly rotates the scapula at the scapulocostal joint. (reverse action 2)

Eccentric Antagonist Functions

1. Restrains/slows arm extension, abduction, and horizontal extension
2. Restrains/slows scapular upward rotation, retraction, and downward tilt

Isometric Stabilization Functions

1. Stabilizes the GH joint
2. Stabilizes the scapula

INNERVATION
☐ The Musculocutaneous Nerve
  ☐ C5, C6, C7

ARTERIAL SUPPLY
☐ The muscular branches of the Brachial Artery (the continuation of the Axillary Artery)
  ☐ and the Anterior Circumflex Humeral Artery (a branch of the Axillary Artery)

Coracobrachialis—cont'd

 PALPATION

1. With the client seated with the arm abducted to 90 degrees and laterally rotated, and the forearm flexed at the elbow joint to 90 degrees, place palpating fingers on the medial side of the humerus, approximately halfway down the shaft.
2. Have the client horizontally flex the arm at the glenohumeral joint against resistance and feel for the contraction of the coracobrachialis. (Note: It can be challenging to discern the coracobrachialis from the short head of the biceps brachii; the biceps brachii also contracts with flexion of the forearm at the elbow joint.)
3. Note: Be careful with palpation in the medial arm because the median and ulnar nerves and brachial artery are superficial here.

■ RELATIONSHIP TO OTHER STRUCTURES

☐ From an anterior perspective, the coracobrachialis lies deep to the deltoid and the pectoralis major.

☐ Proximally, the coracobrachialis lies medial to the short head of the biceps brachii. More distally, the coracobrachialis is deep to the short head of the biceps brachii.
☐ The coracobrachialis attaches onto the shaft of the humerus on the medial side between the attachments of the brachialis and the triceps brachii (medial head).
☐ The proximal attachment of the coracobrachialis is the coracoid process of the scapula. The short head of the biceps brachii and the pectoralis minor also attach to the coracoid process.
☐ The coracobrachialis is located within the deep front arm line myofascial meridian.

■ MISCELLANEOUS

1. The proximal attachment of the coracobrachialis blends with the proximal attachment of the short head of the biceps brachii.
2. The musculocutaneous nerve pierces through the coracobrachialis.

Pectoralis Major

The name, pectoralis major, *tells us that this muscle is located in the pectoral (chest) region and is large (larger than the pectoralis minor).*

Derivation	☐ pectoralis: L. *refers to the chest.*
	major: L. *larger.*
Pronunciation	☐ PEK-to-ra-lis, MAY-jor

■ ATTACHMENTS

☐ **Medial Clavicle, Sternum, and the Costal Cartilages of Ribs One through Seven**
  ☐ the medial ½ of the clavicle, and the aponeurosis of the external abdominal oblique

to the

☐ **Lateral Lip of the Bicipital Groove of the Humerus**

■ FUNCTIONS

CONCENTRIC (SHORTENING) MOVER ACTIONS	
Standard Mover Actions	**Reverse Mover Actions**
☐ **1. Adducts the arm at the GH joint**	☐ 1. Laterally deviates the trunk
☐ **2. Medially rotates the arm at the GH joint**	
☐ **3. Flexes the arm at the GH joint**	☐ 2. Flexes the trunk at the spinal joints
☐ **4. Extends the arm at the GH joint**	☐ 3. Anteriorly translates the trunk
☐ 5. Abducts the arm at the GH joint	☐ 4. Downwardly rotates the scapula at the GH and ScC joints
☐ 6. Horizontally flexes the arm at the GH joint	☐ 5. Ipsilaterally rotates the trunk
☐ 7. Protracts the scapula at the ScC joint	
☐ 8. Retracts the scapula at the ScC joint	
☐ 9. Depresses the scapula at the ScC joint	☐ 6. Elevates the trunk

GH joint = glenohumeral joint; ScC joint = scapulocostal joint

Standard Mover Action Notes

• The pectoralis major crosses the GH joint anteriorly, from medial on the trunk to lateral on the humerus (with the fibers running horizontally in the frontal plane and crossing below the center of the GH joint). When the pectoralis major contracts, it pulls the humerus medially toward the trunk; therefore the pectoralis major adducts the arm at the

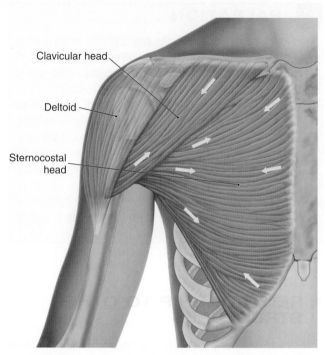

Figure 5-8 Anterior view of the right pectoralis major. The deltoid has been ghosted in.

GH joint. Adduction is performed primarily by the sternocostal head whose fibers are more horizontal in orientation and located within the frontal plane. (action 1)

• The pectoralis major crosses the GH joint anteriorly from the trunk to the humerus. However, the pectoralis major does not attach to the most medial aspect of the humerus but rather wraps around the humerus to attach onto the lateral lip of the bicipital groove (with its fibers running horizontally in the transverse plane). When the pectoralis major contracts, it pulls the humeral attachment posteromedially, causing the anterior surface of the arm to face medially. Therefore the pectoralis major medially rotates the arm at the GH joint. Medial rotation is performed primarily by the sternocostal head whose fibers are more horizontal in orientation and located in the transverse plane. (action 2)

• The clavicular head of the pectoralis major crosses the GH joint anteriorly with the fibers running somewhat vertically (in the sagittal plane); therefore it flexes the arm at the GH joint. The clavicular head of the pectoralis major can only flex the arm up to a position of approximately 60 degrees. (action 3)

• The sternocostal head of the pectoralis major crosses the GH joint in such a way (with its fibers running in the sagittal plane) that if the arm is already in a position of flexion, these fibers can pull the arm, which is more anterior, posteriorly back toward the chest. Therefore the pectoralis major can extend the arm at the GH joint. The pectoralis major cannot extend the arm at the GH joint beyond anatomic position. (action 4)

- If the arm is in a position of approximately 100 degrees of abduction or more, the line of pull of the clavicular head of the pectoralis major relative to the GH joint shifts from being below the center of the joint to being above it, changing its action from adduction to abduction of the arm at the GH joint. (action 5)
- When the arm is first abducted 90 degrees, the fibers of the pectoralis major are lined up in front of the GH joint and can create a powerful horizontal flexion (horizontal adduction) force on the arm at the GH joint. (action 6)
- When the pectoralis major pulls on the arm, if the scapula is fixed to the humerus, the scapula will also be moved and will move at the scapulocostal joint. A pulling force of flexion and medial rotation on the arm can result in protraction of the scapula. A pulling force of extension on the arm can result in retraction of the scapula. If the arm is overhead, pulling the humerus and scapula toward the chest will cause depression of the scapula. Note: This will also result in the clavicle performing the same movement at the sternoclavicular joint. (actions 7, 8, 9)
- Protraction of the scapula is especially important when performing pushing and throwing actions. Retraction of the scapula is important with pulling motions. (actions 7, 8)

Reverse Mover Action Notes

- Reverse actions of the trunk moving relative to the arm can occur at the GH joint if the scapula is fixed to the trunk (so that the trunk and scapula move as a unit relative to the arm), or at the scapulocostal joint if the scapula is fixed to the humerus (so that the trunk moves relative to the scapula/arm as a unit). (reverse actions 1, 2, 3, 5, 6)
- The reverse actions of the trunk moving relative to the arm are often performed by people using handicap bars to pull themselves up from a seated position, or by people pulling themselves up stairs using a banister. (reverse actions 1, 2, 3, 5, 6)
- If the arm is in an abducted position and fixed, the pectoralis major can pull the trunk laterally toward the arm in the frontal plane. This will result in the trunk laterally deviating toward the same-side arm. (reverse action 1)
- If the arm is fixed, the clavicular head of the pectoralis major can pull the trunk down toward the humerus. This will result in flexion of the trunk at the spinal joints (as well as moving the scapula (with the trunk) relative to the humerus at the GH joint). (reverse action 2)
- If the arm is in a position of flexion and fixed, the sternocostal head can pull the trunk anteriorly toward the humeral attachment. (reverse action 3)
- When the arm is fixed and the pectoralis major contracts, it pulls indirectly on the scapula by pulling on the clavicle,

pulling the acromion process inferiorly toward the humerus. This causes the glenoid fossa to orient downward. Therefore the pectoralis major downwardly rotates the scapula relative to the humerus at the GH joint and relative to the rib cage at the scapulocostal joint. (reverse action 4)

- When the humerus is fixed, the pectoralis major can pull the trunk toward the arm in the transverse plane. This will result in the trunk ipsilaterally rotating toward the humeral attachment. (reverse action 5)
- The reverse action of depressing the scapula (via the pectoralis major's pull on the humerus) relative to a fixed trunk is to pull the trunk up toward the scapula. (reverse action 6)

Eccentric Antagonist Functions

1. Restrains/slows arm abduction, lateral rotation, extension, horizontal extension, flexion, and adduction
2. Restrains/slows scapular retraction, protraction, elevation, and upward rotation
3. Restrains/slows contralateral rotation. Extension, opposite-side lateral deviation, posterior translation, and depression of the trunk

Isometric Stabilization Functions

1. Stabilizes the GH joint
2. Stabilizes the clavicle and scapula

Additional Note on Actions

- The pectoralis major and the latissimus dorsi are both large, powerful muscles that attach from the trunk to the arm. These two muscles are synergistic to each other with respect to their arm actions in that they both adduct and medially rotate the arm at the GH joint. They are both synergistic and antagonistic to each other with respect to their sagittal plane arm actions; the sternocostal head of the pectoralis major extends the arm at the GH joint and the clavicular head flexes the arm at the GH joint, and the latissimus dorsi extends the arm at the GH joint.

INNERVATION

- ☐ The Medial and Lateral Pectoral Nerves
  - ☐ **C5**, C6, **C7**, C8, T1

ARTERIAL SUPPLY

- ☐ The Pectoral branches of the Thoracoacromial Trunk (a branch of the Axillary Artery)
  - ☐ and the Posterior Intercostal Arteries (branches of the Aorta) and the Lateral Thoracic Artery (a branch of the Axillary Artery)

Pectoralis Major—*cont'd*

 PALPATION

1. With the client seated with the arm raised to 90 degrees of abduction at the glenohumeral joint, place palpating hand on the belly of the pectoralis major.
2. Have the client horizontally flex the arm against resistance and feel for the contraction of the pectoralis major.
3. Continue palpating the pectoralis major medially and superiorly toward its attachments on the trunk and distally toward its humeral attachment.
4. Note: The *anterior axillary fold* of tissue is created by the pectoralis major.

■ RELATIONSHIP TO OTHER STRUCTURES

☐ The pectoralis major is superficial in the chest.
☐ The pectoralis minor and the subclavius, as well as the proximal attachments of the coracobrachialis and the short and long heads of the biceps brachii, are deep to the pectoralis major.
☐ Lateral to the clavicular head of the pectoralis major is the anterior deltoid.
☐ The pectoralis major is located within the superficial front arm line and front functional line myofascial meridians.

■ MISCELLANEOUS

1. Sources differ on how the pectoralis major is divided into parts. Some say that it has clavicular, sternal, costal, and abdominal heads; others lump the sternal and costal heads into a sternocostal head; others omit the abdominal head altogether. Regardless of how it is divided, what is most important to realize is that the pectoralis major has upper fibers and lower fibers that cross the shoulder joint differently and therefore have different actions at the shoulder joint.
2. The pectoralis major has layers: the clavicular fibers are the most superficial (anterior); the sternal fibers are deep to the clavicular fibers; and the costal and abdominal fibers are the deepest (most posterior).
3. The clavicular fibers attach more distally on the humerus; the sternocostal fibers attach more proximally on the humerus.
4. The fibers of the sternocostal head of the pectoralis major twist so that the more superior fibers attach further distally on the humerus; the more inferior fibers attach more proximally on the humerus. Note: The fibers of the latissimus dorsi also twist so that the superior fibers attach distally on the humerus and the inferior fibers attach proximally on the humerus.
5. The pectoralis major makes up the vast majority of the *anterior axillary fold* of tissue, which borders the axilla (the armpit) anteriorly.

Latissimus Dorsi ("Lat")

The name, latissimus dorsi, *tells us that this muscle is a wide muscle of the back.*

Derivation	□ latissimus: L. *wide.*
	dorsi: L. *of the back.*
Pronunciation	□ la-TIS-i-mus, DOOR-si

■ ATTACHMENTS

□ **Spinous processes of T7-L5, Posterior Sacrum, and the Posterior Iliac Crest**
  □ all via the thoracolumbar fascia
  □ and the lowest three to four ribs and the inferior angle of the scapula

to the

□ **Medial Lip of the Bicipital Groove of the Humerus**

■ FUNCTIONS

CONCENTRIC (SHORTENING) MOVER ACTIONS	
Standard Mover Actions	**Reverse Mover Actions**
□ **1. Medially rotates the arm at the GH joint**	□ 1. Contralaterally rotates the pelvis and trunk at the spinal joints
□ **2. Adducts the arm at the GH joint**	□ 2. Elevates the same-side pelvis at the LS joint
□ **3. Extends the arm at the GH joint**	□ 3. Anteriorly tilts the pelvis at the LS joint and extends the trunk at the spinal joints
□ **4. Depresses the scapula at the scapulocostal joint**	□ 4. Elevates the trunk

GH joint = glenohumeral joint; LS joint = lumbosacral joint

Standard Mover Actions Notes

- The latissimus dorsi crosses the GH joint from medial on the pelvis and trunk to lateral on the humerus (with its fibers oriented somewhat horizontally in the transverse plane). However, it does not attach onto the first aspect on the humerus that it reaches but rather wraps around to the anterior side of the humerus to attach onto the medial lip of the bicipital groove of the humerus. When the latissimus dorsi contracts, it pulls the medial lip of the bicipital groove posteromedially, causing the anterior surface of the humerus to face medially. Therefore the latissimus dorsi medially rotates the arm at the GH joint. (action 1)
- The latissimus dorsi crosses the GH joint posteriorly from medial on the trunk to lateral on the humerus (with fibers running horizontally in the frontal plane). Therefore when the lateral attachment, the humerus, is pulled toward the medial attachment, the scapula, the humerus is pulled

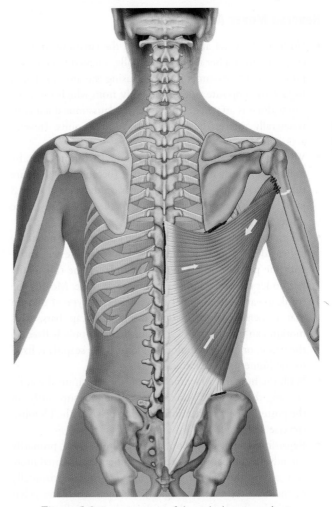

Figure 5-9 Posterior view of the right latissimus dorsi.

toward the midline. Therefore the latissimus dorsi adducts the arm at the GH joint. (action 2)
- The latissimus dorsi crosses the GH joint posteriorly (with the fibers running vertically in the sagittal plane); therefore it extends the arm at the GH joint. (action 3)
- The latissimus dorsi attaches from inferiorly on the trunk to superiorly on the humerus (with its fibers running vertically). When the humerus is fixed to the scapula and the latissimus dorsi contracts, it pulls the humerus and the scapula inferiorly. Therefore when the humerus is fixed to the scapula, the latissimus dorsi depresses the scapula at the scapulocostal joint. (action 4)
- Because the latissimus dorsi often has an attachment onto the inferior angle of the scapula, it can have the ability to act directly on the scapula. When the trunk is fixed, the fibers between the spine and scapula may depress, retract (i.e., adduct), and/or downwardly rotate the scapula at the scapulocostal joint. When the arm is fixed, the fibers between the arm and scapula may elevate, protract (i.e., abduct), and/or upwardly rotate the scapula at the scapulocostal joint. (action 4)

5

Reverse Mover Action Notes

- With the humeral attachment fixed, the latissimus dorsi—especially the higher more horizontally oriented fibers—will pull the trunk toward the arm, causing the anterior trunk to face the opposite side of the body from which the latissimus dorsi is attached. Therefore, the latissimus dorsi contralaterally rotates the trunk at the spinal joints. (reverse action 1)
- With the humeral attachment fixed, the latissimus dorsi, by pulling superiorly on the lateral pelvis (because the fibers are running vertically), elevates the pelvis on that side at the LS joint. Note: Elevation of one side of the pelvis causes the other side to depress. (reverse action 2)
- When the pelvis elevates, because the LS joint does not allow a great deal of motion, the lower lumbar spine will move with the pelvis, causing the lower lumbar spine to laterally flex under the upper lumbar and thoracic spine. Moving the trunk toward a fixed upper extremity is the type of motion that is performed by people using handicap bars. This motion can occur at the GH joint if the scapula is fixed to the trunk, or at the scapulocostal joint if the scapula is fixed to the humerus. (reverse action 2)
- With the humeral attachment fixed, the latissimus dorsi, by crossing the LS joint posteriorly and pulling superiorly on the posterior pelvis, anteriorly tilts the pelvis at the LS joint. (reverse action 3)
- Regarding spinal extension, the latissimus dorsi primarily extends the lumbar spine because its fibers are oriented more vertically in the lumbar region (they are more horizontally oriented in the thoracic region). Further, when the pelvis anteriorly tilts, because the LS joint does not allow a great deal of motion, the lower lumbar spine will move with the pelvis, causing the lower lumbar spine to extend under the upper lumbar and thoracic spine. (reverse action 3)
- If the arm is first in an elevated position (whether it is flexed, extended, abducted, or adducted) above the trunk and the humeral attachment of the latissimus dorsi is fixed, then, when the latissimus dorsi contracts, it pulls the trunk superiorly toward the humerus (because the fibers are running vertically). Therefore the latissimus dorsi elevates the trunk at the scapulocostal joint. This movement of the trunk relative to the scapula at the scapulocostal joint requires the scapula to be fixed to the arm. This type of motion is performed by people using handicap bars, doing a pull-up, or mountain climbing. This motion can occur at the GH joint if the scapula is fixed to the trunk. (reverse action 4)

Eccentric Antagonist Functions

1. Restrains/slows arm lateral rotation, abduction, and flexion
2. Restrains/slows ipsilateral rotation, same-side depression, and posterior tilt of the pelvis
3. Restrains/slows ipsilateral rotation, flexion, and depression of the trunk
4. Restrains/slows elevation of the scapula

Isometric Stabilization Functions

1. Stabilizes the GH joint
2. Stabilizes the spinal joints
3. Stabilizes the scapula

Additional Notes on Actions

1. The latissimus dorsi does all three GH joint actions necessary to swim the crawl (i.e., freestyle stroke), namely, extension, adduction, and medial rotation of the arm at the GH joint. For this reason, it is sometimes called the *swimmer's muscle*.
2. Note the similarity of the direction of fibers of the latissimus dorsi to the direction of fibers of the teres major. They have the same actions of the arm at the GH joint.
3. The latissimus dorsi and the pectoralis major are both large, powerful muscles that attach from the trunk to the arm. These two muscles are synergistic to each other with respect to their arm actions in that they both adduct and medially rotate the arm at the GH joint. They are both synergistic and antagonistic to each other with respect to their sagittal plane arm actions; the latissimus dorsi extends the arm at the GH joint; the sternocostal head of the pectoralis major also extends the arm, but the clavicular head flexes the arm at the GH joint.

INNERVATION
☐ The Thoracodorsal Nerve
  ☐ C6, **C7**, C8

ARTERIAL SUPPLY
☐ The Thoracodorsal Artery (a branch of the Subscapular Artery) and the dorsal branches of the Posterior Intercostal Arteries (branches of the Aorta)

✋ PALPATION

1. Both the client and therapist are standing; the therapist is standing to the front and side of the client.
2. Have the client place his or her arm on your shoulder and place your palpating hand on the client's posterior axillary fold.
3. Have the client attempt to adduct and extend the arm at the glenohumeral joint with your shoulder providing resistance, and feel for the contraction of the latissimus dorsi.
4. Continue palpating the latissimus dorsi distally into the axilla toward the humeral attachment and inferiorly toward the lumbar/pelvic attachment.

Latissimus Dorsi ("Lat")—*cont'd*

■ RELATIONSHIP TO OTHER STRUCTURES

☐ The latissimus dorsi is superficial except for a small portion that is deep to the lower trapezius.

☐ The distal tendon of the latissimus dorsi runs parallel to the distal tendon of the teres major.

☐ The teres major and the latissimus dorsi both attach onto the medial lip of the bicipital groove of the humerus. On the medial lip, the latissimus dorsi attaches more anteriorly, with the teres major attaching directly posterior to it.

☐ The latissimus dorsi's attachments onto the ribs meet with and are approximately perpendicular to the external abdominal oblique's attachments onto the ribs (inferior to the interdigitation of the serratus anterior with the external abdominal oblique).

☐ Deep to the latissimus dorsi in the lumbar region are the serratus posterior inferior, the most posterior attachments of the external and internal abdominal obliques, the erector spinae, and the quadratus lumborum.

☐ From the posterior perspective, the serratus anterior is deep to the latissimus dorsi in the axillary region.

☐ From the anterior perspective, the humeral attachment of the latissimus dorsi is deep to the pectoralis major, the short head of the biceps brachii, and the coracobrachialis.

☐ The attachment of the distal tendon of the latissimus dorsi onto the humerus is between the teres major's humeral attachment (which is posterior to it) and the pectoralis major's humeral attachment (which is anterior to it). A saying to help one remember this is "the lady between two majors." The *lady* (pronounce it *laty*) refers to the *lat*issimus dorsi; the *two majors* refer to the teres *major* and the pectoralis *major*.

☐ The latissimus dorsi is located within the superficial front arm line and back functional line myofascial meridians.

■ MISCELLANEOUS

1. The fibers of the latissimus dorsi twist in such a way that the superior fibers attach distally on the humerus and the inferior fibers attach proximally on the humerus (the distal fibers of the sternocostal head of the pectoralis major also twist so that the superior fibers attach most distally at the humeral attachment and the inferior fibers attach most proximally at the humeral attachment).

2. The latissimus dorsi and the teres major make up vast the majority of the *posterior axillary fold* of tissue, which borders the axilla (armpit) posteriorly.

3. Sometimes the latissimus dorsi blends with the teres major.

4. The scapular attachment of the latissimus dorsi is often absent.

5. Because the humeral attachment of the latissimus dorsi is on the inside of the medial lip at the bicipital groove, it is often described as being in the bicipital groove of the humerus instead of being on the medial lip.

6. The spinal and pelvic attachments of the latissimus dorsi are all via the thoracolumbar fascia, a layer of fascia that covers the deeper muscles of the thoracic and lumbar regions. The thoracolumbar fascia is especially thick in the lumbar region, where it divides into three layers, investing and enveloping the deep muscles of the lumbar region and eventually attaching onto the posterior iliac crest and the spinous processes and transverse processes of the lumbar vertebrae.

5

5

Teres Major

The name, teres major, tells us that this muscle is round and large (larger than the teres minor).

Derivation	☐ teres: L. *round.*
	major: L. *larger.*
Pronunciation	☐ TE-reez, MAY-jor

■ ATTACHMENTS

☐ **Inferior Angle and Inferior Lateral Border of the Scapula**
  ☐ the inferior ⅓ on the dorsal surface

to the

☐ **Medial Lip of the Bicipital Groove of the Humerus**

■ FUNCTIONS

CONCENTRIC (SHORTENING) MOVER ACTIONS	
Standard Mover Actions	**Reverse Mover Actions**
☐ **1. Medially rotates the arm at the GH joint**	☐ 1. Upwardly rotates the scapula at the GH and ScC joints
☐ **2. Adducts the arm at the GH joint**	
☐ **3. Extends the arm at the GH joint**	☐ 2. Downwardly tilts the scapula at the GH and ScC joints

GH joint = glenohumeral joint; ScC joint = scapulocostal joint

Standard Mover Action Notes

- The teres major crosses the GH joint from medial on the scapula to lateral on the humerus (with its fibers oriented somewhat horizontally in the transverse plane). However, it does not attach onto the first aspect on the humerus that it reaches, but rather it wraps around to the anterior side of the humerus to attach onto the medial lip of the bicipital groove of the humerus. Therefore when the teres major contracts and the humeral attachment is pulled toward the scapular attachment, the anterior side of the humerus moves medially. This movement is called medial rotation of the arm at the GH joint, because the anterior side of the humerus rotates medially. (action 1)

- The teres major crosses the GH joint posteriorly, from medial on the scapula to lateral on the humerus (with fibers running horizontally in the frontal plane). Therefore when the lateral humeral attachment is pulled toward the medial scapular attachment, the humerus is pulled toward the midline. Therefore the teres major adducts the arm at the GH joint. (action 2)

- The teres major crosses the GH joint posteriorly (with the fibers running somewhat vertically in the sagittal plane); therefore it extends the arm at the GH joint. (action 3)

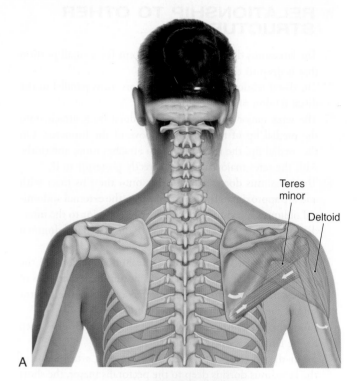

A

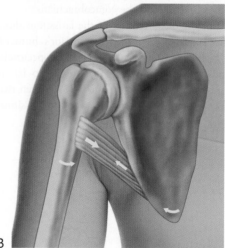

B

Figure 5-10 Views of the right teres major. **A,** Posterior view. The deltoid has been ghosted in. **B,** Anterior view.

Reverse Mover Actions Notes

- If the arm is fixed and the teres major contracts, the inferior angle of the scapula is pulled up toward the humerus, resulting in upward rotation of the scapula at the GH joint. When the scapula moves relative to the arm at the GH joint, it also moves relative to the rib cage at the scapulocostal joint. (reverse action 1)

- Because the humeral attachment is anterior to the scapular attachment, when the humeral attachment is fixed, the teres

Teres Major—cont'd

major can pull the inferior angle of the scapula anteriorly against the rib cage wall. This motion is called downward tilt of the scapula. (reverse action 2)

Eccentric Antagonist Functions

1. Restrains/slows arm lateral rotation, abduction, and flexion
2. Restrains/slows scapular downward rotation and upward tilt

Eccentric Antagonist Function Note

- Upward tilt of the scapula is a motion in which the inferior angle of the scapula lifts posteriorly away from the rib cage wall.

Isometric Stabilization Functions

1. Stabilizes the GH joint
2. Stabilizes the scapula

Additional Note on Actions

1. The teres major is sometimes called the *little brother* or the *little helper* of the latissimus dorsi, because they run together between the scapula and the humerus, they attach together onto the medial lip of the bicipital groove of the humerus, and they have the same direction of muscle fibers and therefore the same actions of the arm at the GH joint (medial rotation, adduction, and extension). Perhaps a better name for the teres major would be the *fat little brother* or *fat little helper*, because this muscle is extremely thick (hence the name teres *major*).

INNERVATION
- The Lower Subscapular Nerve
  - C5, **C6**, C7

ARTERIAL SUPPLY
- The Circumflex Scapular Artery (a branch of the Subscapular Artery)
  - and the Thoracodorsal Artery (a continuation of the Subscapular Artery)

PALPATION

1. With the client prone with the arm on the table and the forearm hanging off the table, place palpating hand just lateral to the inferior lateral border of the scapula.
2. Have the client medially rotate the arm at the glenohumeral joint (this requires the client's hand to swing posteriorly and up) and feel for the contraction of the teres major. Resistance can be added.
3. Continue palpating the teres major distally into the axilla toward the medial lip of the bicipital groove on the anterior surface of the humerus.

■ RELATIONSHIP TO OTHER STRUCTURES

- The teres major lies inferior to the infraspinatus and the teres minor.
- The long head of the triceps brachii runs between the teres minor and the teres major.
- The distal tendon of the teres major runs parallel to the distal tendon of the latissimus dorsi.
- The teres major and the latissimus dorsi both attach onto the medial lip of the bicipital groove of the humerus. On the medial lip, the teres major attaches posterior to the latissimus dorsi.
- Deep to the teres major is the scapula.
- The teres major is located within the superficial front arm line and involved with the deep back arm line myofascial meridians.

■ MISCELLANEOUS

1. Although the teres major and the teres minor share the word *teres* in their name (because they are both round in shape) and sit next to each other, they wrap around the humerus in opposite directions and therefore have opposite rotary actions. The teres major wraps around to the anterior side of the glenohumeral (GH) joint to attach onto the humerus and therefore medially rotates the arm at the GH joint; the teres minor wraps around to the posterior side of the GH joint to attach onto the humerus and therefore laterally rotates the arm at the GH joint.
2. The teres major and the teres minor, because of their different rotary actions of the arm, are in different functional groups. These two muscles are also innervated by different nerves.
3. The latissimus dorsi and the teres major make up the vast majority of the *posterior axillary fold* of tissue that borders the axilla (armpit) posteriorly.
4. The belly and/or distal tendon of the teres major sometimes blend with the latissimus dorsi.

Rotator Cuff Group

The rotator cuff is a group of four muscles that attach from the scapula to the humerus. The four rotator cuff muscles are the supraspinatus, infraspinatus, teres minor, and subscapularis.

■ ATTACHMENTS

☐ These four muscles are grouped together as the rotator *cuff* group, because their distal tendons all conjoin to form a cuff across the greater and lesser tubercles of the humerus.

☐ The supraspinatus, infraspinatus, and teres minor all attach to the greater tubercle of the humerus.

☐ The subscapularis attaches to the lesser tubercle of the humerus.

■ FUNCTIONS

☐ These four muscles are designated as the *rotator* cuff group, because when they act as movers of the humerus, three of the four muscles rotate the humerus.

☐ Functionally, as a group, the rotator cuff muscles are extremely important, because they act to fix (stabilize) the head of the humerus into the glenoid fossa of the scapula whenever the distal end of the humerus is elevated from anatomic position (which can occur with flexion, extension, abduction, and adduction of the arm). When elevating the humerus, it is desirable to elevate only the distal end, so that the hand can be brought to a higher position. When this occurs, the proximal end of the humerus, the head of the humerus, must be stabilized down into the glenoid fossa of the scapula. This is accomplished principally by the rotator cuff group. Given that flexion, extension, abduction, and adduction of the humerus may all involve elevation of the distal humerus, the rotator cuff muscles are more active as stabilizers of the humerus than as movers. Of the four rotator cuff muscles, the two most active in this regard are the infraspinatus and the subscapularis.

☐ Their role as fixators (stabilizers) is especially important and necessary, because the ligamentous structure of the shoulder joint is very lax, so stability must be principally provided by the muscles.

■ MISCELLANEOUS

• There is a bursa located between the supraspinatus portion of the rotator cuff tendon and the acromion process of the scapula and deltoid muscle superior to it. This bursa is known as the *subacromial bursa* and/or the *subdeltoid bursa*.

INNERVATION

☐ The rotator cuff muscles are innervated by the suprascapular, axillary, and upper and lower subscapular nerves.

ARTERIAL SUPPLY

☐ The rotator cuff muscles receive their arterial supply almost entirely from the suprascapular and circumflex scapular arteries.

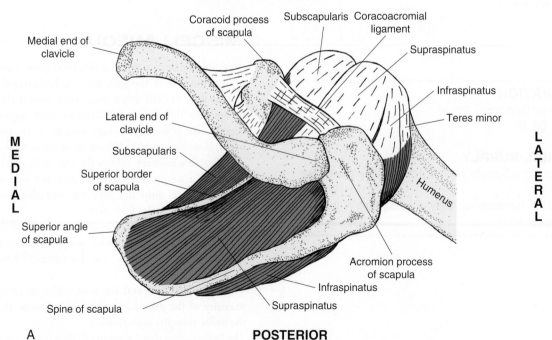

ANTERIOR

Coracoid process of scapula
Subscapularis
Coracoacromial ligament
Medial end of clavicle
Suprascapularis
Infraspinatus
Teres minor
Lateral end of clavicle
Subscapularis
Superior border of scapula
M E D I A L
Humerus
L A T E R A L
Superior angle of scapula
Acromion process of scapula
Infraspinatus
Spine of scapula
Supraspinatus

A
POSTERIOR

Figure 5-11 Views of the right rotator cuff group of muscles. **A,** Superior view of the right scapula.

Rotator Cuff Group—*cont'd*

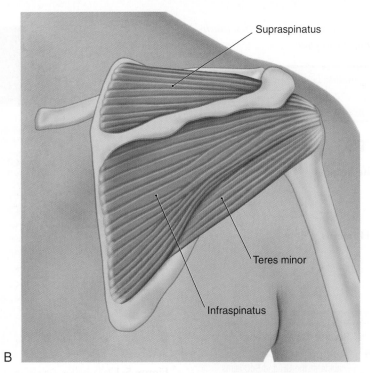

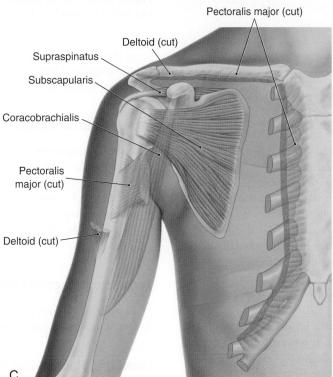

Figure 5-11, cont'd B, Posterior view showing the supraspinatus, infraspinatus, and teres minor. **C,** Anterior view showing the subscapularis. The coracobrachialis and cut deltoid and pectoralis major have been ghosted in.

Supraspinatus (of Rotator Cuff Group)

The name, supraspinatus, *tells us that one of this muscle's attachments is the supraspinous fossa of the scapula.*

Derivation	☐ supraspinatus: L. *above the spine* (of the scapula).
Pronunciation	☐ SOO-pra-spy-NAY-tus

■ ATTACHMENTS

☐ **Supraspinous Fossa of the Scapula**
   ☐ the medial ⅔

to the

☐ **Greater Tubercle of the Humerus**
   ☐ the superior facet

■ FUNCTIONS

CONCENTRIC (SHORTENING) MOVER ACTIONS	
Standard Mover Actions	**Reverse Mover Actions**
☐ **1. Abducts the arm at the GH joint**	☐ 1. Downwardly rotates the scapula at the GH and ScC joints
☐ **2. Flexes the arm at the GH joint**	

GH joint = glenohumeral joint; ScC joint = scapulocostal joint

Standard Mover Action Notes

• The supraspinatus crosses the GH joint over the top of the joint (with its fibers running first horizontally and then vertically in the frontal plane); therefore it abducts the arm at the GH joint. Note the similarity of the direction of fibers of the supraspinatus to the direction of fibers of the middle deltoid. For quite some time it was believed that the supraspinatus could only initiate abduction of the arm at the GH joint and that the deltoid would have to complete this motion. However, recent research has shown that the supraspinatus is capable of moving the arm through the entire range of motion of abduction at the GH joint. Of course, the supraspinatus does not have the strength of the deltoid. (action 1)

• The supraspinatus pulls the arm up into the plane of the scapula. Given that the scapula is approximately 35 degrees off the frontal plane toward the sagittal plane, the arm is not pulled purely into abduction in the frontal plane, but somewhat into flexion in the sagittal plane. It is worth noting that if a person has rounded shoulders, the scapulae lie even farther from the frontal plane and closer to the sagittal plane, increasing the component of flexion action by the supraspinatus (and commensurately decreasing the amount of pure abduction in the frontal plane). Some texts refer to the action of the supraspinatus not as abduction, but as *scaption*

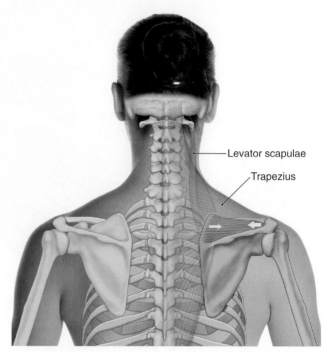

Figure 5-12 Posterior view of the right supraspinatus. The trapezius and levator scapulae have been ghosted in.

to describe the fact that the arm is moved in the plane of the scapula, which is a combination of abduction and flexion. (action 2)

Reverse Mover Action Notes

• If the supraspinatus contracts and the humerus is fixed, it pulls on the scapula, causing the glenoid fossa to orient downward. Therefore it downwardly rotates the scapula relative to the humerus at the GH joint. When the scapula moves relative to the arm at the GH joint, it also moves relative to the rib cage at the scapulocostal joint. (reverse action 1)

Eccentric Antagonist Functions

1. Restrains/slows arm adduction and extension
2. Restrains/slows scapular upward rotation

Isometric Stabilization Function

1. Stabilizes the GH joint
2. Stabilizes the scapula

Isometric Stabilization Function Note

• The rotator cuff muscles (supraspinatus, infraspinatus, teres minor, and subscapularis) are extremely important as stabilizers of the humeral head at the GH joint.

Supraspinatus (of Rotator Cuff Group)—*cont'd*

Additional Notes on Actions

1. Some sources state that the supraspinatus can also contribute to horizontal extension (horizontal abduction) of the arm at the GH joint.
2. The supraspinatus is the only one of the four rotator cuff muscles that does not contribute to a transverse plane rotation action of the arm at the GH joint.

INNERVATION
- The Suprascapular Nerve
  - **C5**, C6

ARTERIAL SUPPLY
- The Suprascapular Artery (a branch of the Thyrocervical Artery)

PALPATION

1. With the client seated and the arm hanging at the side, place palpating hand just superior to the spine of the scapula.
2. Have the client perform a short, gentle range of motion of the arm at the glenohumeral joint that is approximately 30 degrees anterior to pure abduction (i.e., an oblique motion that is a combination of abduction and flexion) and feel for the contraction of the supraspinatus. (Note: If the client is prone, a short, gentle range of pure abduction of the arm can be done.)
3. Palpate the entirety of the belly in the supraspinous fossa and then palpate the distal tendon on the greater tubercle of the humerus (note: the portion deep to the acromion process cannot be palpated).

■ RELATIONSHIP TO OTHER STRUCTURES

- The supraspinatus is superior to the spine of the scapula.
- The proximal attachment of the supraspinatus is deep to the trapezius.
- The distal tendon of the supraspinatus courses deep to the acromion process of the scapula to then attach distally onto the greater tubercle of the humerus, deep to the deltoid.
- The supraspinatus is located within the deep back arm line and may be involved with the deep front arm line myofascial meridians.

■ MISCELLANEOUS

1. The supraspinatus is one of the four rotator cuff muscles. The rotator cuff muscles are the supraspinatus, infraspinatus, teres minor, and subscapularis. Sometimes the rotator cuff muscles are called the *SITS* muscles; each of the four letters stands for the first letter of the four rotator cuff muscles. *S*upraspinatus is the first *S* of *SITS*.
2. The supraspinatus is one of three muscles that attach onto the greater tubercle of the humerus. The two other muscles that attach here are the infraspinatus and the teres minor.
3. The distal tendon of the supraspinatus adheres to the capsule of the glenohumeral joint, which is deep to the supraspinatus.
4. The acromion process and the deltoid are superior to the supraspinatus. There is a bursa called the *subacromial* and/or *subdeltoid bursa* that is located between the supraspinatus and these two other structures.
5. Because of its location between the acromion process of the scapula and the greater tubercle of the humerus, the supraspinatus' distal tendon is the most commonly injured tendon of the rotator cuff musculature. In fact, the distal tendon of the supraspinatus is sometimes referred to as the *critical zone* of the rotator cuff tendon.
6. The supraspinatus is pennate.

Infraspinatus (of Rotator Cuff Group)

The name, infraspinatus, *tells us that one of this muscle's attachments is the infraspinous fossa of the scapula.*

Derivation	☐ infraspinatus: L. *below the spine* (of the scapula).
Pronunciation	☐ IN-fra-spy-NAY-tus

■ ATTACHMENTS

☐ **Infraspinous Fossa of the Scapula**
   ☐ the medial ⅔

to the

☐ **Greater Tubercle of the Humerus**
   ☐ the middle facet

■ FUNCTIONS

CONCENTRIC (SHORTENING) MOVER ACTIONS	
Standard Mover Actions	**Reverse Mover Actions**
☐ **1. Laterally rotates the arm at the GH joint**	☐ 1. Laterally tilts the scapula at the GH and ScC joints
☐ 2. Horizontally extends the arm at the GH joint	

GH joint = glenohumeral joint; ScC joint = scapulocostal joint

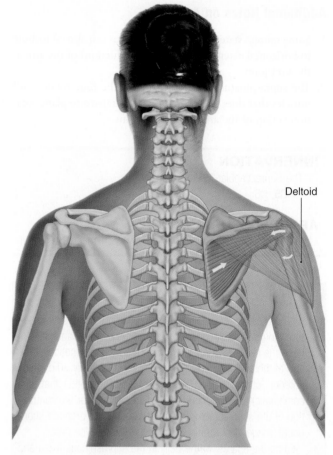

Figure 5-13 Posterior view of the right infraspinatus. The deltoid has been ghosted in.

Standard Mover Action Notes

• The infraspinatus crosses the GH joint posteriorly from medial to lateral (with its fibers running horizontally in the transverse plane). However, it does not attach onto the first aspect of the humerus that it reaches, but rather it wraps around the humerus to attach onto the greater tubercle. Therefore when the infraspinatus contracts and the humeral attachment is pulled toward the scapular attachment, the posterior side of the humerus moves medially. This movement is called lateral rotation of the arm at the GH joint, because the anterior side of the humerus rotates laterally. Note the similarity of the direction of fibers of the infraspinatus to the direction of fibers of the teres minor. (action 1)
• The infraspinatus is a very active muscle because so many arm movements also involve lateral rotation of the arm at the GH joint. (action 1)
• When the arm is in a position of 90 degrees of abduction, the infraspinatus' line of pull is horizontal and can pull the arm directly posteriorly. This motion is called horizontal extension (or horizontal abduction) of the arm at the GH joint. (action 2)

Reverse Mover Action Notes

• When the infraspinatus contracts and the humerus is fixed, the scapula is pulled toward the humerus. This causes the medial border of the scapula to lift away from the rib cage wall. This motion is called lateral tilt of the scapula. (reverse action 1)
• When the scapula moves relative to the arm at the GH joint, it also moves relative to the rib cage at the scapulocostal joint. (reverse action 1)

Eccentric Antagonist Functions

1. Restrains/slows arm medial rotation and horizontal flexion
2. Restrains/slows scapular medial tilt

Eccentric Antagonist Action Note

• Medial tilt of the scapula is a motion in which the medial border of the scapula moves toward the rib cage wall.

Isometric Stabilization Functions

1. Stabilizes the GH joint
2. Stabilizes the scapula

Isometric Stabilization Function Note

- The rotator cuff muscles (supraspinatus, infraspinatus, teres minor, and subscapularis) are extremely important as stabilizers of the head of the humerus at the GH joint.

Additional Note on Actions

1. There is controversy regarding whether the infraspinatus can abduct or adduct the arm at the GH joint. Some sources state that the upper fibers can abduct the arm and the lower fibers can adduct the arm. Other sources state that whether one or the other occurs is due to the position of the GH joint at the time. In either case, because of the poor lever arm, the infraspinatus has little strength as an abductor or adductor of the arm at the GH joint.

INNERVATION
- ☐ The Suprascapular Nerve
  - ☐ **C5**, C6

ARTERIAL SUPPLY
- ☐ The Suprascapular Artery (a branch of the Thyrocervical Artery)
- ☐ and the Circumflex Scapular Artery (a branch of the Subscapular Artery)

PALPATION

1. With the client prone with the arm on the table and the forearm hanging off the table, place palpating hand on the infraspinous fossa. (Make sure you are inferior to the deltoid.)
2. Have the client laterally rotate the arm at the glenohumeral joint (this requires the client's hand to swing anteriorly and up) through a small range of motion and feel for the contraction of the infraspinatus. Resistance can be given. (Note: It can be challenging to discern the infraspinatus from the teres minor.)
3. Palpate the infraspinatus in the infraspinous fossa and then follow it distally to the greater tubercle of the humerus.

■ RELATIONSHIP TO OTHER STRUCTURES

- ☐ The infraspinatus is inferior to the spine of the scapula.
- ☐ Inferior to the infraspinatus are the teres minor and teres major.
- ☐ Most of the infraspinatus is superficial in the infraspinous fossa.
- ☐ Medially, a small portion of the infraspinatus lies deep to the trapezius. Distally, the infraspinatus is deep to the deltoid.
- ☐ The infraspinatus is located within the deep back arm line myofascial meridian.

■ MISCELLANEOUS

1. The infraspinatus is one of the four rotator cuff muscles. The rotator cuff muscles are the supraspinatus, infraspinatus, teres minor, and subscapularis. Sometimes the rotator cuff muscles are called the *SITS* muscles; each of the four letters stands for the first letter of the four rotator cuff muscles. *I*nfraspinatus is the *I* of *SITS*.
2. The infraspinatus is one of three muscles that attach onto the greater tubercle of the humerus. The two other muscles that attach here are the supraspinatus and the teres minor.
3. The distal tendon of the infraspinatus adheres to the capsule of the glenohumeral joint, which is deep to the infraspinatus.
4. Sometimes there is a bursa located between the infraspinatus and the glenohumeral joint capsule.
5. There is usually a thick layer of fascia overlying the infraspinatus muscle.
6. Sometimes the infraspinatus blends with the teres minor.
7. The infraspinatus is pennate.

5

Teres Minor (of Rotator Cuff Group)

The name, teres minor, *tells us that this muscle is round and small (smaller than the teres major).*

Derivation	☐ teres: L. *round.* minor: L. *smaller.*
Pronunciation	☐ TE-reez, MY-nor

■ ATTACHMENTS

☐ **Superior Lateral Border of the Scapula**
  ☐ the superior ⅔ of the dorsal surface

to the

☐ **Greater Tubercle of the Humerus**
  ☐ the inferior facet

■ FUNCTIONS

CONCENTRIC (SHORTENING) MOVER ACTIONS	
Standard Mover Actions	**Reverse Mover Actions**
☐ **1. Laterally rotates the arm at the GH joint**	☐ 1. Laterally tilts the scapula at the GH and ScC joints
☐ 2. Adducts the arm at the GH joint	☐ 2. Upwardly rotates the scapula at the GH and ScC joints
☐ 3. Horizontally extends the arm at the GH joint	☐ 3. Laterally tilts the scapula at the GH and ScC joints

GH joint = glenohumeral joint; ScC joint = scapulocostal joint

Standard Mover Action Notes

- The teres minor crosses the GH joint posteriorly from medial to lateral (with its fibers running horizontally in the transverse plane). However, it does not attach onto the first aspect of the humerus that it reaches; rather it wraps around the humerus to attach onto the greater tubercle. Therefore when the teres minor contracts and the humeral attachment is pulled toward the scapular attachment, the posterior side of the humerus moves medially. This movement is called lateral rotation of the arm at the GH joint, because the anterior side of the humerus rotates laterally. Note the similarity of the direction of fibers of the teres minor to the direction of fibers of the infraspinatus. (action 1)
- The teres minor is a very active muscle because so many arm movements also involve lateral rotation of the arm at the GH joint. (action 1)
- There is some controversy regarding whether or not the teres minor can adduct the arm at the GH joint. However, the humeral attachment seems clearly distal enough for it to be below the center of the joint and therefore perform adduction. (action 2)

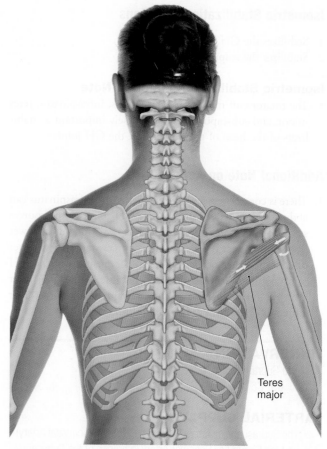

Figure 5-14 Posterior view of the right teres minor. The teres major has been ghosted in.

- When the arm is in a position of 90 degrees of abduction, the teres minor's line of pull is horizontal and can pull the arm directly posteriorly. This motion is called horizontal extension (or horizontal abduction) of the arm at the GH joint. (action 3)

Reverse Mover Action Notes

- If the arm is fixed and the teres minor contracts, the scapula is pulled toward the humerus, causing the medial border to lift away from the rib cage wall. This motion is called lateral tilt of the scapula and occurs at the GH joint. (reverse actions 1, 3)
- If the arm is fixed and the teres minor contracts, the inferior angle of the scapula is pulled up toward the humerus, resulting in upward rotation of the scapula at the GH joint. (reverse action 2)
- When the scapula moves relative to the arm at the GH joint, it also moves relative to the rib cage at the scapulocostal joint. (reverse actions 1, 2, 3)

Teres Minor (of Rotator Cuff Group)—*cont'd*

Eccentric Antagonist Functions

1. Restrains/slows arm medial rotation, abduction, and horizontal flexion
2. Restrains/slows scapular medial tilt and downward rotation

Eccentric Antagonist Function Note

- Medial tilt of the scapula is a motion in which the medial border of the scapula moves toward the rib cage wall.

Isometric Stabilization Functions

1. Stabilizes the GH joint
2. Stabilizes the scapula

Isometric Stabilization Function Note

- The rotator cuff muscles (supraspinatus, infraspinatus, teres minor, and subscapularis) are extremely important as stabilizers of the head of the humerus at the GH joint. However, some sources claim that the stabilization function of the teres minor is not as important as that of the other rotator cuff muscles. Perhaps this is because the teres minor has an adduction action that would oppose any abduction movement, and its posterior location would oppose flexion movements as well. However, its vertical direction of fibers makes it ideal to hold the head of the humerus down into the glenoid fossa as the distal end elevates.

INNERVATION
- The Axillary Nerve
  - **C5**, C6

ARTERIAL SUPPLY
- The Circumflex Scapular Artery (a branch of the Subscapular Artery)
  - and the Posterior Circumflex Humeral Artery (a branch of the Axillary Artery)

✋ PALPATION

1. With the client prone with the arm on the table and the forearm hanging off the table, place palpating hand just lateral to the superior lateral border of the scapula and feel for the round belly of the teres minor.
2. Have the client laterally rotate the arm at the glenohumeral joint (this requires the client's hand to swing anteriorly and up) and feel for its contraction. Resistance can be given. (Note: It can be challenging to discern the teres minor from the infraspinatus.)
3. Palpate the teres minor distally to the greater tubercle of the humerus.

■ RELATIONSHIP TO OTHER STRUCTURES

- The medial portion of the teres minor is superficial and is located at the lateral border of the scapula. The lateral portion of the teres minor is deep to the deltoid.
- On the scapula the teres minor attaches just superior to the attachment of the teres major.
- The teres minor lies between the infraspinatus (which is superior to it) and the teres major (which is inferior to it).
- The teres minor is located within the deep back arm line myofascial meridian.

■ MISCELLANEOUS

1. The teres minor is one of the four rotator cuff muscles. The rotator cuff muscles are the supraspinatus, infraspinatus, teres minor, and subscapularis. Sometimes the rotator cuff muscles are called the *SITS* muscles; each of the four letters stands for the first letter of the four rotator cuff muscles. *T*eres minor is the *T* of *SITS*.
2. The teres minor is one of three muscles that attach onto the greater tubercle of the humerus. The other two muscles that attach here are the supraspinatus and the infraspinatus.
3. Although the teres minor and the teres major share the word *teres* in their name (because they are both round in shape) and sit next to each other, they wrap around the humerus in opposite directions and therefore have opposite rotary actions. The teres minor wraps around to the posterior side of the glenohumeral (GH) joint to attach onto the humerus and therefore laterally rotates the arm at the GH joint; the teres major wraps around to the anterior side of the shoulder joint to attach onto the humerus and therefore medially rotates the arm at the GH joint.
4. The teres major and the teres minor, because of their different rotary actions of the arm, are in different functional groups. These two muscles are also innervated by different nerves.
5. The distal tendon of the teres minor adheres to the capsule of the glenohumeral joint, which is deep to the teres minor.
6. Sometimes the teres minor blends with the infraspinatus.
7. The teres minor is longitudinal (nonpennate).

5

Subscapularis (of Rotator Cuff Group)

The name, subscapularis, *tells us that one of this muscle's attachments is the subscapular fossa of the scapula.*

Derivation	☐ subscapularis: L. *refers to the subscapular fossa.*
Pronunciation	☐ sub-skap-u-LA-ris

■ ATTACHMENTS

☐ **Subscapular Fossa of the Scapula**

to the

☐ **Lesser Tubercle of the Humerus**

■ FUNCTIONS

CONCENTRIC (SHORTENING) MOVER ACTIONS	
Standard Mover Actions	**Reverse Mover Actions**
☐ **1. Medially rotates the arm at the GH joint**	☐ 1. Medially tilts the scapula at the GH and ScC joints

GH joint = glenohumeral joint; ScC joint = scapulocostal joint

Standard Mover Action Note

- The subscapularis crosses the GH joint anteriorly from medial to lateral (with its fibers running horizontally in the transverse plane). However, it does not attach onto the first aspect of the humerus that it reaches, but rather wraps around the humerus to attach onto the lesser tubercle. Therefore when the subscapularis contracts and the humeral attachment is pulled toward the scapular attachment, the anterior side of the humerus moves medially. This movement is called medial rotation of the arm at the GH joint, because the anterior side of the humerus rotates medially. Note the similarity of the direction of fibers of the subscapularis to the direction of fibers of the latissimus dorsi and teres major. (action 1)

Reverse Mover Action Note

- If the subscapularis contracts and the humerus is fixed, the subscapularis pulls the medial border of the scapula against the rib cage wall. This is called medial tilt of the scapula and occurs relative to the humerus at the GH joint. When the scapula moves relative to the arm at the GH joint, it also moves relative to the rib cage at the scapulocostal joint. (reverse action 1)

Eccentric Antagonist Functions

1. Restrains/slows arm lateral rotation and scapular lateral tilt

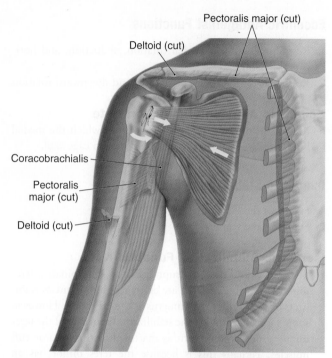

Figure 5-15 Anterior view of the right subscapularis. Most of the rib cage has been removed. The coracobrachialis has been ghosted in. The pectoralis major and deltoid have been cut and ghosted in.

Eccentric Antagonist Function Note

- Lateral tilt of the scapula is a motion in which the medial border of the scapula lifts away from the rib cage wall.

Isometric Stabilization Functions

1. Stabilizes the GH joint
2. Stabilizes the scapula

Isometric Stabilization Function Note

- The rotator cuff muscles (supraspinatus, infraspinatus, teres minor, and subscapularis) are extremely important as stabilizers of the head of the humerus at the GH joint.

Additional Notes on Actions

1. There is controversy regarding whether or not the subscapularis can perform other actions of the arm at the GH joint. Some sources state that depending on the position of the arm, the subscapularis adducts, abducts, flexes, or extends the arm. However, given that its attachment site is so far proximal on the humerus, its lever arm would be poor. If these actions did occur, they would be very weak.
2. Because the lower fibers of the subscapularis are below the axis of motion of the GH joint, they may contribute to the

Subscapularis (of Rotator Cuff Group)—*cont'd*

reverse action of upward rotation of the scapula at the GH and scapulocostal joints.

INNERVATION
☐ The Upper and Lower Subscapular Nerves
   ☐ C5, **C6**

ARTERIAL SUPPLY
☐ The Circumflex Scapular Artery (a branch of the Subscapular Artery) and the Dorsal Scapular and Suprascapular Arteries (both either direct or indirect branches of the Subclavian Artery)
   ☐ and the Lateral Thoracic Artery (a branch of the Axillary Artery)

✋ PALPATION

1. Have the client supine with the arm that is on the side of the target muscle being palpated crossed on the chest such that the elbow is lying on the abdomen and the hand is holding onto the opposite-side shoulder (the arm will be slightly flexed and adducted at the glenohumeral joint, and the forearm will be flexed at the elbow joint). Further, have the client place the opposite-side hand on top of the elbow of the arm that is crossed on the chest, gently holding the elbow down.
2. Place your superior (cephalad) hand under the scapula, grasping the medial border of the scapula and pulling the scapula laterally (protracting the scapula at the scapulocostal joint).
3. With your (inferior) palpating hand, press in between the scapula and the ribcage of the client and then press with your finger pads against the anterior surface of the scapula for the subscapularis.
4. To engage the subscapularis, have the client medially rotate the arm at the glenohumeral joint by simply pressing the forearm against the chest.
5. Palpate as much of the subscapularis as possible.

■ RELATIONSHIP TO OTHER STRUCTURES

☐ From the posterior perspective, the subscapularis is deep to the scapula and superficial to the rib cage. From the anterior perspective, the subscapularis is deep to the entire rib cage and superficial to the scapula.
☐ The anterior wall of the subscapularis faces the serratus anterior. Both the subscapularis and the serratus anterior are located between the scapula and the rib cage.
☐ The distal tendon of the subscapularis is deep to the proximal tendons of the short head of the biceps brachii and the coracobrachialis.
☐ The distal tendon of the subscapularis attaches onto the humerus directly proximal to the distal tendons of the latissimus dorsi and teres major.
☐ The subscapularis is involved with the deep back arm line myofascial meridian.

■ MISCELLANEOUS

1. The subscapularis is one of the four rotator cuff muscles. The rotator cuff muscles are the supraspinatus, infraspinatus, teres minor, and subscapularis. Sometimes the rotator cuff muscles are called the *SITS* muscles; each of the four letters stands for the first letter of the four rotator cuff muscles. *S*ubscapularis is the last *S* of *SITS.*
2. The subscapularis (along with the latissimus dorsi and teres major) is located in the *posterior axillary fold* of tissue, which borders the axilla (armpit) posteriorly.
3. The distal tendon of the subscapularis adheres to the capsule of the glenohumeral joint, which is deep to the subscapularis.
4. There is a bursa located between the subscapularis muscle and the scapula called the *subscapular bursa.*
5. The subscapularis is pennate.

5

CHAPTER

6

Muscles of the Elbow and Radioulnar Joints

CHAPTER **OVERVIEW**

The muscles addressed in this chapter are the muscles whose principal function is usually considered to be movement of the elbow and radioulnar joints. Other muscles in the body can also move the elbow and radioulnar joints, but they are placed in different chapters because their primary function is usually considered to be at another joint. These muscles cross the wrist joint and/or finger joints and are covered in Chapters 7 and 8.

Overview of Structure
Structurally, muscles that flex the elbow joint are located anteriorly. The biceps brachii and brachialis have their bellies in the arm; the brachioradialis has its belly in the forearm. In all cases, they cross the elbow joint anteriorly. The muscles that extend the elbow joint are located posteriorly. The triceps brachii has its belly in the arm and the anconeus has its belly in the forearm; they both cross the elbow joint posteriorly.

Structurally, the pronator teres and pronator quadratus are located anteriorly and the supinator is located posteriorly.

Note: Some muscles covered in this chapter cross and move both the elbow and radioulnar joints.

Overview of Function
The following general rules regarding actions can be stated for the functional groups of muscles of the elbow and radioulnar joints:

☐ If a muscle crosses the elbow joint anteriorly with a vertical direction to its fibers, it can flex the forearm at the elbow joint by moving the anterior surface of the forearm toward the anterior surface of the arm.
☐ If a muscle crosses the elbow joint posteriorly with a vertical direction to its fibers, it can extend the forearm at the elbow joint by moving the posterior surface of the forearm toward the posterior surface of the arm.
☐ Reverse actions at the elbow joint involve moving the arm toward the forearm at the elbow joint. This usually occurs when the hand (and therefore the forearm) is fixed by holding onto an immovable object.
☐ If a muscle crosses the radioulnar joints anteriorly with a horizontal orientation to its fibers, it will pronate the forearm at the radioulnar joints.
☐ If a muscle crosses the radioulnar joints posteriorly with a horizontal direction to its fibers, it will supinate the forearm at the radioulnar joints.
☐ Reverse actions of these standard mover actions at the radioulnar joints involve moving the ulna toward the radius at the radioulnar joints. This usually occurs when the hand (and therefore the radius) is fixed by holding onto an immovable object.

Review the muscles and bones from this chapter on the enclosed CD!

Anterior Views of the Muscles of the Right Elbow Joint

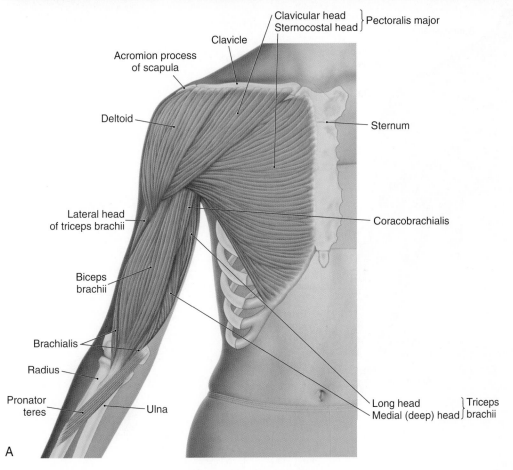

- Clavicular head
- Sternocostal head } Pectoralis major
- Clavicle
- Acromion process of scapula
- Deltoid
- Sternum
- Lateral head of triceps brachii
- Coracobrachialis
- Biceps brachii
- Brachialis
- Radius
- Pronator teres
- Ulna
- Long head
- Medial (deep) head } Triceps brachii

A

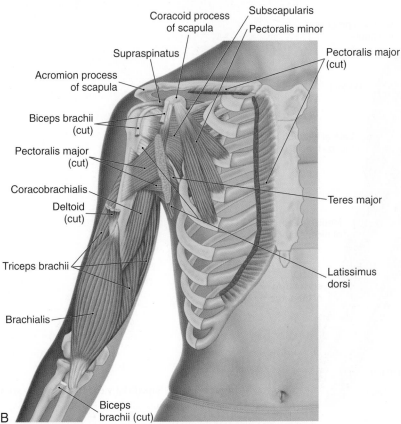

- Coracoid process of scapula
- Subscapularis
- Pectoralis minor
- Supraspinatus
- Pectoralis major (cut)
- Acromion process of scapula
- Biceps brachii (cut)
- Pectoralis major (cut)
- Coracobrachialis
- Deltoid (cut)
- Teres major
- Triceps brachii
- Latissimus dorsi
- Brachialis
- Biceps brachii (cut)

B

Figure 6-1 A, Superficial view. **B,** Deep view with the pectoralis major, deltoid, and biceps brachii cut and/or removed.

Posterior Views of the Muscles of the Right Elbow Joint

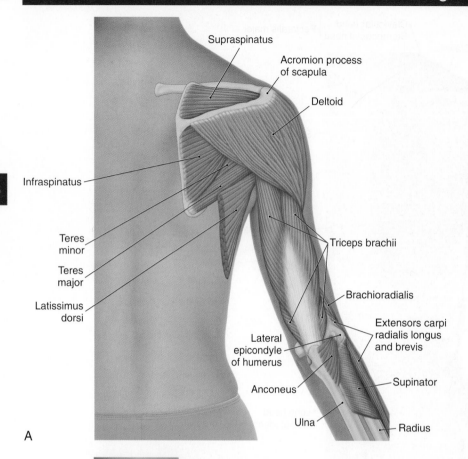

A

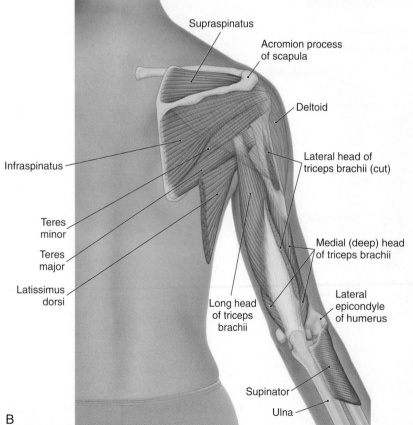

B

Figure 6-2 A, Superficial view. **B,** Deep view with deltoid ghosted in.

Lateral View of the Muscles of the Right Elbow Joint

6

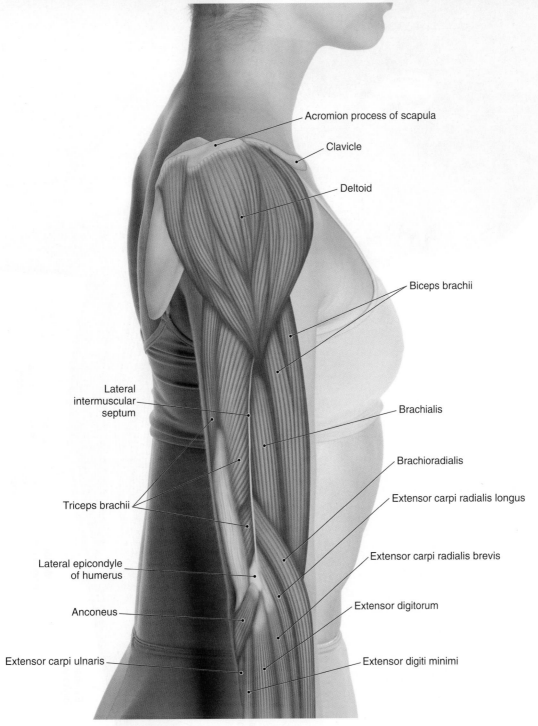

Acromion process of scapula

Clavicle

Deltoid

Biceps brachii

Lateral intermuscular septum

Brachialis

Brachioradialis

Triceps brachii

Extensor carpi radialis longus

Extensor carpi radialis brevis

Lateral epicondyle of humerus

Extensor digitorum

Anconeus

Extensor digiti minimi

Extensor carpi ulnaris

Figure 6-3

Medial View of the Muscles of the Right Elbow Joint

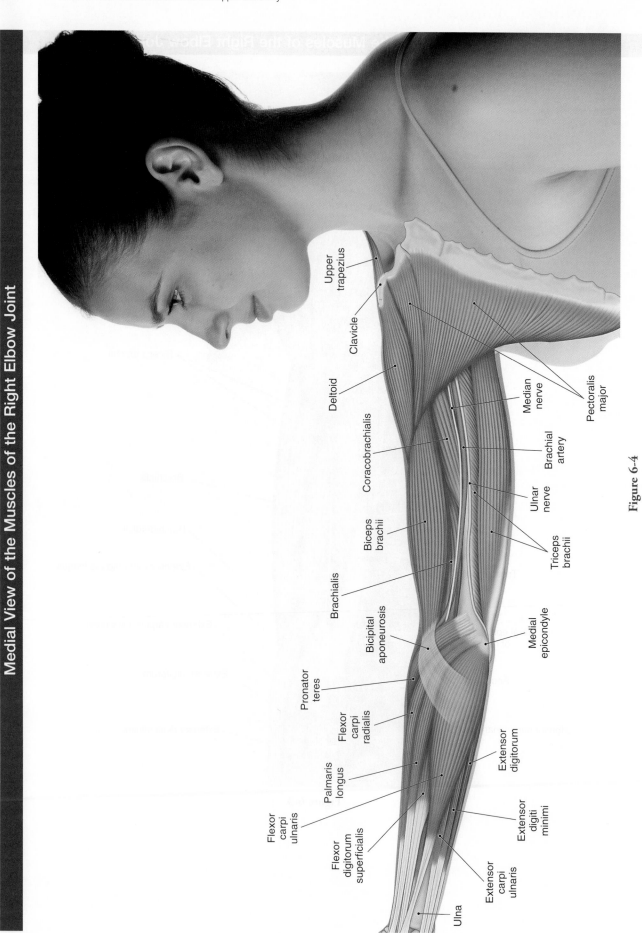

Upper trapezius

Clavicle

Deltoid

Coracobrachialis

Biceps brachii

Brachialis

Bicipital aponeurosis

Pronator teres

Flexor carpi radialis

Palmaris longus

Flexor carpi ulnaris

Flexor digitorum superficialis

Extensor carpi ulnaris

Extensor digiti minimi

Extensor digitorum

Medial epicondyle

Triceps brachii

Ulnar nerve

Brachial artery

Median nerve

Pectoralis major

Ulna

Figure 6-4

Views of the Muscles of the Right Radioulnar Joints

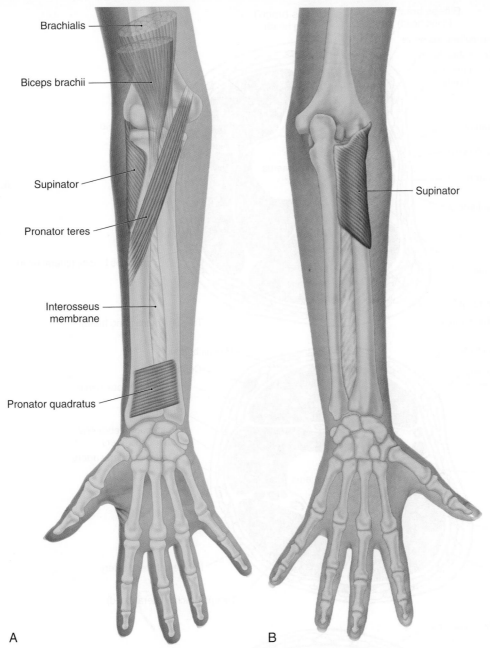

Brachialis

Biceps brachii

Supinator

Pronator teres

Interosseus membrane

Pronator quadratus

Supinator

A

B

Figure 6-5 A, Anterior view. The biceps brachii and brachialis have been cut and ghosted in. **B,** Posterior view.

6

Transverse Plane Cross Sections of the Right Arm

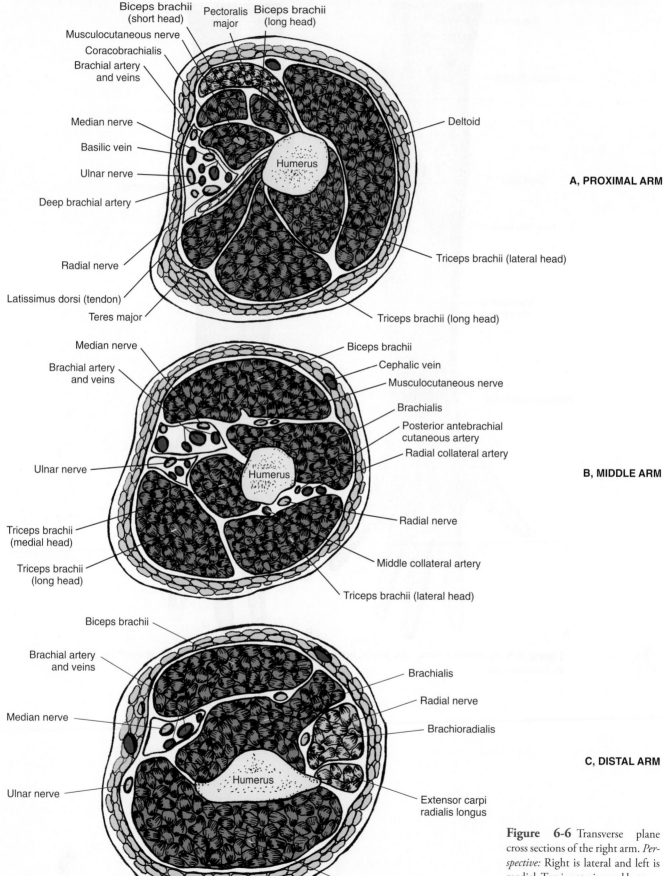

Biceps brachii (short head)
Pectoralis major
Biceps brachii (long head)
Musculocutaneous nerve
Coracobrachialis
Brachial artery and veins
Median nerve
Basilic vein
Ulnar nerve
Deep brachial artery
Deltoid
Humerus
Radial nerve
Triceps brachii (lateral head)
Latissimus dorsi (tendon)
Teres major
Triceps brachii (long head)

A, PROXIMAL ARM

Median nerve
Brachial artery and veins
Ulnar nerve
Biceps brachii
Cephalic vein
Musculocutaneous nerve
Brachialis
Posterior antebrachial cutaneous artery
Radial collateral artery
Humerus
Triceps brachii (medial head)
Triceps brachii (long head)
Radial nerve
Middle collateral artery
Triceps brachii (lateral head)

B, MIDDLE ARM

Biceps brachii
Brachial artery and veins
Median nerve
Ulnar nerve
Brachialis
Radial nerve
Brachioradialis
Humerus
Extensor carpi radialis longus
Triceps brachii

C, DISTAL ARM

Figure 6-6 Transverse plane cross sections of the right arm. *Perspective:* Right is lateral and left is medial. Top is anterior and bottom is posterior.

Biceps Brachii

The name, biceps brachii, *tells us that this muscle has two heads and lies over the brachium (the arm).*

Derivation	☐ biceps: L. *two heads.*
	brachii: L. *of the arm.*
Pronunciation	☐ BY-seps, BRAY-key-eye

■ ATTACHMENTS

☐ **LONG HEAD: Supraglenoid Tubercle of the Scapula**
☐ **SHORT HEAD: Coracoid Process of the Scapula**
  ☐ the apex

  to the

☐ **Radial Tuberosity**
  ☐ and the bicipital aponeurosis into deep fascia overlying the common flexor tendon

■ FUNCTIONS

CONCENTRIC (SHORTENING) MOVER ACTIONS	
Standard Mover Actions	**Reverse Mover Actions**
☐ **1. Flexes the forearm at the elbow joint**	☐ 1. Flexes the arm at the elbow joint
☐ **2. Supinates the forearm at the RU joints**	☐ 2. Supinates the ulna at the RU joints and medially rotates the arm at the GH joint
☐ **3. Flexes the arm at the GH joint**	☐ 3. Upwardly tilts the scapula at the GH and ScC joints
☐ 4. Abducts the arm at the GH joint (long head)	☐ 4. Downwardly rotates the scapula at the GH and ScC joints
☐ 5. Adducts the arm at the GH joint (short head)	☐ 5. Downwardly rotates and laterally tilts the scapula at the GH and ScC joints
☐ 6. Horizontally flexes the arm at the GH joint	☐ 6. Protracts the scapula at the GH and ScC joints

RU joints = radioulnar joints; GH joint = glenohumeral joint; ScC joint = scapulocostal joint

Standard Mover Action Notes

• The biceps brachii crosses the elbow joint anteriorly (with its fibers running vertically in the sagittal plane); therefore it flexes the forearm at the elbow joint. (action 1)

• When the forearm is pronated, the biceps brachii attachment onto the radial tuberosity is deep between the radius and the ulna. Thus the fibers wrap around the medial side of the proximal radius. When the biceps brachii pulls at the radial tuberosity, the head of the radius will laterally rotate and the distal radius will move around the distal ulna. This movement of the radius is called *supination.* Therefore the biceps brachii supinates the forearm at the RU joints. (action 2)

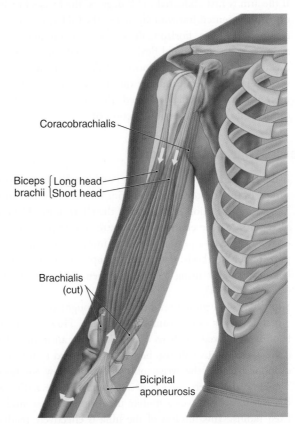

Figure 6-7 Anterior view of the right biceps brachii. The coracobrachialis and distal end of the brachialis have been ghosted in.

• The biceps brachii is a supinator in addition to being a flexor of the forearm. For this reason, engaging and palpating the biceps brachii is best accomplished by having the client flex the forearm when it is fully supinated. The biceps brachii can supinate the forearm at the RU joints regardless of the position of flexion/extension of the elbow joint. However, the biceps brachii is strongest with regard to supination of the forearm when the forearm is partially flexed. (actions 1, 2)

• The biceps brachii crosses the shoulder joint anteriorly (with its fibers running vertically in the sagittal plane); therefore it flexes the arm at the shoulder joint. (action 3)

• Similar to the middle deltoid, the long head of the biceps brachii crosses over the top of the GH joint. Therefore, it abducts the arm at the GH joint. Its ability to abduct increases if the arm is in a position of lateral rotation. Laterally rotating the arm places the long head's tendon more in the frontal plane for abduction. (action 4)

• The short head of the biceps brachii crosses the GH joint from medial to lateral (with its fibers running horizontally in the frontal plane) below the center of the joint. Therefore, it adducts the arm at the GH joint. It makes sense that the short head of the biceps brachii can adduct the arm at the GH joint because it has the same line of pull relative to the shoulder joint as the coracobrachialis. (action 5)

- If the arm is first abducted to 90 degrees, the biceps brachii fibers are oriented horizontally across the GH joint so they can pull the arm horizontally toward the midline. This action is called horizontal flexion (horizontal adduction) of the arm at the GH joint. Horizontal flexion of the arm by the biceps brachii is primarily due to the short head. The more the arm is medially rotated, the more the long head can contribute to this action. (action 6)

Reverse Mover Action Notes

- If the forearm is fixed, the biceps brachii pulls the anterior surface of the arm toward the anterior surface of the forearm. This action is flexion of the arm at the elbow joint. Flexion of the arm at the elbow joint is extremely important and occurs whenever a person grasps an immovable object and pulls his or her body toward it (examples include using a handicap bar or using a handrail when going up stairs). (reverse action 1)
- Supination and pronation are usually thought of as having a mobile radius move around a fixed ulna. However, if the hand is held fixed (perhaps by holding onto an immovable object), the radius will also be fixed with regard to rotation motions because the wrist joint does not allow rotation. Therefore the reverse action of supination of the radius at the RU joints involves a mobile ulna supinating around a fixed radius. This motion of the ulna is effectively medial rotation. However, when the ulna medially rotates around the radius, because the elbow joint also does not allow rotation motions, the humerus moves with the ulna; this results in medial rotation of the arm at the GH joint. (reverse action 2)
- If the biceps brachii contracts and the arm and forearm are fixed, the scapula is pulled forward in the sagittal plane toward the arm. This causes the scapula to upwardly tilt relative to the arm at the GH joint by lifting its inferior angle away from the rib cage wall. When the scapula moves relative to the arm at the GH joint, it also moves relative to the rib cage at the scapulocostal joint. (reverse action 3)
- The reverse action of the long head moving the arm into abduction relative to the scapula in the frontal plane is to move the scapula into downward rotation relative to the arm in the frontal plane. This motion occurs at the GH joint. When the scapula moves at the GH joint, it also moves relative to the rib cage at the scapulocostal joint. (reverse action 4)
- The reverse action of adduction of the arm at the GH joint is also to downwardly rotate the scapula at the GH and scapulocostal joints because the line of pull of the short head is on the same side of the axis for scapular rotation as is the long head's line of pull. (reverse action 5)
- Because the short head crosses the GH joint more anteriorly than the long head, it will also tend to pull the medial border of the scapula away from the rib cage wall. This is known as lateral tilt of the scapula. (reverse action 5)

- Protraction of the scapula relative to the humerus is not a very likely reverse action. (reverse action 6)

Eccentric Antagonist Functions

1. Restrains/slows elbow joint extension
2. Restrains/slows RU joint pronation
3. Restrains/slows arm extension, horizontal extension, adduction, abduction, and lateral rotation
4. Restrains/slows scapular upward rotation, downward tilt, medial tilt, and retraction.

Eccentric Antagonist Function Notes

- Restraining/slowing extension of the forearm at the elbow joint is extremely important when lowering an object in a careful and controlled manner.
- Restraining/slowing reverse actions occur when the distal attachment of the biceps brachii is fixed, usually by the hand holding onto an immovable object.

Isometric Stabilization Functions

1. Stabilizes the elbow, RU, and GH joints
2. Stabilizes the scapula

INNERVATION
☐ The Musculocutaneous Nerve
  ☐ C5, C6

ARTERIAL SUPPLY
☐ The muscular branches of the Brachial Artery (the continuation of the Axillary Artery)
  ☐ and the Anterior Circumflex Humeral Artery (a branch of the Axillary Artery)

✋ PALPATION

1. With the client seated or supine and the forearm supinated, place palpating hand on the anterior arm and feel for the biceps brachii.
2. Have the client flex the forearm at the elbow joint and feel for the contraction of the biceps brachii. Resistance can be added.
3. Continue palpating the biceps brachii proximally and distally toward its attachments.
4. Note: Be careful with palpation in the medial arm, because the median and ulnar nerves and brachial artery are superficial here.

Biceps Brachii—*cont'd*

■ RELATIONSHIP TO OTHER STRUCTURES

☐ Proximally, the biceps brachii is deep to the deltoid and deep to the distal tendon of the pectoralis major. The remainder of the biceps brachii is superficial.

☐ From an anterior perspective, the brachialis lies deep to the biceps brachii.

☐ The short head of the biceps brachii lies lateral to the coracobrachialis.

☐ The proximal attachment of the short head of the biceps brachii is the coracoid process of the scapula. The coracobrachialis and the pectoralis minor also attach to the coracoid process.

☐ The long head of the biceps brachii courses through the bicipital groove of the humerus. The long head of the biceps brachii then courses through the joint cavity of the glenohumeral joint; therefore it is intra-articular.

☐ Directly medial to the belly and distal tendon of the biceps brachii are the brachial artery and the median nerve.

☐ The bicipital aponeurosis is superficial to the common flexor tendon, and does not attach into bone.

☐ The biceps brachii is located within the deep front arm line and involved with the superficial front arm line myofascial meridians.

■ MISCELLANEOUS

1. The bicipital groove of the humerus is named the *bicipital* groove, because the long head of the biceps brachii courses through it. (The bicipital groove of the humerus is also known as the *intertubercular groove,* because it is located between the two tubercles of the humerus.)

2. The proximal attachment of the short head of the biceps brachii blends with the proximal attachment of the coracobrachialis at the coracoid process of the scapula.

3. The bicipital aponeurosis is also known as the *lacertus fibrosis.*

Brachialis

The name, brachialis, *tells us that this muscle attaches to the brachium (the arm).*

Derivation	☐ brachialis: L. *refers to the arm.*
Pronunciation	☐ BRAY-key-AL-is

■ ATTACHMENTS

☐ **Distal ½ of the Anterior Shaft of the Humerus**

to the

☐ **Ulnar Tuberosity**
  ☐ and the coronoid process of the ulna

■ FUNCTIONS

CONCENTRIC (SHORTENING) MOVER ACTIONS	
Standard Mover Actions	**Reverse Mover Actions**
☐ 1. Flexes the forearm at the elbow joint	☐ 1. Flexes the arm at the elbow joint

Standard Mover Action Notes

- The brachialis crosses the elbow joint anteriorly (with its fibers running vertically in the sagittal plane); therefore it flexes the forearm at the elbow joint. (action 1)
- Even though the biceps brachii is more well known for flexing the elbow joint, the brachialis is actually the prime mover (most powerful mover) of flexion of the elbow joint. (action 1)
- The brachialis is especially engaged with elbow joint flexion if the forearm is fully pronated (because the biceps brachii and brachioradialis would supinate a fully pronated forearm in addition to flexing it). For this reason, the brachialis is best engaged and palpated by asking the client to flex the forearm when it is fully pronated. (action 1)

Reverse Mover Action Note

- If the forearm is fixed, the brachialis pulls the anterior surface of the arm toward the anterior surface of the forearm. This action is flexion of the arm at the elbow joint. The reverse action of flexion of the arm at the elbow joint is extremely important and occurs whenever a person grasps an immovable object and pulls his or her body toward it. Examples include using a handicap bar or using a handrail when going up stairs. (reverse action 1)

Eccentric Antagonist Function

1. Restrains/slows elbow joint extension

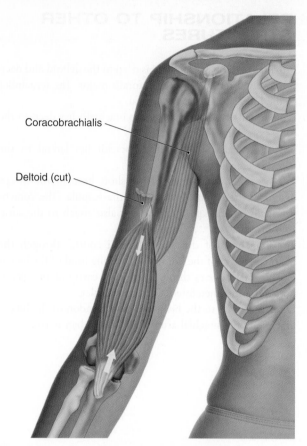

Figure 6-8 Anterior view of the right brachialis; the coracobrachialis and distal end of the deltoid have been ghosted in.

Eccentric Antagonist Function Note

- Restraining/slowing extension of the forearm at the elbow joint is extremely important when lowering an object in a careful and controlled manner.

Isometric Stabilization Function

1. Stabilizes the elbow joint

INNERVATION
☐ The Musculocutaneous Nerve
  ☐ C5, **C6**, C7

ARTERIAL SUPPLY
☐ Muscular branches of the Brachial Artery (the continuation of the Axillary Artery)

Brachialis—*cont'd*

✋ PALPATION

1. With the client seated or supine and the forearm fully pronated at the radioulnar joints, place palpating hand on the distal lateral arm.
2. Have the client flex the forearm further with a short, gentle range of motion and feel for the contraction of the brachialis. If resistance is added, add only gentle resistance.
3. The brachialis can be palpated on the lateral side of the arm and the medial side of the arm. It can also be palpated anteriorly through the biceps brachii.
4. Note: Be careful with palpation in the distal medial arm, because the median and ulnar nerves and brachial artery are superficial here.

■ RELATIONSHIP TO OTHER STRUCTURES

☐ Although most of the brachialis is deep to the biceps brachii, the lateral margin of the brachialis is superficial between the biceps brachii and the triceps brachii. More distally, the brachialis is superficial on both sides of the biceps brachii's distal tendon.

☐ Deep to the brachialis is the shaft of the humerus.

☐ The proximal attachment of the brachialis forms a V shape and surrounds the distal attachment of the deltoid.

☐ On the medial side, the triceps brachii is posterior to the brachialis.

☐ On the lateral side, the triceps brachii is posterior to the brachialis proximally; the brachioradialis is posterior to the brachialis distally.

☐ The brachialis is located within the deep front arm line myofascial meridian.

■ MISCELLANEOUS

1. The brachialis is a strong and fairly large muscle, which accounts for much of the contour of the biceps brachii being so visible. ("Behind every great biceps brachii is a great brachialis." ☺)

Brachioradialis (of Radial Group)

The name, brachioradialis, *tells us that this muscle attaches onto the brachium (the arm) and the radius.*

Derivation	☐ brachio: L. *refers to the arm.*
	radialis: L. *refers to the radius.*
Pronunciation	☐ BRAY-key-o-RAY-dee-AL-is

■ ATTACHMENTS

☐ **Lateral Supracondylar Ridge of the Humerus**
  ☐ the proximal ⅔

  to the

☐ **Styloid Process of the Radius**
  ☐ the lateral side

■ FUNCTIONS

CONCENTRIC (SHORTENING) MOVER ACTIONS	
Standard Mover Actions	**Reverse Mover Actions**
☐ **1. Flexes the forearm at the elbow joint**	☐ 1. Flexes the arm at the elbow joint
☐ **2. Supinates the forearm at the RU joints**	☐ 2. Supinates the ulna at the RU joints and medially rotates the arm at the GH joint
☐ **3. Pronates the forearm at the RU joints**	☐ 3. Pronates the ulna at the RU joints and laterally rotates the arm at the GH joint

RU joints = radioulnar joints; GH joint = glenohumeral joint

Standard Mover Action Notes

- The brachioradialis crosses the elbow joint anteriorly (with its fibers running vertically in the sagittal plane); therefore it flexes the forearm at the elbow joint. (action 1)
- The brachioradialis is most effective as a forearm flexor when the forearm is in a position that is halfway between full pronation and full supination. (action 1)
- The brachioradialis is unusual in that it can both supinate and pronate the forearm at the RU joints. If the forearm is fully supinated, the brachioradialis can pronate the forearm to a position that is approximately halfway between full pronation and full supination because that position will have the two attachments of the brachioradialis, the styloid process of the radius and the lateral supracondylar ridge of the humerus, as close to each other as possible. Similarly, if the forearm is fully pronated, the brachioradialis can supinate the forearm to a position that is halfway between full pronation and full supination for the same reason. The brachioradialis is an excellent example of a muscle in the

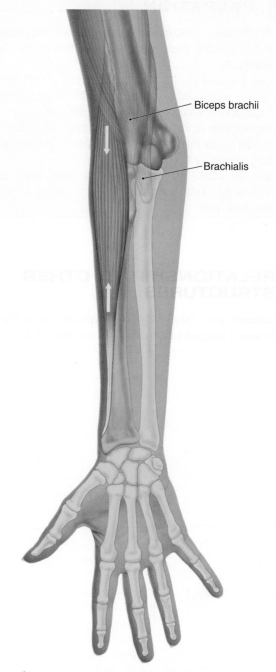

Figure 6-9 Anterior view of the right brachioradialis. The biceps brachii and brachialis have been ghosted in.

— Biceps brachii

— Brachialis

human body that has one line of pull but can have two opposite actions at the same joint (pronation and supination at the radioulnar joints) based on the position that the joint is in when the muscle contracts.

Brachioradialis (of Radial Group)—*cont'd*

Reverse Mover Action Notes

- If the forearm is fixed, the brachioradialis pulls the anterior surface of the arm toward the anterior surface of the forearm. This action is flexion of the arm at the elbow joint. The reverse action of flexion of the arm at the elbow joint is extremely important and occurs whenever a person grasps an immovable object and pulls his or her body toward it. Examples include using a handicap bar or using a handrail when going up stairs. (reverse action 1)
- Supination and pronation are usually thought of as having a mobile radius move around a fixed ulna. However, if the hand is held fixed (perhaps by holding onto an immovable object), the radius will also be fixed with regard to rotation motions because the wrist joint does not allow rotation. Therefore the reverse action of supination of the forearm at the RU joints involves a mobile ulna supinating around a fixed radius. This supination motion of the ulna is effectively medial rotation. When the ulna medially rotates around the radius, because the elbow joint also does not allow rotation motions, the humerus moves with the ulna; this results in medial rotation of the arm at the GH joint. Similarly, the reverse action of pronation of the forearm at the RU joints involves a mobile ulna pronating around a fixed radius. This pronation motion of the ulna is effectively lateral rotation. This results in lateral rotation of the arm at the GH joint. (reverse actions 2, 3)

Eccentric Antagonist Functions

1. Restrains/slows elbow joint extension
2. Restrains/slows RU joints pronation and supination

Eccentric Antagonist Function Notes

- Restraining/slowing extension of the forearm at the elbow joint is extremely important when lowering an object in a careful and controlled manner.
- The brachioradialis can only restrain/slow pronation when the forearm is between a fully supinated position and the position that is halfway between full supination and full pronation. Similarly, it can only restrain/slow supination when the forearm is between a fully pronated position and the position that is halfway between full supination and full pronation.

Isometric Stabilization Functions

1. Stabilizes the elbow and RU joints

INNERVATION
- The Radial Nerve
  - C5, **C6**

ARTERIAL SUPPLY
- Branches of the Brachial Artery (the continuation of the Axillary Artery) and the Radial Artery (a terminal branch of the Brachial Artery)

✋ PALPATION

1. With the client seated or supine and the forearm flexed at the elbow joint to 90 degrees and in a position halfway between full pronation and full supination, place palpating hand on the lateral anterior forearm.
2. Resist the client from further flexing the forearm and look and feel for the contraction of the brachioradialis.
3. Continue palpating the brachioradialis proximally toward the lateral supracondylar ridge of the humerus and distally toward the styloid process of the radius.

■ RELATIONSHIP TO OTHER STRUCTURES

- The brachioradialis is superficial in the lateral forearm, except at its distal end, where the abductor pollicis longus and the extensor pollicis brevis cross over it superficially.
- The proximal tendon of the brachioradialis is found between the brachialis and the triceps brachii.
- The belly of the brachioradialis is directly anterior to the extensor carpi radialis longus.
- The radial attachment of the pronator teres lies deep to the brachioradialis.
- The brachioradialis is involved with the superficial back arm line and the deep back arm line myofascial meridians.

■ MISCELLANEOUS

1. The brachioradialis, the extensor carpi radialis longus, and the extensor carpi radialis brevis are often grouped together as the *radial group* of forearm muscles. They are also sometimes known as the *wad of three*.
2. The brachioradialis is sometimes nicknamed the *hitchhiker muscle* for the characteristic action of flexing the forearm in a position halfway between full pronation and full supination (with the thumb up) when hitchhiking. (Keep in mind that the brachioradialis has no action on the thumb itself.)
3. The brachioradialis is a flexor of the forearm at the elbow joint, but it is innervated by the radial nerve, which innervates all the forearm extensors.

Triceps Brachii

The name, triceps brachii, *tells us that this muscle has three heads and attaches to the brachium (the arm).*

Derivation	☐ triceps: L. *three heads.*
	brachii: L. *of the arm.*
Pronunciation	☐ TRY-seps, BRAY-key-eye

■ ATTACHMENTS

☐ **LONG HEAD: Infraglenoid Tubercle of the Scapula**
☐ **LATERAL HEAD: Posterior Shaft of the Humerus**
   ☐ the proximal ⅓
☐ **MEDIAL HEAD: Posterior Shaft of the Humerus**
   ☐ the distal ⅔

to the

☐ **Olecranon Process of the Ulna**

■ FUNCTIONS

CONCENTRIC (SHORTENING) MOVER ACTIONS

Standard Mover Actions	Reverse Mover Actions
☐ **1. Extends the forearm at the elbow joint**	☐ 1. Extends the arm at the elbow joint
☐ **2. Extends the arm at the GH joint (long head)**	☐ 2. Downwardly rotates the scapula at the GH and ScC joints
☐ 3. Adducts the arm at the GH joint (long head)	
☐ 4. Horizontally extends the arm at the GH joint (long head)	☐ 3. Protracts and laterally tilts the scapula at the GH and ScC joints

GH joint = glenohumeral joint; ScC joint = scapulocostal joint

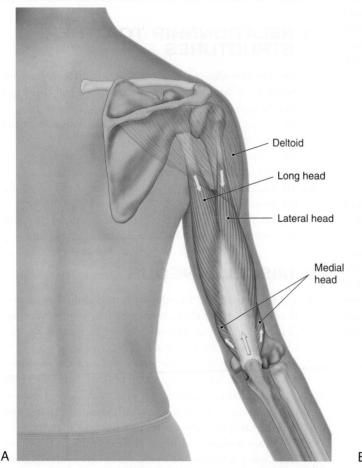

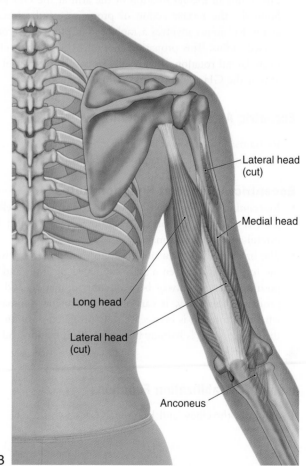

Figure 6-10 Views of the right triceps brachii. **A,** Superficial view. The deltoid has been ghosted in. **B,** The lateral head has been cut to better show the medial head. The anconeus has been ghosted in.

Triceps Brachii—*cont'd*

Standard Mover Action Notes

- The triceps brachii crosses the elbow joint posteriorly (with its fibers running vertically in the sagittal plane); therefore it extends the forearm at the elbow joint. (action 1)
- The triceps brachii is the prime mover (most powerful mover) of elbow joint extension. (action 1)
- The long head of the triceps brachii crosses the shoulder joint posteriorly (with the fibers running vertically in the sagittal plane); therefore it extends the arm at the GH joint. (action 2)
- The long head of the triceps brachii crosses the shoulder joint medially (with the fibers running horizontally in the frontal plane); therefore it adducts the arm at the GH joint. Note: the horizontal component to its fiber direction increases as the arm is abducted in the frontal plane. Therefore, if the arm is first abducted, the adduction action of the triceps brachii becomes more prominent. (action 3)
- If the arm is abducted to 90 degrees, the triceps brachii's long head is oriented horizontally across the GH joint posteriorly. Therefore it can horizontally extend (horizontally abduct) the arm at the GH joint. (action 4)

Reverse Mover Action Notes

- If the distal attachment of the triceps brachii is fixed, the posterior surface of the arm will be pulled toward the posterior surface of the forearm. Therefore, the triceps brachii extends the arm at the elbow joint. (reverse action 1)
- When the long head of the triceps brachii pulls downward on the scapula, the glenoid fossa will be oriented downward. Therefore the long head downwardly rotates the scapula at the GH joint. (reverse action 2)
- When the scapula moves relative to the arm at the GH joint, it also moves relative to the rib cage at the ScC joint. (reverse actions 2, 3)
- Pulling the scapula laterally toward the abducted arm results in protraction of the scapula. (reverse action 3)
- The long head of the triceps brachii can only laterally tilt the scapula (pulling the medial border of the scapula away from the rib cage wall) when horizontally extending the arm if the arm is in front of the body. (reverse action 3)

Eccentric Antagonist Functions

1. Restrains/slows elbow joint flexion
2. Restrains/slows arm flexion, abduction, and horizontal flexion
3. Restrains/slows scapular upward rotation, retraction, and medial tilt

Eccentric Antagonist Function Note

- Medial tilt of the scapula is a motion in which the medial border of the scapula moves toward the rib cage wall. Given that the long head of the triceps brachii can only laterally tilt the scapula if the arm is in front of the body, it can only restrain/slow medial tilt if the arm is in front of the body.

Isometric Stabilization Functions

1. Stabilizes the elbow and GH joints.
2. Stabilizes the scapula.

INNERVATION
- ☐ The Radial Nerve
  - ☐ C6, **C7**, C8

ARTERIAL SUPPLY
- ☐ The Deep Brachial Artery (a branch of the Brachial Artery)
  - ☐ and the Circumflex Scapular Artery (a branch of the Subscapular Artery)

🖐 PALPATION

1. With the client seated, place palpating hand on the distal, posterior arm, just proximal to the olecranon process of the ulna.
2. Have the client extend the forearm at the elbow joint against resistance and feel for the contraction of the triceps brachii.
3. Continue palpating the triceps brachii proximally toward the infraglenoid tubercle of the scapula, deep to the posterior deltoid.

■ RELATIONSHIP TO OTHER STRUCTURES

- ☐ The triceps brachii is superficial in the posterior arm except for the proximal attachments of the long head and the lateral head, which are deep to the deltoid.
- ☐ On the lateral side, the triceps brachii borders the brachialis proximally and the brachioradialis and extensor carpi radialis longus distally.
- ☐ On the medial side, the triceps brachii borders the coracobrachialis and the brachialis.
- ☐ The long head of the triceps brachii runs between the teres minor and the teres major.
- ☐ The triceps brachii is located within the deep back arm line myofascial meridian.

■ MISCELLANEOUS

1. From the posterior perspective, the medial head of the triceps brachii lies deep to the other two heads. For this reason, the medial head of the triceps brachii is sometimes known as the *deep head* (which probably is a better name for this head of the triceps brachii).

Triceps Brachii—*cont'd*

2. At its proximal end, the medial head of the triceps brachii attaches to the medial proximal humerus. However, more distally, the medial head crosses over to also attach to the lateral shaft of the humerus.

3. The medial head of the triceps brachii is the most active of the three heads, meaning it is engaged most often by the nervous system; but the lateral head is the strongest.

4. The radial nerve runs between the medial and lateral heads of the triceps brachii. Because of its location here, the radial nerve is often injured.

Anconeus

The name, anconeus, *tells us that this muscle is involved with the elbow.*

Derivation	☐ anconeus: Gr. *elbow.*
Pronunciation	☐ an-KO-nee-us

■ ATTACHMENTS

☐ **Lateral Epicondyle of the Humerus**

  to the

☐ **Posterior Proximal Ulna**
  ☐ the lateral side of the olecranon process of the ulna and the proximal ¼ of the posterior ulna

■ FUNCTIONS

CONCENTRIC (SHORTENING) MOVER ACTIONS	
Standard Mover Actions	**Reverse Mover Actions**
☐ **1. Extends the forearm at the elbow joint**	☐ 1. Extends the arm at the elbow joint

Standard Mover Action Note

• The anconeus crosses the elbow joint posteriorly (with its fibers running vertically in the sagittal plane); therefore it extends the forearm at the elbow joint. (action 1)

Reverse Mover Action Note

• If the distal attachment of the anconeus is fixed, the posterior surface of the arm will be pulled toward the posterior surface of the forearm. Therefore, the anconeus extends the arm at the elbow joint. (reverse action 1)

Eccentric Antagonist Function

1. Restrains/slows elbow joint flexion

Isometric Stabilization Function

1. Stabilizes the ulna and elbow joint

Isometric Stabilization Function Note

• Some sources state that the major function of the anconeus is to stabilize the ulna from being moved medially (adducted) at the elbow joint during pronation of the forearm at the radioulnar joints.

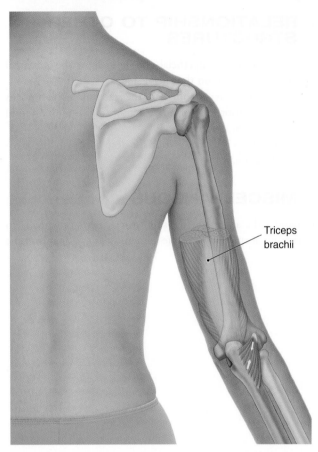

Triceps brachii

Figure 6-11 Posterior view of the right anconeus. The triceps brachii has been cut and ghosted in.

INNERVATION
☐ The Radial Nerve
  ☐ C6, C7, C8

ARTERIAL SUPPLY
☐ The Deep Brachial Artery (a branch of the Brachial Artery)

✋ PALPATION

1. With the client seated, locate the point halfway between the olecranon process of the ulna and the lateral epicondyle of the humerus, and then place your palpating finger approximately ½ inch (1 cm) distal to that point.
2. Have the client actively extend the forearm at the elbow joint against resistance and feel for the contraction of the anconeus.
3. Palpate the entirety of the anconeus.

6

RELATIONSHIP TO OTHER STRUCTURES

☐ The anconeus is superficial and located in the proximal posterior forearm on the lateral side.

☐ The anconeus is proximal to the extensor carpi radialis brevis, extensor digitorum, extensor digiti minimi, and extensor carpi ulnaris.

☐ The anconeus is located within the deep back arm line myofascial meridian.

MISCELLANEOUS

1. Besides the anconeus, the supinator attaches proximally to the lateral epicondyle of the humerus. Also arising from the lateral epicondyle are four other muscles that share the common extensor tendon attachment onto the lateral epicondyle of the humerus (the extensor carpi radialis brevis, extensor digitorum, extensor digiti minimi, and extensor carpi ulnaris).

2. The anconeus often blends with the triceps brachii.

3. Irritation and/or inflammation of the lateral epicondyle and/or the common extensor tendon is known as *lateral epicondylitis*, *lateral epicondylosis*, or *tennis elbow*.

Pronator Teres

The name, pronator teres, *tells us that this muscle pronates the forearm and is round in shape.*

Derivation	□ pronator: L. *a muscle that pronates a body part.*
	□ teres: L. *round.*
Pronunciation	□ pro-NAY-tor, TE-reez

■ ATTACHMENTS

□ **HUMERAL HEAD: Medial Epicondyle of the Humerus (via the Common Flexor Tendon)**
  □ and the medial supracondylar ridge of the humerus
□ **ULNAR HEAD: Coronoid Process of the Ulna**
  □ the medial surface

to the

□ **Lateral Radius**
  □ the middle ⅓

■ FUNCTIONS

CONCENTRIC (SHORTENING) MOVER ACTIONS	
Standard Mover Actions	**Reverse Mover Actions**
□ **1. Pronates the forearm at the RU joints**	□ 1. Pronates the ulna at the RU joints and laterally rotates the arm at the GH joint
□ **2. Flexes the forearm at the elbow joint**	□ 2. Flexes the arm at the elbow joint

RU joints = radioulnar joints; GH joint = glenohumeral joint

Standard Mover Action Notes

- The pronator teres crosses from the medial elbow region to the lateral (radial) side of the forearm onto the radius (with its fibers running somewhat horizontally in the transverse plane), crossing the radioulnar joints anteriorly. When it contracts, it pulls the radial attachment anteromedially. This causes the head of the radius to medially rotate and the distal radius to cross in front of the ulna. This movement of the radius is called pronation. Therefore the pronator teres pronates the forearm at the RU joints. (action 1)
- Pronation of the forearm at the RU joints usually involves motion of the radius around a fixed ulna. (action 1)
- The pronator teres crosses the elbow joint anteriorly (with its fibers running vertically in the sagittal plane); therefore it flexes the forearm at the elbow joint. (action 2)

Reverse Mover Action Notes

- Pronation is usually thought of as having a mobile radius move around a fixed ulna. However, if the hand is held fixed

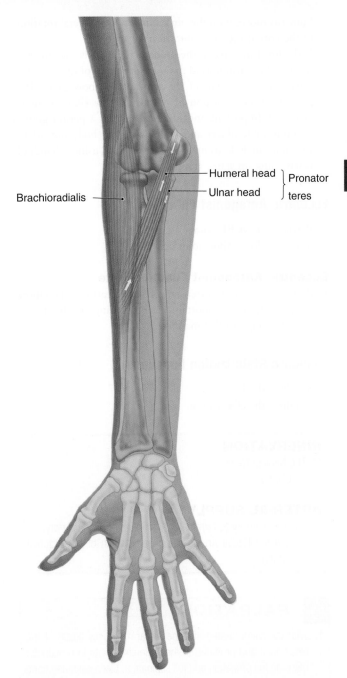

Figure 6-12 Anterior view of the right pronator teres. The brachioradialis has been ghosted in.

(perhaps by holding onto an immovable object), the radius will also be fixed with regard to rotation motions because the wrist joint does not allow rotation. Therefore the reverse action of pronation of the forearm at the RU joints involves a mobile ulna pronating around a fixed radius. This pronation motion of the ulna is effectively lateral rotation. When the ulna laterally rotates around the radius, because the elbow joint also does not allow rotation motions, the

Pronator Teres—*cont'd*

6

humerus moves with the ulna; this results in lateral rotation of the arm at the GH joint. (reverse action 1)

- If the forearm is fixed, the pronator teres pulls the anterior surface of the arm toward the anterior surface of the forearm. This action is flexion of the arm at the elbow joint. The reverse action of flexion of the arm at the elbow joint is extremely important and occurs whenever a person grasps an immovable object and pulls his or her body toward it. Examples include using a handicap bar or using a handrail when going up stairs. (reverse action 2)

Eccentric Antagonist Functions

1. Restrains/slows RU joints supination
2. Restrains/slows elbow joint extension

Eccentric Antagonist Function Note

- Restraining/slowing extension of the forearm at the elbow joint is extremely important when lowering an object in a careful and controlled manner.

Isometric Stabilization Functions

1. Stabilizes the RU joints
2. Stabilizes the elbow joint

INNERVATION
□ The Median Nerve
  □ C6, **C7**

ARTERIAL SUPPLY
□ The Ulnar Artery (a terminal branch of the Brachial Artery)
  □ and the Radial Artery (a terminal branch of the Brachial Artery)

✋ PALPATION

1. With the client seated and the forearm partially flexed at the elbow joint and pronated at the radioulnar joints to a midpoint between full pronation and full supination, place palpating hand on the proximal anterior forearm and place resistance hand on the distal anterior forearm.
2. Have the client further pronate the forearm against resistance and feel for the contraction of the pronator teres.
3. Continue palpating the pronator teres proximally toward the medial epicondyle of the humerus and distally toward the lateral radius.

■ RELATIONSHIP TO OTHER STRUCTURES

□ The proximal part of the pronator teres is superficial in the proximal anterior forearm, but the distal attachment is deep to the brachioradialis.
□ The ulnar head of the pronator teres is entirely deep or nearly entirely deep to the humeral head of the pronator teres.
□ The pronator teres is lateral to the flexor carpi radialis.
□ The pronator teres is largely superficial to the flexor digitorum superficialis.
□ The pronator teres is involved with the deep front arm line and superficial back arm line myofascial meridians.

■ MISCELLANEOUS

1. The humeral head of the pronator teres arises proximally from the medial epicondyle of the humerus via the common flexor tendon. The common flexor tendon is the common proximal attachment of five muscles: the pronator teres, flexor carpi radialis, palmaris longus, flexor carpi ulnaris, and flexor digitorum superficialis.
2. Although the humeral head of the pronator teres is part of the common flexor tendon, the actual attachment site of the humeral head onto the medial epicondyle of the humerus is slightly more proximal than the attachment of the other four muscles of the common flexor tendon.
3. The humeral head of the pronator teres is by far the larger of the two heads.
4. The median nerve courses between the humeral head and the ulnar head of the pronator teres, making it a possible entrapment site of the median nerve. When the median nerve is entrapped there, it is termed *pronator teres syndrome* (and may mimic symptoms of carpal tunnel syndrome or a pathologic cervical disc).
5. Overuse of the pronator teres can cause irritation and/or inflammation of the medial epicondyle and/or the common flexor tendon. This is known as *medial epicondylitis, medial epicondylosis,* or *golfer's elbow.*

Pronator Quadratus

The name, pronator quadratus, *tells us that this muscle pronates the forearm and has a square shape.*

Derivation	☐ pronator: L. *a muscle that pronates a body part.*
	quadratus: L. *squared.*
Pronunciation	☐ pro-NAY-tor, kwod-RAY-tus

■ ATTACHMENTS

☐ **Anterior Distal Ulna**
  ☐ the distal ¼

to the

☐ **Anterior Distal Radius**
  ☐ the distal ¼

■ FUNCTIONS

CONCENTRIC (SHORTENING) MOVER ACTIONS	
Standard Mover Actions	**Reverse Mover Actions**
☐ **1. Pronates the forearm at the RU joints**	☐ 1. Pronates the ulna at the RU joints and laterally rotates the arm at the GH joint

RU joints = radioulnar joints; GH joint = glenohumeral joint

Standard Mover Action Notes

* The pronator quadratus crosses the distal anterior forearm from the ulna to the radius (with its fibers running horizontally in the transverse plane). When the pronator quadratus contracts, it pulls the distal radius anteromedially. This causes the distal radius to cross in front of the distal ulna (and the head of the radius to medially rotate). This movement of the radius is called pronation. Therefore the pronator quadratus pronates the forearm at the RU joints. (action 1)
* Pronation of the forearm at the RU joints usually involves motion of the radius around a fixed ulna. (action 1)
* According to most sources, the pronator quadratus is the prime mover of forearm pronation at the RU joints even though the pronator teres is much larger. This is due to the pronator quadratus' excellent leverage at the distal radius. (action 1)

Reverse Mover Action Note

* Pronation is usually thought of as having a mobile radius move around a fixed ulna. However, if the hand is held fixed (perhaps by holding onto an immovable object), the radius will also be fixed with regard to rotation motions because the wrist joint does not allow rotation. Therefore the reverse

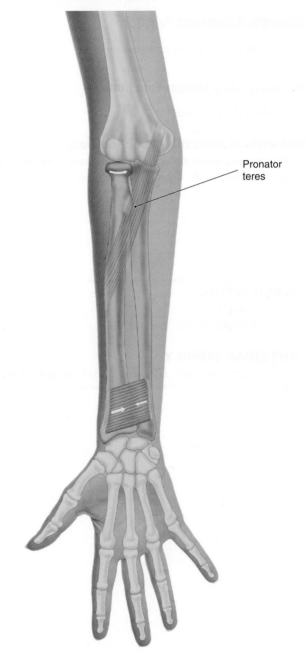

Figure 6-13 Anterior view of the right pronator quadratus. The pronator teres has been ghosted in.

action of pronation of the forearm at the RU joints involves a mobile ulna pronating around a fixed radius. This pronation motion of the ulna is effectively lateral rotation. When the ulna laterally rotates around the radius, because the elbow joint also does not allow rotation motions, the humerus moves with the ulna; this results in lateral rotation of the arm at the GH joint.

Pronator Quadratus—*cont'd*

Eccentric Antagonist Function

1. Restrains/slows RU joints supination

Isometric Stabilization Function

1. Stabilizes the RU joints

Isometric Stabilization Function Note

- The pronator quadratus is especially important for preventing separation of the distal radius and ulna.

INNERVATION
- ☐ The Median Nerve
  - ☐ anterior interosseus nerve, C7, **C8**

ARTERIAL SUPPLY
- ☐ The Anterior Interosseus Artery (a branch of the Ulnar Artery)

PALPATION

1. With the client seated or supine, place palpating hand distally on the distal anterolateral forearm.
2. Find the radial pulse to locate the radial artery and then palpate on either side of it to locate the pronator quadratus. The pronator quadratus is very deep and can be difficult to palpate and discern.
3. Resist the client from actively pronating the forearm at the radioulnar joints and feel for the contraction of the pronator quadratus.

■ RELATIONSHIP TO OTHER STRUCTURES

- ☐ The pronator quadratus is the deepest muscle in the anterior forearm.
- ☐ Every structure that crosses the wrist on the anterior side is superficial to the pronator quadratus.
- ☐ Deep to the pronator quadratus are the radius, the ulna, and the interosseus membrane.
- ☐ The pronator quadratus is involved with the deep front arm line and deep back arm line myofascial meridians.

Supinator

The name, supinator, *tells us that this muscle supinates the forearm.*

Derivation	☐ supinator: L. *a muscle that supinates a body part.*
Pronunciation	☐ SUE-pin-AY-tor

■ ATTACHMENTS

☐ **Lateral Epicondyle of the Humerus and the Proximal Ulna**
  ☐ the supinator crest of the ulna

  to the

☐ **Proximal Radius**
  ☐ the proximal ⅓ of the posterior, lateral, and anterior sides

■ FUNCTIONS

CONCENTRIC (SHORTENING) MOVER ACTIONS	
Standard Mover Actions	**Reverse Mover Actions**
☐ 1. Supinates the forearm at the RU joints	☐ 1. Supinates the ulna at the RU joints and medially rotates the arm at the GH joint
☐ 2. Flexes the forearm at the elbow joint	☐ 2. Flexes the arm at the elbow joint

RU joints = radioulnar joints; GH joint = glenohumeral joint

Standard Mover Action Notes

- The supinator crosses from the proximal posterior ulna to the proximal posterolateral radius; thus it wraps around the posterior forearm. When the supinator pulls the radius toward the ulna on the posterior side, it causes the head of the radius to laterally rotate and the distal radius to move posterolaterally around the distal ulna. This movement of the radius is called *supination.* Therefore the supinator supinates the forearm at the RU joints. (action 1)
- The supinator has a few fibers that run vertically and are located anterior to the elbow joint; therefore the supinator can flex the elbow joint. However, given how few fibers are oriented in this manner, this action of the supinator is very weak. (action 2)

Reverse Mover Action Notes

- Supinaton and pronation are usually thought of as having a mobile radius move around a fixed ulna. However, if the hand is held fixed (perhaps by holding onto an immovable object), the radius will also be fixed with regard to rotation motions because the radiocarpal joint does not allow rotation. Therefore the reverse action of supination of the forearm at the RU joints involves a mobile ulna supinating around a fixed radius. This supination motion of the ulna is

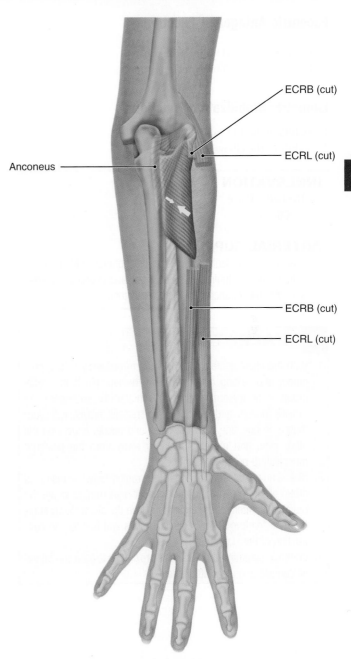

Figure 6-14 Posterior view of the right supinator. The anconeus has been ghosted in. The extensor carpi radialis longus (ECRL) and extensor carpi radialis brevis (ECRB) have been cut and ghosted in.

effectively medial rotation. When the ulna medially rotates around the radius, because the elbow joint also does not allow rotation motions, the humerus moves with the ulna; this results in medial rotation of the arm at the GH joint. (reverse action 1)
- The reverse action of flexing the forearm toward the arm at the elbow joint is flexing the arm toward the forearm at the elbow joint. (reverse action 2)

6

Eccentric Antagonist Functions

1. Restrains/slows RU joint pronation
2. Restrains/slows elbow joint extension

Isometric Stabilization Functions

1. Stabilizes the RU joints
2. Stabilizes the elbow joint

INNERVATION
- [ ] The Radial Nerve
  - [ ] **C6**, C7

ARTERIAL SUPPLY
- [ ] Branches of the Radial Artery (a terminal branch of the Brachial Artery) and the Interosseus Recurrent and Posterior Interosseus Arteries (branches of the Ulnar Artery)

PALPATION

1. With the client seated and the forearm passively flexed, pronated, and resting comfortably on the lap, pinch the radial group of the forearm muscles (brachioradialis, extensor carpi radialis longus, and extensor carpi radialis brevis) with your thumb on one side and your index and middle fingers on the other side, and move it anteriorly away from the posterior musculature of the forearm.
2. Sink in an palpate deeper against the radius (between the radial group of the forearm and the extensor digitorum) to locate the radial attachment of the supinator. Have the client slowly supinate the forearm at the radioulnar joints and feel for the contraction of the supinator.
3. Continue palpating the supinator proximally toward the lateral epicondyle and ulnar attachment.

■ RELATIONSHIP TO OTHER STRUCTURES

- [ ] The supinator is a deep muscle in the proximal posterior forearm. The supinator lies deep to the anconeus, extensor digitorum, extensor digiti minimi, extensor carpi radialis brevis, extensor carpi radialis longus, and brachioradialis.
- [ ] The distal tendon of the supinator attaches onto the radius next to the distal attachment of the pronator teres.
- [ ] The supinator is located within the deep front arm line myofascial meridian.

■ MISCELLANEOUS

1. Besides the supinator, the anconeus attaches proximally to the lateral epicondyle of the humerus. Also arising from the lateral epicondyle are four other muscles that share the common extensor tendon attachment onto the lateral epicondyle of the humerus (the extensor carpi radialis brevis, extensor digitorum, extensor digiti minimi, and extensor carpi ulnaris).
2. Proximally, the supinator muscle has two layers: a superficial layer and a deep layer.
3. The posterior interosseus nerve, a deep branch of the radial nerve, runs between the two layers of the supinator and may be entrapped there. (Most sources state that the posterior interosseus nerve can also be called the deep branch of the radial nerve. However, other sources state that the posterior interosseus nerve is the continuation of the deep branch of the radial nerve after it has emerged from the supinator muscle.)
4. The supinator crest is located deep between the two bones of the forearm on the lateral side of the ulna.
5. Irritation and/or inflammation of the lateral epicondyle and/or the common extensor tendon is known as *lateral epicondylitis*, *lateral epicondylosis*, or *tennis elbow*.

7

Muscles of the Wrist Joint

CHAPTER **OUTLINE**

CHAPTER **OVERVIEW**

The muscles addressed in this chapter are the muscles whose principal function is usually considered to be movement of the wrist joint. Other muscles in the body can also move the wrist joint, but they are placed in different chapters because their primary function is usually considered to be at another joint. These muscles are the extrinsic finger joint muscles and are covered in Chapter 8.

Overview of Structure

☐ Structurally, muscles of the wrist joint are divided into two superficial groups, each one containing three muscles.

☐ The wrist flexor group is located anteriorly and attaches proximally to the medial epicondyle of the humerus via the common flexor tendon.

☐ The wrist extensor group is located posteriorly and two of the three muscles in this group attach proximally to the lateral epicondyle of the humerus via the common extensor tendon. The third one attaches proximally to the lateral supracondylar ridge of the humerus, just proximal to the lateral epicondyle.

☐ The wrist flexor group is composed of the flexor carpi radialis, palmaris longus, and flexor carpi ulnaris. The wrist extensor group is composed of the extensor carpi radialis longus, extensor carpi radialis brevis, and extensor carpi ulnaris. The extensors carpi radialis longus and brevis (along with the brachioradialis) are also part of the *radial group* of forearm muscles, sometimes referred to as the *wad of three*.

Overview of Function

The following general rules regarding actions can be stated for the functional groups of muscles of the wrist joint:

☐ If a muscle crosses the wrist joint anteriorly with a vertical direction to its fibers, it can flex the hand at the wrist joint by moving the palmar (anterior) surface of the hand toward the anterior surface of the forearm.

☐ If a muscle crosses the wrist joint posteriorly with a vertical direction to its fibers, it can extend the hand at the wrist joint by moving the dorsal (posterior) surface of the hand toward the posterior surface of the forearm.

☐ If a muscle crosses the wrist joint on the radial side (laterally) with a vertical direction to its fibers, it can radially deviate (abduct) the hand at the wrist joint by moving the radial side of the hand toward the radial side of the forearm.

☐ If a muscle crosses the wrist joint on the ulnar side (medially) with a vertical direction to its fibers, it can ulnar deviate (adduct) the hand at the wrist joint by moving the ulnar side of the hand toward the ulnar side of the forearm.

☐ Reverse actions of these standard mover actions involve the forearm being moved toward the hand at the wrist joint. These reverse actions usually occur when the hand is fixed, such as when holding onto an immovable object.

Review the muscles and bones from this chapter on the enclosed CD!

7

Anterior View of the Muscles of the Right Wrist Joint—Superficial View

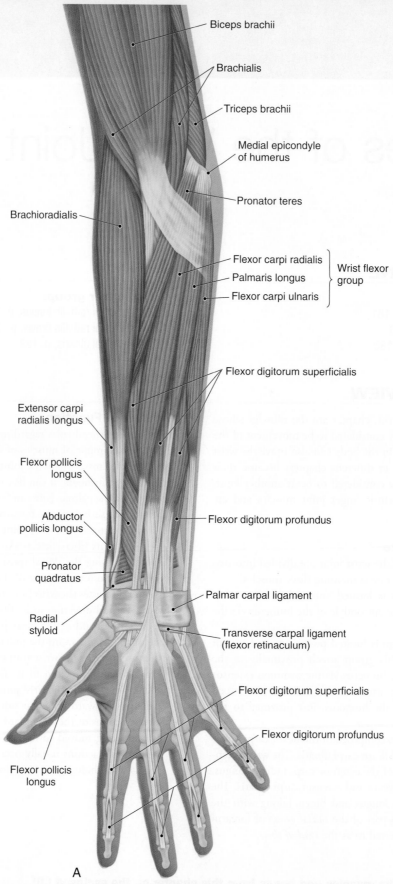

Biceps brachii

Brachialis

Triceps brachii

Medial epicondyle
of humerus

Pronator teres

Brachioradialis

Flexor carpi radialis
Palmaris longus   Wrist flexor
                         group
Flexor carpi ulnaris

Flexor digitorum superficialis

Extensor carpi
radialis longus

Flexor pollicis
longus

Abductor
pollicis longus

Flexor digitorum profundus

Pronator
quadratus

Palmar carpal ligament

Radial
styloid

Transverse carpal ligament
(flexor retinaculum)

Flexor digitorum superficialis

Flexor digitorum profundus

Flexor pollicis
longus

A

Figure 7-1 Anterior views of the muscles of the right wrist joint. **A,** Superficial view.

Anterior View of the Muscles of the Right Wrist Joint—Intermediate View

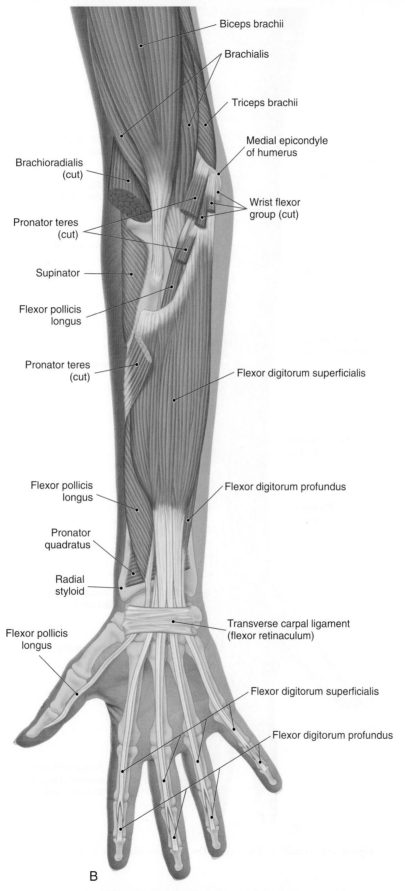

Biceps brachii

Brachialis

Triceps brachii

Medial epicondyle of humerus

Brachioradialis (cut)

Wrist flexor group (cut)

Pronator teres (cut)

Supinator

Flexor pollicis longus

Pronator teres (cut)

Flexor digitorum superficialis

Flexor pollicis longus

Flexor digitorum profundus

Pronator quadratus

Radial styloid

Transverse carpal ligament (flexor retinaculum)

Flexor pollicis longus

Flexor digitorum superficialis

Flexor digitorum profundus

B

Figure 7-1, cont'd B, Intermediate view.

7

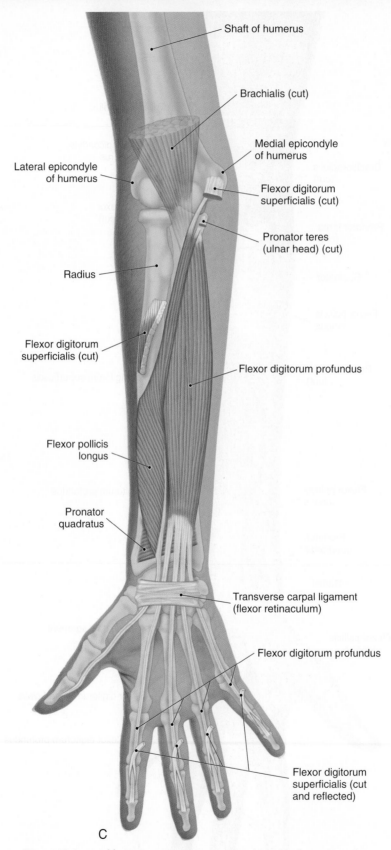

Shaft of humerus

Brachialis (cut)

Medial epicondyle of humerus

Lateral epicondyle of humerus

Flexor digitorum superficialis (cut)

Pronator teres (ulnar head) (cut)

Radius

Flexor digitorum superficialis (cut)

Flexor digitorum profundus

Flexor pollicis longus

Pronator quadratus

Transverse carpal ligament (flexor retinaculum)

Flexor digitorum profundus

Flexor digitorum superficialis (cut and reflected)

C

Figure 7-1, cont'd C, Deep view. The (cut) brachialis has been ghosted in.

Anterior View of the Right Wrist Flexor Group of Muscles

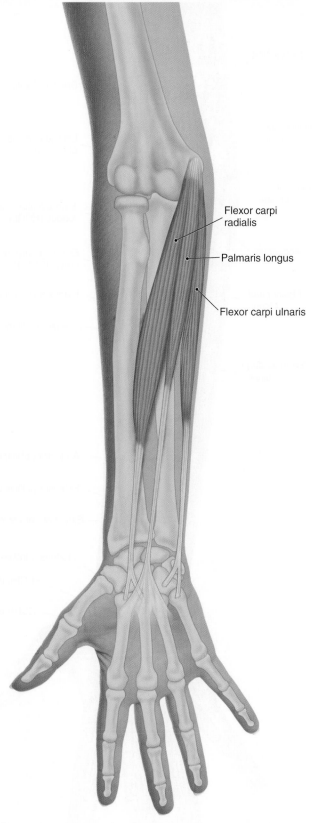

Flexor carpi radialis

Palmaris longus

Flexor carpi ulnaris

Figure 7-2 Anterior view of the right wrist flexor group of muscles.

Posterior View of the Muscles of the Right Wrist Joint—Superficial View

7

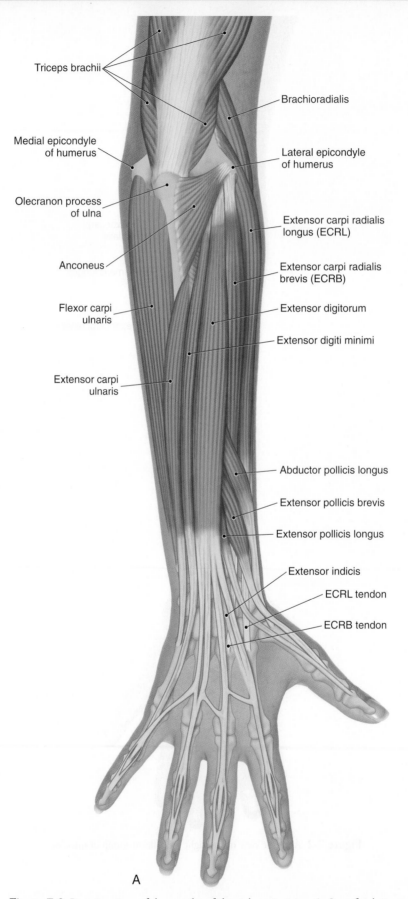

Figure 7-3 Posterior views of the muscles of the right wrist joint. **A,** Superficial view.

Posterior Views of the Muscles of the Right Wrist Joint—Deep Views

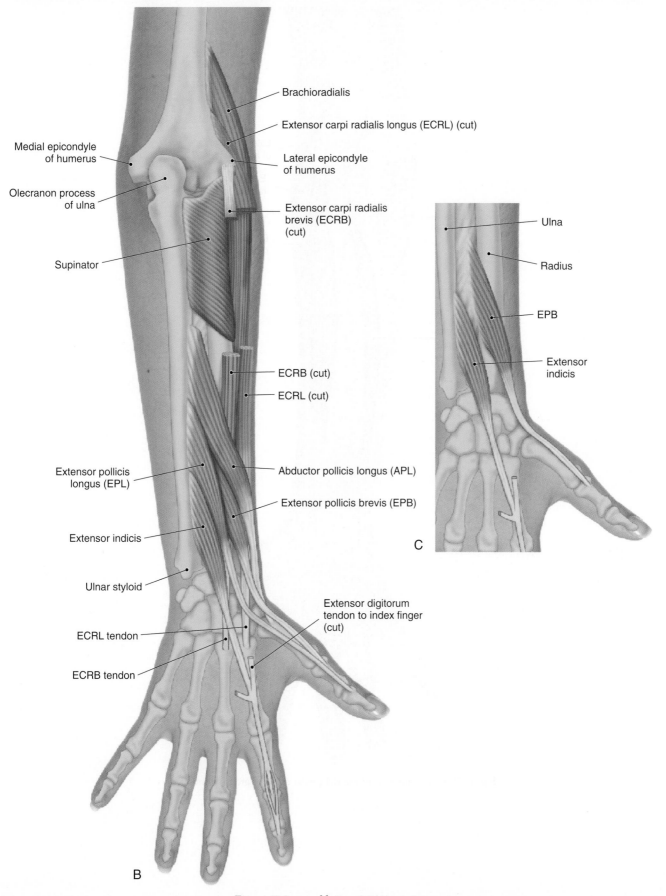

Brachioradialis

Extensor carpi radialis longus (ECRL) (cut)

Medial epicondyle
of humerus

Lateral epicondyle
of humerus

Olecranon process
of ulna

Extensor carpi radialis
brevis (ECRB)
(cut)

Supinator

Ulna

Radius

ECRB (cut)

ECRL (cut)

EPB

Extensor
indicis

Extensor pollicis
longus (EPL)

Abductor pollicis longus (APL)

Extensor pollicis brevis (EPB)

Extensor indicis

C

Ulnar styloid

Extensor digitorum
tendon to index finger
(cut)

ECRL tendon

ECRB tendon

B

Figure 7-3, cont'd B and **C**, Deep views.

7

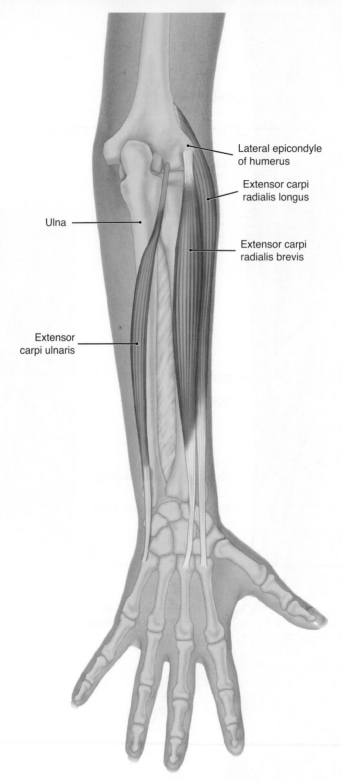

Lateral epicondyle
of humerus

Extensor carpi
radialis longus

Ulna

Extensor carpi
radialis brevis

Extensor
carpi ulnaris

Figure 7-4 Posterior view of the right wrist extensor group of muscles.

Medial View of the Muscles of the Right Wrist Joint

7

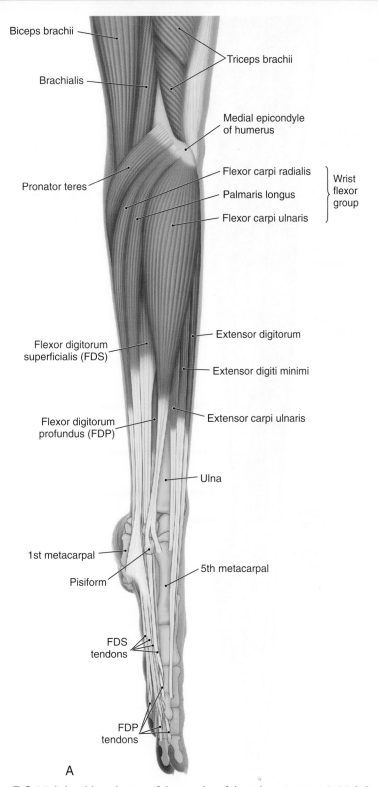

Biceps brachii

Triceps brachii

Brachialis

Medial epicondyle
of humerus

Pronator teres

Flexor carpi radialis ⎤
Palmaris longus ⎬ Wrist flexor group
Flexor carpi ulnaris ⎦

Flexor digitorum
superficialis (FDS)

Extensor digitorum

Extensor digiti minimi

Flexor digitorum
profundus (FDP)

Extensor carpi ulnaris

Ulna

1st metacarpal

5th metacarpal

Pisiform

FDS
tendons

FDP
tendons

A

Figure 7-5 Medial and lateral views of the muscles of the right wrist joint. **A,** Medial view.

Lateral View of the Muscles of the Right Wrist Joint

7

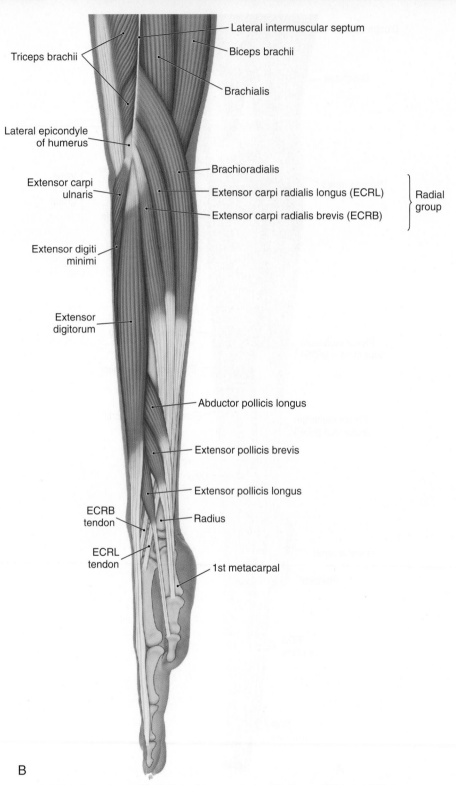

Triceps brachii

Lateral intermuscular septum

Biceps brachii

Brachialis

Lateral epicondyle of humerus

Brachioradialis

Extensor carpi ulnaris

Extensor carpi radialis longus (ECRL)

Extensor carpi radialis brevis (ECRB)

Radial group

Extensor digiti minimi

Extensor digitorum

Abductor pollicis longus

Extensor pollicis brevis

Extensor pollicis longus

ECRB tendon

Radius

ECRL tendon

1st metacarpal

B

Figure 7-5, cont'd B, Lateral view with the elbow joint fully extended.

Lateral View of the Muscles of the Right Wrist Joint—*cont'd*

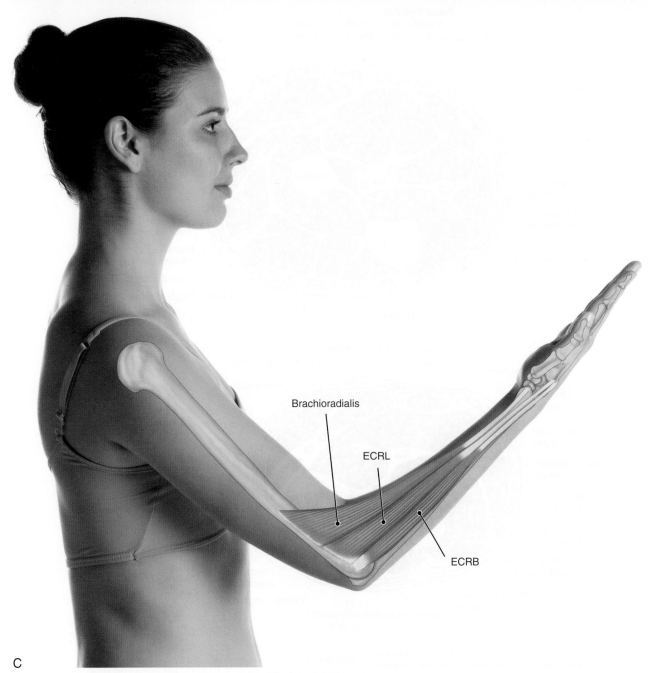

Brachioradialis

ECRL

ECRB

Figure 7-5, cont'd C, Lateral view with the elbow joint flexed. The three muscles of the radial group are shown. ECRL = extensor carpi radialis longus, ECRB = extensor carpi radialis brevis.

Transverse Plane Cross Sections of the Right Forearm

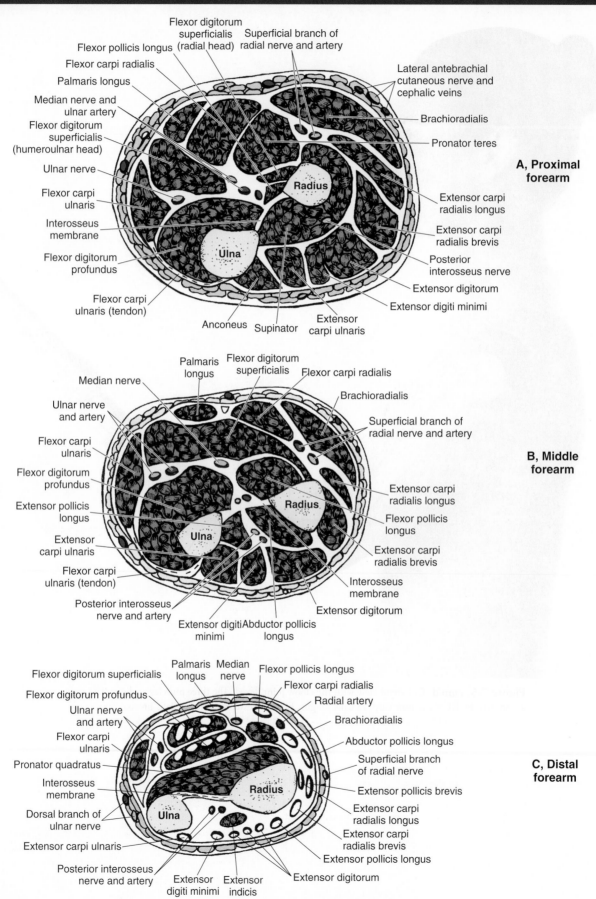

Figure 7-6 A, Proximal. **B,** Middle. **C,** Distal.

Flexor Carpi Radialis (of Wrist Flexor Group)

The name, flexor carpi radialis, *tells us two of its actions:* flexor *tells us that this muscle performs flexion, and* radialis *tells us that this muscle performs radial deviation (abduction). Both of these actions occur at the wrist joint;* carpi *means wrist.*

Derivation	☐ flexor: L. *a muscle that flexes a body part.*
	carpi: L. *of the wrist.*
	radialis: L. *refers to the radial side (of the forearm).*
Pronunciation	☐ FLEKS-or, KAR-pie, RAY-dee-A-lis

■ ATTACHMENTS

☐ **Medial Epicondyle of the Humerus via the Common Flexor Tendon**

to the

☐ **Anterior Hand on the Radial Side**
  ☐ the anterior side of the bases of the second and third metacarpals

■ FUNCTIONS

CONCENTRIC (SHORTENING) MOVER ACTIONS	
Standard Mover Actions	**Reverse Mover Actions**
☐ **1. Flexes the hand at the wrist joint**	☐ 1. Flexes the forearm at the wrist joint
☐ **2. Radially deviates the hand at the wrist joint**	☐ 2. Radially deviates the forearm at the wrist joint
☐ 3. Flexes the forearm at the elbow joint	☐ 3. Flexes the arm at the elbow joint
☐ 4. Pronates the forearm at the RU joints	☐ 4. Pronates the ulna at the RU joints and laterally rotates the arm at the GH joint

RU joints = radioulnar joints; GH joint = glenohumeral joint

Standard Mover Action Notes

- The flexor carpi radialis crosses the wrist joint on the anterior side to attach onto the hand (with its fibers running vertically in the sagittal plane); therefore it flexes the hand at the wrist joint. (action 1)
- The flexor carpi radialis crosses the wrist joint on the radial (lateral) side (with its fibers running vertically in the frontal plane); therefore it radially deviates (abducts) the hand at the wrist joint. (action 2)
- Motion at the wrist joint occurs at the radiocarpal and midcarpal joints. (actions 1, 2)
- All three members of the wrist flexor group (flexor carpi radialis, palmaris longus, and flexor carpi ulnaris) can flex the forearm at the elbow joint because they cross it anteriorly

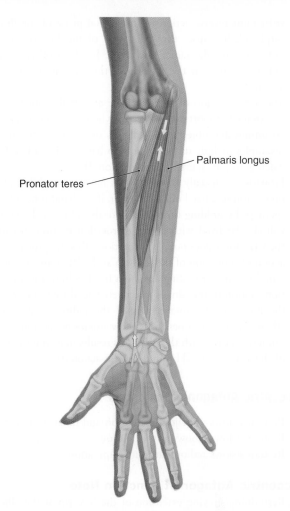

Pronator teres

Palmaris longus

Figure 7-7 Anterior view of the right flexor carpi radialis. The pronator teres and palmaris longus have been ghosted in.

(with their fibers running vertically in the sagittal plane). (action 3)
- Pronation of the forearm at the RU joints usually involves motion of the radius around a fixed ulna. The flexor carpi radialis crosses the RU joints anteriorly in such a way that when it pulls at the lateral hand attachment, it pulls the radial side of the hand anteromedially, thereby pulling the distal radius around the distal ulna. Therefore, the flexor carpi radialis pronates the forearm at the RU joints. Note the similar line of pull to the pronator teres. (action 4)

Reverse Mover Action Notes

- Reverse actions at the wrist joint occur when the hand is fixed by holding onto an immovable object and the forearm moves relative to the fixed hand. The wrist joint reverse action in the sagittal plane of the flexor carpi radialis causes the anterior forearm to be pulled toward the anterior hand, in other words, flexion of the forearm at the wrist joint. The

Flexor Carpi Radialis (of Wrist Flexor Group)—*cont'd*

wrist joint reverse action in the frontal plane of the flexor carpi radialis causes the radial side of the forearm to be pulled toward the radial side of the hand, in other words, radial deviation of the forearm at the wrist joint. (reverse actions 1, 2)

- The reverse action of flexion of the arm at the elbow joint is extremely important and occurs whenever a person grasps an immovable object and pulls his or her body toward it (examples include using a handicap bar or using a handrail when going up stairs). (reverse action 3)
- Pronation is usually thought of as having a mobile radius move around a fixed ulna. However, if the hand is held fixed (perhaps by holding onto an immovable object), the radius will also be fixed with regard to rotation motions because the wrist joint does not allow rotation. Therefore the reverse action of pronation of the forearm at the RU joints involves a mobile ulna pronating around a fixed radius. This pronation motion of the ulna is effectively lateral rotation. When the ulna laterally rotates around the radius, because the elbow joint also does not allow rotation motions, the humerus moves with the ulna; this results in lateral rotation of the arm at the GH joint. (reverse action 4)

Eccentric Antagonist Functions

1. Restrains/slows wrist joint extension and ulnar deviation
2. Restrains/slows elbow joint extension
3. Restrains/slows radioulnar joints supination

Eccentric Antagonist Function Note

- Restraining/slowing extension of the forearm at the elbow joint is extremely important when lowering an object in a careful and controlled manner.

Isometric Stabilization Functions

1. Stabilizes the wrist joint
2. Stabilizes the elbow joint
3. Stabilizes the RU joints

INNERVATION
- The Median Nerve
  - C6, C7

ARTERIAL SUPPLY
- The Ulnar and Radial Arteries (terminal branches of the Brachial Artery)

PALPATION

1. With the client seated or supine, place palpating hand across the anterior wrist.
2. Have the client actively flex and/or radially deviate (abduct) the hand at the wrist joint and look and feel for the distal tendon of the flexor carpi radialis on the radial (lateral) side (slightly lateral to the distal tendon of the palmaris longus, which is located dead center in the anterior wrist). Resistance can be added.
3. Continue palpating the flexor carpi radialis proximally toward the medial epicondyle of the humerus.
4. To distinguish the flexor carpi radialis from the palmaris longus and the other muscles of the common flexor tendon, radial deviation is the best action to ask the client to perform.

■ RELATIONSHIP TO OTHER STRUCTURES

- The flexor carpi radialis is superficial in the anterior forearm.
- Proximally, the flexor carpi radialis is medial to the pronator teres. More distally, the flexor carpi radialis is medial to the brachioradialis.
- The flexor carpi radialis is lateral to the palmaris longus.
- The flexor carpi radialis is superficial to the flexor digitorum superficialis.
- The flexor carpi radialis is located within the superficial front arm line myofascial meridian.

■ MISCELLANEOUS

1. The flexor carpi radialis, palmaris longus, and flexor carpi ulnaris are often grouped together as the *wrist flexor group* of the forearm.
2. The flexor carpi radialis arises proximally from the medial epicondyle of the humerus via the common flexor tendon. The common flexor tendon is the common proximal attachment of five muscles: the pronator teres, flexor carpi radialis, palmaris longus, flexor carpi ulnaris, and the flexor digitorum superficialis.
3. Overuse of the flexor carpi radialis can cause irritation and/or inflammation of the medial epicondyle and/or the common flexor tendon. This is known as *medial epicondylitis, medial epicondylosis,* or *golfer's elbow.*

Palmaris Longus (of Wrist Flexor Group)

The name, palmaris longus, *tells us that this muscle attaches into the palm of the hand and is long (longer than the palmaris brevis).*

Derivation	☐ palmaris: L. *refers to the palm.*
	☐ longus: L. *longer.*
Pronunciation	☐ pall-MA-ris, LONG-us

■ ATTACHMENTS

☐ **Medial Epicondyle of the Humerus via the Common Flexor Tendon**

to the

☐ **Palm of the Hand**
   ☐ the palmar aponeurosis and the flexor retinaculum

■ FUNCTIONS

CONCENTRIC (SHORTENING) MOVER ACTIONS	
Standard Mover Actions	**Reverse Mover Actions**
☐ **1. Flexes the hand at the wrist joint**	☐ 1. Flexes the forearm at the wrist joint
☐ 2. Wrinkles the skin of the palm	
☐ 3. Flexes the forearm at the elbow joint	☐ 2. Flexes the arm at the elbow joint
☐ 4. Pronates the forearm at the RU joints	☐ 3. Pronates the ulna at the RU joints and laterally rotates the arm at the GH joint
☐ 5. Ulnar deviates the hand at the wrist joint	☐ 4. Ulnar deviates the forearm at the wrist joint
☐ 6. Radially deviates the hand at the wrist joint	☐ 5. Radially deviates the forearm at the wrist joint

RU joints = radioulnar joints; GH joint = glenohumeral joint

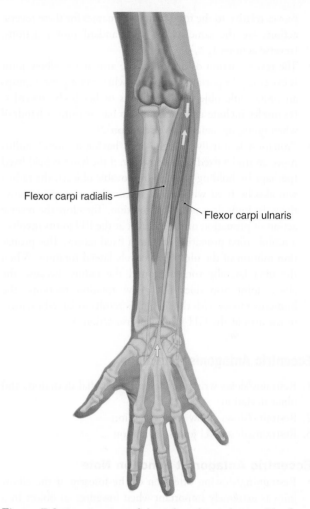

Flexor carpi radialis

Flexor carpi ulnaris

Figure 7-8 Anterior view of the right palmaris longus. The flexor carpi radialis and flexor carpi ulnaris have been ghosted in.

Standard Mover Action Notes

- The palmaris longus crosses the wrist on the anterior side to attach onto the hand (with its fibers running vertically in the sagittal plane); therefore it flexes the hand at the wrist joint. (action 1)
- When the palmaris longus pulls on its distal attachment, if the wrist joint does not flex (perhaps because it is stabilized by a wrist joint extensor muscle), it pulls on the palmar aponeurosis, causing the skin of the palm to wrinkle. This helps to create a slightly stronger grip on an object that is being held. (action 2)
- All three members of the wrist flexor group (flexor carpi radialis, palmaris longus, and flexor carpi ulnaris) can flex the forearm at the elbow joint because they cross it anteriorly (with their fibers running vertically in the sagittal plane). (action 3)
- Pronation of the forearm at the RU joints usually involves motion of the radius around a fixed ulna. The palmaris

longus crosses from the medial elbow region to attach more laterally into the palm of the hand. It crosses the RU joints anteriorly in such a way that when it pulls at the more lateral hand attachment, it pulls the radial side of the hand antero-medially, thereby pulling the distal radius around the distal ulna, in other words, pronation of the forearm at the RU joints. (action 4)
- The palmaris longus can only ulnar deviate (adduct) the wrist joint if it is first in radial deviation. The palmaris longus can only radially deviate (abduct) the wrist joint if it is first in ulnar deviation. (actions 5, 6)
- Motion at the wrist joint occurs at the radiocarpal and midcarpal joints. (actions 1, 5, 6)

Reverse Mover Action Notes

- Reverse actions at the wrist joint occur when the hand is fixed by holding onto an immovable object and the forearm

Palmaris Longus (of Wrist Flexor Group)—*cont'd*

moves relative to the fixed hand. The names for these reverse actions are the same as for the standard mover actions. (reverse actions 1, 4, 5)

- The reverse action of flexion of the arm at the elbow joint is extremely important and occurs whenever a person grasps an immovable object and pulls his or her body toward it (examples include using a handicap bar or using a handrail when going up stairs). (reverse action 2)
- Pronation is usually thought of as having a mobile radius move around a fixed ulna. However, if the hand is held fixed (perhaps by holding onto an immovable object), the radius will also be fixed with regard to rotation motions because the wrist joint does not allow rotation. Therefore the reverse action of pronation of the forearm at the RU joints involves a mobile ulna pronating around a fixed radius. This pronation motion of the ulna is effectively lateral rotation. When the ulna laterally rotates around the radius, because the elbow joint also does not allow rotation motions, the humerus moves with the ulna; this results in lateral rotation of the arm at the GH joint. (reverse action 3)

Eccentric Antagonist Functions

1. Restrains/slows wrist joint extension, radial deviation, and ulnar deviation
2. Restrains/slows elbow joint extension
3. Restrains/slows RU joints supination

Eccentric Antagonist Function Note

- Restraining/slowing extension of the forearm at the elbow joint is extremely important when lowering an object in a careful and controlled manner.

Isometric Stabilization Functions

1. Stabilizes the wrist joint
2. Stabilizes the elbow joint
3. Stabilizes the RU joints

INNERVATION
- ☐ The Median Nerve
  - ☐ C7, C8

ARTERIAL SUPPLY
- ☐ The Ulnar Artery (a terminal branch of the Brachial Artery)

✋ PALPATION

1. The palmaris longus is superficial and easy to palpate.
2. With the client seated or supine, place palpating hand on the anterior wrist.
3. Ask the client to cup the hand (by bringing the thenar eminence toward the hypothenar eminence) and/or flex the hand at the wrist joint against resistance with the fingers fully extended, and look and feel for the distal tendon of the palmaris longus in the center of the anterior wrist. Resistance can be added.
4. Continue palpating the palmaris longus distally into the palmar fascia and proximally toward the medial epicondyle of the humerus. It is difficult to distinguish the proximal tendon of the palmaris longus from the proximal tendons of the other muscles of the common flexor tendon.

■ RELATIONSHIP TO OTHER STRUCTURES

- ☐ The palmaris longus is superficial in the anteromedial forearm.
- ☐ The palmaris longus is medial to the flexor carpi radialis.
- ☐ Proximally, the palmaris longus is lateral to the flexor carpi ulnaris. More distally, the palmaris longus is lateral to the flexor digitorum superficialis.
- ☐ The palmaris longus is located within the superficial front arm line myofascial meridian.

■ MISCELLANEOUS

1. The flexor carpi radialis, palmaris longus, and flexor carpi ulnaris are often grouped together as the *wrist flexor group* of the forearm.
2. The palmaris longus arises proximally from the medial epicondyle of the humerus via the common flexor tendon. The common flexor tendon is the common proximal attachment of five muscles: the pronator teres, flexor carpi radialis, palmaris longus, flexor carpi ulnaris, and flexor digitorum superficialis.
3. The palmaris longus is the only muscle of the anterior forearm with a tendon that is superficial to the flexor retinaculum.
4. Irritation and/or inflammation of the medial epicondyle and/or the common flexor tendon is known as *medial epicondylitis*, *medial epicondylosis*, or *golfer's elbow*.
5. In many individuals, the palmaris longus is bilaterally or unilaterally absent.

Flexor Carpi Ulnaris (of Wrist Flexor Group)

The name, flexor carpi ulnaris, *tells us two of its actions:* flexor *tells us that this muscle performs flexion, and* ulnaris *tells us that this muscle performs ulnar deviation (adduction). Both of these actions occur at the wrist joint;* carpi *means wrist.*

Derivation	☐ flexor: L. *a muscle that flexes a body part.*
	carpi: L. *of the wrist.*
	ulnaris: L. *refers to the ulnar side* (of the forearm).
Pronunciation	☐ FLEKS-or, KAR-pie, ul-NA-ris

■ ATTACHMENTS

☐ **Medial Epicondyle of the Humerus via the Common Flexor Tendon, and the Ulna**
  ☐ the medial margin of the olecranon and the posterior proximal ⅔ of the ulna

to the

☐ **Anterior Hand on the Ulnar Side**
  ☐ the pisiform, the hook of the hamate, and the base of the fifth metacarpal

■ FUNCTIONS

CONCENTRIC (SHORTENING) MOVER ACTIONS	
Standard Mover Actions	**Reverse Mover Actions**
☐ **1. Flexes the hand at the wrist joint**	☐ 1. Flexes the forearm at the wrist joint
☐ **2. Ulnar deviates the hand at the wrist joint**	☐ 2. Ulnar deviates the forearm at the wrist joint
☐ 3. Flexes the forearm at the elbow joint	☐ 3. Flexes the arm at the elbow joint

Standard Mover Action Notes

- The flexor carpi ulnaris crosses the wrist joint on the anterior side to attach onto the hand (with its fibers running vertically in the sagittal plane); therefore it flexes the hand at the wrist joint. (action 1)
- The flexor carpi ulnaris crosses the wrist joint on the ulnar (medial) side (with its fibers running vertically in the frontal plane); therefore it ulnar deviates (adducts) the hand at the wrist joint. (action 2)
- Motion at the wrist joint occurs at the radiocarpal and midcarpal joints. (actions 1, 2)
- All three members of the wrist flexor group (flexor carpi radialis, palmaris longus, and flexor carpi ulnaris) can flex the forearm at the elbow joint because they cross it anteriorly (with their fibers running vertically in the sagittal plane). (action 3)

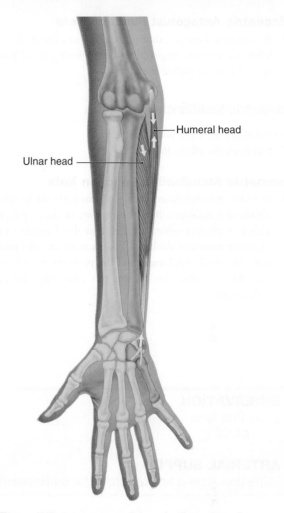

Figure 7-9 Anterior view of the right flexor carpi ulnaris.

Reverse Mover Action Notes

- Reverse actions at the wrist joint occur when the hand is fixed by holding onto an immovable object and the forearm moves relative to the fixed hand. The flexor carpi ulnaris' sagittal plane reverse action is flexion of the forearm at the wrist joint. Its frontal plane reverse action is ulnar deviation of the forearm at the wrist joint. (reverse actions 1, 2)
- The reverse action of flexion of the arm at the elbow joint is extremely important and occurs whenever a person grasps an immovable object and pulls his or her body toward it (examples include using a handicap bar or using a handrail when going up stairs). (reverse action 3)

Eccentric Antagonist Functions

1. Restrains/slows wrist joint extension and radial deviation
2. Restrains/slows elbow joint extension

Flexor Carpi Ulnaris (of Wrist Flexor Group)—*cont'd*

Eccentric Antagonist Function Note

- Restraining/slowing extension of the forearm at the elbow joint is extremely important when lowering an object in a careful and controlled manner.

Isometric Stabilization Functions

1. Stabilizes the wrist joint
2. Stabilizes the elbow joint

Isometric Stabilization Function Note

- In addition to stabilizing the wrist joint itself, the flexor carpi ulnaris also stabilizes the pisiform bone of the carpal group. This is important when the abductor digiti minimi manus (intrinsic muscle of the hand) contracts because the pisiform is its proximal attachment and the pisiform must be stabilized/fixed so that this muscle can efficiently abduct the little finger.

INNERVATION

- The Ulnar Nerve
  - **C7**, C8

ARTERIAL SUPPLY

- The Ulnar Artery (a terminal branch of the Brachial Artery)

 PALPATION

1. With the client seated or supine, place palpating hand across the anterior wrist.
2. Have the client actively flex and/or ulnar deviate (adduct) the hand at the wrist joint and feel for the distal tendon of the flexor carpi ulnaris on the ulnar (medial) side of the anterior wrist. Resistance can be added.
3. Continue palpating the flexor carpi ulnaris distally toward the pisiform, and proximally toward the medial epicondyle of the humerus and the posterior ulna.
4. To distinguish the flexor carpi ulnaris from the palmaris longus and the other muscles of the common flexor tendon, ulnar deviation is the best action to ask the client to perform.

■ RELATIONSHIP TO OTHER STRUCTURES

- The flexor carpi ulnaris is superficial in the medial forearm.
- The flexor carpi ulnaris is anterior to the extensor carpi ulnaris.
- Proximally, the flexor carpi ulnaris is medial to the palmaris longus. More distally, the flexor carpi ulnaris is medial to the flexor digitorum superficialis.
- From the medial perspective, the flexor carpi ulnaris is superficial to the flexor digitorum superficialis and the flexor digitorum profundus.
- The flexor carpi ulnaris is located within the superficial front arm line myofascial meridian.

■ MISCELLANEOUS

1. The flexor carpi radialis, palmaris longus, and flexor carpi ulnaris are often grouped together as the *wrist flexor group* of the forearm.
2. The flexor carpi ulnaris arises proximally from the medial epicondyle of the humerus via the common flexor tendon. The common flexor tendon is the common proximal attachment of five muscles: the pronator teres, flexor carpi radialis, palmaris longus, flexor carpi ulnaris, and flexor digitorum superficialis.
3. The flexor carpi ulnaris has two heads: a humeral head and an ulnar head. The humeral head is much larger in mass than the ulnar head (the ulnar head is very thin).
4. The ulnar head attachment of the flexor carpi ulnaris blends with the ulnar attachments of the extensor carpi ulnaris and the flexor digitorum profundus.
5. Some sources describe the distal tendon of the flexor carpi ulnaris ending at the pisiform, with the pull of its contraction passing onto the hamate and the fifth metacarpal via the pisohamate and pisometacarpal ligaments.
6. The ulnar nerve passes between the two heads of the flexor carpi ulnaris. Compression of the ulnar nerve between the two heads of the flexor carpi ulnaris is called *cubital tunnel syndrome*.
7. The flexor carpi ulnaris is the only muscle of the anterior forearm that is innervated by the ulnar nerve instead of the median nerve. (The flexor digitorum profundus is innervated by both the median and ulnar nerves [and the brachioradialis is innervated by the radial nerve].)
8. Overuse of the flexor carpi ulnaris can cause irritation and/or inflammation of the medial epicondyle and/or the common flexor tendon. This is known as *medial epicondylitis*, *medial epicondylosis*, or *golfer's elbow*.

Extensor Carpi Radialis Longus (of Wrist Extensor and Radial Groups)

The name, extensor carpi radialis longus, *tells us two of its actions:* extensor *tells us that this muscle performs extension, and* radialis *tells us that this muscle performs radial deviation (abduction). Both of these actions occur at the wrist joint;* carpi *means wrist.* Longus *tells us that this muscle is long (longer than the extensor carpi radialis brevis).*

Derivation	□ extensor: L. *a muscle that extends a body part.*
	carpi: L. *of the wrist.*
	radialis: L. *refers to the radial side (of the forearm).*
	longus: L. *longer.*
Pronunciation	□ eks-TEN-sor, KAR-pie, RAY-dee-A-lis, LONG-us

■ ATTACHMENTS

□ **Lateral Supracondylar Ridge of the Humerus**
  □ the distal ⅓

to the

□ **Posterior Hand on the Radial Side**
  □ the posterior side of the base of the second metacarpal

■ FUNCTIONS

CONCENTRIC (SHORTENING) MOVER ACTIONS	
Standard Mover Actions	**Reverse Mover Actions**
□ **1. Extends the hand at the wrist joint**	□ 1. Extends the forearm at the wrist joint
□ **2. Radially deviates the hand at the wrist joint**	□ 2. Radially deviates the forearm at the wrist joint
□ 3. Flexes the forearm at the elbow joint	□ 3. Flexes the arm at the elbow joint
□ 4. Pronates the forearm at the RU joints	□ 4. Pronates the ulna at the RU joints and laterally rotates the arm at the GH joint
□ 5. Supinates the forearm at the RU joints	□ 5. Supinates the ulna at the RU joints and medially rotates the arm at the GH joint

RU joints = radioulnar joints; GH joint = glenohumeral joint

Standard Mover Action Notes

- The extensor carpi radialis longus crosses the wrist joint posteriorly to attach onto the hand (with its fibers running vertically in the sagittal plane); therefore it extends the hand at the wrist joint. (action 1)
- The extensor carpi radialis longus crosses the wrist joint on the radial (lateral) side (with its fibers running vertically in the frontal plane). Therefore the extensor carpi radialis

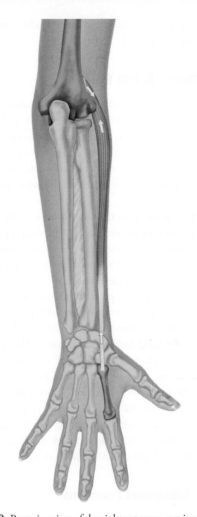

Figure 7-10 Posterior view of the right extensor carpi radialis longus.

longus radially deviates (abducts) the hand at the wrist joint. (action 2)

- The extensor carpi radialis longus crosses the wrist joint posteriorly, so it is an extensor of the wrist joint. However, it crosses the elbow joint anteriorly, so it flexes the elbow joint. (actions 1, 3)
- Similar to the nearby brachioradialis, the extensor carpi radialis longus can both pronate and supinate the forearm at the RU joints. However, it can only pronate a supinated forearm to a position that is approximately halfway between full supination and full pronation; and it can only supinate a pronated forearm to a position that is approximately halfway between full supination and full pronation. This halfway position is the position that has its attachments closest to each other. This is an example of a muscle that has one line of pull but can have two opposite actions at the same joint based on the position of the joint when the muscle contracts. (actions 4, 5)
- Pronation/supination of the forearm at the radioulnar joints usually involves motion of the radius around a fixed ulna. (actions 4, 5)

Extensor Carpi Radialis Longus (of Wrist Extensor and Radial Groups)—*cont'd*

- Motion at the wrist joint occurs at the radiocarpal and mid-carpal joints. (actions 1, 2)

Reverse Mover Action Notes

- Reverse actions at the wrist joint occur when the hand is fixed by holding onto an immovable object and the forearm moves relative to the fixed hand. The extensor carpi radialis longus' sagittal plane reverse action is extension of the forearm at the wrist joint. Its frontal plane reverse action is radial deviation of the forearm at the wrist joint. (reverse actions 1, 2)
- The reverse action of flexion of the arm at the elbow joint is extremely important and occurs whenever a person grasps an immovable object and pulls his or her body toward it (examples include using a handicap bar or using a handrail when going up stairs). (reverse action 3)
- The reverse actions of pronation/supination of the ulna around a fixed radius usually occurs only if the hand is fixed by holding onto an immovable object and the ulna moves relative to the fixed radius. Pronation of the ulna is effectively lateral rotation; supination of the ulna is effectively medial rotation. Because the elbow joint does not allow rotation, the humerus will have to move with the ulna. For this reason, the reverse action of forearm pronation causes the arm to laterally rotate at the GH joint; and the reverse action of forearm supination causes the arm to medially rotate at the GH joint. (reverse actions 4, 5)

Eccentric Antagonist Functions

1. Restrains/slows wrist joint flexion and ulnar deviation
2. Restrains/slows elbow joint extension
3. Restrains/slows RU joints supination and pronation

Eccentric Antagonist Function Note

- Restraining/slowing extension of the forearm at the elbow joint is extremely important when lowering an object in a careful and controlled manner.

Isometric Stabilization Functions

1. Stabilizes the wrist joint
2. Stabilizes the elbow joint
3. Stabilizes the RU joints

Isometric Stabilization Function Note

- Stabilizing the wrist joint is an important action of the extensor carpi radialis longus. Whenever the flexors digitorum superficialis and profundus contract to make a fist, wrist joint extensor muscles such as the extensor carpi radialis longus must contract to prevent these finger flexor muscles from also flexing the hand at the wrist joint.

INNERVATION
- ☐ The Radial Nerve
  - ☐ C5, **C6**

ARTERIAL SUPPLY
- ☐ Branches of the Brachial Artery (the continuation of the Axillary Artery) and the Radial Artery (a terminal branch of the Brachial Artery)

✋ PALPATION

1. With the client seated or supine, place palpating hand posterior to the belly of the brachioradialis.
2. Ask the client to radially deviate the hand at the wrist joint and feel for the contraction of the extensor carpi radialis longus.
3. Continue palpating the extensor carpi radialis longus proximally toward the lateral supracondylar ridge of the humerus and distally to the second metacarpal. (Note: Discerning between the extensor carpi radialis longus and extensor carpi radialis brevis is challenging.)

■ RELATIONSHIP TO OTHER STRUCTURES

- ☐ The extensor carpi radialis longus lies directly posterior to the brachioradialis and directly anterior to the extensor carpi radialis brevis.
- ☐ The extensor carpi radialis longus is superficial, except for a small part that is deep to the brachioradialis proximally and a portion of its distal tendon that is deep to the abductor pollicis longus, extensor pollicis brevis, and extensor pollicis longus.
- ☐ The extensor carpi radialis longus is located within the superficial back arm line myofascial meridian.

■ MISCELLANEOUS

1. The extensor carpi radialis longus, extensor carpi radialis brevis, and extensor carpi ulnaris are often grouped together as the *wrist extensor group* of the forearm.
2. The extensor carpi radialis longus, the extensor carpi radialis brevis, and the brachioradialis are often grouped together as the *radial group* of forearm muscles. This group is also known as the *wad of three*.

Extensor Carpi Radialis Brevis (of Wrist Extensor and Radial Groups)

The name, extensor carpi radialis brevis, *tells us two of its actions:* extensor *tells us that this muscle performs extension, and* radialis *tells us that this muscle performs radial deviation (abduction). Both of these actions occur at the wrist joint;* carpi *means wrist.* Brevis *tells us that this muscle is short (shorter than the extensor carpi radialis longus).*

Derivation	☐ extensor: L. *a muscle that extends a body part.*
	carpi: L. *of the wrist.*
	radialis: L. *refers to the radial side (of the forearm).*
	brevis: L. *shorter.*
Pronunciation	☐ eks-TEN-sor, KAR-pie, RAY-dee-A-lis, BRE-vis

■ ATTACHMENTS

☐ **Lateral Epicondyle of the Humerus via the Common Extensor Tendon**

to the

☐ **Posterior Hand on the Radial Side**
  ☐ the posterior side of the base of the third metacarpal

■ FUNCTIONS

CONCENTRIC (SHORTENING) MOVER ACTIONS	
Standard Mover Actions	**Reverse Mover Actions**
☐ **1. Extends the hand at the wrist joint**	☐ 1. Extends the forearm at the wrist joint
☐ **2. Radially deviates the hand at the wrist joint**	☐ 2. Radially deviates the forearm at the wrist joint
☐ 3. Flexes the forearm at the elbow joint	☐ 3. Flexes the arm at the elbow joint
☐ 4. Pronates the forearm at the RU joints	☐ 4. Pronates the ulna at the RU joints and laterally rotates the arm at the GH joint
☐ 5. Supinates the forearm at the RU joints	☐ 5. Supinates the ulna at the RU joints and medially rotates the arm at the GH joint

RU joints = radioulnar joints; GH joints = glenohumeral joints

Standard Mover Action Notes

- The extensor carpi radialis brevis crosses the wrist joint posteriorly to attach onto the hand (with its fibers running vertically in the sagittal plane); therefore it extends the hand at the wrist joint. (action 1)
- The extensor carpi radialis brevis crosses the wrist joint on the radial (lateral) side (with its fibers running vertically in

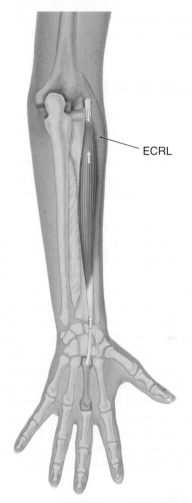

Figure 7-11 Posterior view of the right extensor carpi radialis brevis. The extensor carpi radialis longus (ECRL) has been ghosted in.

the frontal plane); therefore it radially deviates (abducts) the hand at the wrist joint. (action 2)
- Motion at the wrist joint occurs at the radiocarpal and midcarpal joints. (actions 1, 2)
- The extensor carpi radialis brevis crosses the wrist joint posteriorly, so it is an extensor of the wrist joint. However, it crosses the elbow joint anteriorly, so it flexes the elbow joint. (actions 1, 3)
- Similar to the nearby brachioradialis, the extensor carpi radialis brevis can both pronate and supinate the forearm at the RU joints. However, it can only pronate a supinated forearm to a position that is approximately halfway between full supination and full pronation; and it can only supinate a pronated forearm to a position that is approximately halfway between full supination and full pronation. This halfway position is the position that has its attachments closest to each other. This is an example of a muscle that has one line of pull but can have two opposite actions at the same joint based on the position of the joint when the muscle contracts. (actions 4, 5)

Extensor Carpi Radialis Brevis (of Wrist Extensor and Radial Groups)—*cont'd*

- Pronation/supination of the forearm at the RU joints usually involves motion of the radius around a fixed ulna. (actions 4, 5)

Reverse Mover Action Notes

- Reverse actions at the wrist joint occur when the hand is fixed by holding onto an immovable object and the forearm moves relative to the fixed hand. The extensor carpi radialis brevis' sagittal plane reverse action is extension of the forearm at the wrist joint. Its frontal plane reverse action is radial deviation of the forearm at the wrist joint. (reverse actions 1, 2)
- The reverse action of flexion of the arm at the elbow joint is extremely important and occurs whenever a person grasps an immovable object and pulls his or her body toward it (examples include using a handicap bar or using a handrail when going up stairs). (reverse action 3)
- The reverse actions of pronation/supination of the ulna around a fixed radius usually occurs only if the hand is fixed by holding onto an immovable object and the ulna moves relative to the fixed radius. Pronation of the ulna is effectively lateral rotation; supination of the ulna is effectively medial rotation. Because the elbow joint does not allow rotation, the humerus will have to move with the ulna. For this reason, the reverse action of forearm pronation causes the arm to laterally rotate at the GH joint; and the reverse action of forearm supination causes the arm to medially rotate at the GH joint. (reverse actions 4, 5)

Eccentric Antagonist Functions

1. Restrains/slows wrist joint flexion and ulnar deviation
2. Restrains/slows elbow joint extension
3. Restrains/slows RU joints supination and pronation

Eccentric Antagonist Function Note

- Restraining/slowing extension of the forearm at the elbow joint is extremely important when lowering an object in a careful and controlled manner.

Isometric Stabilization Functions

1. Stabilizes the wrist joint
2. Stabilizes the elbow joint
3. Stabilizes the RU joints

Isometric Stabilization Function Note

- Stabilizing the wrist joint is an important action of the extensor carpi radialis brevis. Whenever the flexors digitorum superficialis and profundus contract to make a fist, wrist joint extensor muscles such as the extensor carpi radialis brevis must contract to prevent these finger flexor muscles from also flexing the hand at the wrist joint. Of all wrist joint extensors, the extensor carpi radialis brevis is usually the most active with regard to stabilizing and thereby preventing flexion of the hand at the wrist joint.

INNERVATION
- The Radial Nerve
  - posterior interosseus nerve, **C7**, C8

ARTERIAL SUPPLY
- Branches of the Brachial Artery (the continuation of the Axillary Artery)
  - and the Radial Artery (a terminal branch of the Brachial Artery)

✋ PALPATION

1. With the client seated or supine, pinch the radial group of the forearm muscles (brachioradialis, extensor carpi radialis longus, and extensor carpi radialis brevis) with your thumb on one side and your index and middle fingers on the other side, and pull it slightly away from the forearm. The fingers on the posterior aspect of the radial group are on the extensor carpi radialis brevis.
2. Have the client radially deviate the hand at the wrist joint and feel for the contraction of the extensor carpi radialis brevis. (Note: Discerning between the extensor carpi radialis brevis and extensor carpi radialis longus is challenging.)
3. The distal tendon of the extensor carpi radialis brevis can be visualized and easily palpated on the radial side of the posterior wrist when the client makes a fist (flexes the fingers) with the wrist in neutral position (or in slight extension).

■ RELATIONSHIP TO OTHER STRUCTURES

- The extensor carpi radialis brevis is superficial, except for a small part that is deep to the brachioradialis and the extensor carpi radialis longus proximally and a portion of its distal tendon, which is deep to the abductor pollicis longus, extensor pollicis brevis, and extensor pollicis longus. The actual distal attachment onto the third metacarpal is deep to the distal tendon of the extensor indicis.
- The extensor carpi radialis brevis lies directly posterior to the extensor carpi radialis longus and directly anterior to the extensor digitorum.
- The extensor carpi radialis brevis is located within the superficial back arm line myofascial meridian.

■ MISCELLANEOUS

1. The extensor carpi radialis longus, extensor carpi radialis brevis, and extensor carpi ulnaris are often grouped together as the *wrist extensor group* of the forearm.

Extensor Carpi Radialis Brevis (of Wrist Extensor and Radial Groups)—*cont'd*

2. The extensor carpi radialis brevis, the extensor carpi radialis longus, and the brachioradialis are often grouped together as the *radial group* of forearm muscles. This group is also known as the *wad of three*.

3. The extensor carpi radialis brevis arises proximally from the lateral epicondyle of the humerus via the common extensor tendon. The common extensor tendon is the common proximal attachment of four muscles: the extensor carpi radialis brevis, extensor digitorum, extensor digiti minimi, and extensor carpi ulnaris. (The anconeus and the supinator also arise from the lateral epicondyle of the humerus, but not from the common extensor tendon.)

4. Overuse of the extensor carpi radialis brevis can cause irritation and/or inflammation of the lateral epicondyle and/or the common extensor tendon. This is known as *lateral epicondylitis*, *lateral epicondylosis*, or *tennis elbow*.

7

Extensor Carpi Ulnaris (of Wrist Extensor Group)

The name, extensor carpi ulnaris, *tells us two of its actions:* extensor *tells us that this muscle performs extension, and* ulnaris *tells us that this muscle performs ulnar deviation (adduction). Both of these actions occur at the wrist joint;* carpi *means wrist.*

Derivation	□ extensor: L. *a muscle that extends a body part.*
	carpi: L. *of the wrist.*
	ulnaris: L. *refers to the ulnar side* (of the forearm).
Pronunciation	□ eks-TEN-sor, KAR-pie, ul-NA-ris

■ ATTACHMENTS

□ **Lateral Epicondyle of the Humerus via the Common Extensor Tendon, and the Ulna**
  □ the posterior middle ⅓ of the ulna

to the

□ **Posterior Hand on the Ulnar Side**
  □ the posterior side of the base of the fifth metacarpal

■ FUNCTIONS

CONCENTRIC (SHORTENING) MOVER ACTIONS	
Standard Mover Actions	**Reverse Mover Actions**
□ **1. Extends the hand at the wrist joint**	□ 1. Extends the forearm at the wrist joint
□ **2. Ulnar deviates the hand at the wrist joint**	□ 2. Ulnar deviates the forearm at the wrist joint
□ 3. Extends the forearm at the elbow joint	□ 3. Extends the arm at the elbow joint
□ 4. Pronates the forearm at the RU joints	□ 4. Pronates the ulna at the RU joints and laterally rotates the arm at the GH joint

RU joints = radioulnar joints; GH joint = glenohumeral joint

Standard Mover Action Notes

- The extensor carpi ulnaris crosses the wrist joint posteriorly to attach onto the hand (with its fibers running vertically in the sagittal plane); therefore it extends the hand at the wrist joint. (action 1)
- The extensor carpi ulnaris crosses the wrist joint on the ulnar (medial) side (with its fibers running vertically in the frontal plane); therefore it ulnar deviates (adducts) the hand at the wrist joint. (action 2)
- Motion at the wrist joint occurs at the radiocarpal and midcarpal joints. (actions 1, 2)
- The extensor carpi ulnaris crosses the elbow joint posteriorly (with its fibers running vertically in the sagittal plane); therefore it extends the forearm at the elbow joint. (action 3)

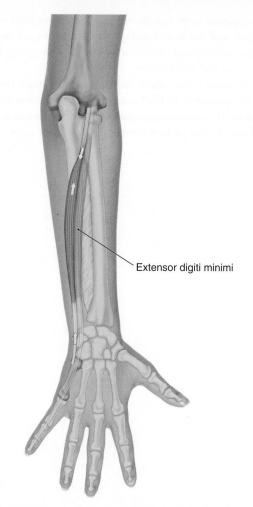

Extensor digiti minimi

Figure 7-12 Posterior view of the right extensor carpi ulnaris. The extensor digiti minimi has been ghosted in.

- The extensor carpi ulnaris can only pronate a supinated forearm to a position that is halfway between full supination and full pronation. Pronation of the forearm at the RU joints usually involves motion of the radius around a fixed ulna. (action 4)

Reverse Mover Action Notes

- Reverse actions at the wrist joint occur when the hand is fixed by holding onto an immovable object and the forearm moves relative to the fixed hand. The extensor carpi ulnaris' sagittal plane reverse action is extension of the forearm at the wrist joint. Its frontal plane reverse action is ulnar deviation of the forearm at the wrist joint. (reverse actions 1, 2)
- The reverse action of pronation of the ulna around a fixed radius usually occurs only if the hand is fixed by holding onto an immovable object and the ulna moves relative to the fixed radius. Pronation of the ulna is effectively lateral rotation. Because the elbow joint does not allow rotation,

Extensor Carpi Ulnaris (of Wrist Extensor Group)—*cont'd*

the humerus will have to move with the ulna. For this reason, the reverse action of forearm pronation causes the arm to laterally rotate at the GH joint. (reverse action 4)

Eccentric Antagonist Functions

1. Restrains/slows wrist joint flexion and radial deviation
2. Restrains/slows elbow joint flexion
3. Restrains/slows RU joints supination

Isometric Stabilization Functions

1. Stabilizes the wrist joint
2. Stabilizes the elbow joint
3. Stabilizes the RU joints

Isometric Stabilization Function Note

• Stabilizing the wrist joint is an important action of the extensor carpi ulnaris. Whenever the flexors digitorum superficialis and profundus contract to make a fist, wrist joint extensor muscles such as the extensor carpi ulnaris must contract to prevent these finger flexor muscles from also flexing the hand at the wrist joint.

INNERVATION
☐ The Radial Nerve
  ☐ posterior interosseus nerve, **C7**, C8

ARTERIAL SUPPLY
☐ The Posterior Interosseus Artery (a branch of the Ulnar Artery)

 PALPATION

1. With the client seated or supine, place palpating hand directly posterior to the shaft of the ulna and feel for the belly of the extensor carpi ulnaris.
2. Continue palpating the extensor carpi ulnaris proximally toward the lateral epicondyle of the humerus and distally toward the fifth metacarpal.
3. To further bring out the extensor carpi ulnaris, have the client ulnar deviate (adduct) the hand at the wrist joint.

■ RELATIONSHIP TO OTHER STRUCTURES

☐ The extensor carpi ulnaris is superficial in the posterior forearm and is medial to the extensor digiti minimi and lateral (posterior) to the medial border of the ulna and the flexor carpi ulnaris.
☐ The anconeus is proximal to the extensor carpi ulnaris.
☐ The extensor carpi ulnaris is superficial to the shaft of the ulna and the deeper layer of posterior forearm muscles, which includes the supinator, abductor pollicis longus, extensor pollicis brevis, extensor pollicis longus, and extensor indicis.
☐ The extensor carpi ulnaris is located within the superficial back arm line myofascial meridian.

■ MISCELLANEOUS

1. The extensor carpi radialis longus, extensor carpi radialis brevis, and extensor carpi ulnaris are often grouped together as the *wrist extensor group* of the forearm.
2. The extensor carpi ulnaris arises proximally from the lateral epicondyle of the humerus via the common extensor tendon. The common extensor tendon is the common proximal attachment of four muscles: the extensor carpi radialis brevis, extensor digitorum, extensor digiti minimi, and extensor carpi ulnaris. (The anconeus and the supinator also arise from the lateral epicondyle of the humerus, but not from the common extensor tendon.)
3. The extensor carpi ulnaris has two heads: a humeral head and an ulnar head. The humeral head is much larger in mass than the ulnar head (the ulnar head is very thin).
4. The attachment of the extensor carpi ulnaris onto the ulna blends with the ulnar attachment of the flexor carpi ulnaris and the flexor digitorum profundus.
5. Overuse of the extensor carpi ulnaris can cause irritation and/or inflammation of the lateral epicondyle and/or the common extensor tendon. This is known as *lateral epicondylitis, lateral epicondylosis,* or *tennis elbow.*

Extrinsic Muscles of the Finger Joints

CHAPTER **OUTLINE**

CHAPTER **OVERVIEW**

The muscles addressed in this chapter are the extrinsic muscles of the hand that move the fingers, including the thumb. Extrinsic muscles of the hand attach proximally to the arm or forearm and then travel distally to enter and attach to the hand. Intrinsic muscles of the hand that also move the fingers are addressed in Chapter 9 (intrinsic muscles of the hand are wholly located within the hand; in other words, they begin and end in the hand).

Note: For cross-sectional views of the forearm, wrist, and hand, see Figures 7-6, 9-3A, and 9-3B, respectively.

Overview of Structure

☐ Structurally, extrinsic muscles of the hand that move the fingers can be divided into three groups: flexors, superficial extensors, and the deep extensors of the deep distal four group.
☐ The flexors are the flexor digitorum superficialis, flexor digitorum profundus, and flexor pollicis longus.
☐ The superficial extensors are the extensor digitorum and extensor digiti minimi.
☐ The deep distal four group is composed of the abductor pollicis longus, extensor pollicis brevis, extensor pollicis longus, and extensor indicis. Three of the four muscles of this group have the word *pollicis* in their name because they move the thumb (*pollicis* means thumb); the extensor indicis moves the index finger.

☐ The finger flexors are located in the anterior forearm and the superficial finger extensors are located in the posterior forearm. The deep distal four muscles are located deep in the distal posterior forearm.

Overview of Function

The following general rules regarding actions can be stated for the functional groups of extrinsic finger muscles:
☐ Fingers two through five can move at three joints: the metacarpophalangeal (MCP), proximal interphalangeal (PIP), and distal interphalangeal (DIP) joints. If a muscle crosses only the MCP joint, it can move the finger only at the MCP joint. If the muscle crosses the MCP and PIP joints, it can move the finger at both of these joints. If the muscle crosses the MCP, PIP, and DIP joints, it can move the finger at all three joints. Note: The little finger can also move at the carpometacarpal (CMC) joint.
☐ The thumb (finger one) can move at three joints: the carpometacarpal (CMC), metacarpophalangeal (MCP), and interphalangeal (IP) joints. Similarly, a muscle can only move the thumb at a joint or joints that it crosses.
☐ If a muscle crosses the MCP, PIP, or DIP joints of fingers two through five on the anterior side, it can flex the finger at the joint(s) crossed; if a muscle crosses the MCP, PIP, or DIP joints of fingers two through five on the posterior side, it can extend the finger at the joint(s) crossed.

- If a muscle crosses the MCP joint of fingers two, three, four, or five on the side that faces the middle finger, it can adduct the finger at the MCP joint; if a muscle crosses the MCP joint of fingers two, three, or four on the side that is away from the middle-finger side, it can abduct the finger at the MCP joint (the middle finger abducts in both directions, radial and ulnar abduction).
- Muscles that cross the CMC, MCP, and IP joints of the thumb on the medial side can flex the thumb at the joint(s) crossed; muscles that cross the CMC, MCP, and IP joints of the thumb on the lateral side can extend the thumb at the joint(s) crossed.
- Muscles that cross the CMC joint of the thumb on the anterior side can abduct the thumb at the CMC joint; muscles that cross the CMC joint of the thumb on the posterior side can adduct the thumb at the CMC joint.

- Reverse actions involve the proximal attachment moving toward the distal one. This would occur when the fingers are holding onto a fixed, immovable object.
- Because extrinsic finger/thumb muscles attach proximally to the arm or forearm, they can also move the wrist, elbow, and/or radioulnar joints.
- If a muscle crosses the elbow or wrist joint anteriorly, it can flex them; if it crosses these joints posteriorly, it can extend.
- If a muscle crosses the wrist joint on the lateral (radial) side, it can radially deviate (abduct) the hand at the wrist joint; if it crosses it on the medial (ulnar) side, it can ulnar deviate (adduct).
- If the muscle crosses the radioulnar joints, it can pronate or supinate the forearm at the radioulnar joints.

Anterior View of the Muscles of the Right Wrist Joint and Extrinsic Finger Muscles— Superficial View

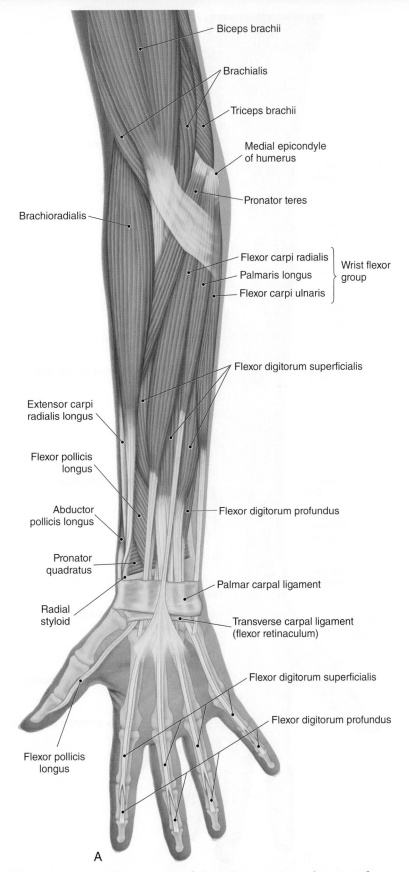

Figure 8-1 Anterior views of the muscles of the right wrist joint and extrinsic finger muscles. **A,** Superficial view.

Anterior View of the Muscles of the Right Wrist Joint and Extrinsic Finger Muscles— Intermediate View

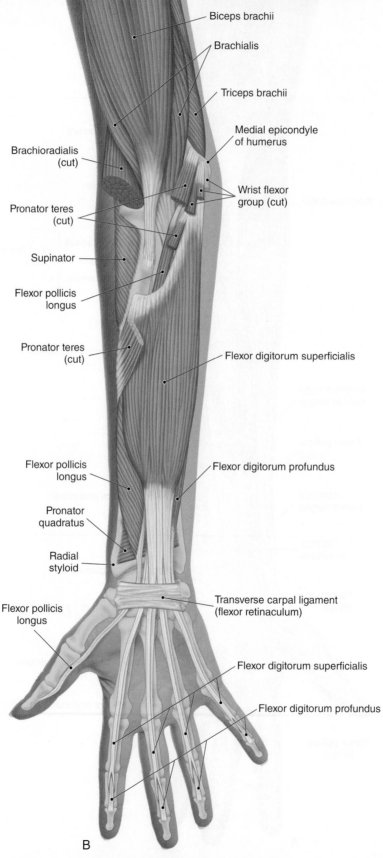

Biceps brachii

Brachialis

Triceps brachii

Medial epicondyle of humerus

Brachioradialis (cut)

Wrist flexor group (cut)

Pronator teres (cut)

Supinator

Flexor pollicis longus

Pronator teres (cut)

Flexor digitorum superficialis

Flexor pollicis longus

Flexor digitorum profundus

Pronator quadratus

Radial styloid

Flexor pollicis longus

Transverse carpal ligament (flexor retinaculum)

Flexor digitorum superficialis

Flexor digitorum profundus

B

Figure 8-1, cont'd B, Intermediate view.

Anterior View of the Muscles of the Right Wrist Joint and Extrinsic Finger Muscles—Deep View

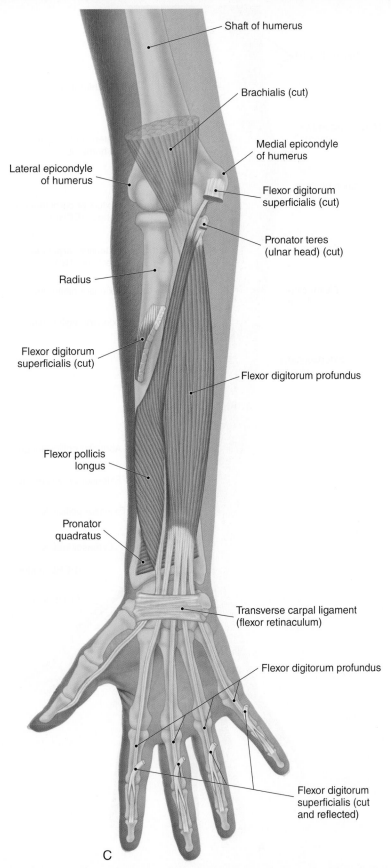

Shaft of humerus

Brachialis (cut)

Medial epicondyle of humerus

Lateral epicondyle of humerus

Flexor digitorum superficialis (cut)

Pronator teres (ulnar head) (cut)

Radius

Flexor digitorum superficialis (cut)

Flexor digitorum profundus

Flexor pollicis longus

Pronator quadratus

Transverse carpal ligament (flexor retinaculum)

Flexor digitorum profundus

Flexor digitorum superficialis (cut and reflected)

C

Figure 8-1, cont'd C, Deep view. The brachialis has been cut and ghosted in.

Posterior View of the Muscles of the Right Wrist Joint and Extrinsic Finger Muscles— Superficial View

8

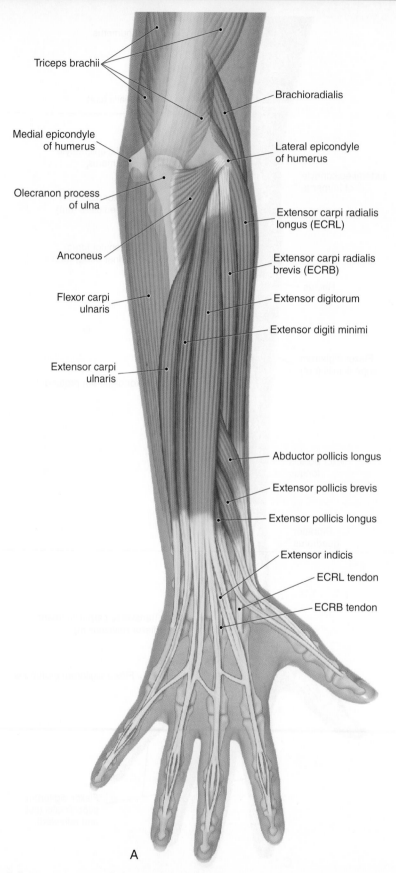

Triceps brachii

Brachioradialis

Medial epicondyle of humerus

Lateral epicondyle of humerus

Olecranon process of ulna

Extensor carpi radialis longus (ECRL)

Anconeus

Extensor carpi radialis brevis (ECRB)

Flexor carpi ulnaris

Extensor digitorum

Extensor digiti minimi

Extensor carpi ulnaris

Abductor pollicis longus

Extensor pollicis brevis

Extensor pollicis longus

Extensor indicis

ECRL tendon

ECRB tendon

A

Figure 8-2 Posterior views of the muscles of the right wrist joint and extrinsic finger muscles. **A,** Superficial view. The triceps brachii has been ghosted in.

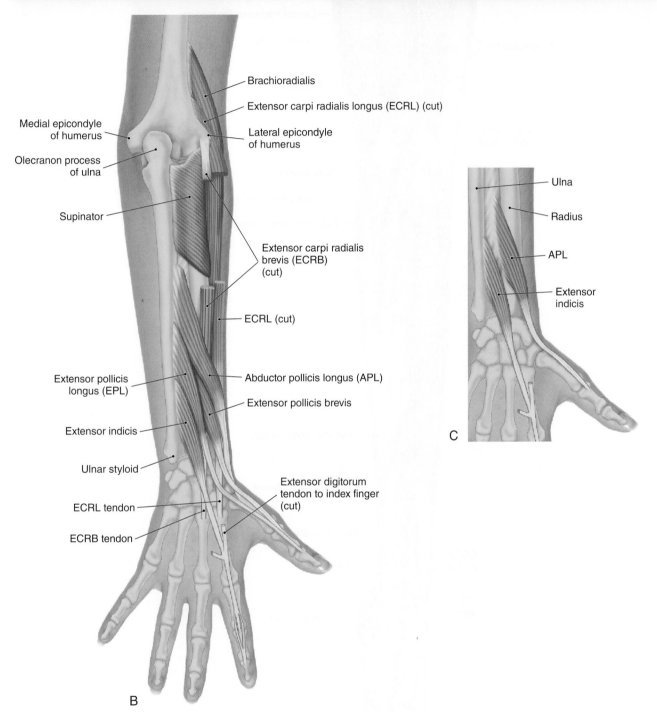

Figure 8-2, cont'd **B,** Intermediate view. **C,** Deep view.

Lateral View of the Muscles of the Right Wrist Joint and Extrinsic Finger Muscles

8

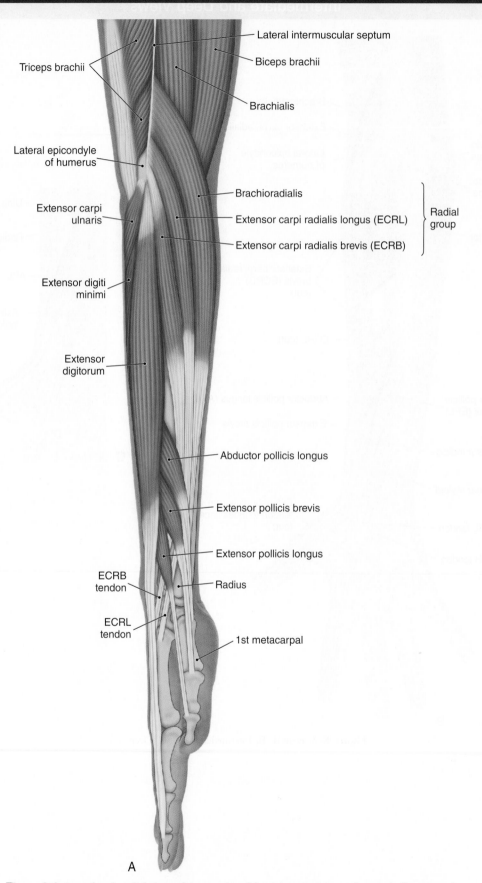

Triceps brachii

Lateral intermuscular septum

Biceps brachii

Brachialis

Lateral epicondyle of humerus

Brachioradialis

Extensor carpi ulnaris

Extensor carpi radialis longus (ECRL)

Extensor carpi radialis brevis (ECRB)

Radial group

Extensor digiti minimi

Extensor digitorum

Abductor pollicis longus

Extensor pollicis brevis

Extensor pollicis longus

ECRB tendon

Radius

ECRL tendon

1st metacarpal

A

Figure 8-3 Lateral and medial views of the muscles of the right wrist joint and extrinsic finger muscles. **A,** Lateral view.

Medial View of the Muscles of the Right Wrist Joint and Extrinsic Finger Muscles

8

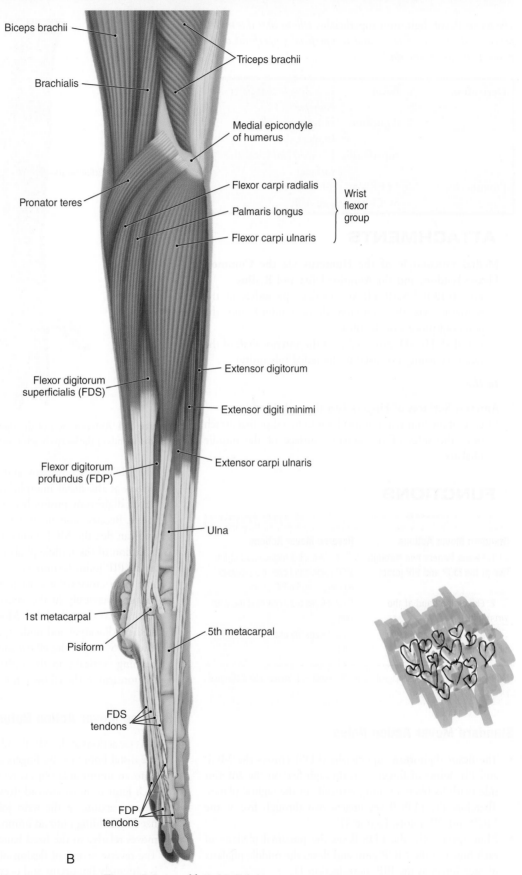

Biceps brachii

Triceps brachii

Brachialis

Medial epicondyle
of humerus

Pronator teres

Flexor carpi radialis ⎫
Palmaris longus   ⎬ Wrist flexor group
Flexor carpi ulnaris ⎭

Extensor digitorum

Flexor digitorum
superficialis (FDS)

Extensor digiti minimi

Extensor carpi ulnaris

Flexor digitorum
profundus (FDP)

Ulna

1st metacarpal

5th metacarpal

Pisiform

FDS
tendons

FDP
tendons

B

Figure 8-3, cont'd B, Medial view.

Flexor Digitorum Superficialis (FDS)

The name, flexor digitorum superficialis, *tells us that this muscle flexes the digits (i.e., fingers) and is superficial (superficial to the flexor digitorum profundus).*

Derivation	☐ flexor:	L. *a muscle that flexes a body part.*
	digitorum:	L. *refers to a digit* (finger).
	superficialis:	L. *superficial* (near the surface).
Pronunciation	☐ FLEKS-or, dij-i-TOE-rum, SOO-per-fish-ee-A-lis

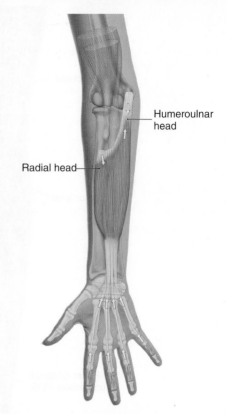

Figure 8-4 Anterior view of the right flexor digitorum superficialis. The distal ends of the biceps brachii and brachialis have been ghosted in.

Labels: Humeroulnar head, Radial head

■ ATTACHMENTS

☐ **Medial Epicondyle of the Humerus via the Common Flexor Tendon, and the Anterior Ulna and Radius**
  ☐ HUMEROULNAR HEAD: medial epicondyle of the humerus (via the common flexor tendon) and the coronoid process of the ulna
  ☐ RADIAL HEAD: proximal ½ of the anterior shaft of the radius (starting just distal to the radial tuberosity)

to the

☐ **Anterior Surfaces of Fingers Two through Five**
  ☐ each of the four tendons divides into two slips that attach onto the sides of the anterior surface of the middle phalanx

■ FUNCTIONS

CONCENTRIC (SHORTENING) MOVER ACTIONS	
Standard Mover Actions	**Reverse Mover Actions**
☐ **1. Flexes fingers two through five at the MCP and PIP joints**	☐ 1. Flexes the metacarpals at the MCP joints and flexes the proximal phalanges at the PIP joints
☐ **2. Flexes the hand at the wrist joint**	☐ 2. Flexes the forearm at the wrist joint
☐ 3. Flexes the forearm at the elbow joint	☐ 3. Flexes the arm at the elbow joint

MCP joints = metacarpophalangeal joints; PIP joints = proximal interphalangeal joints

Standard Mover Action Notes

- The flexor digitorum superficialis (FDS) crosses the MCP and PIP joints of fingers two through five on the anterior side (with its fibers running vertically in the sagittal plane). Therefore the FDS flexes fingers two through five at the MCP and PIP joints. (action 1)
- More specifically, the FDS flexes the proximal phalanx of each finger at the MCP joint and flexes the middle phalanx of each finger at the PIP joint. (action 1)

- The FDS does not cross and therefore cannot move the fingers at the distal interphalangeal (DIP) joints; only the flexor digitorum profundus crosses and can flex the DIP joints. Because so many other (intrinsic hand) muscles cross and can flex the MCP joints, the major action of the FDS is flexion of the middle phalanx of fingers two through five at the PIP joint. (action 1)
- The FDS crosses the wrist joint anteriorly (with its fibers running vertically in the sagittal plane); therefore it flexes the hand at the wrist joint. Motion at the wrist joint occurs at the radiocarpal and midcarpal joints. (action 2)
- The FDS crosses the elbow joint anteriorly (with its fibers running vertically in the sagittal plane); therefore it flexes the forearm at the elbow joint. (action 3)

Reverse Mover Action Notes

- Reverse actions at the MCP and IP joints usually occur when the distal bones of the fingers are fixed, usually by holding onto an immovable object, requiring the proximal bone at each joint to move instead. (reverse action 1)
- Reverse actions at the wrist joint occur when the hand is fixed by holding onto an immovable object and the forearm moves relative to the fixed hand. (reverse action 2)
- The reverse action of flexion of the arm at the elbow joint is extremely important and occurs whenever a person grasps

Flexor Digitorum Superficialis (FDS)—*cont'd*

an immovable object and pulls his or her body toward it (examples include using a handicap bar or using a handrail when going up stairs). (reverse action 3)

Eccentric Antagonist Functions

1. Restrains/slows MCP and PIP joint extension
2. Restrains/slows wrist joint extension
3. Restrains/slows elbow joint extension

Eccentric Antagonist Function Note

- Restraining/slowing extension of the forearm at the elbow joint is extremely important when lowering an object in a careful and controlled manner.

Isometric Stabilization Functions

1. Stabilizes the MCP and PIP joints
2. Stabilizes the wrist joint
3. Stabilizes the elbow joint
4. Stabilizes the RU joints

Isometric Stabilization Function Note

- Even though the FDS has little or no action across the radioulnar (RU) joints because the direction of its fibers is vertical, given that it does cross the RU joints, it can help stabilize these joints.

Additional Note on Functions

1. The FDS and flexor digitorum profundus may contribute to adduction of fingers two, four, and five at the MCP joints.

INNERVATION
- The Median Nerve
  - C7, **C8**, T1

ARTERIAL SUPPLY
- The Ulnar and Radial Arteries (terminal branches of the Brachial Artery)

✋ PALPATION

1. With the client seated or supine, place palpating hand on the medial side of the proximal anterior forearm approximately ½ inch (1 cm) anterior to the medial border of the shaft of the ulna.
2. Have the client actively flex fingers two through five at the metacarpophalangeal joints (keep the fingers extended at the interphalangeal joints) and feel for the contraction of the flexor digitorum superficialis (FDS).
3. Continue palpating the FDS proximally toward the humeral attachment and distally toward the fingers.

■ RELATIONSHIP TO OTHER STRUCTURES

- The flexor digitorum superficialis (FDS) is located in the anterior forearm, directly deep to the flexor carpi radialis, palmaris longus, and flexor carpi ulnaris.
- From the medial perspective, the FDS is deep to the ulnar head of the flexor carpi ulnaris.
- Deep to the flexor FDS are the flexor digitorum profundus and flexor pollicis longus.
- The four tendons of the FDS travel through the carpal tunnel medial to the median nerve and superficial to the four tendons of the flexor digitorum profundus.
- The flexor digitorum superficialis is located within the superficial front arm line myofascial meridian.

■ MISCELLANEOUS

1. The flexor digitorum superficialis (FDS) is also known as the *flexor digitorum sublimis*.
2. The humeral attachment of the FDS arises from the medial epicondyle of the humerus via the common flexor tendon. The common flexor tendon is the common proximal attachment of five muscles: the pronator teres, flexor carpi radialis, palmaris longus, flexor carpi ulnaris, and the FDS.
3. The four distal tendons of the FDS are arranged in two layers, with the tendons going to the middle and ring fingers superficially and the tendons going to the little finger and index finger deeply. (If you take your own little finger and index finger and you make them touch behind the middle and ring fingers, you will have the arrangement that these tendons are in when they travel through the carpal tunnel.)
4. The distal tendons of the FDS attach onto the middle phalanges in an unusual manner. Because the distal tendons of the flexor digitorum profundus are deeper and yet they must ultimately attach further distally onto the distal phalanges, the tendons of the FDS must split to allow passage of the tendons of the flexor digitorum profundus through to the distal phalanges. Each one of the split distal tendons of the FDS then attaches onto both sides of the anterior surface of the middle phalanx. (This arrangement is essentially identical to that of the splitting of each of the distal tendons of the flexor digitorum brevis' distal tendon to allow passage of the flexor digitorum longus' distal tendon onto the distal phalanx of toes two through five in the lower extremity.)
5. The median nerve and ulnar artery travel between the two heads of the FDS.
6. Irritation of the synovial sheaths of the FDS and/or the flexor digitorum profundus in the carpal tunnel can press on the median nerve and cause *carpal tunnel syndrome*.
7. Irritation and/or inflammation of the medial epicondyle and/or the common flexor tendon is known as *medial epicondylitis*, *medial epicondylosis*, or *golfer's elbow*.

Flexor Digitorum Profundus (FDP)

The name, flexor digitorum profundus, *tells us that this muscle flexes the digits (i.e., fingers) and is deep (deep to the flexor digitorum superficialis).*

Derivation	☐ flexor:	L. *a muscle that flexes a body part.*
	digitorum:	L. *refers to a digit* (finger).
	profundus:	L. *deep.*
Pronunciation	☐ FLEKS-or, dij-i-TOE-rum, pro-FUN-dus	

■ ATTACHMENTS

☐ **Medial and Anterior Ulna**
    ☐ the proximal ½ (starting just distal to the ulnar tuberosity) and the interosseus membrane

to the

☐ **Anterior Surfaces of Fingers Two through Five**
    ☐ the distal phalanges

■ FUNCTIONS

CONCENTRIC (SHORTENING) MOVER ACTIONS	
Standard Mover Actions	**Reverse Mover Actions**
☐ 1. Flexes fingers two through five at the MCP, PIP, and DIP joints	☐ 1. Flexes the metacarpals at the MCP joints, flexes the proximal phalanges at the PIP joints, and flexes the middle phalanges at the DIP joints
☐ 2. Flexes the hand at the wrist joint	☐ 2. Flexes the forearm at the wrist joint

MCP joints = metacarpophalangeal joints; PIP joints = proximal interphalangeal joints; DIP joints = distal interphalangeal joints

Standard Mover Action Notes

- The flexor digitorum profundus (FDP) crosses the MCP and the PIP and DIP joints of fingers two through five on the anterior side (with its fibers running vertically in the sagittal plane). Therefore the FDP flexes fingers two through five at the MCP and the PIP and DIP joints. (action 1)
- More specifically, the FDP flexes the proximal phalanx of each finger at the MCP joint, flexes the middle phalanx of each finger at the PIP joint, and flexes the distal phalanx of each finger at the DIP joint. (action 1)
- The FDP crosses and can flex fingers two through five at the MCP, PIP, and DIP joints. However, because it is the only muscle that can flex the DIP joints, it is especially important for this action. (action 1)
- The tautness (passive elastic recoil force) of the FDP is responsible for the partially flexed position of fingers two through five at the MCP, PIP, and DIP joints.

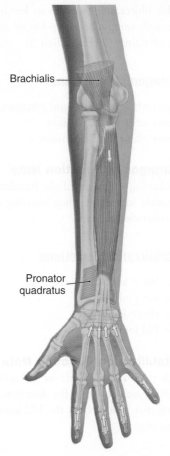

Figure 8-5 Anterior view of the right flexor digitorum profundus. The pronator quadratus and distal end of the brachialis have been ghosted in.

- The muscle bellies for each individual finger of the FDP are not well separated (except for the index finger). Therefore it is difficult to isolate DIP joint flexion of one finger. (action 1)
- The FDP crosses the wrist joint anteriorly (with its fibers running vertically in the sagittal plane); therefore it flexes the hand at the wrist joint. Motion at the wrist joint occurs at the radiocarpal and midcarpal joints. (action 2)

Reverse Mover Action Notes

- Reverse actions at the MCP and interphalangeal joints usually occur when the distal bones of the fingers are fixed, usually by holding onto an immovable object, requiring the proximal bone at each joint to move instead. (reverse action 1)
- Reverse actions at the wrist joint occur when the hand is fixed by holding onto an immovable object and the forearm moves relative to the fixed hand. (reverse action 2)

Flexor Digitorum Profundus (FDP)—*cont'd*

Eccentric Antagonist Functions

1. Restrains/slows MCP, PIP, and DIP joint extension
2. Restrains/slows wrist joint extension

Isometric Stabilization Functions

1. Stabilizes the MCP, PIP, and DIP joints
2. Stabilizes the wrist joint

Additional Note on Functions

1. The FDP and flexor digitorum superficialis may contribute to adduction of fingers two, four, and five at the MCP joints.

INNERVATION
- ☐ The Median and the Ulnar Nerves
  - ☐ C8, T1
  - ☐ the anterior interosseus branch of the median nerve

ARTERIAL SUPPLY
- ☐ The Ulnar and Radial Arteries (terminal branches of the Brachial Artery) and the Anterior Interosseus Artery (a branch of the Ulnar Artery)

✋ PALPATION

1. With the client seated or supine, place palpating hand on the medial side of the proximal forearm just anterior to the medial border of the shaft of the ulna.
2. Have the client flex the fingers at the interphalangeal joints (keep the metacarpophalangeal joints extended) and feel for the contraction of the flexor digitorum profundus.
3. Continue palpating the flexor digitorum profundus as far proximally and distally as possible.

■ RELATIONSHIP TO OTHER STRUCTURES

- ☐ From the anterior perspective, the FDP is deep to the flexor digitorum superficialis.
- ☐ From the medial perspective, the FDP is deep to the ulnar head of the flexor carpi ulnaris.
- ☐ The FDP is medial to the flexor pollicis longus.
- ☐ Deep to the FDP are the ulna and the interosseus membrane.
- ☐ The flexor digitorum profundus is located within the superficial front arm line myofascial meridian.

■ MISCELLANEOUS

1. The distal tendons of the FDP reach their attachment site on the distal phalanges in an unusual manner. The tendons of the flexor digitorum superficialis are superficial and split; the tendons of the FDP then pass through these splits to continue onto the distal phalanges. (This is essentially identical to the arrangement of the flexor digitorum longus and the flexor digitorum brevis of the lower extremity.)
2. Irritation of the synovial sheaths of the flexor digitorum superficialis and/or the FDP in the carpal tunnel can press on the median nerve and cause *carpal tunnel syndrome*.

8

Flexor Pollicis Longus

The name, flexor pollicis longus, *tells us that this muscle flexes the thumb and is long (longer than the flexor pollicis brevis).*

Derivation	☐ flexor: L. *a muscle that flexes a body part.*
	pollicis: L. *thumb.*
	longus: L. *long.*
Pronunciation	☐ FLEKS-or, POL-i-sis, LONG-us

■ ATTACHMENTS

☐ **Anterior Surface of the Radius**
  ☐ and the interosseus membrane, the medial epicondyle of the humerus, and the coronoid process of the ulna

  to the

☐ **Thumb**
  ☐ the anterior aspect of the base of the distal phalanx

■ FUNCTIONS

CONCENTRIC (SHORTENING) MOVER ACTIONS	
Standard Mover Actions	**Reverse Mover Actions**
☐ 1. Flexes the thumb at the CMC, MCP, and IP joints	☐ 1. Flexes the metacarpal at the MCP joint and flexes the proximal phalanx at the IP joint
☐ 2. Flexes the hand at the wrist joint	☐ 2. Flexes the forearm at the wrist joint
☐ 3. Radially deviates the hand at the wrist joint	☐ 3. Radially deviates the forearm at the wrist joint
☐ 4. Flexes the forearm at the elbow joint	☐ 4. Flexes the arm at the elbow joint
☐ 5. Pronates the forearm at the RU joints	☐ 5. Pronates the ulna and laterally rotates the arm

CMC joint = carpometacarpal joint; MCP joint = metacarpophalangeal joint; IP joint = interphalangeal joint; RU joints = radioulnar joints

Standard Mover Action Notes

- The flexor pollicis longus crosses the CMC joint of the thumb medially (on the ulnar side) to attach onto the distal phalanx of the thumb (with its fibers running vertically in the frontal plane). When the flexor pollicis longus contracts, it pulls the thumb medially (in an ulnar direction) within the plane of the palm of the hand (frontal plane) toward the index finger. This action is called flexion of the thumb. Therefore the flexor pollicis longus flexes the thumb by flexing the metacarpal of the thumb at the first CMC joint. The flexor pollicis longus also crosses the MCP and the IP joints of the thumb medially (on the ulnar side) to attach onto the distal phalanx of the thumb. Therefore the flexor pollicis longus also flexes the proximal and distal phalanges of the thumb at these joints as well. Because of the rotational

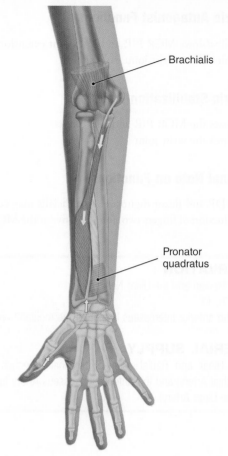

Figure 8-6 Anterior view of the right flexor pollicis longus. The pronator quadratus and distal end of the brachialis have been ghosted in.

development of the thumb embryologically, the named actions of flexion and extension of the thumb occur within the frontal plane. (action 1)

- The flexor pollicis longus is the only muscle that can flex the thumb at the IP joint, therefore this action best engages it. (action 1)
- The flexor pollicis longus crosses the wrist joint anteriorly (with its fibers running vertically in the sagittal plane); therefore it flexes the hand at the wrist joint. Motion at the wrist joint occurs at the radiocarpal and midcarpal joints. (action 2)
- The flexor pollicis longus crosses the wrist joint on the radial (lateral) side to attach onto the hand (with its fibers running vertically in the frontal plane); therefore it radially deviates (abducts) the hand at the wrist joint. (action 3)
- Because the humeroulnar head of the flexor pollicis longus is small or even absent, the actions of elbow joint flexion and pronation of the radioulnar joints are weak or absent. (actions 4, 5)
- Pronation of the forearm at the RU joints usually involves motion of the radius around a fixed ulna. (action 5)

Flexor Pollicis Longus—*cont'd*

Reverse Mover Action Notes

- Reverse actions involve moving the proximal attachment toward the distal one. This usually occurs when the distal attachment is fixed, perhaps because it is holding onto an immovable object. (reverse actions 1, 2, 3, 4)
- Another reverse action would be to move (flex) the trapezium toward the metacarpal of the thumb at the CMC joint; this would occur if the distal end (the metacarpal) is fixed, perhaps because the thumb is gripping an immovable object. Movement of the trapezium would likely involve movement of the entire carpus (wrist) and forearm relative to the hand. (reverse action 1)
- Reverse actions at the wrist joint occur when the hand is fixed by holding onto an immovable object and the forearm moves relative to the fixed hand. (reverse actions 2, 3)
- The reverse action, flexion of the arm at the elbow joint, is extremely important and occurs whenever a person grasps an immovable object and pulls his or her body toward it (examples include using a handicap bar or using a handrail when going up stairs). However, because the humeroulnar head of the flexor pollicis longus is very small or even absent, this function would be very weak or absent. (reverse action 4)
- The reverse action of pronation of the ulna around a fixed radius usually occurs only if the hand is fixed by holding onto an immovable object and the ulna moves relative to the fixed radius. Because the elbow joint does not allow rotation, this will cause the arm to laterally rotate at the glenohumeral joint. However, because the humeroulnar head of the flexor pollicis longus is very small or even absent, this function would be very weak or absent. (reverse action 5)

Eccentric Antagonist Functions

1. Restrains/slows CMC, MCP, and IP joint extension
2. Restrains/slows wrist joint extension
3. Restrains/slows wrist joint ulnar deviation
4. Restrains/slows elbow joint extension
5. Restrains/slows supination of RU joints

Eccentric Antagonist Function Note

- Restraining/slowing extension of the forearm at the elbow joint is extremely important when lowering an object in a careful and controlled manner.

Isometric Stabilization Functions

1. Stabilizes the CMC, MCP, and IP joints of the thumb
2. Stabilizes the wrist joint
3. Stabilizes the elbow joint
4. Stabilizes the RU joints

Isometric Stabilization Function Note

- Because the humeroulnar head of the flexor pollicis longus is small or even absent, the stabilization force across the elbow and RU joints would be weak or absent.

INNERVATION
- The Median Nerve
  - the anterior interosseus branch of the median nerve; C7, **C8**

ARTERIAL SUPPLY
- The Radial Artery (a terminal branch of the Brachial Artery) and the Anterior Interosseus Artery (a branch of the Ulnar Artery)

✋ PALPATION

1. With the client seated or supine, place palpating fingers on the distal anterolateral (anteroradial) forearm.
2. Have the client actively flex the distal phalanx of the thumb at the interphalangeal joint and feel for the contraction of the flexor pollicis longus.
3. Continue palpating the flexor pollicis longus as far proximally and distally as possible.

■ RELATIONSHIP TO OTHER STRUCTURES

- The flexor pollicis longus is a deep muscle of the anterior forearm. The majority of it is directly deep to the flexor digitorum superficialis. However, a small part of the flexor pollicis longus is superficial in the distal forearm on the medial side (and to a lesser extent, the lateral side) of the distal tendon of the flexor carpi radialis.
- The flexor pollicis longus is found lateral to the flexor digitorum profundus.
- Deep to the flexor pollicis longus are the radius and the interosseus membrane.
- The flexor pollicis longus is located within the superficial front arm line myofascial meridian.

■ MISCELLANEOUS

1. The distal tendon of the flexor pollicis longus travels through the carpal tunnel lateral to the median nerve.
2. Irritation of the synovial sheath of the flexor pollicis longus in the carpal tunnel can press on the median nerve and cause/contribute to *carpal tunnel syndrome.*
3. The proximal attachments of the flexor pollicis longus are variable. The medial epicondylar attachment is often missing. Sometimes the coronoid process attachment is on the medial side of the coronoid process; sometimes it is on the lateral side, and other times it is missing altogether.

8

Extensor Digitorum

The name, extensor digitorum, *tells us that this muscle extends the digits (i.e., fingers).*

Derivation	☐ extensor: L. *a muscle that extends a body part.*
	digitorum: L. *refers to a digit* (finger).
Pronunciation	☐ eks-TEN-sor, dij-i-TOE-rum

■ ATTACHMENTS

☐ **Lateral Epicondyle of the Humerus via the Common Extensor Tendon**

to the

☐ **Phalanges of Fingers Two through Five**
    ☐ via its dorsal digital expansion onto the posterior surfaces of the middle and distal phalanges

■ FUNCTIONS

CONCENTRIC (SHORTENING) MOVER ACTIONS	
Standard Mover Actions	**Reverse Mover Actions**
☐ **1. Extends fingers two through five at the MCP, PIP, and DIP joints**	☐ 1. Extends the metacarpals at the MCP joints, extends the proximal phalanges at the PIP joints, and extends the middle phalanges at the DIP joints
☐ **2. Extends the hand at the wrist joint**	☐ 2. Extends the forearm at the wrist joint
☐ 3. Medially rotates the little finger at the CMC joint	☐ 3. Lateral rotation of the hamate (carpus) at the CMC joint
☐ 4. Extends the forearm at the elbow joint	☐ 4. Extends the arm at the elbow joint

MCP joints = metacarpophalangeal joints; PIP joints = proximal interphalangeal joints; DIP joints = distal interphalangeal joints; CMC = carpometacarpal joint

Standard Mover Action Notes

• The extensor digitorum crosses the MCP joint and the PIP and DIP joints posteriorly to finally attach onto the distal phalanges of fingers two through five (with its fibers running vertically in the sagittal plane). Therefore the extensor digitorum extends fingers two through five at the MCP, PIP, and DIP joints. (action 1)

• More specifically, the extensor digitorum extends the proximal phalanx of each finger at the MCP joint, extends the middle phalanx of each finger at the PIP joint, and extends the distal phalanx of each finger at the DIP joint. (action 1)

• Distally the tendons of the extensor digitorum are somewhat tied together by intertendinous connections, making independent movement of an individual finger more difficult. (action 1)

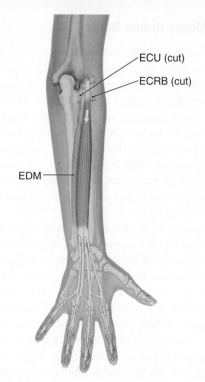

Figure 8-7 Posterior view of the right extensor digitorum. The extensor digiti minimi (EDM) and the cut extensor carpi ulnaris (ECU) and cut extensor carpi radialis brevis (ECRB) have been ghosted in.

• The extensor digitorum crosses the wrist joint posteriorly (with its fibers running vertically in the sagittal plane); therefore it extends the hand at the wrist (radiocarpal and midcarpal) joint. (action 2)

• The tendon of the extensor digitorum that goes to the little finger (finger five) crosses the fifth CMC joint posteriorly from lateral on the lateral epicondyle to attach more medially onto the phalanges of the little finger (with its fibers running slightly horizontally in the transverse plane). When the extensor digitorum contracts, it pulls the posterior side of the little finger laterally. This is medial rotation of the little finger, because the anterior surface of the little finger rotates medially. Therefore the extensor digitorum medially rotates the metacarpal of the little finger at the fifth CMC joint. (action 3)

• Medial rotation of the little finger at the CMC joint is an important part of repositioning the little finger back to anatomic position from a position of opposition to the thumb. (action 3)

• The extensor digitorum crosses the elbow joint posteriorly (with its fibers running vertically in the sagittal plane); therefore it extends the forearm at the elbow joint. (action 4)

Reverse Mover Action Notes

• Reverse actions at the MCP, PIP, and DIP joints usually occurs when the distal bones of the fingers are fixed, usually

Extensor Digitorum—*cont'd*

by holding onto an immovable object, requiring the proximal bone at each joint to move instead of the distal bone. (reverse action 1)

- Reverse actions at the wrist joint occur when the hand is fixed by holding onto an immovable object and the forearm moves relative to the fixed hand. (reverse action 2)
- Lateral rotation of the hamate bone of the carpus (wrist) at the CMC joint only occurs if the metacarpal of the little finger is stabilized and the hamate (and entire carpus and radius) moves relative to the fifth metacarpal. This causes supination of the radius at the radioulnar joints. (reverse action 3)
- The extensor digitorum crosses the elbow joint posteriorly; therefore it extends the elbow joint. If the distal attachment is fixed, the arm will extend toward the forearm instead of the forearm extending toward the arm. (reverse action 4)

Eccentric Antagonist Functions

1. Restrains/slows MCP, PIP, and DIP joint flexion
2. Restrains/slows wrist joint flexion
3. Restrains/slows lateral rotation of the little finger
4. Restrains/slows elbow joint flexion

Eccentric Antagonist Function Note

- The extensor digitorum also restrains/slows medial rotation of the hamate (carpus and radius) at the fifth CMC joint, and pronation of the radius at the radioulnar joints.

Isometric Stabilization Functions

1. Stabilizes the MCP, PIP, and DIP joints
2. Stabilizes the wrist joint
3. Stabilizes the fifth CMC and radioulnar joints
4. Stabilizes the elbow joint

Additional Note on Functions

1. Whenever the extensor digitorum contracts forcefully to extend the fingers at the MCP and IP joints, the wrist flexors also contract, creating a force of flexion of the hand at the wrist joint to fix (stabilize) the hand so that the extensor digitorum does not cause extension of the hand at the wrist joint. This can be easily felt by palpating the common flexor tendon at the medial epicondyle of the humerus while forcefully extending the fingers.

INNERVATION
- The Radial Nerve
  - posterior interosseus nerve, C7, C8

ARTERIAL SUPPLY
- The Posterior Interosseus Artery (a branch of the Ulnar Artery)

PALPATION

1. With the client seated or supine, place palpating hand in the middle of the posterior forearm.
2. Have the client actively extend fingers two through five (at the metacarpophalangeal and interphalangeal joints) and feel for the contraction of the extensor digitorum. Resistance can be added.
3. Palpate the extensor digitorum proximally and distally as far as possible.

■ RELATIONSHIP TO OTHER STRUCTURES

- The extensor digitorum is located medial to the extensor carpi radialis brevis and extensor carpi radialis longus, and lateral to the extensor digiti minimi and extensor carpi ulnaris.
- The extensor digitorum is superficial. Deep to the extensor digitorum is the deeper layer of posterior forearm muscles, which includes the supinator, abductor pollicis longus, extensor pollicis brevis, extensor pollicis longus, and extensor indicis.
- The extensor digitorum is located within the superficial back arm line myofascial meridian.

■ MISCELLANEOUS

1. The extensor digitorum is sometimes called the *extensor digitorum communis*.
2. The extensor digitorum arises proximally from the lateral epicondyle of the humerus via the common extensor tendon. The common extensor tendon is the common proximal attachment of four muscles: the extensor carpi radialis brevis, extensor digitorum, extensor digiti minimi, and the extensor carpi ulnaris. (The anconeus and the supinator also arise from the lateral epicondyle of the humerus, but not from the common extensor tendon.)
3. The distal attachment of the extensor digitorum spreads out to become a fibrous aponeurotic expansion that covers the posterior, medial, and lateral sides of the proximal phalanx. It then continues distally to attach onto the posterior sides of the middle and distal phalanges. This structure is called the *dorsal digital expansion*.
4. The dorsal digital expansion is also known as the *extensor expansion* and/or the *dorsal hood*. The term *dorsal hood* is used because one of its purposes is to serve as a movable hood of tissue when the fingers flex and extend.
5. The dorsal digital expansion also serves as an attachment site for the lumbricals manus, palmar interossei, dorsal interossei manus, and abductor digiti minimi manus muscles. Given that the dorsal digital expansion crosses the proximal and distal interphalangeal joints posteriorly, these muscles can extend the middle and distal phalanges at these joints.
6. Irritation and/or inflammation of the lateral epicondyle and/or the common extensor tendon is known as *lateral epicondylitis*, *lateral epicondylosis*, or *tennis elbow*.

8

Extensor Digiti Minimi

The name, extensor digiti minimi, *tells us that this muscle extends the little finger.*

Derivation	☐ extensor: L. *a muscle that extends a body part.*
	digiti: L. *refers to a digit* (finger).
	minimi: L. *least.*
Pronunciation	☐ eks-TEN-sor, DIJ-i-tee, MIN-i-mee

■ ATTACHMENTS

☐ **Lateral Epicondyle of the Humerus via the Common Extensor Tendon**

to the

☐ **Phalanges of the Little Finger (Finger Five)**
  ☐ attaches into the ulnar side of the tendon of the extensor digitorum muscle (to attach onto the posterior surface of the middle and distal phalanges of the little finger via the dorsal digital expansion)

■ FUNCTIONS

CONCENTRIC (SHORTENING) MOVER ACTIONS	
Standard Mover Actions	**Reverse Mover Actions**
☐ 1. Extends the little finger (finger five) at the MCP, PIP, and DIP joints	☐ 1. Extends the fifth metacarpal at the MCP joint, extends the fifth proximal phalanx at the PIP joint, and extends the fifth middle phalanx at the DIP joint
☐ 2. Extends the hand at the wrist joint	☐ 2. Extends the forearm at the wrist joint
☐ 3. Medially rotates the little finger at the CMC joint	☐ 3. Lateral rotation of the hamate (carpus) at the CMC joint
☐ 4. Extends the forearm at the elbow joint	☐ 4. Extends the arm at the elbow joint

MCP joint = metacarpophalangeal joint; PIP joint = proximal interphalangeal joint; DIP joint = distal interphalangeal joint; CMC joint = carpometacarpal joint

Standard Mover Action Notes

• The extensor digiti minimi crosses the fifth MCP joint (of the little finger) before it attaches into the distal tendon of the extensor digitorum muscle of the little finger. Because the extensor digiti minimi crosses this joint posteriorly (with its fibers running vertically in the sagittal plane), it extends the little finger at the fifth MCP joint. Further, by attaching into the distal tendon of the extensor digitorum, the extensor digiti minimi pulls on that tendon the same as if the belly of the extensor digitorum muscle itself had contracted and pulled on its own tendon. Therefore the extensor digiti minimi has the same actions at the little finger as the extensor digitorum muscle has, namely, extension of the little finger at the PIP and DIP joints. (action 1)

• More specifically, the extensor digiti minimi extends the proximal phalanx of the little finger at the MCP joint,

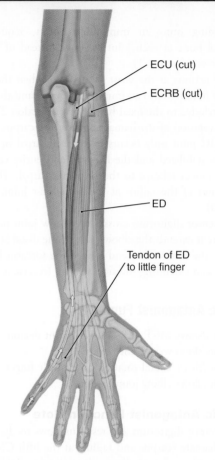

Figure 8-8 Posterior view of the right extensor digiti minimi. The extensor digitorum (ED) and the cut extensor carpi ulnaris (ECU) and cut extensor carpi radialis brevis (ECRB) have been ghosted in.

extends the middle phalanx of the little finger at the PIP joint, and extends the distal phalanx of the little finger at the DIP joint. (action 1)

• The extensor digiti minimi crosses the wrist joint posteriorly (with its fibers running vertically in the sagittal plane); therefore it extends the hand at the wrist (radiocarpal and midcarpal) joint. (action 2)

• The extensor digiti minimi crosses the fifth CMC joint posteriorly from lateral on the lateral epicondyle of the humerus to attach more medially onto the little finger (with its fibers running slightly horizontally in the transverse plane). When the extensor digiti minimi contracts, it pulls the posterior side of the little finger laterally. This is medial rotation of the little finger, because the anterior surface of the little finger rotates medially. Therefore the extensor digiti minimi medially rotates the metacarpal of the little finger at the fifth CMC joint. (action 3)

• Medial rotation of the little finger at the CMC joint is an important part of repositioning the little finger back to anatomic position from a position of opposition to the thumb. (action 3)

• The extensor digiti minimi crosses the elbow joint posteriorly (with its fibers running vertically in the sagittal

Extensor Digiti Minimi—*cont'd*

plane); therefore it extends the forearm at the elbow joint. (action 4)

Reverse Mover Action Notes

• Reverse actions at the MCP, PIP, and DIP joints occur when the distal bones of the fingers are fixed, usually by holding onto an immovable object, requiring the proximal bone at each joint to move instead. (reverse action 1)
• Reverse actions at the wrist joint occur when the hand is fixed by holding onto an immovable object and the forearm moves relative to the fixed hand. (reverse action 2)
• Lateral rotation of the hamate bone of the carpus (wrist) at the CMC joint occurs only if the metacarpal of the little finger is stabilized and the hamate (and entire carpus and radius) moves relative to the fifth metacarpal. This causes supination of the radius at the radioulnar joints. (reverse action 3)
• The extensor digiti minimi crosses the elbow joint posteriorly; therefore it extends the elbow joint. If the distal attachment is fixed, the arm will extend toward the forearm instead of the forearm extending toward the arm. (reverse action 4)

Eccentric Antagonist Functions

1. Restrains/slows fifth MCP, PIP, and DIP joint flexion
2. Restrains/slows wrist joint flexion
3. Restrains/slows lateral rotation of the little finger
4. Restrains/slows elbow joint flexion

Eccentric Antagonist Function Note

• The extensor digiti minimi also restrains/slows medial rotation of the hamate (carpus and radius) at the fifth CMC joint, and pronation of the radius at the radioulnar joints.

Isometric Stabilization Functions

1. Stabilizes the fifth MCP, PIP, and DIP joints
2. Stabilizes the wrist joint
3. Stabilizes the fifth CMC and radioulnar joints
4. Stabilizes the elbow joint

Additional Note on Functions

1. The extensor digiti minimi, by attaching into the distal tendon of the extensor digitorum, exerts a pull on the dorsal digital expansion of the little finger.

INNERVATION
☐ The Radial Nerve
  ☐ posterior interosseus nerve; **C7**, C8

ARTERIAL SUPPLY
☐ The Posterior Interosseus Artery (a branch of the Ulnar Artery)

✋ PALPATION

1. With the client seated or supine, place palpating hand on the posterior forearm toward the ulnar side.
2. Have the client actively extend the little finger at the fifth metacarpophalangeal and interphalangeal joints and feel for the contraction of the extensor digiti minimi. Resistance can be added.
3. Note: It is challenging to discern the extensor digiti minimi from the extensor digitorum fibers that go to the little finger. These extensor digitorum fibers are located more laterally (radially); the extensor digiti minimi fibers are located more medially (ulnar side).

◼ RELATIONSHIP TO OTHER STRUCTURES

☐ The extensor digiti minimi is superficial and located between the extensor digitorum (which is lateral to it) and the extensor carpi ulnaris (which is medial to it).
☐ The extensor digiti minimi is superficial to the deeper layer of posterior forearm muscles, which includes the supinator, abductor pollicis longus, extensor pollicis brevis, extensor pollicis longus, and extensor indicis.
☐ The extensor digiti minimi is located within the superficial back arm line myofascial meridian.

◼ MISCELLANEOUS

1. The extensor digiti minimi arises proximally from the lateral epicondyle of the humerus via the common extensor tendon. The common extensor tendon is the common proximal attachment of four muscles: the extensor carpi radialis brevis, extensor digitorum, extensor digiti minimi, and extensor carpi ulnaris. (The anconeus and the supinator also arise from the lateral epicondyle of the humerus, but not from the common extensor tendon.)
2. The belly of the extensor digiti minimi sometimes blends with the belly of the extensor digitorum.
3. Both the extensor digiti minimi and extensor indicis attach into the ulnar side of the extensor digitorum tendon to which they attach.
4. Other than the little finger and the thumb, only the index finger has a second extensor muscle (the extensor indicis).
5. Irritation and inflammation of the lateral epicondyle and/or the common extensor tendon is known as *lateral epicondylitis*, *lateral epicondylosis*, or *tennis elbow*.

8

Deep Distal Four Group

The deep distal four group is a group of four muscles that are located deep in the distal posterior forearm. Three of them move the thumb and therefore have the word *pollicis* in their name (*pollicis* means thumb). These are the abductor pollicis longus and extensor pollicis brevis that border the anatomic snuffbox on the lateral (radial) side, and the extensor pollicis longus that borders the anatomic snuffbox on the medial (ulnar) side. The fourth muscle in the group is the extensor indicis, which extends the index finger, as its name implies.

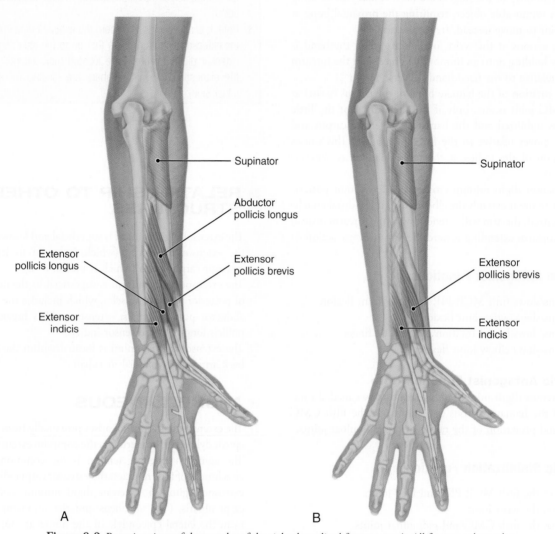

Figure 8-9 Posterior views of the muscles of the right deep distal four group. **A,** All four muscles with the supinator ghosted in. **B,** Same illustration with the abductor pollicis longus and extensor pollicis longus ghosted in.

Abductor Pollicis Longus (of Deep Distal Four Group)

The name, abductor pollicis longus, *tells us that this muscle abducts the thumb and is long (longer than the abductor pollicis brevis).*

Derivation	□ abductor: L. *a muscle that abducts a body part.*
	pollicis: L. *thumb.*
	longus: L. *longer.*
Pronunciation	□ ab-DUK-tor, POL-i-sis, LONG-us

■ ATTACHMENTS

□ **Posterior Radius and Ulna**
  □ approximately the middle ⅓ of the radius, ulna, and interosseus membrane

to the

□ **Thumb**
  □ the lateral side of the base of the first metacarpal

■ FUNCTIONS

CONCENTRIC (SHORTENING) MOVER ACTIONS	
Standard Mover Actions	**Reverse Mover Actions**
□ **1. Abducts the thumb at the CMC joint**	□ 1. Abducts the carpal bone (trapezium) at the CMC joint
□ **2. Extends the thumb at the CMC joint**	□ 2. Extends the carpal bone (trapezium) at the CMC joint
□ 3. Laterally rotates the thumb at the CMC joint	□ 3. Medially rotates the carpal bone (trapezium) at the CMC joint
□ 4. Radially deviates the hand at the wrist joint	□ 4. Radially deviates the forearm at the wrist joint
□ 5. Flexes the hand at the wrist joint	□ 5. Flexes the forearm at the wrist joint
□ 6. Supinates the forearm at the radioulnar joints	□ 6. Supinates the ulna and medially rotates the arm

CMC joint = carpometacarpal joint (of the thumb; saddle joint of the thumb)

Standard Mover Action Notes

- The abductor pollicis longus crosses the first CMC joint anteriorly to attach onto the metacarpal of the thumb (with its fibers running vertically in the sagittal plane). When the abductor pollicis longus contracts, it pulls the metacarpal of the thumb anteriorly (in the sagittal plane, in a direction that is perpendicular to and away from the plane of the palm of the hand). This action is called *abduction of the thumb.* Therefore the abductor pollicis longus abducts the thumb by abducting the metacarpal of the thumb at the first CMC joint. (Note: Because of the rotational development of the thumb embryologically, the named actions of abduction and

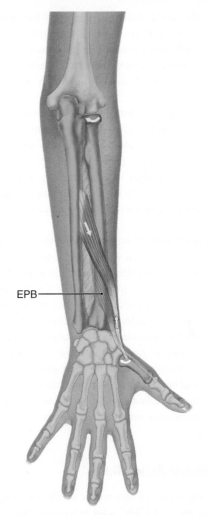

Figure 8-10 Posterior view of the abductor pollicis longus. The extensor pollicis brevis (EPB) has been ghosted in.

EPB

adduction of the thumb occur within the sagittal plane.) (action 1)
- The abductor pollicis longus crosses the first CMC joint laterally (radially) to attach onto the metacarpal of the thumb (with its fibers running vertically in the frontal plane). When the abductor pollicis longus contracts, it pulls the metacarpal of the thumb laterally (i.e., radially, in the frontal plane, within the plane of the palm of the hand away from the index finger). This action is called *extension of the thumb.* Therefore the abductor pollicis longus extends the thumb by extending the metacarpal of the thumb at the first CMC joint. (Note: Because of the rotational development of the thumb embryologically, the named actions of flexion and extension of the thumb occur within the frontal plane.) (action 2)
- The abductor pollicis longus crosses the first CMC joint posteriorly from medial in the forearm to attach more laterally onto the thumb (with its fibers running slightly

Abductor Pollicis Longus (of Deep Distal Four Group)—*cont'd*

horizontally in the transverse plane). When the abductor pollicis longus contracts, it pulls the thumb posterolaterally. This is lateral rotation of the thumb, because the anterior side of the thumb rotates laterally. Therefore the abductor pollicis longus laterally rotates the thumb at the first CMC joint. (action 3)

- The abductor pollicis longus crosses the wrist joint on the radial (lateral) side (with it fibers running vertically in the frontal plane); therefore it radially deviates (abducts) the hand at the wrist joint. (action 4)
- The abductor pollicis longus crosses the wrist joint slightly anteriorly (with its fibers running vertically in the sagittal plane); therefore it flexes the hand at the wrist joint. (action 5)
- The abductor pollicis longus crosses the ulna and radius in the posterior forearm with an ulnar-to-radial orientation to its fibers (hence its fibers are running somewhat horizontally in the transverse plane). When the thumb and the hand are fixed to the radius of the forearm, and the abductor pollicis longus pulls at its distal attachment, the distal radius moves. If the forearm is in a position of pronation, the abductor pollicis longus' line of pull causes the distal radius to be pulled in a posterolateral direction around the distal ulna (and the head of the radius to laterally rotate). This movement of the radius is called *supination*. Therefore the abductor pollicis longus supinates the forearm at the radioulnar joints. (action 6)

Reverse Mover Action Notes

- The reverse action of movement of the metacarpal of the thumb at the first CMC joint is to move the carpal bone (trapezium) toward the metacarpal of the thumb at the CMC joint; this would occur if the distal end (the metacarpal) is fixed, perhaps because the thumb is gripping an immovable object. Movement of the trapezium would likely involve movement of the entire carpus (wrist) and forearm relative to the hand. (reverse actions 1, 2, 3)
- Reverse actions at the wrist joint occur when the hand is fixed by holding onto an immovable object and the forearm moves relative to the fixed hand. (reverse actions 4, 5)
- Supination of the forearm usually involves a mobile radius moving around a fixed ulna. The reverse action in which the ulna supinates around a fixed radius usually occurs if the hand is fixed by holding onto an immovable object. Because the elbow joint does not allow rotation, supination of the ulna causes the arm to move with it, causing medial rotation of the arm at the glenohumeral joint. (reverse action 6)

Eccentric Antagonist Functions

1. Restrains/slows adduction, flexion, and medial rotation of the metacarpal at the CMC joint of the thumb

2. Restrains/slows adduction, flexion, and lateral rotation of the carpal bone (trapezium) at the CMC joint of the thumb
3. Restrains/slows wrist joint ulnar deviation and extension
4. Restrains/slows pronation of the radioulnar joints

Isometric Stabilization Functions

1. Stabilizes the first CMC joint
2. Stabilizes the wrist joint
3. Stabilizes the radioulnar joints

Additional Notes on Functions

1. Whenever the abductor pollicis longus contracts quickly or powerfully to perform extension of the thumb at the CMC joint, it would also radially deviate the hand at the wrist joint. To prevent this, an ulnar deviator of the hand at the wrist joint (i.e., flexor carpi ulnaris or extensor carpi ulnaris) must contract to create an ulnar deviation force, stabilizing the hand so that it does not radially deviate. Palpate the ulnar side of the forearm when extending the thumb and this can be felt.
2. All three deep distal muscles of the posterior forearm that move the thumb (abductor pollicis longus, extensor pollicis brevis, and extensor pollicis longus) can do radial deviation (abduction) of the hand at the wrist joint.

INNERVATION
- ☐ The Radial Nerve
  - ☐ the posterior interosseus nerve, **C7**, C8

ARTERIAL SUPPLY
- ☐ The Posterior Interosseus Artery (a branch of the Ulnar Artery)
  - ☐ and the perforating branches of the Anterior Interosseus Artery (a branch of the Ulnar Artery)

🖐 PALPATION

1. With the client seated and the forearm in a position halfway between full pronation and full supination, place palpating hand on the lateral wrist.
2. Have the client actively abduct and extend the thumb at the first carpometacarpal joint and feel for the distal tendons of the abductor pollicis longus and extensor pollicis brevis. (They are usually visible bordering the anatomic snuffbox on the radial [lateral] side, but may appear as one tendon because they are right next to each other.)
3. Continue palpating the abductor pollicis longus proximally and distally as far as possible.

Abductor Pollicis Longus (of Deep Distal Four Group)—*cont'd*

■ RELATIONSHIP TO OTHER STRUCTURES

☐ The abductor pollicis longus is one of four deep muscles found in the distal posterior forearm (the abductor pollicis longus, extensor pollicis brevis, extensor pollicis longus, and extensor indicis). Most of the belly of the abductor pollicis longus is deep to the extensor digitorum, extensor digiti minimi, and extensor carpi ulnaris.

☐ The belly of the abductor pollicis longus is directly lateral to the extensor pollicis longus and the extensor pollicis brevis.

☐ The distal belly and tendon of the abductor pollicis longus become superficial (along with the extensor pollicis brevis) in the distal posterolateral forearm and lie superficial to the radial group of muscles (the brachioradialis, extensor carpi radialis longus, and extensor carpi radialis brevis).

☐ The abductor pollicis longus and extensor pollicis brevis pass immediately anterior to the styloid process of the radius.

☐ The abductor pollicis longus is involved with the superficial back arm line and deep front arm line myofascial meridians.

■ MISCELLANEOUS

1. The abductor pollicis longus is one of the four muscles that make up the deep distal four group of the posterior forearm (the four muscles of this group are the abductor pollicis longus, extensor pollicis brevis, extensor pollicis longus, and extensor indicis).

2. The distal tendon of the abductor pollicis longus and the distal tendon of the extensor pollicis brevis make up the lateral border of the anatomic snuffbox. These two tendons are very close together and can be difficult to distinguish from each other. The abductor pollicis longus is the more anterolateral of the two. (Note: The anatomic snuffbox is bordered on the medial side by the extensor pollicis longus.)

3. The distal tendon of the abductor pollicis longus often splits to also attach onto the trapezium.

4. The abductor pollicis longus and the extensor pollicis brevis share a common synovial sheath. With excessive movements of the thumb, the friction between the tendons of the abductor pollicis longus and/or the extensor pollicis brevis and the styloid process of the radius can cause a tenosynovitis (inflammation of the synovial sheath). This condition is known as *de Quervain's disease.*

8

Extensor Pollicis Brevis (of Deep Distal Four Group)

The name, extensor pollicis brevis, *tells us that this muscle extends the thumb and is short (shorter than the extensor pollicis longus).*

Derivation	☐ extensor: L. *a muscle that extends a body part.*
	pollicis: L. *thumb.*
	brevis: L. *shorter.*
Pronunciation	☐ eks-TEN-sor, POL-i-sis, BRE-vis

■ ATTACHMENTS

☐ **Posterior Radius**
  ☐ the distal ⅓ and the adjacent interosseus membrane

to the

☐ **Thumb**
  ☐ the posterolateral base of the proximal phalanx

■ FUNCTIONS

CONCENTRIC (SHORTENING) MOVER ACTIONS	
Standard Mover Actions	**Reverse Mover Actions**
☐ **1. Extends the thumb at the CMC and MCP joints**	☐ 1. Extends the carpal bone (trapezium) at the CMC joint and extends the first metacarpal at the MCP joint
☐ **2. Abducts the thumb at the CMC joint**	☐ 2. Abducts the carpal bone (trapezium) at the CMC joint
☐ 3. Laterally rotates the thumb at the CMC joint	☐ 3. Medially rotates the carpal bone (trapezium) at the CMC joint
☐ 4. Radially deviates the hand at the wrist joint	☐ 4. Radially deviates the forearm at the wrist joint

CMC joint = carpometacarpal joint (of the thumb; saddle joint of the thumb); MCP joint = metacarpophalangeal joint

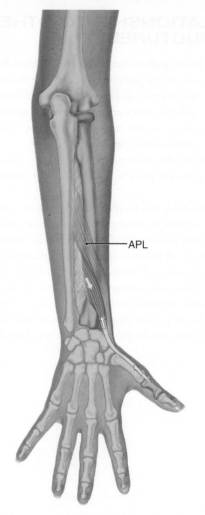

Figure 8-11 Posterior view of the extensor pollicis brevis. The abductor pollicis longus (APL) has been ghosted in.

Standard Mover Action Notes

- The extensor pollicis brevis crosses the first CMC joint of the thumb laterally (radially) to attach onto the proximal phalanx of the thumb (with its fibers running vertically in the frontal plane). When the extensor pollicis brevis contracts, it pulls the proximal phalanx of the thumb laterally (radially) within the plane of the palm of the hand (frontal plane), away from the index finger. This action is called extension of the thumb. Therefore the extensor pollicis brevis extends the thumb by extending the metacarpal of the thumb at the first CMC joint. Additionally, the extensor pollicis brevis also crosses the first MCP joint of the thumb laterally (radially). Therefore it extends the proximal phalanx of the thumb at this joint as well. (Note: Because of the rotational development of the thumb embryologically, the named actions of flexion and extension of the thumb occur within the frontal plane.) (action 1)

- The extensor pollicis brevis crosses the first CMC joint of the thumb anteriorly to attach onto the proximal phalanx of the thumb (with its fibers running vertically in the sagittal plane). When the extensor pollicis brevis contracts, it pulls the proximal phalanx of the thumb in a direction that is perpendicular to and away from the plane of the palm of the hand (moving it within the sagittal plane). This action is called abduction of the thumb. Therefore the extensor pollicis brevis abducts the thumb by abducting the metacarpal of the thumb at the first CMC joint. (Note: Because of the rotational development of the thumb embryologically, the named actions of abduction and adduction of the thumb occur within the sagittal plane.) The extensor pollicis brevis also crosses the first MCP joint of the thumb anteriorly; however, this joint does not allow abduction. (action 2)

- The extensor pollicis brevis crosses the first CMC joint posteriorly from medial in the forearm to attach more laterally onto the thumb (with its fibers running slightly horizontally

Extensor Pollicis Brevis (of Deep Distal Four Group)—*cont'd*

in the transverse plane). When the extensor pollicis brevis contracts, it pulls the thumb posterolaterally. This is lateral rotation of the thumb, because the anterior side of the thumb rotates laterally. Therefore the extensor pollicis brevis laterally rotates the thumb at the first CMC joint. (action 3)

- The extensor pollicis brevis crosses the wrist joint on the radial (lateral) side (with it fibers running vertically in the frontal plane); therefore it radially deviates (abducts) the hand at the wrist joint. (action 4)

Reverse Mover Action Notes

- The reverse action of movement of the metacarpal of the thumb at the first CMC joint is to move the carpal bone (trapezium) toward the metacarpal of the thumb at the CMC joint; this would occur if the distal end (the metacarpal) is fixed, perhaps because the thumb is gripping an immovable object. Movement of the trapezium would likely involve movement of the entire carpus (wrist) and forearm relative to the hand. (reverse actions 1, 2, 3)
- The reverse action of movement of the proximal phalanx of the thumb at the MCP joint is to move the metacarpal of the thumb toward the proximal phalanx at the MCP joint; this would occur if the distal end (the proximal phalanx) is fixed, perhaps because the thumb is gripping an immovable object. (reverse action 1)
- Reverse actions at the wrist joint occur when the hand is fixed by holding onto an immovable object and the forearm moves relative to the fixed hand. (reverse action 4)

Eccentric Antagonist Functions

1. Restrains/slows flexion of the CMC and MCP joints of the thumb
2. Restrains/slows adduction of the CMC joint of the thumb
3. Restrains/slows medial rotation of the metacarpal and lateral rotation of the carpal bone (trapezium) at the CMC joint of the thumb
4. Restrains/slows wrist joint ulnar deviation

Isometric Stabilization Functions

1. Stabilizes the CMC and MCP joints of the thumb
2. Stabilizes the wrist joint

Additional Notes on Functions

1. Whenever the extensor pollicis brevis contracts quickly or powerfully to perform extension and/or abduction of the thumb at the CMC joint, it would also radially deviate the hand at the wrist joint. To prevent this, an ulnar deviator of the hand at the wrist joint (i.e., flexor carpi ulnaris or extensor carpi ulnaris) must contract to create an ulnar deviation

force, stabilizing the hand so that it does not radially deviate. Palpate the ulnar side of the forearm when extending and/ or abducting the thumb and this can be felt.

2. The extensor pollicis brevis is the only muscle of the deep distal four group that cannot supinate the forearm at the radioulnar joints because it does not cross the radioulnar joints.

3. All three deep distal muscles of the posterior forearm that move the thumb (abductor pollicis longus, extensor pollicis brevis, and extensor pollicis longus) can do radial deviation (abduction) of the hand at the wrist joint.

INNERVATION
☐ The Radial Nerve
  ☐ the posterior interosseus nerve, **C7**, C8

ARTERIAL SUPPLY
☐ The Posterior Interosseus Artery (a branch of the Ulnar Artery)
  ☐ and the perforating branches of the Anterior Interosseus Artery (a branch of the Ulnar Artery)

✋ PALPATION

1. With the client seated and the forearm in a position halfway between full pronation and full supination, place palpating hand on the lateral wrist.
2. Have the client actively abduct and extend the thumb at the first carpometacarpal joint and feel for the distal tendons of the extensor pollicis brevis and abductor pollicis longus. (They are usually visible bordering the anatomic snuffbox on the radial (lateral) side, but may appear as one tendon because they are right next to each other.)
3. Continue palpating the extensor pollicis brevis proximally and distally as far as possible.

■ RELATIONSHIP TO OTHER STRUCTURES

☐ The extensor pollicis brevis is one of four deep muscles found in the distal posterior forearm (the abductor pollicis longus, extensor pollicis brevis, extensor pollicis longus, and extensor indicis). Most of the belly of the extensor pollicis brevis is deep to the extensor digitorum.

☐ The extensor pollicis brevis lies directly medial to the abductor pollicis longus and directly lateral to the extensor pollicis longus.

☐ The distal belly and tendon of the extensor pollicis brevis become superficial (along with the abductor pollicis longus) in the distal posterolateral forearm and lie superficial to the radial group of muscles (the brachioradialis and extensors carpi radialis longus and brevis).

☐ The extensor pollicis brevis and abductor pollicis longus pass immediately anterior to the styloid process of the radius.

☐ The extensor pollicis brevis is involved with the superficial back arm line and deep front arm line myofascial meridians.

■ MISCELLANEOUS

1. The extensor pollicis brevis is one of the four muscles that make up the deep distal four group of the posterior forearm (the four muscles of this group are the abductor pollicis longus, extensor pollicis brevis, extensor pollicis longus, and extensor indicis).

2. The distal tendon of the extensor pollicis brevis and the distal tendon of the abductor pollicis longus make up the lateral border of the anatomic snuffbox. These two tendons are very close together and can be difficult to distinguish from each other. The extensor pollicis brevis is the more posteromedial of the two. (Note: The anatomic snuffbox is bordered medially by the extensor pollicis longus.)

3. The extensor pollicis brevis and the abductor pollicis longus share a common synovial sheath. With excessive movements of the thumb, the friction between the tendons of the extensor pollicis brevis and/or the abductor pollicis longus and the styloid process of the radius can cause a tenosynovitis (inflammation of the synovial sheath). This condition is known as *de Quervain's disease.*

8

Extensor Pollicis Longus (of Deep Distal Four Group)

The name, extensor pollicis longus, *tells us that this muscle extends the thumb and is long (longer than the extensor pollicis brevis).*

Derivation	☐ extensor: L. *a muscle that extends a body part.*
	pollicis: L. *thumb.*
	longus: L. *longer.*
Pronunciation	☐ eks-TEN-sor, POL-i-sis, LONG-us

■ ATTACHMENTS

☐ **Posterior Ulna**
    ☐ the middle ⅓ and the adjacent interosseus membrane

to the

☐ **Thumb**
    ☐ via its dorsal digital expansion onto the posterior surface of the distal phalanx of the thumb

■ FUNCTIONS

CONCENTRIC (SHORTENING) MOVER ACTIONS	
Standard Mover Actions	**Reverse Mover Actions**
☐ **1. Extends the thumb at the CMC, MCP, and IP joints**	☐ 1. Extends the carpal bone (trapezium) at the CMC joint; extends the first metacarpal at the MCP joint and extends the proximal phalanx at the IP joint
☐ 2. Laterally rotates the thumb at the CMC joint	☐ 2. Medially rotates the carpal bone (trapezium) at the CMC joint
☐ 3. Extends the hand at the wrist joint	☐ 3. Extends the forearm at the wrist joint
☐ 4. Radially deviates the hand at the wrist joint	☐ 4. Radially deviates the forearm at the wrist joint
☐ 5. Supinates the forearm at the radioulnar joints	☐ 5. Supinates the ulna and medially rotates the arm
☐ 6. Adducts the thumb at the CMC joint	☐ 6. Adducts the carpal bone (trapezium) at the CMC joint

CMC joint = carpometacarpal joint (of the thumb; saddle joint of the thumb); MCP joint = metacarpophalangeal joint; IP joint = interphalangeal joint

Standard Mover Action Notes

- The extensor pollicis longus crosses the CMC joint of the thumb laterally (radially) to attach onto the distal phalanx of the thumb (with its fibers running vertically in the frontal plane). When the extensor pollicis longus contracts, it pulls the distal phalanx of the thumb laterally (radially) within the plane of the palm of the hand (frontal plane), away from the index finger. This action is called *extension of the thumb.* Therefore the extensor pollicis longus extends the thumb by extending the metacarpal of the thumb at the first CMC joint. (Note: Because of the rotational development of the

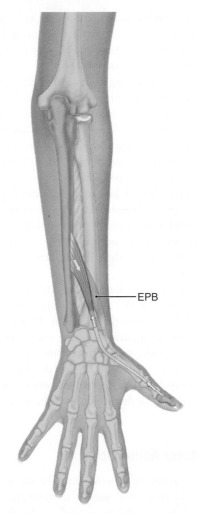

Figure 8-12 Posterior view of the extensor pollicis longus. The extensor pollicis brevis (EPB) has been ghosted in.

thumb embryologically, the named actions of flexion and extension of the thumb occur within the frontal plane.) Additionally, the extensor pollicis longus crosses the MCP and IP joints of the thumb laterally (radially). Therefore it also extends the phalanges of the thumb at these joints. (action 1)

- The extensor pollicis longus crosses the first CMC joint posteriorly from medial in the forearm to attach more laterally onto the thumb (with its fibers running slightly horizontally in the transverse plane). When the extensor pollicis longus contracts, it pulls the thumb posterolaterally. This is lateral rotation of the thumb, because the anterior side of the thumb rotates laterally. Therefore the extensor pollicis longus laterally rotates the thumb at the first CMC joint. (action 2)

- The extensor pollicis longus crosses the wrist joint posteriorly (with its fibers running vertically in the sagittal plane); therefore it extends the hand at the wrist joint. (action 3)

Extensor Pollicis Longus (of Deep Distal Four Group)—cont'd

- The extensor pollicis longus crosses the wrist joint on the radial (lateral) side (with it fibers running vertically in the frontal plane); therefore it radially deviates (abducts) the hand at the wrist joint. (action 4)
- The extensor pollicis longus crosses the ulna and radius in the posterior forearm with an ulnar-to-radial orientation to its fibers (hence its fibers are running somewhat horizontally in the transverse plane). When the thumb and the hand are fixed to the radius of the forearm, and the extensor pollicis longus pulls at its distal attachment, the distal radius moves. If the forearm is in a position of pronation, the extensor pollicis longus' line of pull causes the distal radius to be pulled in a posterolateral direction around the distal ulna (and the head of the radius to laterally rotate). This movement of the radius is called *supination*. Therefore the extensor pollicis longus supinates the forearm at the radioulnar joints. (action 5)
- The extensor pollicis longus can adduct the thumb at the CMC joint if the thumb is first in an abducted position. Adduction of the thumb at the CMC joint is a movement of the metacarpal of the thumb in the sagittal plane, perpendicular to and toward the palm of the hand. (Note: Because of the rotational development of the thumb embryologically, the named actions of abduction and adduction of the thumb occur within the sagittal plane.) (action 6)

Reverse Mover Action Notes

- The reverse action of movement of the metacarpal of the thumb at the first CMC joint is to move the carpal bone (trapezium) toward the metacarpal of the thumb at the CMC joint; this would occur if the distal end (the metacarpal) is fixed, perhaps because the thumb is gripping an immovable object. Movement of the trapezium would likely involve movement of the entire carpus (wrist) and forearm relative to the hand. (reverse actions 1, 2, 6)
- Reverse actions at the wrist joint occur when the hand is fixed by holding onto an immovable object and the forearm moves relative to the fixed hand. (reverse actions 3, 4)
- Supination of the forearm usually involves a mobile radius moving around a fixed ulna. The reverse action in which the ulna supinates around a fixed radius usually occurs if the hand is fixed by holding onto an immovable object. Because the elbow joint does not allow rotation, supination of the ulna causes the arm to move with it, causing medial rotation of the arm at the glenohumeral joint. (reverse action 5)

Eccentric Antagonist Functions

1. Restrains/slows flexion of the CMC, MCP, and IP joints of the thumb

2. Restrains/slows medial rotation of the metacarpal and lateral rotation of the carpal bone (trapezium) at the CMC joint of the thumb
3. Restrains/slows wrist joint flexion and ulnar deviation
4. Restrains/slows pronation of the radioulnar joints
5. Restrains/slows abduction of the CMC joint of the thumb

Isometric Stabilization Functions

1. Stabilizes the CMC, MCP, and IP joints of the thumb
2. Stabilizes the wrist joint
3. Stabilizes the radioulnar joints

Additional Notes on Functions

1. Whenever the extensor pollicis longus contracts quickly or powerfully to perform extension of the thumb at the CMC joint, it would also radially deviate the hand at the wrist joint. To prevent this, an ulnar deviator of the hand at the wrist joint (i.e., flexor carpi ulnaris or extensor carpi ulnaris) must contract to create an ulnar deviation force, stabilizing the hand so that it does not radially deviate. Palpate the ulnar side of the forearm when extending the thumb and this can be felt.
2. All three deep distal muscles of the posterior forearm that move the thumb (abductor pollicis longus, extensor pollicis brevis, and extensor pollicis longus) can do radial deviation (abduction) of the hand at the wrist joint.

INNERVATION
- ☐ The Radial Nerve
  - ☐ the posterior interosseus nerve, **C7**, C8

ARTERIAL SUPPLY
- ☐ The Posterior Interosseus Artery (a branch of the Ulnar Artery)
  - ☐ and the perforating branches of the Anterior Interosseus Artery (a branch of the Ulnar Artery)

✋ PALPATION

1. With the client seated and the forearm in a position halfway between full pronation and full supination, place palpating hand on the posterolateral wrist.
2. Have the client actively extend the thumb at the carpometacarpal, metacarpophalangeal, and interphalangeal joints and feel for tensing of the distal tendon of the extensor pollicis longus. It is usually visible bordering the anatomic snuffbox on the ulnar (medial) side.
3. Continue palpating the extensor pollicis longus distally to the thumb and proximally to the attachment on the radial (lateral) surface of the ulna.

Extensor Pollicis Longus (of Deep Distal Four Group)—*cont'd*

■ RELATIONSHIP TO OTHER STRUCTURES

☐ The extensor pollicis longus is one of four deep muscles found in the distal posterior forearm (the abductor pollicis longus, extensor pollicis brevis, extensor pollicis longus, and extensor indicis). Most of the belly of the extensor pollicis longus is deep to the extensor digitorum, extensor digiti minimi, and extensor carpi ulnaris.

☐ The extensor pollicis longus' proximal attachment onto the posterior ulna is located between the abductor pollicis longus and the extensor indicis; it is distal to the abductor pollicis longus and proximal to the extensor indicis.

☐ The extensor pollicis longus is superficial to the proximal attachment of the extensor pollicis brevis.

☐ The bellies of the abductor pollicis longus and the extensor pollicis brevis lie just lateral to the belly of the extensor pollicis longus.

☐ The distal belly and tendon of the extensor pollicis longus become superficial in the posterior wrist. They are superficial to the extensor carpi radialis longus and the extensor carpi radialis brevis.

☐ The distal tendon of the extensor pollicis longus turns around a bony fulcrum on the radius called the *dorsal tubercle* (also known as *Lister's tubercle*) that alters its line of pull.

☐ The extensor pollicis longus is involved with the superficial back arm line myofascial meridian.

■ MISCELLANEOUS

1. The extensor pollicis longus is one of the four muscles that make up the deep distal four group of the posterior forearm (the four muscles of this group are the abductor pollicis longus, extensor pollicis brevis, extensor pollicis longus, and extensor indicis).

2. The distal tendon of the extensor pollicis longus makes up the medial border of the anatomic snuffbox. (Note: The anatomic snuffbox is bordered laterally by the abductor pollicis longus and extensor pollicis brevis.)

3. The distal attachment of the extensor pollicis longus spreads out to become a fibrous aponeurotic expansion that covers the posterior, medial, and lateral sides of the proximal phalanx of the thumb. It then continues distally to attach onto the posterior side of the distal phalanx. This structure is called the *dorsal digital expansion*.

4. The dorsal digital expansion is also known as the *extensor expansion* and/or the *dorsal hood*. The name dorsal hood is given because it serves as a movable hood of tissue when the thumb flexes and extends.

5. The dorsal digital expansion of the thumb also serves as an attachment site for the abductor pollicis brevis and adductor pollicis (and the palmar interosseus muscle of the thumb, if present). Given that the dorsal digital expansion of the thumb crosses the interphalangeal joint posteriorly, these muscles can all extend the distal phalanx of the thumb at this joint.

8

Extensor Indicis (of Deep Distal Four Group)

The name, extensor indicis, *tells us that this muscle extends the index finger.*

Derivation	☐ extensor: L. *a muscle that extends a body part.*
	indicis: L. *index finger* (finger two).
Pronunciation	☐ eks-TEN-sor, IN-di-sis

■ ATTACHMENTS

☐ **Posterior Ulna**
  ☐ the distal ⅓ and the interosseus membrane

to the

☐ **Index Finger (Finger Two)**
  ☐ attaches into the ulnar side of the tendon of the extensor digitorum muscle (to attach onto the posterior surface of the middle and distal phalanges of the index finger via the dorsal digital expansion)

■ FUNCTIONS

CONCENTRIC (SHORTENING) MOVER ACTIONS	
Standard Mover Actions	**Reverse Mover Actions**
☐ **1. Extends the index finger at the MCP, PIP, and DIP joints**	☐ 1. Extends the second metacarpal at the MCP joint; extends the proximal phalanx at the PIP joint; extends the middle phalanx at the DIP joint
☐ **2. Extends the hand at the wrist joint**	☐ 2. Extends the forearm at the wrist joint
☐ 3. Adducts the index finger at the MCP joint	☐ 3. Adducts the second metacarpal at the MCP joint
☐ 4. Supinates the forearm at the radioulnar joints	☐ 4. Supinates the ulna and medially rotates the arm

MCP joint = metacarpophalangeal joint; PIP joint = proximal interphalangeal joint; DIP joint = distal interphalangeal joint

Standard Mover Action Notes

• The extensor indicis crosses the second MCP joint (of the index finger) before it attaches into the distal tendon of the extensor digitorum muscle of the index finger. Because the extensor indicis crosses this joint posteriorly (with its fibers running vertically in the sagittal plane), it extends the index finger at the second MCP joint. Further, by attaching into the distal tendon of the extensor digitorum, the extensor indicis pulls on that tendon the same as if the belly of the extensor digitorum muscle itself had contracted and pulled on its own tendon. Therefore the extensor indicis has the same actions at the index finger as the extensor digitorum muscle has, namely, extension of the index finger at the PIP and DIP joints. (action 1)

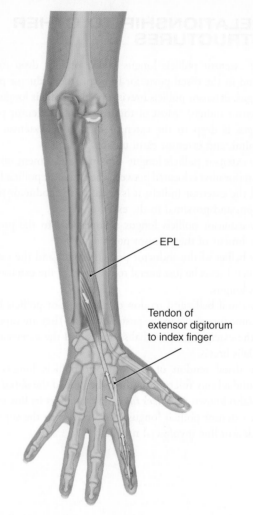

Figure 8-13 Posterior view of the extensor indicis. The extensor pollicis longus (EPL) has been ghosted in.

• More specifically, it extends the proximal phalanx of the index finger at the MCP joint, extends the middle phalanx at the PIP joint, and extends the distal phalanx at the DIP joint. (action 1)
• The extensor indicis crosses the wrist posteriorly (with its fibers running vertically in the sagittal plane); therefore it extends the hand at the wrist joint. (action 2)
• The extensor indicis attaches from the ulna to the index finger, crossing the second MCP joint from medial to lateral (with its fibers running somewhat horizontally in the frontal plane). When the extensor indicis pulls on the index finger, it pulls the index finger medially toward the ulna (i.e., toward the middle finger). Therefore the extensor indicis can adduct the index finger at the second MCP joint. (action 3)
• The extensor indicis crosses the ulna and radius in the posterior forearm with an ulnar-to-radial orientation to its fibers (hence its fibers are running somewhat horizontally in the transverse plane). When the index finger and the hand are fixed to the radius of the forearm, and the extensor indicis pulls at its distal attachment, the distal radius moves. If the

Extensor Indicis (of Deep Distal Four Group)—*cont'd*

forearm is in a position of pronation, the extensor indicis' line of pull causes the distal radius to be pulled in a postero-lateral direction around the distal ulna (and the head of the radius to laterally rotate). This movement of the radius is called supination. Therefore the extensor indicis supinates the forearm at the radioulnar joints. (action 4)

Reverse Mover Action Notes

• The reverse actions move the more proximal bone at each joint. This would occur when the distal bone is fixed, usually when the index finger is gripping an immovable object. (reverse actions 1, 2, 3, 4)
• Reverse actions at the wrist joint occur when the hand is fixed by holding onto an immovable object and the forearm moves relative to the fixed hand. (reverse action 2)
• Supination of the forearm usually involves a mobile radius moving around a fixed ulna. The reverse action in which the ulna supinates around a fixed radius usually occurs if the hand is fixed by holding onto an immovable object. Because the elbow joint does not allow rotation, supination of the ulna causes the arm to move with it, causing medial rotation of the arm at the glenohumeral joint. (reverse action 4)

Eccentric Antagonist Functions

1. Restrains/slows flexion of the index finger at the MCP, PIP, and DIP joints
2. Restrains/slows wrist joint flexion
3. Restrains/slows abduction of the index finger
4. Restrains/slows pronation of the radioulnar joints

Isometric Stabilization Functions

1. Stabilizes the MCP, PIP, and DIP joints of the index finger
2. Stabilizes the wrist joint
3. Stabilizes the radioulnar joints

Additional Note on Functions

1. The extensor indicis, by attaching into the distal tendon of the extensor digitorum, exerts its pull on the dorsal digital expansion of the index finger.

INNERVATION

□ The Radial Nerve
  □ posterior interosseus nerve, C7, C8

ARTERIAL SUPPLY

□ The Posterior Interosseus Artery (a branch of the Ulnar Artery)
  □ and the perforating branches of the Anterior Interosseus Artery (a branch of the Ulnar Artery)

✋ PALPATION

1. With the client seated and the forearm fully pronated at the radioulnar joints, place palpating fingers on the distal ⅓ of the ulna on the posterior side.
2. Have the client actively extend the index finger at the metacarpophalangeal and interphalangeal joints and feel for the contraction of the extensor indicis.
3. Continue palpating the extensor indicis distally and proximally as far as possible. Note: It may be difficult to distinguish the distal tendon of the extensor indicis from the distal tendon of the extensor digitorum that goes to the index finger. If the two can be felt, the extensor indicis will be the more medial (ulnar) of the two.

■ RELATIONSHIP TO OTHER STRUCTURES

□ The extensor indicis is one of four deep muscles found in the distal posterior forearm (the abductor pollicis longus, extensor pollicis brevis, extensor pollicis longus, and extensor indicis). Most of the belly of the extensor indicis is deep to the extensor digitorum, the extensor digiti minimi, and the extensor carpi ulnaris.
□ The extensor indicis attaches onto the posterior ulna just distal to the attachment of the extensor pollicis longus.
□ The belly of the extensor indicis lies just medial to the belly of the extensor pollicis longus.
□ The distal tendon of the extensor indicis becomes superficial in the posterior hand and lies just medial (ulnar) to the tendon of the extensor digitorum that attaches onto the index finger.
□ The extensor indicis is involved with the superficial back arm line myofascial meridian.

■ MISCELLANEOUS

1. The extensor indicis is one of the four muscles that make up the deep distal four group of the posterior forearm (the four muscles of this group are the abductor pollicis longus, extensor pollicis brevis, extensor pollicis longus, and extensor indicis). The extensor indicis is the only muscle of this group that moves the index finger instead of the thumb.
2. The extensor indicis is another extensor muscle (besides the extensor digitorum) of the index finger. This muscle helps us to point at things (or indicate, hence the name *indicis*).
3. Other than the index finger and the thumb, only the little finger has a second extensor muscle (extensor digiti minimi).
4. Both the extensor indicis to the index finger and extensor digiti minimi to the little finger attach into the ulnar side of the extensor digitorum tendon to which they attach.

Intrinsic Muscles of the Finger Joints

CHAPTER OUTLINE

CHAPTER OVERVIEW

The muscles addressed in this chapter are the intrinsic muscles of the hand that move the fingers, including the thumb. Intrinsic muscles of the hand are wholly located within the hand; in other words, they begin and end in the hand. Extrinsic muscles of the hand that also move the fingers are covered in Chapter 8 (extrinsic muscles of the hand attach proximally to the arm or forearm and then travel distally to enter and attach to the hand).

Overview of Structure

☐ Structurally, intrinsic muscles of the hand that move the fingers can be divided into three groups: thenar eminence muscles, hypothenar eminence muscles, and central compartment muscles. There is one other muscle, the palmaris brevis, that does not belong to these groups (although it is occasionally placed into the hypothenar group because it overlies the hypothenar group).

☐ The thenar group is located on the lateral (radial) side of the proximal hand and creates the eminence there. The three thenar eminence group muscles are the abductor pollicis brevis, flexor pollicis brevis, and opponens pollicis. All three thenar eminence muscles attach onto and move the thumb; *pollicis* means thumb.

☐ The hypothenar group is located on the medial (ulnar) side of the proximal hand and creates the eminence there. The three hypothenar eminence group muscles are the abductor digiti minimi manus, flexor digiti minimi manus, and opponens digiti minimi. All three hypothenar eminence muscles attach onto and move the little finger; *digiti minimi* means little finger (or little toe in the foot).

Note the symmetry between the thenar and hypothenar groups. Each group contains three muscles, which include an abductor, a flexor, and an opponens.

☐ The central compartment group is located in the center of the hand between the thenar and hypothenar groups. The muscles of the central compartment are the adductor pollicis, lumbricals manus, palmar interossei, and dorsal interossei manus. The lumbricals manus, palmar interossei, and dorsal interossei manus all attach into the dorsal digital expansion of the hand.

Overview of Function

The following general rules regarding actions can be stated for the functional groups of intrinsic finger muscles:

Review the muscles and bones from this chapter on the enclosed CD!

☐ Fingers two through five can move at three joints: the metacarpophalangeal (MCP), proximal interphalangeal (PIP), and distal interphalangeal (DIP) joints (the little finger can also move at the carpometacarpal [CMC] joint). If a muscle crosses only the MCP joint, it can move the finger only at the MCP joint. If the muscle crosses the MCP and PIP joints, it can move the finger at both of these joints. If the muscle crosses the MCP, PIP, and DIP joints, it can move the finger at all three joints.

☐ The thumb (finger one) can move at three joints: the carpometacarpal (CMC), metacarpophalangeal (MCP), and interphalangeal (IP) joints. Similarly, a muscle can only move the thumb at a joint or joints that it crosses.

☐ If a muscle crosses the MCP, PIP, or DIP joints of fingers two through five on the anterior side, it can flex the finger at the joint(s) crossed; if a muscle crosses the MCP, PIP, or DIP joints of fingers two through five on the posterior side, it can extend the finger at the joint(s) crossed.

☐ If a muscle crosses the MCP joint of fingers two, four, or five on the side that faces the middle finger, it can adduct the finger at the MCP joint; if a muscle crosses the MCP joint of fingers two, three, or four on the side that faces away from the center of the middle finger, it can abduct the finger at the MCP joint (the middle finger abducts in both directions, radial and ulnar abduction).

☐ Regarding motion of the fingers, to be more specific, the proximal phalanx of the finger moves at the MCP joint, the middle phalanx moves at the PIP joint, and the distal phalanx moves at the DIP joint.

☐ Muscles that cross the CMC, MCP, and IP joints of the thumb on the medial side can flex the thumb at the joint(s) crossed; muscles that cross the CMC, MCP, and IP joints of the thumb on the lateral side can extend the thumb at the joint(s) crossed.

☐ Muscles that cross the CMC joint of the thumb on the anterior side can abduct the thumb at the CMC joint; muscles that cross the CMC joint of the thumb on the posterior side can adduct the thumb at the CMC joint.

☐ To be more specific, the metacarpal of the thumb moves at the CMC joint, the proximal phalanx moves at the MCP joint, and the distal phalanx moves at the IP joint.

☐ Note: Because of the rotational development of the thumb embryologically, the named actions of flexion and extension of the thumb occur within the frontal plane (not the sagittal plane); and abduction and adduction of the thumb occur within the sagittal plane (not the frontal plane).

☐ Every muscle that attaches into the dorsal digital expansion of the hand flexes at the MCP and extends at the IP joints.

☐ Reverse actions involve the proximal attachment moving toward the distal one. This would occur when the fingers are holding onto a fixed immovable object.

☐ Therefore reverse actions for all fingers involve the metacarpal moving at the MCP joint (relative to a fixed proximal phalanx). For fingers two through five, reverse actions involve the proximal phalanx moving at the PIP joint (relative to a fixed middle phalanx), and the middle phalanx moving at the DIP joint (relative to a fixed distal phalanx). For the thumb, reverse actions involve the proximal phalanx moving at the IP joint (relative to a fixed distal phalanx).

BOX 9-1

Note Regarding the Palmar Interossei Muscles

There is a great deal of confusion regarding the naming of the intrinsic hand muscles of the thumb. Some sources state that there are four palmar interossei muscles, one of which goes to the thumb; other sources state that there are only three palmar interossei muscles, none of which attach to the thumb. Some sources state that the flexor pollicis brevis has only one part to it; others state that it has superficial and deep heads. Although all sources agree that the adductor pollicis has a transverse head and an oblique head, some state the deep head of the flexor pollicis brevis is actually part of the oblique head of the adductor pollicis; others state that the deep head of the flexor pollicis brevis is separate from the adductor pollicis. This confusion is caused by the great deal of variation that occurs in this region. From one body to another, the anatomy of the musculature varies, leading to confusion as to how to name the structures that are present. This book adheres to the following organization: there are three palmar interossei muscles, and the flexor pollicis brevis has two parts—a superficial head and a deep head. When another fasciculus (group of muscle fibers) is present in this region, it may be a true fourth palmar interosseus muscle (known as the *palmar interosseus of Henle*). It may also be another fasciculus of the deep head of the flexor pollicis brevis or another fasciculus of the oblique head of the adductor pollicis.

Anterior (Palmar) View of the Musculature of the Right Hand—Superficial View with Palmar Aponeurosis

9

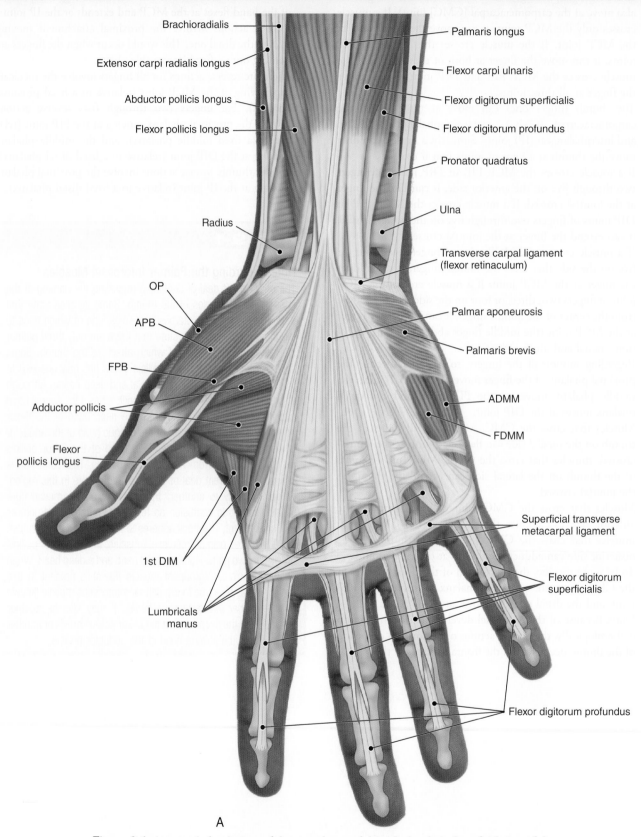

A

Figure 9-1 Anterior (palmar) views of the musculature of the right hand. **A,** Superficial view of the hand with the palmar aponeurosis. ADMM, Abductor digiti minimi manus; APB, abductor pollicis brevis; DIM, dorsal interosseus manus; FDMM, flexor digiti minimi manus; FPB, flexor pollicis brevis; OP, opponens pollicis.

Anterior (Palmar) View of the Musculature of the Right Hand—Superficial Muscular View

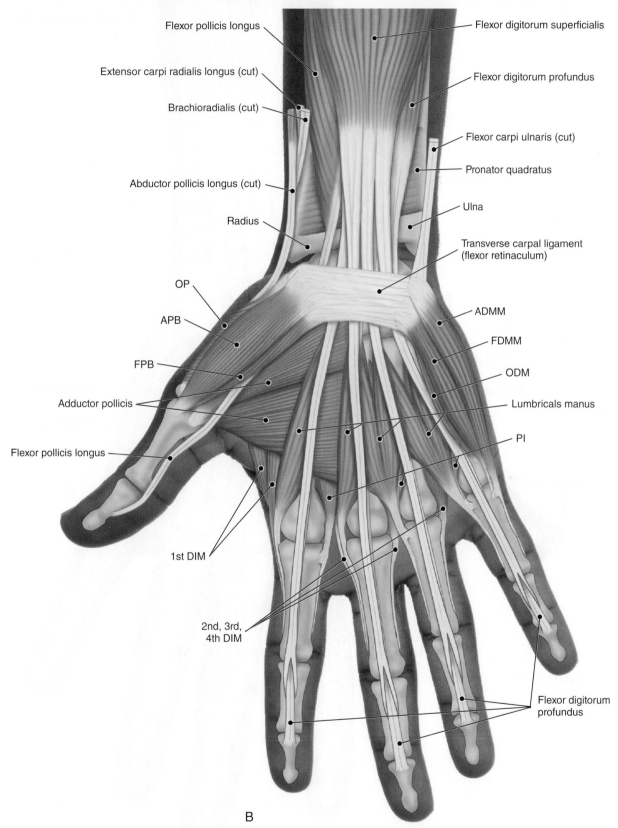

Flexor pollicis longus

Extensor carpi radialis longus (cut)

Brachioradialis (cut)

Abductor pollicis longus (cut)

Radius

OP

APB

FPB

Adductor pollicis

Flexor pollicis longus

1st DIM

2nd, 3rd, 4th DIM

Flexor digitorum superficialis

Flexor digitorum profundus

Flexor carpi ulnaris (cut)

Pronator quadratus

Ulna

Transverse carpal ligament (flexor retinaculum)

ADMM

FDMM

ODM

Lumbricals manus

PI

Flexor digitorum profundus

B

Figure 9-1, cont'd B, Superficial view of the musculature of the hand with the palmar aponeurosis removed. ADMM, Abductor digiti minimi manus; APB, abductor pollicis brevis; DIM, dorsal interossei manus; FDMM, flexor digiti minimi manus; FPB, flexor pollicis brevis; ODM, opponens digiti minimi; OP, opponens pollicis; PI, palmar interossei.

Anterior (Palmar) View of the Musculature of the Right Hand—Intermediate Muscular View

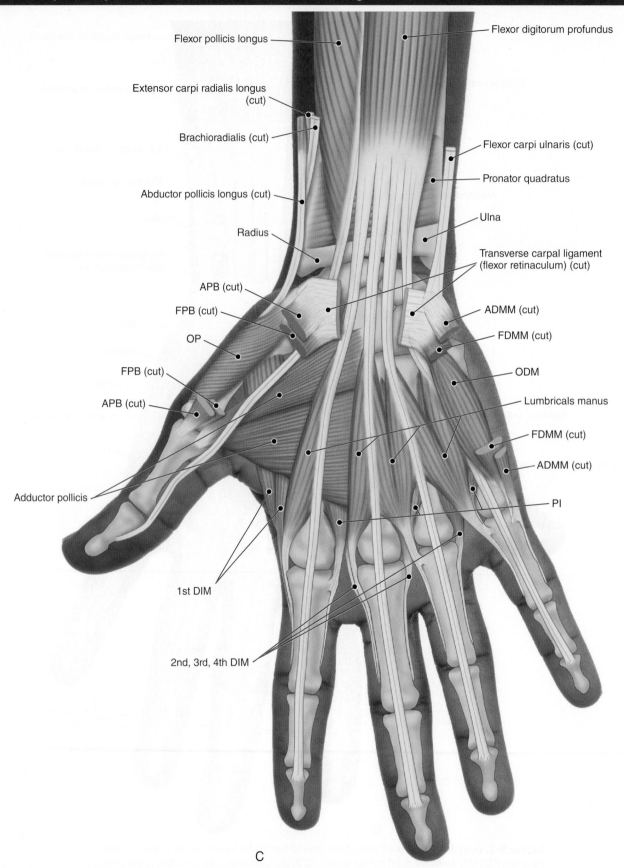

Figure 9-1, cont'd C, Intermediate view with the more superficial thenar and hypothenar muscles cut. *ADMM,* Abductor digiti minimi manus; *APB,* abductor pollicis brevis; *DIM,* dorsal interosseus/interossei manus; *FDMM,* flexor digiti minimi manus; *FPB,* flexor pollicis brevis; *ODM,* opponens digiti minimi; *OP,* opponens pollicis; *PI,* palmar interossei.

Anterior (Palmar) View of the Musculature of the Right Hand—Deep Muscular View

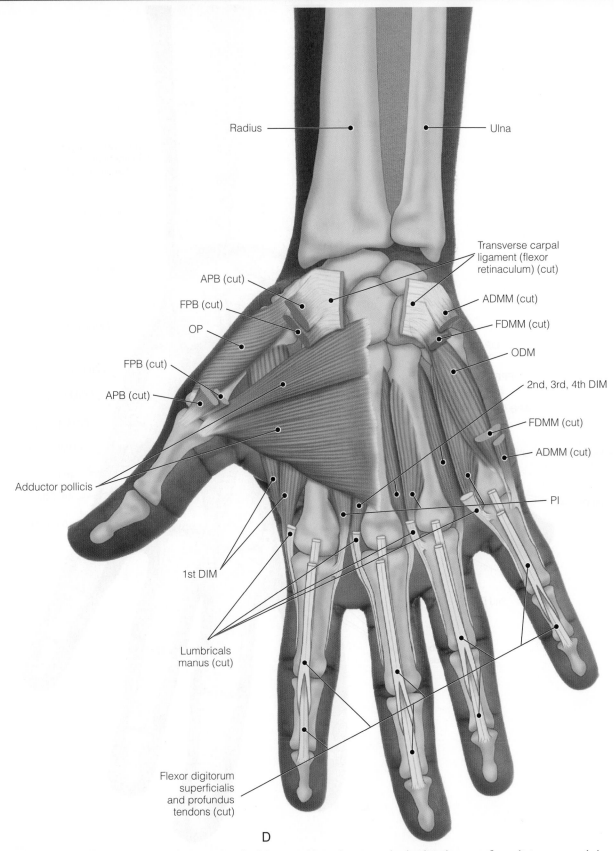

Radius

Ulna

Transverse carpal ligament (flexor retinaculum) (cut)

APB (cut)

ADMM (cut)

FPB (cut)

FDMM (cut)

OP

ODM

FPB (cut)

2nd, 3rd, 4th DIM

APB (cut)

FDMM (cut)

ADMM (cut)

Adductor pollicis

PI

1st DIM

Lumbricals manus (cut)

Flexor digitorum superficialis and profundus tendons (cut)

D

Figure 9-1, cont'd D, Deep view with the more superficial thenar and hypothenar muscles, lumbricals manus, flexor digitorum muscles' tendons, and all forearm muscles cut and/or removed. *ADMM,* Abductor digiti minimi manus; *APB,* abductor pollicis brevis; *DIM,* dorsal interosseus/interossei manus; *FDMM,* flexor digiti minimi manus; *FPB,* flexor pollicis brevis; *ODM,* opponens digiti minimi; *OP,* opponens pollicis; *PI,* palmar interossei.

9

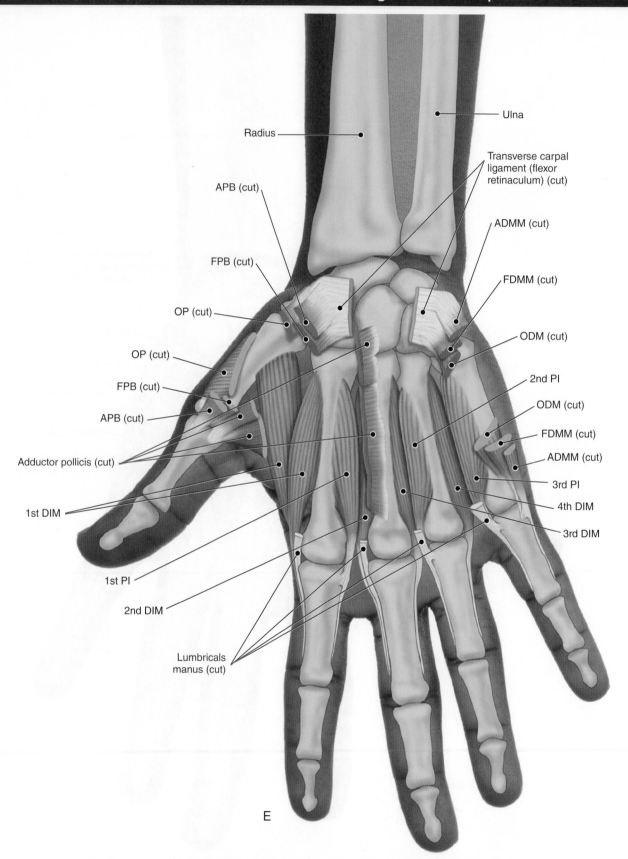

E

Figure 9-1, cont'd E, Deepest view of the palmar musculature. *ADMM,* Abductor digiti minimi manus; *APB,* abductor pollicis brevis; *DIM,* dorsal interosseus manus; *FDMM,* flexor digiti minimi manus; *FPB,* flexor pollicis brevis; *ODM,* opponens digiti minimi; *OP,* opponens pollicis; *PI,* palmar interosseus.

Posterior (Dorsal) View of the Musculature of the Right Hand

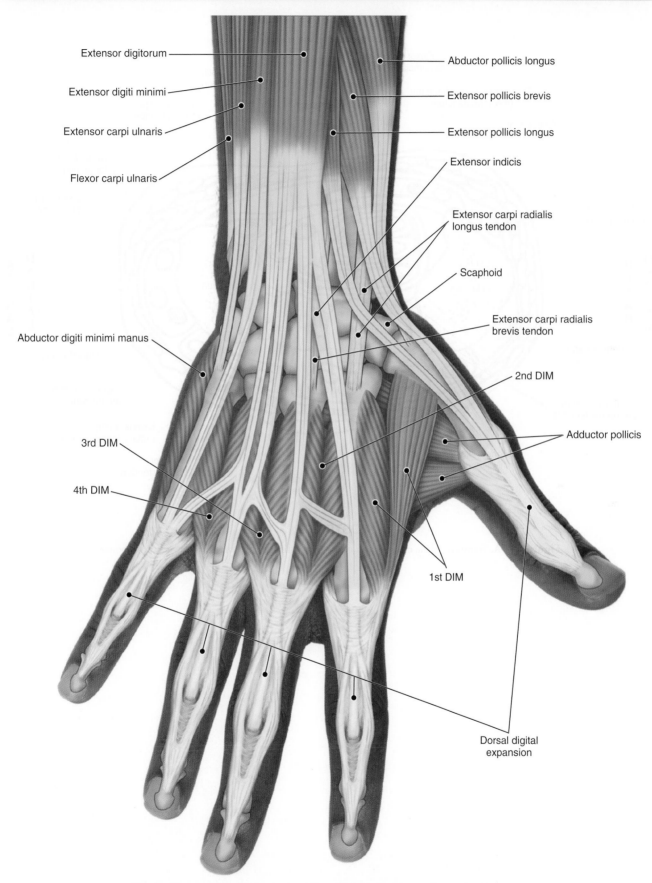

Extensor digitorum

Extensor digiti minimi

Extensor carpi ulnaris

Flexor carpi ulnaris

Abductor digiti minimi manus

3rd DIM

4th DIM

Abductor pollicis longus

Extensor pollicis brevis

Extensor pollicis longus

Extensor indicis

Extensor carpi radialis longus tendon

Scaphoid

Extensor carpi radialis brevis tendon

2nd DIM

Adductor pollicis

1st DIM

Dorsal digital expansion

9

Figure 9-2 Posterior (dorsal) view of the right hand. DIM, Dorsal interosseus manus.

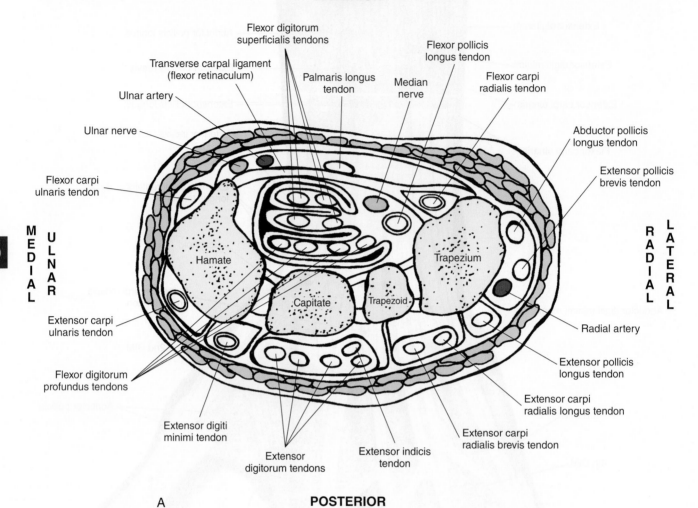

Figure 9-3 A, Transverse plane cross section of the right wrist through the distal row of carpal bones.

Transverse Plane Cross Section of the Right Hand through the Metacarpal Bones

ANTERIOR

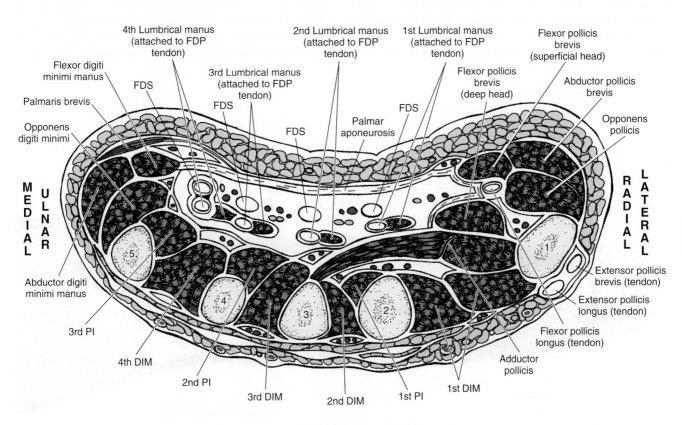

POSTERIOR

B

Figure 9-3, cont'd B, Cross-sectional view of the right hand through the metacarpal bones. DIM, dorsal interosseus manus; FDP, flexor digitorum profundus; FDS, flexor digitorum superficialis; LM, lumbrical manus; PI, palmar interosseus.

Dorsal Digital Expansion

The dorsal digital expansion is an attachment site for the lumbricals manus, palmar interossei, dorsal interossei manus, and abductor digiti minimi manus muscles, which attach into it from the sides. The dorsal digital expansion is actually a fibrous aponeurotic expansion of the distal attachment of the extensor digitorum muscle on the fingers (index, middle, ring, and little fingers) that serves as a movable hood of tissue when the fingers flex and extend. The dorsal digital expansion begins on the dorsal, lateral, and medial sides of the proximal phalanx of each finger and then ultimately attaches onto the dorsal side of the

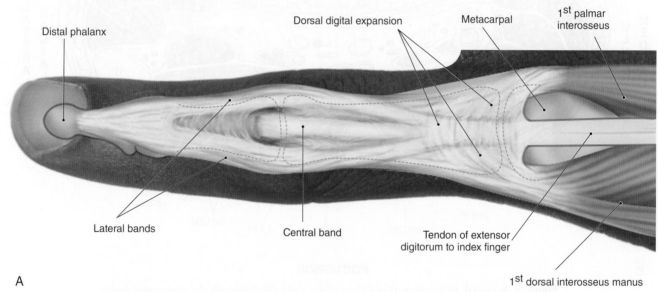

Distal phalanx

Dorsal digital expansion

Metacarpal

1st palmar interosseus

Lateral bands

Central band

Tendon of extensor digitorum to index finger

1st dorsal interosseus manus

A

Figure 9-4 Views of the dorsal digital expansion of the index finger of the right hand. Dotted lines represent borders of underlying bones. **A,** Dorsal view.

Dorsal Digital Expansion—*cont'd*

middle and distal phalanges. Because the dorsal digital expansion eventually attaches onto the dorsal (posterior) side of the middle and distal phalanges, any muscle that attaches into the dorsal digital expansion can create extension of these phalanges at the interphalangeal joints. There is also a dorsal digital expansion of the thumb formed by the distal tendon of the extensor pollicis longus. The dorsal digital expansion is also known as the *extensor expansion* and/or the *dorsal hood.*

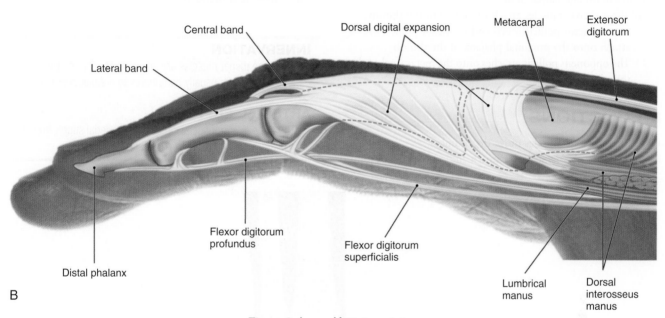

Figure 9-4, cont'd B, Lateral view.

Thenar Eminence Group

■ ORGANIZATION OF THE THENAR MUSCLES

The thenar eminence is an eminence of soft tissue located on the radial side of the palm of the hand. There are three muscles in the thenar eminence group: the abductor pollicis brevis, flexor pollicis brevis, and opponens pollicis.

■ ATTACHMENTS

☐ All three thenar muscles attach proximally onto the flexor retinaculum and carpal bones.
☐ All three thenar muscles attach distally onto the thumb.
  ☐ The abductor pollicis brevis and the flexor pollicis brevis attach onto the proximal phalanx of the thumb.
  ☐ The opponens pollicis attaches onto the metacarpal of the thumb.

■ FUNCTIONS

☐ All three thenar muscles move the thumb.
☐ In each case, the name of the muscle indicates its major joint action.

■ MISCELLANEOUS

☐ The layering of the thenar muscles is approximately as follows: The abductor pollicis brevis is the most superficial of the three. The flexor pollicis brevis is intermediate. The opponens pollicis is the deepest of the three.
☐ There are three muscles located in the hypothenar eminence that are analogous to the thenar muscles. The three hypothenar muscles are the abductor digiti minimi manus, flexor digiti minimi manus, and opponens digiti minimi.
☐ The thenar muscles are located within the deep front arm line myofascial meridian.

INNERVATION
☐ The three thenar muscles are innervated by the median nerve. (The ulnar nerve usually contributes to a small degree.)

ARTERIAL SUPPLY
☐ The three thenar muscles receive their arterial supply from the radial artery.

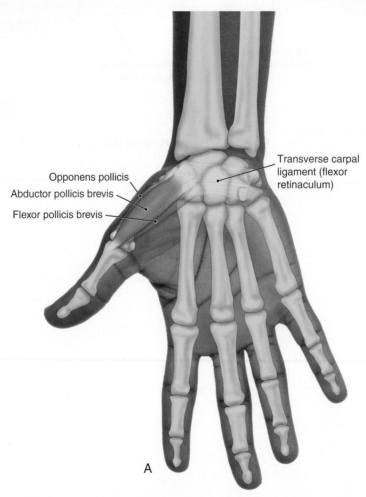

A

Figure 9-5 Anterior views of the right thenar group muscles. **A,** Superficial view.

9

Thenar Eminence Group—*cont'd*

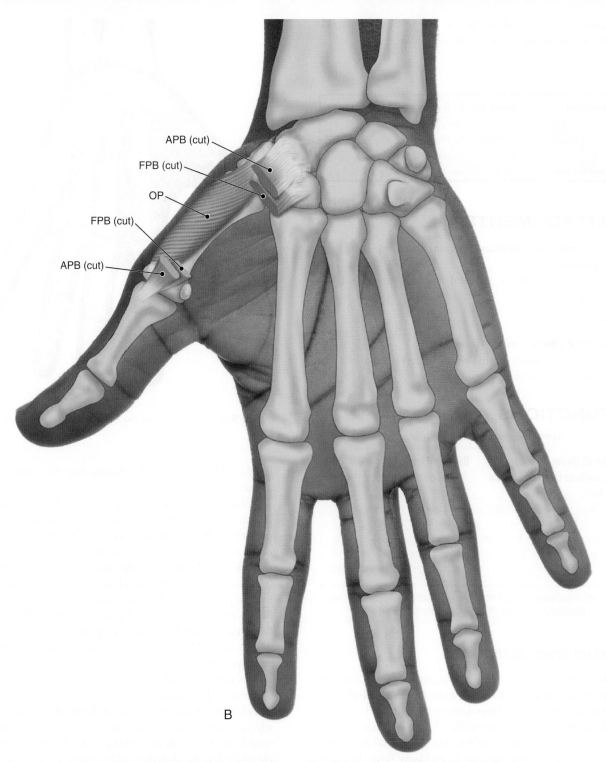

Figure 9-5, cont'd B, Deep view. The abductor pollicis brevis and flexor pollicis brevis have been cut. APB, abductor pollicis brevis; FPB, flexor pollicis brevis; OP, opponens pollicis.

Abductor Pollicis Brevis

The name, abductor pollicis brevis, *tells us that this muscle abducts the thumb and is short (shorter than the abductor pollicis longus).*

Derivation	☐ abductor: L. *a muscle that abducts a body part.*
	pollicis L. *thumb.*
	brevis: L. *shorter.*
Pronunciation	☐ ab-DUK-tor, POL-i-sis, BRE-vis

■ ATTACHMENTS

☐ **The Flexor Retinaculum and the Scaphoid and the Trapezium**
  ☐ the tubercle of the scaphoid and the tubercle of the trapezium

to the

☐ **Proximal Phalanx of the Thumb**
  ☐ the radial (lateral) side of the base of the proximal phalanx and the dorsal digital expansion

■ FUNCTIONS

Concentric (Shortening) Mover Actions	
Standard Mover Actions	**Reverse Mover Actions**
☐ **1. Abducts the thumb at the CMC joint**	☐ 1. Abducts the trapezium at the CMC joint
☐ 2. Flexes the thumb at the MCP joint	☐ 2. Flexes the metacarpal of the thumb at the MCP joint
☐ 3. Extends the thumb at the CMC and IP joints	☐ 3. Extends the trapezium at the CMC joint; extends the proximal phalanx of the thumb at the IP joint.

CMC joint = carpometacarpal joint (of the thumb; saddle joint of the thumb); MCP joint = metacarpophalangeal joint; IP joint = interphalangeal joint

Standard Mover Action Notes

• The abductor pollicis brevis crosses the first CMC joint of the thumb anteriorly to attach onto the proximal phalanx of the thumb (with its fibers running vertically in the sagittal plane). When the abductor pollicis brevis contracts, it pulls the metacarpal of the thumb within the sagittal plane in a direction that is perpendicular to and away from the plane of the palm of the hand. This action is called *abduction of the thumb.* Therefore the abductor pollicis brevis abducts the thumb by abducting the metacarpal of the thumb at the first CMC joint. (Note: Because of the rotational development of the thumb embryologically, the named actions of abduction and adduction of the thumb occur within the sagittal plane). Additionally, the abductor pollicis brevis also crosses

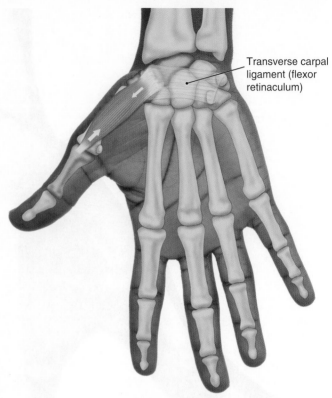

Transverse carpal ligament (flexor retinaculum)

Figure 9-6 Anterior view of the right abductor pollicis brevis.

the first MCP joint of the thumb, but this joint cannot abduct. (action 1)

• The abductor pollicis brevis crosses the MCP joint of the thumb medially (ulnar side) to attach onto the proximal phalanx of the thumb (with its fibers running vertically in the frontal plane). When the abductor pollicis brevis contracts, it pulls the proximal phalanx of the thumb in a medial (ulnar) direction within the plane of the palm of the hand (frontal plane), toward the index finger. This action is called flexion of the thumb. Therefore the abductor pollicis brevis flexes the thumb by flexing the proximal phalanx of the thumb at the MCP joint. (Note: Because of the rotational development of the thumb embryologically, the named actions of flexion and extension of the thumb occur within the frontal plane. (action 2)

• The abductor pollicis brevis crosses the first CMC joint laterally (radially) to attach onto the proximal phalanx of the thumb (with its fibers running vertically in the frontal plane). When the abductor pollicis brevis contracts, it pulls the metacarpal of the thumb in a lateral (radial) direction within the plane of the palm of the hand (frontal plane), away from the index finger. This action is called *extension of the thumb.* Therefore the abductor pollicis brevis extends the thumb by extending the metacarpal of the thumb at the first CMC joint. Additionally, because of its attachment into the dorsal digital expansion of the thumb, the abductor

Abductor Pollicis Brevis—*cont'd*

pollicis brevis also crosses the IP joint of the thumb laterally (radially). Therefore the abductor pollicis brevis extends the distal phalanx of the thumb at the IP joint of the thumb as well. (action 3)

Reverse Mover Action Notes

- The reverse action of motion at the first CMC joint occurs when the carpal bone (trapezium) moves toward the metacarpal of the thumb at the CMC joint. This occurs when the distal end (the metacarpal) is fixed, perhaps because the thumb is gripping an immovable object. Movement of the trapezium would likely involve movement of the entire carpus (wrist) and forearm relative to the hand. (reverse actions 1, 3)
- The reverse action of the thumb at the MCP joint occurs when the metacarpal moves relative to the proximal phalanx of the thumb at the MCP joint. This occurs when the distal segment, the proximal phalanx, is fixed, such as when the thumb is gripping an immovable object. (reverse action 2)
- The reverse action of IP joint extension involves the proximal phalanx moving instead of the distal phalanx. This occurs if the distal phalanx is fixed, usually because the thumb is gripping an immovable object. (reverse action 3)

Eccentric Antagonist Functions

1. Restrains/slows adduction of the CMC joint of the thumb
2. Restrains/slows extension of the MCP joint of the thumb
3. Restrains/slows flexion of the CMC and IP joints of the thumb

Isometric Stabilization Functions

1. Stabilizes the CMC joint of the thumb
2. Stabilizes the MCP joint of the thumb
3. Stabilizes the IP joint of the thumb

Additional Note on Functions

1. All three thenar muscles attach onto and move the thumb. (Note: All three hypothenar muscles attach onto and move the little finger.)

INNERVATION

- ☐ The Median Nerve
  - ☐ C8, **T1**

ARTERIAL SUPPLY

- ☐ Branches of the Radial Artery (a terminal branch of the Brachial Artery)

✋ PALPATION

1. With the client seated or supine, place palpating fingers over the lateral (radial) aspect of the thenar eminence.
2. Ask the client to abduct the thumb at the first carpometacarpal joint against resistance and feel for the contraction of the abductor pollicis brevis. (Note: Distinguishing the ulnar [medial] border of the abductor pollicis brevis from the adjacent flexor pollicis brevis can be difficult.)

■ RELATIONSHIP TO OTHER STRUCTURES

- ☐ The abductor pollicis brevis is superficial in the thenar eminence.
- ☐ The abductor pollicis brevis is lateral to the flexor pollicis brevis. Where they overlap, the abductor pollicis brevis is superficial; the lateral portion of the flexor pollicis brevis is covered by the abductor pollicis brevis.
- ☐ The abductor pollicis brevis is also superficial to the opponens pollicis.
- ☐ The abductor pollicis brevis is located within the deep front arm line myofascial meridian.

■ MISCELLANEOUS

1. The three muscles of the thenar eminence are the abductor pollicis brevis, the flexor pollicis brevis, and the opponens pollicis. (Note: There are three analogous hypothenar muscles. They are the abductor digiti minimi manus, the flexor digiti minimi manus, and the opponens digiti minimi.)

Flexor Pollicis Brevis

The name, flexor pollicis brevis, *tells us that this muscle flexes the thumb and is short (shorter than the flexor pollicis longus).*

Derivation	□ flexor: L. *a muscle that flexes a body part.*
	pollicis: L. *thumb.*
	brevis: L. *shorter.*
Pronunciation	□ FLEKS-or, POL-i-sis, BRE-vis

■ ATTACHMENTS

□ **The Flexor Retinaculum and the Trapezium**

   to the

□ **Proximal Phalanx of the Thumb**
   □ the radial (lateral) side of the base of the proximal phalanx

■ FUNCTIONS

Concentric (Shortening) Mover Actions	
Standard Mover Actions	**Reverse Mover Actions**
□ **1. Flexes the thumb at the CMC and MCP joints**	□ 1. Flexes the trapezium at the CMC joint; flexes the metacarpal of the thumb at the MCP joint
□ 2. Abducts the thumb at the CMC joint	□ 2. Abducts the trapezium at the CMC joint

CMC joint = carpometacarpal joint (of the thumb; saddle joint of the thumb); MCP joint = metacarpophalangeal joint

Standard Mover Action Notes

• The flexor pollicis brevis crosses the CMC joint of the thumb medially (on the ulnar side) to attach onto the proximal phalanx of the thumb (with its fibers running vertically in the frontal plane). When the flexor pollicis brevis contracts, it pulls the metacarpal of the thumb in a medial (ulnar) direction within the plane of the palm of the hand (frontal plane), toward the index finger. This action is called flexion of the thumb. Therefore the flexor pollicis brevis flexes the thumb by flexing the metacarpal of the thumb at the first CMC joint. (Note: Because of the rotational development of the thumb embryologically, the named actions of flexion and extension of the thumb occur within the frontal plane.) Additionally, the flexor pollicis brevis crosses the MCP joint of the thumb medially. Therefore the flexor pollicis brevis flexes the thumb by flexing the proximal phalanx of the thumb at the MCP joint as well. (action 1)

• The flexor pollicis brevis crosses the CMC joint of the thumb anteriorly to attach onto the proximal phalanx of the

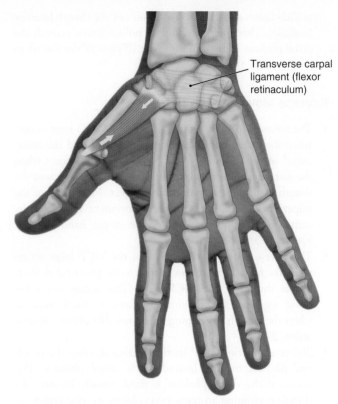

Transverse carpal ligament (flexor retinaculum)

Figure 9-7 Anterior view of the right flexor pollicis brevis.

thumb (with its fibers running vertically in the sagittal plane). When the flexor pollicis brevis contracts, it pulls the metacarpal of the thumb within the sagittal plane in a direction that is perpendicular to and away from the plane of the palm of the hand. This action is called *abduction of the thumb*. Therefore the flexor pollicis brevis abducts the thumb by abducting the metacarpal of the thumb at the first CMC joint. (Note: Because of the rotational development of the thumb embryologically, the named actions of abduction and adduction of the thumb occur within the sagittal plane.) Additionally, the flexor pollicis brevis crosses the MCP joint of the thumb, but this joint cannot abduct. (action 2)

Reverse Mover Action Notes

• The reverse action of motion at the first CMC joint occurs when the carpal bone (trapezium) moves toward the metacarpal of the thumb at the CMC joint. This occurs when the distal end (the metacarpal) is fixed, perhaps because the thumb is gripping an immovable object. Movement of the trapezium would likely involve movement of the entire carpus (wrist) and forearm relative to the hand. (reverse actions 1, 2)

• The reverse action of motion at the MCP joint occurs when the metacarpal moves relative to the proximal phalanx of the

Flexor Pollicis Brevis—*cont'd*

thumb. This occurs when the distal segment, the proximal phalanx, is fixed, usually because the thumb is gripping an immovable object. (reverse action 1)

Eccentric Antagonist Functions

1. Restrains/slows extension of the CMC and MCP joints of the thumb
2. Restrains/slows adduction of the CMC joint of the thumb

Isometric Stabilization Functions

1. Stabilizes the CMC and MCP joints of the thumb

Additional Note on Functions

1. All three thenar muscles attach onto and move the thumb. (Note: All three hypothenar muscles attach onto and move the little finger.)

INNERVATION
- The Median and Ulnar Nerves
  - C8, **T1** (superficial head: the median nerve; deep head: the ulnar nerve)

ARTERIAL SUPPLY
- Branches of the Radial Artery (a terminal branch of the Brachial Artery)

 PALPATION

1. With the client seated or supine, place palpating hand on the medial (ulnar) aspect of the thenar eminence.
2. Ask the client to flex the thumb at the first carpometacarpal joint and feel for the contraction of the medial portion of the flexor pollicis brevis.
3. Continue palpating the flexor pollicis brevis more laterally, deep to the abductor pollicis brevis. (Note: Discerning the lateral portion of the flexor pollicis brevis from the superficial abductor pollicis brevis can be difficult.)

■ RELATIONSHIP TO OTHER STRUCTURES

- The medial portion of the flexor pollicis brevis is superficial in the thenar eminence. The lateral portion of the flexor pollicis brevis is deep to the abductor pollicis brevis.
- The superficial head of the flexor pollicis brevis is superficial to the medial portion of the opponens pollicis. The deep head of the flexor pollicis brevis is deep to the medial portion of the opponens pollicis. Hence the medial portion of the opponens pollicis is sandwiched between the two heads of the flexor pollicis brevis.
- The distal tendon of the flexor pollicis longus is sandwiched between the two heads of the flexor pollicis brevis.
- The flexor pollicis brevis is located within the deep front arm line myofascial meridian.

■ MISCELLANEOUS

1. The three muscles of the thenar eminence are the abductor pollicis brevis, the flexor pollicis brevis, and the opponens pollicis. (Note: There are three analogous hypothenar muscles. They are the abductor digiti minimi manus, the flexor digiti minimi manus, and the opponens digiti minimi.)
2. The flexor pollicis brevis is usually considered to have a superficial and deep head.
3. Some sources state that the flexor pollicis brevis does not have a superficial and deep head but rather has only one part to it. What is called the *deep head of the flexor pollicis brevis* is considered by some sources to be part of the oblique head of the adductor pollicis and by other sources to be a palmar interosseus muscle of the thumb.
4. There is a sesamoid bone in the distal tendon of the flexor pollicis brevis. (Note: There is a second sesamoid bone of the thumb located in the distal tendon of the adductor pollicis.)

9

Opponens Pollicis

The name, opponens pollicis, *tells us that this muscle opposes the thumb.*

Derivation	☐ opponens: L. *opposing.*
	pollicis: L. *thumb.*
Pronunciation	☐ op-PO-nens, POL-i-sis

■ ATTACHMENTS

☐ **The Flexor Retinaculum and the Trapezium**
   ☐ the tubercle of the trapezium

to the

☐ **First Metacarpal (of the Thumb)**
   ☐ the anterior surface and radial (lateral) border

■ FUNCTIONS

Concentric (Shortening) Mover Actions	
Standard Mover Actions	**Reverse Mover Actions**
☐ **1. Opposes the thumb at the CMC joint**	☐ 1. Flexes, laterally rotates, and abducts the trapezium at the CMC joint
☐ 2. Flexes the thumb at the CMC joint	☐ 2. Flexes the trapezium at the CMC joint
☐ 3. Medially rotates the thumb at the CMC joint	☐ 3. Laterally rotates the trapezium at the CMC joint
☐ 4. Abducts the thumb at the CMC joint	☐ 4. Abducts the trapezium at the CMC joint

CMC joint = carpometacarpal joint (of the thumb; saddle joint of the thumb)

Standard Mover Action Notes

- Opposition is not a specific cardinal plane action, but rather is the term given to an oblique plane motion that is a combination of three cardinal plane actions that occur at the CMC joint of the thumb, which are required to bring the pad of the thumb against the pad of another finger. Opposition involves flexion, medial rotation, and abduction of the metacarpal of the thumb. (actions 1, 2, 3, 4)
- The opponens pollicis crosses the first CMC joint of the thumb medially (on the ulnar side) to attach onto the metacarpal of the thumb (with its fibers running vertically in the frontal plane). When the opponens pollicis contracts, it pulls the metacarpal of the thumb in a medial (ulnar) direction within the plane of the palm of the hand (frontal plane), toward the index finger. This action is called *flexion of the thumb.* Therefore the opponens pollicis flexes the thumb by flexing the metacarpal of the thumb at the first CMC joint. (Note: Because of the rotational development of the thumb embryologically, the named actions of flexion and extension of the thumb occur within the frontal plane.) The action of

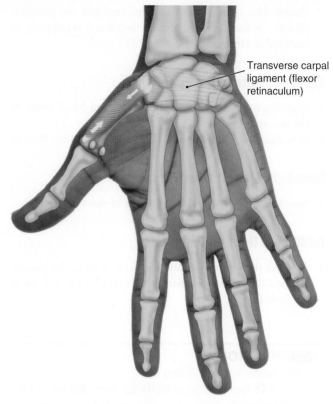

Transverse carpal ligament (flexor retinaculum)

Figure 9-8 Anterior view of the right opponens pollicis.

CMC joint flexion always couples with CMC joint medial rotation. (action 2)

- The opponens pollicis crosses the first CMC joint on the anterior side from slightly medial on the flexor retinaculum to attach more laterally onto the metacarpal of the thumb (with its fibers running somewhat horizontally in the transverse plane). When the opponens pollicis contracts, it rotates the first metacarpal posteriorly toward the little finger (finger five), causing the medial surface of the thumb to face somewhat posteriorly. Therefore the opponens pollicis medially rotates the thumb by medially rotating the metacarpal of the thumb at the CMC joint. The action of CMC joint medial rotation always couples with CMC joint flexion. (action 3)
- The opponens pollicis crosses the first CMC joint of the thumb anteriorly to attach onto the metacarpal of the thumb (with its fibers running vertically in the sagittal plane). When the opponens pollicis contracts, it pulls the metacarpal of the thumb within the sagittal plane in a direction that is perpendicular to and away from the plane of the palm of the hand. This action is called *abduction of the thumb.* Therefore the opponens pollicis abducts the thumb by abducting the metacarpal of the thumb at the first CMC joint. Note: Because of the rotational development of the thumb embryologically, the named actions of abduction and adduction of the thumb occur within the sagittal plane. (action 3)

Opponens Pollicis—*cont'd*

Reverse Mover Action Notes

- Given that opposition is an oblique plane motion that is a combination of three cardinal plane actions, the reverse action of opposition involves the reverse actions of all three of these cardinal plane components of opposition. (reverse actions 1, 2, 3, 4)
- The reverse action of motion at the first CMC occurs when the carpal bone (trapezium) moves toward the metacarpal of the thumb at the CMC joint. This occurs when the distal end (the metacarpal) is fixed, usually because the thumb is gripping an immovable object. Movement of the trapezium would likely involve movement of the entire carpus (wrist) and forearm relative to the hand. (reverse actions 1, 2, 3, 4)

Eccentric Antagonist Functions

1. Restrains/slows reposition of the thumb at the CMC joint
2. Restrains/slows extension of the CMC joint of the thumb
3. Restrains/slows lateral rotation of the metacarpal and medial rotation of the trapezium at the CMC joint of the thumb
4. Restrains/slows adduction of the CMC joint of the thumb

Isometric Stabilization Function

1. Stabilizes the CMC joint of the thumb

Additional Notes on Functions

1. All three thenar muscles attach onto and move the thumb. (Note: All three hypothenar muscles attach onto and move the little finger.)
2. Some sources state that the opponens pollicis can also extend the thumb at the first metacarpophalangeal joint. If this were true, it would have to be the most lateral fibers that would create this action by pulling the thumb radially (laterally) away from the other fingers within the plane of the palm of the hand (the frontal plane).

INNERVATION
- ☐ The Median and Ulnar Nerves
  - ☐ C8, **T1**

ARTERIAL SUPPLY
- ☐ Branches of the Radial Artery (a terminal branch of the Brachial Artery)

 PALPATION

1. With the client seated or supine, place palpating fingers over the lateral portion of the thenar eminence against the shaft of the metacarpal of the thumb (i.e., deep to the abductor pollicis brevis).
2. Have the client flex the thumb at the first carpometacarpal joint against resistance and feel for the contraction of the lateral portion of the opponens pollicis.
3. Continue palpating the opponens pollicis more medially, deep to the abductor and flexor pollicis brevis. (Note: Discerning the opponens pollicis from these two more superficial thenar eminence muscles can be difficult because they both can flex and/or abduct the metacarpal of the thumb at the first carpometacarpal joint.)

■ RELATIONSHIP TO OTHER STRUCTURES

- ☐ The opponens pollicis is the deepest of the three thenar muscles.
- ☐ The opponens pollicis is deep to the abductor pollicis brevis and the flexor pollicis brevis.
- ☐ Deep to the opponens pollicis is the distal attachment of the abductor pollicis longus.
- ☐ The opponens pollicis is located within the deep front arm line myofascial meridian.

■ MISCELLANEOUS

1. The three muscles of the thenar eminence are the abductor pollicis brevis, the flexor pollicis brevis, and the opponens pollicis. (Note: There are three analogous hypothenar muscles. They are the abductor digiti minimi manus, the flexor digiti minimi manus, and the opponens digiti minimi.)
2. Both the opponens pollicis and the opponens digiti minimi attach onto their respective metacarpal bone (first and fifth) and not onto the phalanges, as do all the other thenar and hypothenar muscles.
3. The ulnar nerve component of the opponens pollicis is often absent.
4. Apes can oppose their thumb, but it is so short that it is not very functional for grasping objects.

9

Hypothenar Eminence Group

The hypothenar eminence is an eminence of soft tissue located on the ulnar side of the palm of the hand. There are three muscles in the hypothenar eminence group: the abductor digiti minimi manus, flexor digiti minimi manus, and opponens digiti minimi.

ATTACHMENTS

☐ All three hypothenar muscles attach proximally onto the flexor retinaculum and/or the carpal bones.
☐ All three hypothenar muscles attach distally onto the little finger (finger five).
　☐ The abductor digiti minimi manus and flexor digiti minimi manus attach onto the proximal phalanx of the little finger.
　☐ The opponens digiti minimi attaches onto the fifth metacarpal (of the little finger).

FUNCTIONS

☐ All three hypothenar muscles move the little finger.
☐ In each case, the name of the muscle indicates its major joint action.

MISCELLANEOUS

The layering of the hypothenar muscles is approximately as follows:
☐ The abductor digiti minimi manus is the most superficial of the three.
☐ The flexor digiti minimi manus is intermediate.
☐ The opponens digiti minimi is the deepest of the three.
☐ There are three muscles located in the thenar eminence that are analogous to the hypothenar muscles. The three thenar muscles are the abductor pollicis brevis, flexor pollicis brevis, and opponens pollicis.
☐ The hypothenar muscles are located within the deep back arm line myofascial meridian.

INNERVATION

☐ The three hypothenar muscles are innervated by the ulnar nerve.

ARTERIAL SUPPLY

☐ The three hypothenar muscles receive their arterial supply from the ulnar artery.

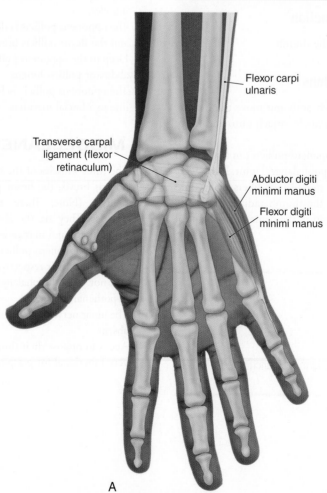

Flexor carpi ulnaris

Transverse carpal ligament (flexor retinaculum)

Abductor digiti minimi manus

Flexor digiti minimi manus

A

Figure 9-9 Anterior views of the right hypothenar group muscles. **A,** Superficial view.

Hypothenar Eminence Group—*cont'd*

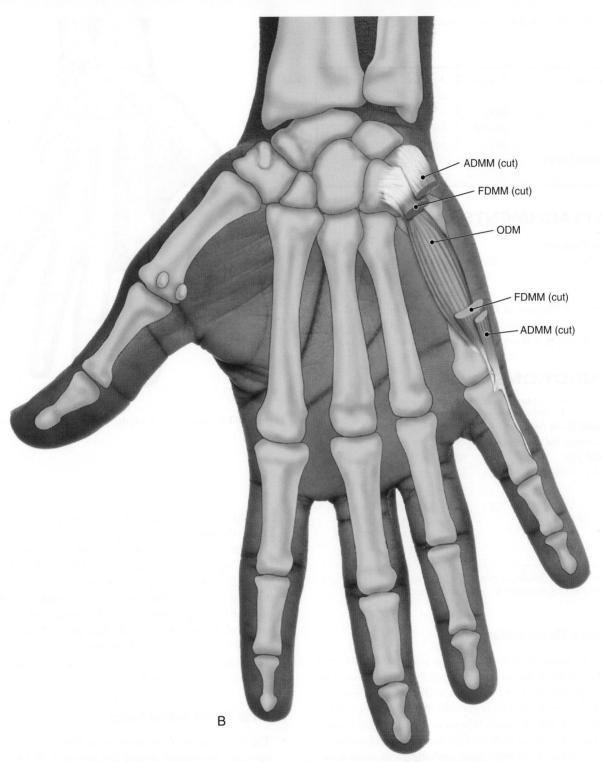

Figure 9-9, cont'd B, Deep view. The abductor digiti minimi manus and flexor digiti minimi manus have been cut. ADMM, abductor digiti minimi manus; FDMM, flexor digiti minimi manus; ODM, opponens digiti minimi.

Abductor Digiti Minimi Manus

The name, abductor digiti minimi manus, *tells us that this muscle abducts the little finger.*

Derivation	☐ abductor: L. *a muscle that abducts a body part.*
	digiti: L. *refers to a digit* (finger).
	minimi: L. *least.*
	manus: L. *refers to the hand.*
Pronunciation	☐ ab-DUK-tor, DIJ-i-tee, MIN-i-mee, MAN-us

■ ATTACHMENTS

☐ **The Pisiform**
  ☐ And the tendon of the flexor carpi ulnaris

to the

☐ **Proximal Phalanx of the Little Finger (Finger Five)**
  ☐ The ulnar (medial) side of the base of the proximal phalanx and the dorsal digital expansion

■ FUNCTIONS

Concentric (Shortening) Mover Actions	
Standard Mover Actions	**Reverse Mover Actions**
☐ **1. Abducts the little finger at the MCP joint**	☐ 1. Abducts the fifth metacarpal at the MCP joint
☐ 2. Abducts the little finger at the CMC joint	☐ 2. Abducts the hamate at the CMC joint of the little finger
☐ 3. Extends the little finger at the PIP and DIP joints	☐ 3. Extends the proximal phalanx of the little finger at the PIP joint; extends the middle phalanx of the little finger at the DIP joint

MCP joint = metacarpophalangeal joint; CMC joint = carpometacarpal joint; PIP joint = proximal interphalangeal joint; DIP joint = distal interphalangeal joint

Standard Mover Action Notes

- The abductor digiti minimi manus crosses the CMC and MCP joints of the little finger medially (on the ulnar side) from proximally at the wrist area to distally onto the proximal phalanx of the little finger (with its fibers running vertically in the frontal plane). When the abductor digiti minimi manus contracts, it pulls the fifth metacarpal and the proximal phalanx of the little finger medially (in an ulnar direction) into abduction. Therefore the abductor digiti minimi manus abducts the little finger by abducting the metacarpal at the CMC joint and the proximal phalanx at the MCP joint. (actions 1, 2)
- Abduction of the little finger at the CMC joint is a motion of the metacarpal of the little finger in the frontal plane that is away from the thumb; this action is a component of

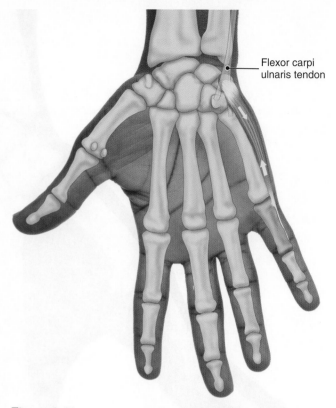

Flexor carpi ulnaris tendon

Figure 9-10 Anterior view of the right abductor digiti minimi manus.

reposition of the little finger (i.e., returning from opposition to the thumb). (action 2)
- The abductor digiti minimi manus attaches into the dorsal digital expansion, which crosses the PIP and DIP joints of the little finger on the posterior side (with the line of pull running vertically in the sagittal plane). Therefore the abductor digiti minimi manus extends the middle and distal phalanges of the little finger at the PIP and DIP joints of the little finger respectively. All muscles that attach into the dorsal digital expansion of the hand extend the interphalangeal (IP) joints. (action 3)

Reverse Mover Action Notes

- The reverse action of motion at the fifth MCP joint is to move the metacarpal toward the proximal phalanx of the little finger. This occurs when the distal end (the proximal phalanx) is fixed, such as when the little finger is holding onto an immovable object. (reverse action 1)
- The reverse action of motion at the fifth CMC joint is to move the hamate toward the metacarpal of the little finger. This occurs if the distal end (the metacarpal) is fixed, perhaps because the little finger is gripping an immovable

object. Movement of the hamate would likely involve movement of the entire carpus (wrist) and forearm relative to the hand. (reverse action 2)

• The reverse action of PIP joint extension of the little finger occurs when the proximal phalanx moves instead of the middle phalanx at the PIP joint. The reverse action of DIP joint extension of the little finger occurs when the middle phalanx moves instead of the distal phalanx at the DIP joint. These reverse actions occur if the distal end is fixed, usually because the little finger is gripping an immovable object. (reverse action 3)

Eccentric Antagonist Functions

1. Restrains/slows adduction of the MCP and CMC joints of the little finger
2. Restrains/slows flexion of the PIP and DIP joints of the little finger

Isometric Stabilization Functions

1. Stabilizes the MCP joint of the little finger
2. Stabilizes the CMC joint of the little finger
3. Stabilizes the PIP and DIP joints of the little finger

Additional Note on Functions

1. All three hypothenar muscles attach onto and move the little finger. (Note: All three thenar muscles attach onto and move the thumb.)

INNERVATION
☐ The Ulnar Nerve
   ☐ C8, **T1**

ARTERIAL SUPPLY
☐ Branches of the Ulnar Artery (A Terminal Branch of the Brachial Artery)

PALPATION

1. With the client seated or supine, place palpating fingers on the medial aspect of the hypothenar eminence.
2. Have the client actively abduct the little finger at the fifth metacarpophalangeal joint and feel for the contraction of the belly of the abductor digiti minimi manus. Resistance can be added.
3. Follow proximally and distally to its attachments.

■ RELATIONSHIP TO OTHER STRUCTURES

☐ The abductor digiti minimi manus is superficial in the medial part of the hypothenar eminence.
☐ The abductor digiti minimi manus is somewhat superficial to, and therefore somewhat overlies, the flexor digiti minimi manus.
☐ The abductor digiti minimi manus is located within the deep back arm line myofascial meridian.

■ MISCELLANEOUS

1. The abductor digiti minimi manus is also known as the *abductor digiti minimi.* However, this allows for confusion with the abductor digiti minimi pedis of the foot, which abducts the little toe of the foot.
2. The three muscles of the hypothenar eminence are the abductor digiti minimi manus, the flexor digiti minimi manus, and the opponens digiti minimi. (Note: There are three analogous thenar muscles. They are the abductor pollicis brevis, the flexor pollicis brevis, and the opponens pollicis.)
3. The dorsal interossei manus muscles cross the metacarpophalangeal joints of the index, middle, and ring fingers (fingers two through four, respectively) on the side away from the middle finger; consequently, the dorsal interossei manus abduct the index, middle, and ring fingers. The abductor digiti minimi manus crosses the metacarpophalangeal joint of the little finger on the side away from the middle finger and abducts the little finger. Therefore the abductor digiti minimi manus can be regarded as an analogous muscle to the dorsal interossei manus with respect to structure and function.
4. Whenever the abductor digiti minimi manus contracts, the flexor carpi ulnaris also contracts to fix (stabilize) the proximal attachment, the pisiform, of the abductor digiti minimi manus. This can be easily palpated at the distal tendon of the flexor carpi ulnaris at the distal antero-ulnar wrist.

Flexor Digiti Minimi Manus

The name, flexor digiti minimi manus, *tells us that this muscle flexes the little finger.*

Derivation	□	flexor:	L. *a muscle that flexes a body part.*
		digiti:	L. *refers to a digit* (finger).
		minimi:	L. *least.*
		manus:	L. *refers to the hand.*
Pronunciation	□	FLEKS-or, DIJ-i-tee, MIN-i-mee, MAN-us	

9

■ ATTACHMENTS

□ **The Flexor Retinaculum and the Hamate**
  □ the hook of the hamate

to the

□ **Proximal Phalanx of the Little Finger (Finger Five)**
  □ the ulnar (medial) side of the base of the proximal phalanx

■ FUNCTIONS

Concentric (Shortening) Mover Actions	
Standard Mover Actions	**Reverse Mover Actions**
□ **1. Flexes the little finger at the MCP joint**	□ 1. Flexes the fifth metacarpal at the MCP joint
□ 2. Flexes the little finger at the CMC joint	□ 2. Flexes the hamate at the fifth CMC joint

MCP joint = metacarpophalangeal joint; CMC joint = carpometacarpal joint

Standard Mover Action Notes

• The flexor digiti minimi manus crosses the MCP joint of the little finger anteriorly (with its fibers running vertically in the sagittal plane), therefore it flexes the little finger at the MCP joint. Flexion of the little finger at the MCP joint involves flexion of the proximal phalanx of the little finger at the MCP joint. (action 1)
• The flexor digiti minimi also crosses the CMC joint of the little finger anteriorly (with its fibers running vertically in the sagittal plane), therefore it also flexes the little finger at the CMC joint. Flexion of the little finger at the CMC joint involves flexion of the metacarpal of the little finger at the CMC joint. (action 2)

Reverse Mover Action Notes

• The reverse action of flexion of the little finger at the MCP joint occurs when the metacarpal flexes relative to the proximal phalanx of the little finger. This occurs when the distal segment, the proximal phalanx, is fixed, such as when

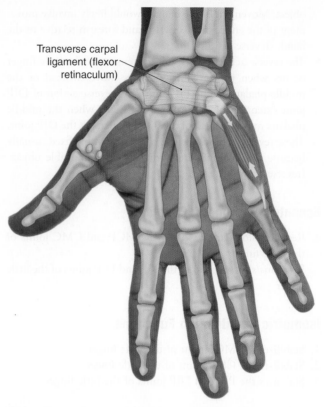

Figure 9-11 Anterior view of the right flexor digiti minimi manus.

the little finger is gripping an immovable object. (reverse action 1)
• The reverse action of flexion of the CMC joint of the little finger occurs when the hamate moves toward the metacarpal of the little finger at the CMC joint. This occurs if the distal end (the metacarpal) is fixed, perhaps because the little finger is gripping an immovable object. Movement of the hamate would likely involve movement of the entire carpus (wrist) and forearm relative to the hand.

Eccentric Antagonist Functions

1. Restrains/slows extension of MCP joint of the little finger
2. Restrains/slows extension of CMC joint of the little finger

Isometric Stabilization Functions

1. Stabilizes the MCP joint of the little finger
2. Stabilizes the CMC joint of the little finger

Additional Note on Functions

1. All three hypothenar muscles attach onto and move the little finger. (Note: All three thenar muscles attach onto and move the thumb.)

Flexor Digiti Minimi Manus—*cont'd*

INNERVATION

- The Ulnar Nerve
  - C8, **T1**

ARTERIAL SUPPLY
- Branches of the Ulnar Artery (a terminal branch of the Brachial Artery)

🖐 PALPATION

1. With the client seated or supine, place palpating fingers toward the lateral edge of the hypothenar eminence.
2. Have the client actively flex the little finger at the fifth metacarpophalangeal joint and feel for the contraction of the lateral aspect of the belly of the flexor digit minimi. Resistance can be added.
3. A part of the medial portion of the flexor digiti minimi manus, deep to the abductor digiti minimi manus, can be palpated as you continue palpating medially as long as the abductor digiti minimi manus is relaxed. (Be sure that the client is not abducting the little finger.)

■ RELATIONSHIP TO OTHER STRUCTURES

- The flexor digiti minimi manus lies in the hypothenar eminence, lateral and partially deep to the abductor digiti minimi manus.
- Partially deep to the flexor digiti minimi manus is the opponens digiti minimi.
- The flexor digiti minimi manus is located within the deep back arm line myofascial meridian.

■ MISCELLANEOUS

1. The flexor digiti minimi manus is also known as the *flexor digiti minimi.* However, this allows for confusion with the flexor digiti minimi pedis of the foot, which flexes the little toe.
2. The flexor digiti minimi manus is also known as the *flexor digiti minimi brevis.* However, the addition of the word *brevis* at the end of the name is not necessary and does not make sense in this case. Usually, the word *brevis* at the end of a muscle's name is added to distinguish the muscle from a longer muscle that does the same action. In this case there is no flexor digiti minimi longus.
3. The three muscles of the hypothenar eminence are the abductor digiti minimi manus, the flexor digiti minimi manus, and the opponens digiti minimi. (Note: There are three analogous thenar muscles. They are the abductor pollicis brevis, the flexor pollicis brevis, and the opponens pollicis.)
4. The flexor digiti minimi manus is the smallest of the three hypothenar muscles.
5. The flexor digiti minimi manus is often very small or entirely absent.

Opponens Digiti Minimi

The name, opponens digiti minimi, *tells us that this muscle opposes the little finger.*

Derivation	☐ opponens: L. *opposing.*
	digiti: L. *refers to a digit* (finger).
	minimi: L. *least.*
Pronunciation	☐ op-PO-nens, DIJ-i-tee, MIN-i-mee

■ ATTACHMENTS

☐ **The Flexor Retinaculum and the Hamate**
   ☐ the hook of the hamate

to the

☐ **Fifth Metacarpal (of the Little Finger)**
   ☐ the anterior surface and the medial (ulnar) border of the fifth metacarpal

■ FUNCTIONS

Concentric (Shortening) Mover Actions	
Standard Mover Actions	**Reverse Mover Actions**
☐ **1. Opposes the little finger at the CMC joint**	☐ 1. Flexes, medially rotates, and adducts the hamate at the fifth CMC joint
☐ 2. Flexes the little finger at the CMC joint	☐ 2. Flexes the hamate at the CMC joint of the little finger
☐ 3. Laterally rotates the little finger at the CMC joint	☐ 3. Medially rotates the hamate at the CMC joint of the little finger
☐ 4. Adducts the little finger at the CMC joint	☐ 4. Adducts the hamate at the CMC joint of the little finger

CMC joint = carpometacarpal joint

Standard Mover Action Notes

- Opposition of the little finger is not a specific cardinal plane action; rather, it is a triplanar oblique plane motion that is composed of flexion, lateral rotation, and adduction of the little finger at the CMC joint, all aimed to bring the pad of the little finger to meet the pad of the thumb. (actions 1, 2, 3, 4)
- The opponens digiti minimi crosses the fifth CMC joint anteriorly to attach onto the metacarpal of the little finger (with its fibers running vertically in the sagittal plane). When the opponens digiti minimi contracts, it pulls the fifth metacarpal anteriorly into flexion. Therefore the opponens digiti minimi flexes the little finger by flexing the metacarpal of the little finger at the CMC joint. (action 2)

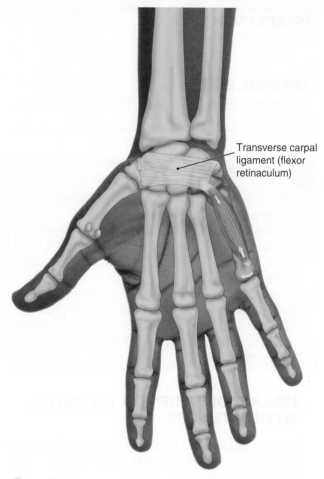

Transverse carpal ligament (flexor retinaculum)

Figure 9-12 Anterior view of the right opponens digiti minimi.

- The opponens digiti minimi crosses the fifth CMC joint anteriorly from slightly more lateral on the flexor retinaculum to attach more medially onto the metacarpal of the little finger (with its fibers running somewhat horizontally in the transverse plane). When the opponens digiti minimi contracts, it rotates the fifth metacarpal anterolaterally toward the thumb, causing the anterior surface of the little finger to face somewhat laterally. Therefore the opponens digiti minimi laterally rotates the little finger by laterally rotating the metacarpal of the little finger at the CMC joint. (action 3)
- The opponens digiti minimi crosses the fifth CMC joint anteriorly from laterally at the wrist area to medially onto the metacarpal of the little finger (with its fibers running slightly horizontally in the frontal plane). When the opponens digiti minimi contracts, it pulls the fifth metacarpal laterally into adduction. Therefore the opponens digiti minimi adducts the little finger by adducting the metacarpal of the little finger at the CMC joint. (action 4)

Opponens Digiti Minimi—*cont'd*

Reverse Mover Action Notes

- Given that opposition is an oblique plane motion that is a combination of three cardinal plane actions, the reverse action of opposition involves the reverse actions of all three of these cardinal plane components of opposition. (reverse actions 1, 2, 3, 4)
- The reverse action of motion at the fifth CMC occurs when the hamate moves toward the metacarpal of the little finger at the CMC joint. This occurs when the distal end (the metacarpal) is fixed, usually because the little finger is gripping an immovable object. Movement of the hamate would likely involve movement of the entire carpus (wrist) and forearm relative to the hand. (reverse actions 1, 2, 3, 4)

Eccentric Antagonist Functions

1. Restrains/slows reposition of the little finger at the CMC joint
2. Restrains/slows extension and abduction of the CMC joint of the little finger
3. Restrains/slows medial rotation of the metacarpal and lateral rotation of the hamate of the CMC joint of the little finger

Isometric Stabilization Function

1. Stabilizes the CMC joint of the little finger

Additional Note on Functions

1. All three hypothenar muscles attach onto and move the little finger. (Note: All three thenar muscles attach onto and move the thumb.)

INNERVATION
- The Ulnar Nerve
  - C8, **T1**

ARTERIAL SUPPLY
- Branches of the Ulnar Artery (a terminal branch of the Brachial Artery)

PALPATION

1. With the client seated or supine, place palpating finger on the lateral aspect of the hypothenar eminence.
2. Have the client actively oppose the little finger at the fifth carpometacarpal joint and feel for the contraction of the belly of the opponens digiti minimi.
3. Continue palpating the opponens digiti minimi medially and try to follow it deep to the flexor digiti minimi manus and the abductor digiti minimi manus.

■ RELATIONSHIP TO OTHER STRUCTURES

- The medial portion of the opponens digiti minimi is deep to the abductor digiti minimi manus and the flexor digiti minimi manus. A small part of the lateral portion of the opponens digiti minimi is superficial in the most lateral aspect of the hypothenar eminence.
- The opponens digiti minimi is superficial to some of the more lateral tendons of the flexor digitorum superficialis and the flexor digitorum profundus.
- The opponens digiti minimi is located within the deep back arm line myofascial meridian.

■ MISCELLANEOUS

1. The three muscles of the hypothenar eminence are the abductor digiti minimi manus, the flexor digiti minimi manus, and the opponens digiti minimi. (Note: There are three analogous thenar muscles. They are the abductor pollicis brevis, the flexor pollicis brevis, and the opponens pollicis.)
2. Both the opponens digiti minimi and the opponens pollicis attach onto their respective metacarpal bone (fifth and first) and not onto the phalanges, as do all the other thenar and hypothenar muscles.
3. The flexor digiti minimi manus, which overlies the opponens digiti minimi, is often very small or entirely absent. When this occurs, the opponens digiti minimi will have relatively more superficial exposure.
4. The opponens digiti minimi is the largest of the three hypothenar muscles.

Central Compartment Group

The central compartment is located between the thenar eminence and hypothenar eminence of the hand. There are four muscles in the central compartment group: the adductor pollicis, lumbricals manus, palmar interossei, and dorsal interossei manus.

■ ATTACHMENTS

☐ The lumbricals manus, palmar interossei, and dorsal interossei manus all attach distally into the dorsal digital expansion of the hand.

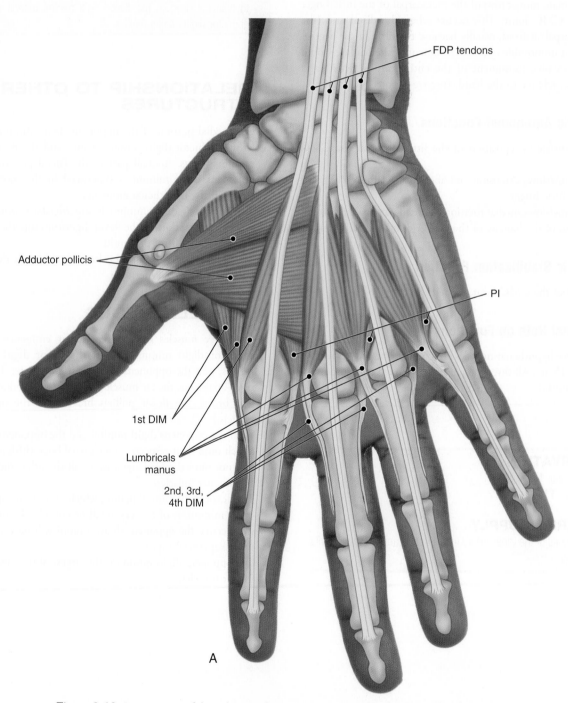

FDP tendons

Adductor pollicis

PI

1st DIM

Lumbricals manus

2nd, 3rd, 4th DIM

A

Figure 9-13 Anterior view of the right central compartment group muscles. DIM, dorsal interosseus/interossei manus; PI, palmar interossei; FDP, flexor digitorum profundus. **A,** Superficial view.

Central Compartment Group—*cont'd*

■ FUNCTIONS

☐ The palmar interossei adduct fingers at the metacarpophalangeal joints.

☐ The dorsal interossei manus abduct fingers at the metacarpophalangeal joints.

☐ A mnemonic to remember the frontal plane actions of the interossei muscles of the hand is DAB PAD: **D**orsals **AB**duct, **P**almars **AD**duct.

☐ The lumbricals manus, palmar interossei, and dorsal interossei manus all flex fingers at the metacarpophalangeal joints and extend fingers at the interphalangeal joints.

INNERVATION

☐ The four central compartment muscles are innervated by the ulnar nerve (two of the lumbricals manus are innervated by the median nerve).

ARTERIAL SUPPLY

☐ The four central compartment muscles receive their arterial supply from branches of the radial and ulnar arteries (terminal branches of the brachial artery).

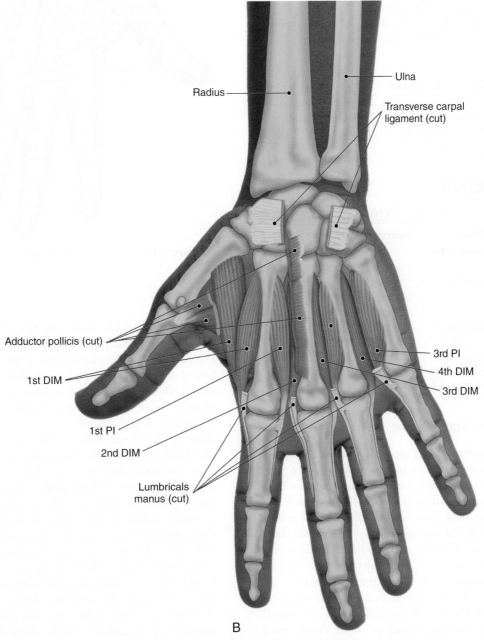

B

Figure 9-13, cont'd B, Deep view. The adductor pollicis and lumbricals manus have been cut.

Adductor Pollicis

The name, adductor pollicis, *tells us that this muscle adducts the thumb.*

Derivation	☐ adductor: L. *a muscle that adducts a body part.*
	pollicis: L. *thumb.*
Pronunciation	☐ ad-DUK-tor, POL-i-sis

■ ATTACHMENTS

☐ **Third Metacarpal**
  ☐ OBLIQUE HEAD: the anterior bases of the second and third metacarpals and the capitate
  ☐ TRANSVERSE HEAD: the distal ⅔ of the anterior surface of the third metacarpal

to the

☐ **Proximal Phalanx of the Thumb**
  ☐ OBLIQUE HEAD: the medial side of the base of the proximal phalanx and the dorsal digital expansion
  ☐ TRANSVERSE HEAD: the medial side of the base of the proximal phalanx

■ FUNCTIONS

Concentric (Shortening) Mover Actions	
Standard Mover Actions	**Reverse Mover Actions**
☐ **1. Adducts the thumb at the CMC joint**	☐ 1. Adducts the trapezium at the CMC joint of the thumb
☐ 2. Flexes the thumb at the CMC and MCP joints	☐ 2. Flexes the trapezium at the CMC joint; flexes the metacarpal of the thumb at the MCP joint
☐ 3. Extends the thumb at the IP joint	☐ 3. Extends the proximal phalanx of the thumb at the IP joint

CMC joint = carpometacarpal joint (of the thumb; saddle joint of the thumb); MCP joint = metacarpophalangeal joint; IP joint = interphalangeal joint.

Standard Mover Action Notes

• The adductor pollicis crosses the CMC joint of the thumb posteriorly by attaching from posteromedially on the palm of the hand to anterolaterally onto the thumb (with its fibers running horizontally in the sagittal plane). When the thumb is first in a position of abduction and the adductor pollicis contracts, it pulls the thumb posteriorly, perpendicularly toward the plane of the palm of the hand. This action is called *adduction of the thumb.* Therefore the adductor pollicis adducts the thumb by adducting the metacarpal of the thumb at the CMC joint. (Note: Because of the rotational development of the thumb embryologically, the named actions of abduction and adduction of the thumb occur within the sagittal plane.) (action 1)

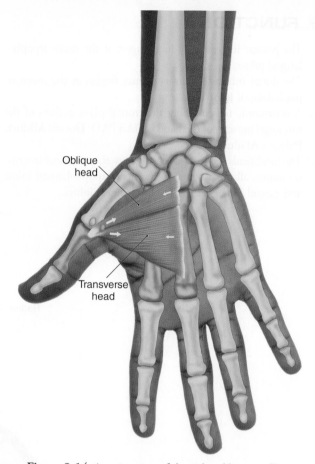

Figure 9-14 Anterior view of the right adductor pollicis.

• The adductor pollicis crosses the first CMC joint of the thumb from medially on the hand to more laterally onto the metacarpal of the thumb (with its fibers running in the frontal plane). When the adductor pollicis contracts, it pulls the thumb medially (in an ulnar direction) within the plane of the palm of the hand (frontal plane), toward its other attachment (the third metacarpal). This action is called *flexion of the thumb.* Therefore the adductor pollicis flexes the thumb by flexing the metacarpal of the thumb at the CMC joint. The adductor pollicis also crosses the first MCP joint of the thumb medially (with it fibers running in the frontal plane). Therefore the adductor pollicis also flexes the proximal phalanx of the thumb at the first MCP joint. (Note: Because of the rotational development of the thumb embryologically, the named actions of flexion and extension of the thumb occur within frontal plane.) (action 2)
• In addition to its major action of adduction of the thumb at the CMC joint, the adductor pollicis is extremely strong at flexing the thumb at the CMC joint. (actions 1, 2)
• Because of its attachment into the dorsal digital expansion, which crosses the IP joint of the thumb on the lateral side

Adductor Pollicis—cont'd

(with its fibers running vertically in the frontal plane), the adductor pollicis can extend the thumb by extending the distal phalanx of the thumb at the IP joint. (action 3)

Reverse Mover Action Notes

- The reverse action of motion at the first CMC joint occurs when the trapezium moves toward the metacarpal of the thumb at the CMC joint. This occurs when the distal end (the metacarpal) is fixed, perhaps because the thumb is gripping an immovable object. Movement of the trapezium would likely involve movement of the entire carpus (wrist) and forearm relative to the hand. (reverse actions 1, 2)
- The reverse action of the thumb at the MCP joint occurs when the metacarpal moves relative to the proximal phalanx of the thumb at the MCP joint. This occurs when the distal segment, the proximal phalanx, is fixed, such as when the thumb is gripping an immovable object. (reverse action 2)
- The reverse action of IP joint extension involves the proximal phalanx moving instead of the distal phalanx. This occurs if the distal phalanx is fixed, usually because the thumb is gripping an immovable object. (reverse action 3)

Eccentric Antagonist Functions

1. Restrains/slows abduction of the CMC joint of the thumb
2. Restrains/slows extension of the CMC and MCP joints of the thumb
3. Restrains/slows flexion of the IP joint of the thumb

Isometric Stabilization Functions

1. Stabilizes the CMC, MCP, and IP joints of the thumb

INNERVATION
- The Ulnar Nerve
  - C8, T1

ARTERIAL SUPPLY
- Branches of the Radial Artery (a terminal branch of the Brachial Artery)

✋ PALPATION

1. With the client seated or supine and the thumb abducted at the carpometacarpal joint, place palpating fingers in the middle of the thumb web of the hand.
2. Have the client actively adduct the thumb at the first carpometacarpal joint against resistance and feel for the contraction of the adductor pollicis.
3. Continue palpating the adductor pollicis as far lateral and medial as possible toward its attachments.

■ RELATIONSHIP TO OTHER STRUCTURES

- Except for the part of the adductor pollicis that is superficial in the thumb web, the adductor pollicis is deeply situated in the hand. All the thenar muscles, the distal tendons of flexors digitorum superficialis and profundus (going to the second and third fingers), the distal tendon of the flexor pollicis longus, and the first and second lumbricals manus are superficial to the adductor pollicis.
- Although somewhat deep to the thenar muscles, the adductor pollicis also lies medial to the flexor pollicis brevis and the opponens pollicis.
- The distal attachment of the flexor carpi radialis and the shaft of the second metacarpal bone are deep to the adductor pollicis.
- From an anterior perspective, the first and second dorsal interossei manus are also deep to the adductor pollicis.
- The adductor pollicis is located within the deep front arm line myofascial meridian.

■ MISCELLANEOUS

1. The adductor pollicis has two heads: an *oblique head* and a *transverse head*. The oblique head runs more obliquely in the hand (i.e., its fiber direction is between vertical and horizontal in orientation). The transverse head runs transversely across the hand (i.e., its fiber direction is horizontal in orientation). (Note: The adductor hallucis of the foot also has two heads: an oblique head and a transverse head.)
2. There is a lot of variation and confusion regarding the region of the oblique head of the adductor pollicis. The oblique head often has a fasciculus (a group of muscle fibers) that joins with the flexor pollicis brevis and is called the *deep head* of the flexor pollicis brevis.
3. The oblique head of the adductor pollicis has a sesamoid bone located within it. (Note: There is a second sesamoid bone of the thumb located in the distal tendon of the flexor pollicis brevis.)
4. The majority of tissue of the thumb web of the hand is made up of the adductor pollicis and the first dorsal interosseus manus.
5. The attachment of the adductor pollicis into the dorsal digital expansion of the thumb is small and often absent. When it is absent, the adductor pollicis does not have the ability to extend the distal phalanx of the thumb at the interphalangeal joint of the thumb.

9

Lumbricals Manus

There are four lumbrical manus muscles, named one, two, three, and four.

The name, lumbricals manus, *tells us that these muscles are shaped like earthworms and are located in the hand.*

Derivation	☐ lumbricals: L. *earthworms.*
	manus: L. *refers to the hand.*
Pronunciation	☐ LUM-bri-kuls, MAN-us

■ ATTACHMENTS

☐ **The Distal Tendons of the Flexor Digitorum Profundus**
  ☐ **One:** the radial (lateral) side of the tendon of the index finger (finger two)
  ☐ **Two:** the radial side of the tendon of the middle finger (finger three)
  ☐ **Three:** the ulnar (medial) side of the tendon of the middle finger (finger three) and the radial side of the tendon of the ring finger (finger four)
  ☐ **Four:** the ulnar side of the tendon of the ring finger (finger four) and the radial side of the tendon of the little finger (finger five)

to the

☐ **Distal Tendons of the Extensor Digitorum (the Dorsal Digital Expansion)**
  ☐ the radial side of the tendons merging into the dorsal digital expansion
  ☐ **One:** into the tendon of the index finger (finger two)
  ☐ **Two:** into the tendon of the middle finger (finger three)
  ☐ **Three:** into the tendon of the ring finger (finger four)
  ☐ **Four:** into the tendon of the little finger (finger five)

■ FUNCTIONS

Concentric (Shortening) Mover Actions	
Standard Mover Actions	**Reverse Mover Actions**
☐ **1. Extend fingers two through five at the PIP and DIP joints**	☐ 1. Extend the more proximal phalanges at the PIP and DIP joints
☐ **2. Flex fingers two through five at the MCP joints**	☐ 2. Flex the metacarpals at the MCP joints
☐ 3. Abduct/adduct fingers two through five	☐ 3. Abduct/adduct the metacarpals at the MCP joints

MCP joints = metacarpophalangeal joints; PIP joints = proximal interphalangeal joints; DIP joints = distal interphalangeal joints

Standard Mover Action Notes

- The lumbricals manus, by attaching into the tendons of the extensor digitorum muscle (after the MCP joint but before the interphalangeal [IP] joints of the fingers), exert their pull on the distal attachments of the extensor digitorum, which

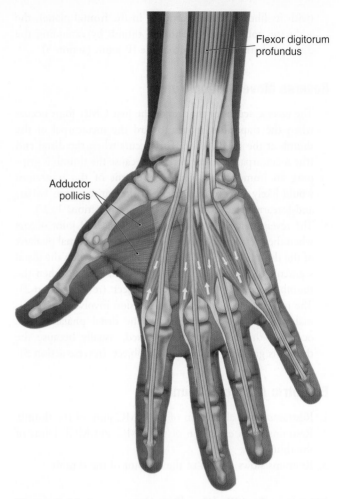

Figure 9-15 Anterior view of the right lumbricals manus. The adductor pollicis has been ghosted in.

are the distal phalanges of fingers two through five. The lumbricals manus, in effect, cross the PIP and DIP joints of fingers two through five posteriorly (with their pull exerted vertically in the sagittal plane) and therefore extend the middle phalanges at the PIP joints and extend the distal phalanges at the DIP joints of fingers two through five. (action 1)

- The lumbricals manus cross the MCP joints of fingers two through five anteriorly (with their fibers running vertically in the sagittal plane); therefore they flex the proximal phalanges of fingers two through five at the MCP joints. (action 2)

- The lumbricals manus cross the MCP joint of each finger to the side; therefore each lumbrical manus has the ability to either abduct or adduct the finger based on whether it pulls the finger toward or away from the reference line for abduction/adduction. The first lumbrical manus abducts the index finger, the second one radially abducts the middle finger, the third one adducts the ring finger, and the fourth one adducts the little finger. (action 3)

Lumbricals Manus—*cont'd*

Reverse Mover Action Notes

☐ Extending the more proximal phalanges at the interphalangeal joints refers to extending the proximal phalanges at the PIP joints and extending the middle phalanges at the DIP joints. (reverse action 1)

☐ The reverse action of a finger at an MCP joint occurs when the metacarpal moves relative to the proximal phalanx of the finger at the MCP joint. This occurs when the distal segment, the proximal phalanx, is fixed, such as when the finger is gripping an immovable object. (reverse actions 2, 3)

Eccentric Antagonist Functions

1. Restrains/slows flexion of fingers two through five at the interphalangeal joints
2. Restrains/slows extension of fingers two through five at the MCP joints
3. Restrains/slows adduction/abduction of two through five fingers at the MCP joints

Isometric Stabilization Functions

1. Stabilizes the MCP and interphalangeal joints of fingers two through five

Additional Notes on Functions

1. The lumbricals pedis of the foot have similar actions in that they flex the toes at the metatarsophalangeal joints and extend the toes at the interphalangeal (IP) joints.
2. By flexing the MCP joint and simultaneously extending the proximal and distal IP joints, the lumbricals manus help to create a strong grip with the fingers opposed to the thumb.
3. In addition to directly contributing to extension of the fingers at the IP joints, the lumbricals manus and the interossei of the hand help create these actions in another manner. Whenever the extensor digitorum contracts, these intrinsic muscles of the hand create a flexion force at the MCP joint to keep the extensor digitorum from excessively extending the MCP joint and thereby losing its ability to create tension and extend the IP joints of the fingers.
4. All muscles that attach into the dorsal digital expansion of the hand flex the MCP joints and extend the IP joints.

🖐 PALPATION

1. With the client seated or supine, place palpating fingers on the lateral side of the anterior shaft of the metacarpal of the little finger.
2. Have the client actively flex the little finger at the fifth metacarpophalangeal joint with the interphalangeal joints fully extended and feel for the contraction of the fourth lumbrical manus.
3. To palpate the third, second, and first lumbricals manus, follow the previously described procedure on the lateral sides of the ring, middle, and index fingers, respectively.

■ RELATIONSHIP TO OTHER STRUCTURES

☐ The lumbricals manus are actually not that deep in the palm of the hand. In the palm, they are deep only to the palmar fascia. As the lumbricals manus approach the phalanges, they dive deeper (more posteriorly) to attach onto the tendons of the extensor digitorum, which are on the posterior sides of the fingers.

☐ The bellies of the lumbricals manus are located between the distal tendons of the flexor digitorum profundus.

☐ Directly deep to the first and second lumbricals manus is the adductor pollicis. Directly deep to the third and fourth lumbricals manus are the metacarpals and the palmar interossei.

☐ The lumbricals manus are located within the superficial front arm line myofascial meridian.

■ MISCELLANEOUS

1. The lumbricals manus are actually four small separate muscles named from lateral to medial: one, two, three, and four.
2. The lumbricals manus are usually known as the *lumbricals*. However, this allows for confusion with the lumbricals pedis of the foot.

INNERVATION

☐ The Median and Ulnar Nerves
  ☐ C8, **T1** (first and second lumbricals manus: the median nerve; third and fourth lumbricals manus: the ulnar nerve)

ARTERIAL SUPPLY

☐ Branches of the Radial and Ulnar Arteries (terminal branches of the Brachial Artery)

There are three palmar interossei, named one, two, and three.

The name, palmar interossei, *tells us that these muscles are located between bones (metacarpals) on the palmar (anterior) side.*

Derivation	☐	palmar: L. *refers to the palm.*
		interossei: L. *between bones.*
Pronunciation	☐	PAL-mar, IN-ter-OSS-ee-I

■ ATTACHMENTS

☐ **The Metacarpals of Fingers Two, Four, and Five**
  ☐ The anterior side and on the "middle finger side" of the metacarpals:
  ☐ **One:** attaches to the metacarpal of the index finger (finger two)
  ☐ **Two:** attaches to the metacarpal of the ring finger (finger four)
  ☐ **Three:** attaches to the metacarpal of the little finger (finger five)

to the

☐ **Proximal Phalanges of Fingers Two, Four, and Five on the "Middle Finger Side"**
  ☐ The base of the proximal phalanx and the dorsal digital expansion:
  ☐ **One:** attaches to the index finger (finger two)
  ☐ **Two:** attaches to the ring finger (finger four)
  ☐ **Three:** attaches to the little finger (finger five)

■ FUNCTIONS

Concentric (Shortening) Mover Actions	
Standard Mover Actions	**Reverse Mover Actions**
☐ **1. Adduct fingers two, four, and five at the MCP joints**	☐ 1. Adduct the metacarpals of fingers two, four, and five at the MCP joints
☐ 2. Flex fingers two, four, and five at the MCP joints	☐ 2. Flex the metacarpals of fingers two, four, and five at the MCP joints
☐ 3. Extend fingers two, four, and five at the PIP and DIP joints	☐ 3. Extend the more proximal phalanges of fingers two, four, and five at the PIP and DIP joints

MCP joints = metacarpophalangeal joints; PIP joint = proximal interphalangeal joint; DIP joint = distal interphalangeal joint

Standard Mover Action Notes

• The palmar interossei are always on the "middle finger side" of the metacarpals and phalanges (with their fibers running vertically in the frontal plane); therefore a palmar interosseus muscle pulls the finger to which it is attached toward the

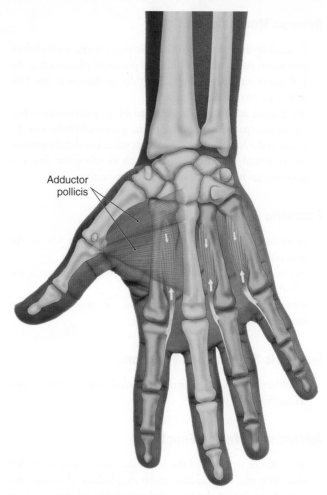

Figure 9-16 Anterior view of the right palmar interossei. The adductor pollicis has been ghosted in.

middle finger. This action is defined as *adduction of the finger.* (action 1)

• The first palmar interosseus muscle crosses the MCP joint of the index finger (finger two) on the medial side and therefore pulls the proximal phalanx of this finger medially, which is toward the middle finger (which is the axis for abduction/adduction in the hand). Therefore the first palmar interosseus adducts the index finger at the MCP joint. The second and third palmar interossei cross the MCP joint of the ring and little fingers (fingers four and five) respectively on the lateral side and therefore pull these fingers laterally, toward the middle finger. Therefore the second and third palmar interossei adduct the ring finger and the little finger at the MCP joint. (action 1)

• The palmar interossei cross the MCP joint on the palmar (anterior) side (with their fibers running vertically in the sagittal plane); therefore they flex the proximal phalanx of fingers two, four, and five at the MCP joint. (action 2)

• Because of their attachment into the dorsal digital expansion of the extensor digitorum, the palmar interossei exert their

Palmar Interossei—*cont'd*

pull through the dorsal digital expansion, which crosses the proximal and distal interphalangeal (IP) joints of the fingers on the posterior side (with the line of pull running vertically in the sagittal plane). Therefore the palmar interossei extend the middle phalanx at the proximal PIP joint and extend the distal phalanx at the DIP joint of fingers two, four, and five. (action 3)

Reverse Mover Action Notes

- The reverse action of a finger at the MCP joint occurs when the metacarpal moves relative to the proximal phalanx of the finger. This occurs when the distal segment, the proximal phalanx, is fixed, such as when the finger is gripping an immovable object. (reverse actions 1, 2)
- Extending the more proximal phalanges at the interphalangeal (IP) joints refers to extending the proximal phalanx at the proximal IP joint and extending the middle phalanx at the distal IP joint. (reverse action 3)

Eccentric Antagonist Functions

1. Restrains/slows abduction of fingers two, four, and five at the MCP joints
2. Restrains/slows extension of fingers two, four, and five at the MCP joints
3. Restrains/slows flexion of fingers two, four, and five at the PIP and DIP joints

Isometric Stabilization Functions

1. Stabilizes the MCP, PIP, and DIP joints of fingers two, four, and five

Additional Notes on Functions

1. A mnemonic for remembering the actions of the palmar interossei and the dorsal interossei manus muscles is DAB and PAD. The **D**orsals **AB**duct, and the **P**almars **AD**duct.
2. There are plantar interossei of the foot that have essentially identical actions (adduction of the toes at the metacarpophalangeal [MCP] joint, flexion of the toes at the MCP joint, and extension of the toes at the proximal and distal interphalangeal [IP] joints) to the palmar interossei of the hand.
3. In addition to directly contributing to extension of the fingers at the IP joints, the interossei of the hand and the lumbricals manus help create these actions in another manner. Whenever the extensor digitorum contracts, these intrinsic muscles of the hand create a flexion force at the MCP joint to keep the extensor digitorum from excessively extending the MCP joint and thereby losing its ability to create tension and extend the IP joints of the fingers.
4. All muscles that attach into the dorsal digital expansion of the hand flex the MCP joints and extend the IP joints.

INNERVATION

- ☐ The Ulnar Nerve
  - ☐ C8, **T1**; deep branch of the ulnar nerve

ARTERIAL SUPPLY

- ☐ Branches of the Radial and Ulnar Arteries (terminal branches of the Brachial Artery)

✋ PALPATION

1. With the client seated or supine, place palpating fingers on the "middle finger side," in this case, the medial (ulnar) side of the second metacarpal in the palm.
2. Have the client squeeze a pencil between the index and middle fingers and feel for the contraction of the first palmar interosseus against the second metacarpal.
3. To palpate the second and third palmar interossei, follow the previously described procedure on the middle finger (lateral/radial) side of the ring and little fingers, respectively.

■ RELATIONSHIP TO OTHER STRUCTURES

- ☐ The palmar interossei are located in a position that is palmar (anterior) on the metacarpals and slightly between the metacarpals.
- ☐ Each palmar interosseus muscle is located on the side of the metacarpal that faces the middle finger. (The middle finger has no palmar interosseus muscle attached to it.)
- ☐ From an anterior perspective, the palmar interossei are deep to all the other muscles of the anterior hand.
- ☐ From the anterior perspective, the metacarpal bones and the dorsal interossei manus are deep to the palmar interossei.
- ☐ The palmar interossei are involved with the superficial back arm line myofascial meridian.

■ MISCELLANEOUS

1. There are three palmar interossei muscles named from lateral to medial: one, two, and three.
2. There are three palmar interossei, one for each finger except the middle finger and the thumb. It makes sense that the middle finger would not have a palmar interosseus muscle. The palmar interossei adduct the fingers, and the middle finger, by definition, cannot adduct, because an imaginary line that runs through it when it is in anatomic position is the axis for abduction/adduction of the fingers. The thumb has its own adductor muscle (the adductor pollicis).
3. Many sources state that there is a fourth palmar interosseus muscle that attaches to the thumb. This would cause the naming of the palmar interossei muscles to change, because

Palmar Interossei—*cont'd*

they are named from radial to ulnar (lateral to medial). Hence the palmar interosseus of the thumb would be one, the second palmar interosseus would attach to the index finger, the third palmar interosseus would attach to the ring finger, and the fourth palmar interosseus would attach to the little finger. This palmar interosseus muscle that attaches to the thumb is also known as the *palmar interosseus of Henle*.

4. Whether or not a true fourth palmar interosseus muscle exists, even some of the time, is controversial. Some sources name this extra muscle, or bundle of muscle fibers, as part of the oblique head of the adductor pollicis or as part of the deep head of the flexor pollicis brevis.

Dorsal Interossei Manus (DIM)

There are four dorsal interossei manus muscles, named one, two, three, and four.

The name, dorsal interossei manus, *tells us that these muscles are located between bones (metacarpals) on the dorsal (posterior) side and located in the hand.*

Derivation	□ dorsal: L. *back.*
	interossei: L. *between bones.*
	manus: L. *refers to the hand.*
Pronunciation	□ DOR-sul, IN-ter-OSS-ee-i, MAN-us

■ ATTACHMENTS

□ **The Metacarpals of Fingers One through Five**
  □ Each one arises from the adjacent sides of two metacarpals:
  □ **One:** attaches onto the metacarpals of the thumb and index finger (fingers one and two)
  □ **Two:** attaches onto the metacarpals of the index and middle fingers (fingers two and three)
  □ **Three:** attaches onto the metacarpals of the middle and ring fingers (fingers three and four)
  □ **Four:** attaches onto the metacarpals of the ring and little fingers (fingers four and five)

to the

□ **Proximal Phalanges of Fingers Two, Three, and Four on the Side That Faces Away from the Center of the Middle Finger**
  □ The base of the proximal phalanx and the dorsal digital expansion:
  □ **One:** attaches to the lateral side of the index finger (finger two)
  □ **Two:** attaches to the lateral side of the middle finger (finger three)
  □ **Three:** attaches to the medial side of the middle finger (finger three)
  □ **Four:** attaches to the medial side of the ring finger (finger four)

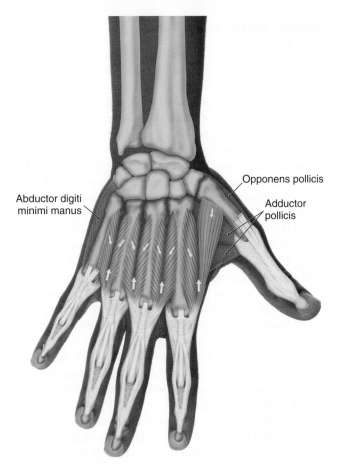

Abductor digiti minimi manus

Opponens pollicis

Adductor pollicis

Figure 9-17 Posterior view of the right dorsal interossei manus. The adductor pollicis, opponens pollicis, and abductor digiti minimi manus have been ghosted in.

■ FUNCTIONS

Concentric (Shortening) Mover Actions	
Standard Mover Actions	**Reverse Mover Actions**
□ **1. Abduct fingers two through four at the MCP joints**	□ 1. Abduct the metacarpals of fingers two through four at the MCP joints; flex and adduct the thumb at the CMC (saddle) joint
□ 2. Flex fingers two through four at the MCP joints	□ 2. Flex the metacarpals of fingers two through four at the MCP joints
□ 3. Extend fingers two through four at the PIP and DIP joints	□ 3. Extend the more proximal phalanges of fingers two through four at the PIP and DIP joints

MCP joints = metacarpophalangeal joints; CMC joints = carpometacarpal joints; PIP joints = proximal interphalangeal joints; DIP joints = distal interphalangeal joints

Dorsal Interossei Manus (DIM)—*cont'd*

Standard Mover Action Notes

- The dorsal interossei manus (DIM) are always on the side of the metacarpals and phalanges (with their fibers running vertically in the frontal plane) that faces away from the axis of abduction/adduction, which is an imaginary line drawn through the center of the middle finger when the middle finger is in anatomic position. Therefore they pull the fingers away from this axis, abducting the fingers. (action 1)

- The first and second DIM cross the MCP joints of the index and middle fingers laterally. They pull the proximal phalanx of these fingers laterally, away from the axis of abduction/adduction. Therefore the first DIM abducts the index finger, and the second DIM "radially abducts" the middle finger at the MCP joints respectively. The third and fourth DIM cross the MCP joints of the middle and ring fingers medially. They pull the proximal phalanx of these fingers medially, away from the axis of abduction/adduction. Therefore the third DIM "ulnar abducts" the middle finger, and the fourth DIM abducts the ring finger at the MCP joints respectively. (action 1)

- The DIM cross the MCP joints anteriorly (with their fibers running vertically in the sagittal plane); therefore they flex the proximal phalanges of the index, middle, and ring fingers at the MCP joints. (action 2)

- The DIM attach into the dorsal digital expansion, which crosses the PIP and DIP joints of the fingers on the posterior side (with the line of pull running vertically in the sagittal plane). Therefore the DIM extend the middle phalanx at the PIP joint and extend the distal phalanx at the DIP joint of the index, middle, and ring fingers. (action 3)

Reverse Mover Action Notes

- The reverse action of a finger at the MCP joint occurs when the metacarpal moves relative to the proximal phalanx of the finger. This occurs when the distal segment, the proximal phalanx, is fixed, such as when the finger is gripping an immovable object. (reverse actions 1, 2)

- When the index finger is fixed (stabilized), the head of the first dorsal interosseus manus that attaches to the thumb pulls its thumb attachment medially and posteriorly toward the index finger, causing flexion and adduction of the thumb at the thumb's CMC (saddle) joint. (reverse action 1)

- Extending the more proximal phalanges at the PIP and DIP joints refers to extending the proximal phalanx at the proximal PIP joint and extending the middle phalanx at the DIP joint. (reverse action 3)

Eccentric Antagonist Functions

1. Restrains/slows adduction of fingers two through four at the MCP joints

2. Restrains/slows extension of fingers two through four at the MCP joints

3. Restrains/slows flexion of fingers two through four at the PIP and DIP joints

Isometric Stabilization Functions

1. Stabilizes the MCP and IP joints of fingers two through four
2. Stabilizes the CMC joint of the thumb

Additional Notes on Functions

1. A mnemonic for remembering the actions of the dorsal interossei manus (DIM) and the palmar interossei muscles is DAB and PAD. The **D**orsals **AB**uct, and the **P**almars **AD**duct.

2. In addition to directly contributing to extension of the fingers at the interphalangeal (IP) joints, the interossei of the hand and the lumbricals manus help create these actions in another manner. Whenever the extensor digitorum contracts, these intrinsic muscles of the hand create a flexion force at the MCP joint to keep the extensor digitorum from excessively extending the MCP joint and thereby losing its ability to create tension and extend the IP joints of the fingers.

3. Regarding reverse actions, the DIM can also adduct metacarpals of fingers four and five at the CMC joints. Similar to how the first DIM can move the metacarpal of the thumb, the fourth DIM can move the metacarpal of the little finger into adduction by pulling it toward the midline of the hand (if the distal ring finger attachment is fixed). The third DIM can move the metacarpal of the ring finger into adduction (if the distal middle finger attachment is fixed). Theoretically, the second DIM can adduct the metacarpal of the index finger in a similar manner; however, the CMC joint of the index finger is fairly locked and does not freely allow this motion.

4. There are four dorsal interossei pedis of the foot that have essentially identical actions (abduction of the toes at the metatarsophalangeal joint, flexion of the toes at the metatarsophalangeal joint, and extension of the toes at the proximal and distal IP joints) to the DIM of the hand.

INNERVATION
☐ The Ulnar Nerve
    ☐ C8, **T1;** deep branch of the ulnar nerve

ARTERIAL SUPPLY
☐ Branches of the Radial and Ulnar Arteries (terminal branches of the Brachial Artery)

Dorsal Interossei Manus (DIM)—*cont'd*

 PALPATION

1. With the client seated or supine, place palpating fingers against the dorsal radial side of the second metacarpal.
2. Have the client abduct the index finger against resistance and feel for the contraction of the first dorsal interosseus manus.
3. To palpate the other three dorsal interossei manus, palpate between the metacarpals from the dorsal side while resisting the client from abducting the finger to which the dorsal interosseus manus is attached.

■ RELATIONSHIP TO OTHER STRUCTURES

☐ The dorsal interossei manus are located between the metacarpals on the dorsal (posterior) side of the hand.
☐ Each dorsal interosseus manus muscle attaches on the side of the proximal phalanx that faces away from the center of the middle finger. (The middle finger has two dorsal interossei manus muscles, one on each side.)
☐ From the anterior perspective, the dorsal interossei manus are deep to the palmar interossei. The first dorsal interosseus manus muscle is mostly deep to the adductor pollicis.
☐ From the posterior perspective, the dorsal interossei manus are superficial and located between the extensor digitorum tendons and between the metacarpal bones. The first dorsal interosseus manus muscle is superficial in the thumb web.
☐ The dorsal interossei manus are involved with the superficial back arm line myofascial meridian.

■ MISCELLANEOUS

1. There are four dorsal interossei manus muscles named from lateral to medial: one, two, three, and four.
2. There are four dorsal interossei manus muscles: one to abduct the index finger, one to abduct the ring finger, and two to abduct the middle finger (the thumb and little finger have their own abductor muscles). The dorsal interosseus manus muscle that attaches onto the radial side of the middle finger "radially abducts" the middle finger at the metacarpophalangeal joint; the dorsal interosseus manus muscle that attaches onto the ulnar side of the middle finger "ulnar abducts" the middle finger at the metacarpophalangeal joint.
3. The first dorsal interosseus manus muscle (the largest) is sometimes known as the *abductor indicis*.
4. The dorsal interossei manus are bipennate in shape.
5. Given that the abductor digiti minimi manus and the abductor pollicis brevis are intrinsic hand muscles that abduct the little finger and the thumb, they can be considered to be analogous to the dorsal interossei manus, which abduct the other three fingers (index, middle, and ring).
6. The majority of tissue of the thumb web of the hand is made up of the first dorsal interosseus manus muscle and the adductor pollicis.

Palmaris Brevis

The name, palmaris brevis, *tells us that this muscle attaches into the palm of the hand and is short (shorter than the palmaris longus).*

Derivation	☐ palmaris: L. *refers to the palm.*
	brevis: L. *shorter.*
Pronunciation	☐ pall-MA-ris, BRE-vis

■ ATTACHMENTS

☐ **The Flexor Retinaculum and the Palmar Aponeurosis**

to the

☐ **Dermis of the Ulnar (Medial) Border of the Hand**

■ FUNCTION

Concentric (Shortening) Mover Actions	
Standard Mover Actions	**Reverse Mover Actions**
☐ **1. Wrinkles the skin of the palm**	☐ 1. Wrinkles the skin of the palm

Standard Mover Action Note

• The palmaris brevis attaches from lateral to medial in the hand (with its fibers running horizontally). When the palmaris brevis contracts, it pulls its medial attachment, the dermis of the ulnar (medial) side of the hand, laterally toward the center of the palm of the hand; this causes the skin of the ulnar side of the hand to wrinkle. This wrinkling of the skin is thought to accentuate or increase the size of the hypothenar eminence. By so doing, it is believed to slightly contribute to the strength and security of the palmar grip. (action 1)

Reverse Mover Action Note

• The reverse action of the palmaris brevis would be if the more central fascia of the hand is moved toward the skin and fascia of the ulnar border of the hand. This still results in wrinkling of the skin of the palm of the hand; in other words, the same action as the standard mover action. (reverse action 1)

Eccentric Antagonist Function

1. Restrains/slows stretching of the skin of the palm

Eccentric Antagonist Function Note

• Restraining/slowing stretching of the skin of the palm restrains the skin from being stretched or lengthened out. This is not a very relevant or important action.

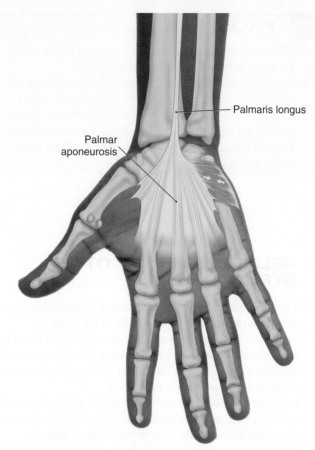

Figure 9-18 Anterior view of the right palmaris brevis.

Isometric Stabilization Function

1. No joint stabilization function

Isometric Stabilization Function Note

• The palmaris brevis is a very thin superficial fascial muscle and does not attach into any bones. Therefore it does not have any significant joint stabilization function.

INNERVATION

☐ The Ulnar Nerve
  ☐ C8, T1

ARTERIAL SUPPLY

☐ The Ulnar Artery (a terminal branch of the Brachial Artery) and the superficial palmar branch of the Radial Artery

Palmaris Brevis—cont'd

 PALPATION

1. The palmaris brevis is located in the dermis proximally on the ulnar side of the palm, superficial to the hypothenar muscle group. However, it is too thin to palpate and distinguish from adjacent tissue.

■ RELATIONSHIP TO OTHER STRUCTURES

☐ The palmaris brevis is superficial in the medial (ulnar) side of the hand.

☐ The hypothenar muscles are all deep to the palmaris brevis.

☐ The palmaris brevis is located within the deep back arm line myofascial meridian.

■ MISCELLANEOUS

1. The palmaris brevis is a very thin, quadrilateral-shaped muscle.
2. The palmaris brevis overlies the hypothenar eminence. Like all the muscles of the hypothenar eminence, it is innervated by the ulnar nerve.
3. Some sources consider the palmaris brevis to be part of the hypothenar group of muscles.

Muscles of the Spinal Joints

CHAPTER OUTLINE

CHAPTER OVERVIEW

The muscles addressed in this chapter are the muscles whose principal function is usually considered to be movement of the trunk, neck, and/or head at the spinal joints. Other muscles in the body can also move the spinal joints, but they are placed in different chapters because their primary function is usually considered to be at another joint. These muscles are located in Chapters 4, 5, 11, 12, 13, and 14.

Overview of Structure

☐ Structurally, muscles of the spinal joints may be categorized based on three factors: the region of the spine, their location,

and their depth. Regionally, they may be divided into three groups: those that run the full length of the spine, those that are primarily located only in the neck, and those that are primarily located only in the low back. Regarding location, they can be described as being anterior or posterior. Regarding their depth, they can be divided based on whether they are superficial or deep.

☐ Beyond these categories, certain spinal muscle groups exist. There are two muscle groups that run the full length of the spine, from the pelvis to the head. These are the erector spinae and transversospinalis groups; collectively, they are

Review the muscles and bones from this chapter on the enclosed CD!

often referred to as the *paraspinal muscles*. In the neck, there are the scalene, prevertebral, and suboccipital groups (the hyoid group is addressed in Chapter 12. The scalene and prevertebral groups are located anteriorly and the suboccipital group is located posteriorly. In the abdominal region, there is the group of anterior abdominal wall muscles.

☐ Generally, the larger, more superficial muscles of the spine are important for creating motion, and the deeper, smaller ones function to stabilize the spine.

Overview of Function

The following general rules regarding actions can be stated for the functional groups of muscles of the spinal joints:

☐ If a muscle crosses the spinal joints anteriorly with a vertical direction to its fibers, it can flex the trunk, neck, and/or head at the spinal joints by moving the superior attachment down toward the inferior attachment in front.

☐ If a muscle crosses the spinal joints posteriorly with a vertical direction to its fibers, it can extend the trunk, neck, and/or head at the spinal joints by moving the superior attachment down toward the inferior attachment in back.

☐ If a muscle crosses the spinal joints laterally, it can laterally flex to that side (ipsilaterally laterally flex) the trunk, neck, and/or head at the spinal joints by moving the superior attachment down toward the inferior attachment on that side of the body.

☐ Right and left rotators of the spine have a horizontal component to their fiber direction and wrap around the body part that they move. Describing a muscle from inferior to superior, ipsilateral (same-side) rotators located posteriorly on the body run from medial to lateral and those located anteriorly on the body run from lateral to medial. Describ-

ing a muscle from inferior to superior, contralateral (opposite-side) rotators located posteriorly on the body run from lateral to medial and those located anteriorly on the body run from medial to lateral.

☐ Reverse actions of these muscles involve the lower spine being moved relative to the upper spine at the spinal joints. These reverse actions usually occur when the client is lying down so the lower attachment is free to move. If the muscle attaches onto the pelvis, the reverse action involves movement of the pelvis at the lumbosacral spinal joint as well.

☐ The reverse action of flexion of the upper spine relative to the lower spine is flexion of the lower spine relative to the upper spine, and posterior tilt of the pelvis if the muscle attaches to it.

☐ The reverse action of extension of the upper spine relative to the lower spine is extension of the lower spine relative to the upper spine, and anterior tilt of the pelvis if the muscle attaches to it.

☐ The reverse action of lateral flexion of the upper spine relative to the lower spine is lateral flexion of the lower spine relative to the upper spine, and elevation of the same side of the pelvis (and therefore depression of the opposite side of the pelvis) if the muscle attaches to it.

☐ The reverse action of ipsilateral rotation of the upper spine relative to the lower spine is contralateral rotation of the lower spine relative to the upper spine, and contralateral rotation of the pelvis if the muscle attaches to it.

☐ The reverse action of contralateral rotation of the upper spine relative to the lower spine is ipsilateral rotation of the lower spine relative to the upper spine, and ipsilateral rotation of the pelvis if the muscle attaches to it.

10

Posterior Views of the Muscles of the Trunk—Superficial and Intermediate Views

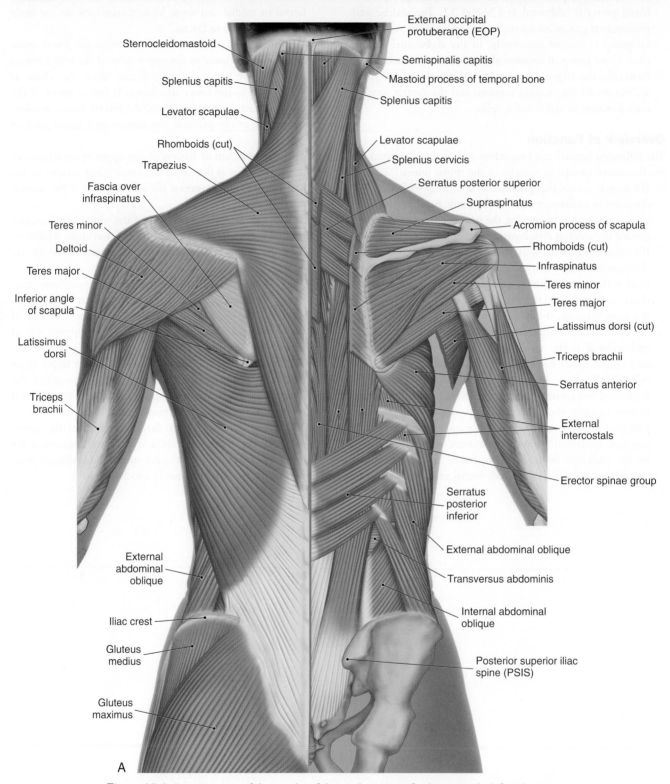

Figure 10-1 Posterior views of the muscles of the trunk. **A,** Superficial view on the left and an intermediate view on the right.

Posterior Views of the Muscles of the Trunk—Deep Views

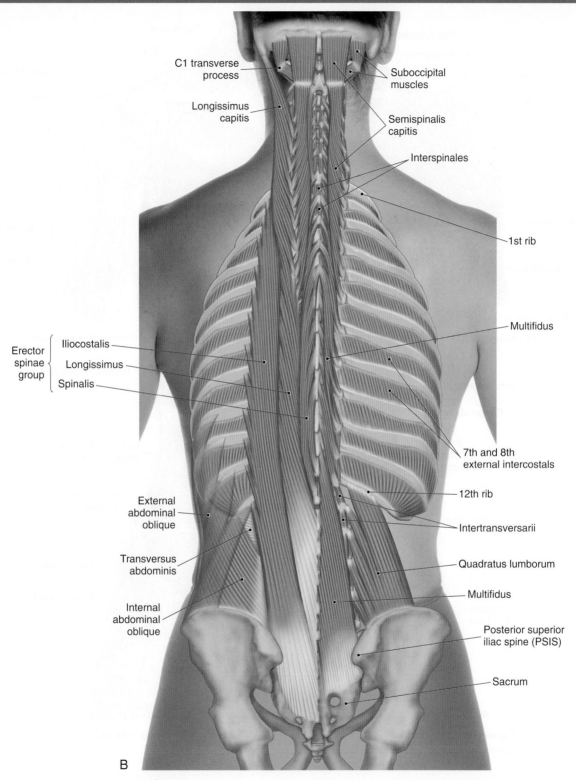

Figure 10-1, cont'd B, Two deep views, the right side deeper than the left. The external abdominal oblique has been ghosted in.

Anterior Views of the Muscles of the Trunk—Superficial and Intermediate Views

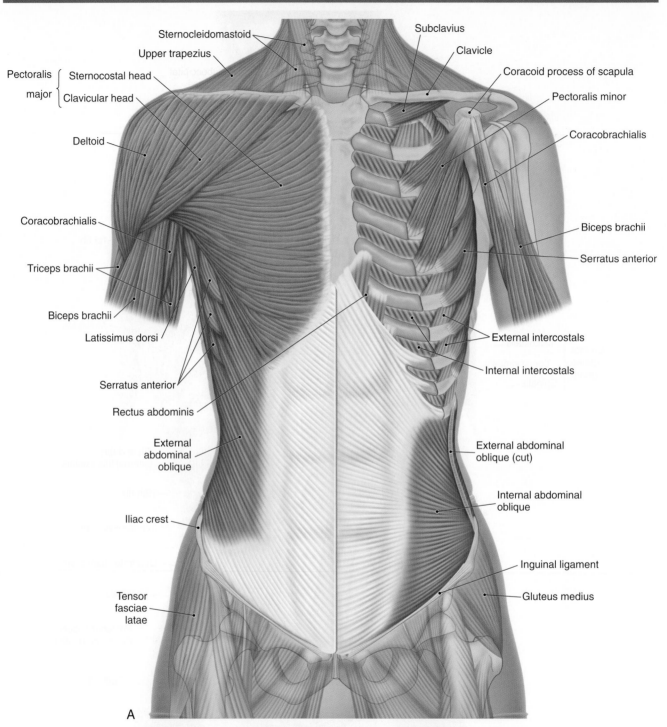

Figure 10-2 Anterior views of the muscles of the trunk. **A,** Superficial view on the right and an intermediate view on the left. The muscles of the neck and thigh have been ghosted in.

Anterior Views of the Muscles of the Trunk—Deep Views

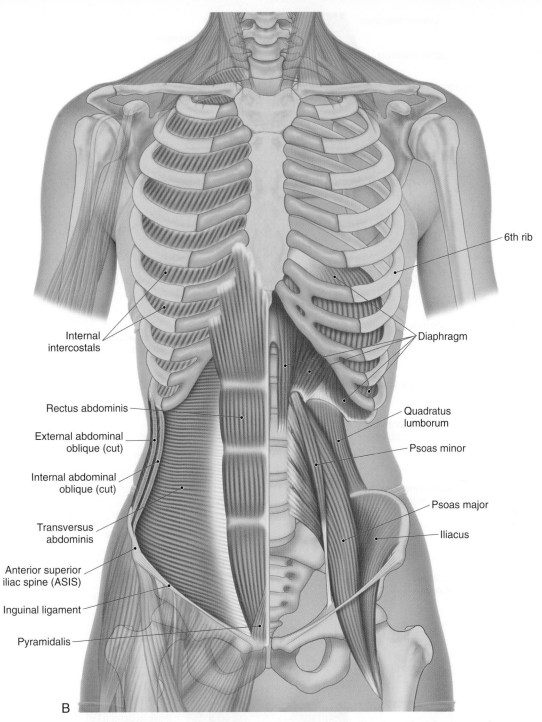

6th rib

Internal
intercostals

Diaphragm

Rectus abdominis

Quadratus
lumborum

External abdominal
oblique (cut)

Psoas minor

Internal abdominal
oblique (cut)

Transversus
abdominis

Psoas major

Anterior superior
iliac spine (ASIS)

Iliacus

Inguinal ligament

Pyramidalis

B

Figure 10-2, cont'd B, Deep views with the posterior abdominal wall seen on the left. The muscles
of the neck, arm, and thigh have been ghosted in.

Right Lateral View of the Muscles of the Trunk

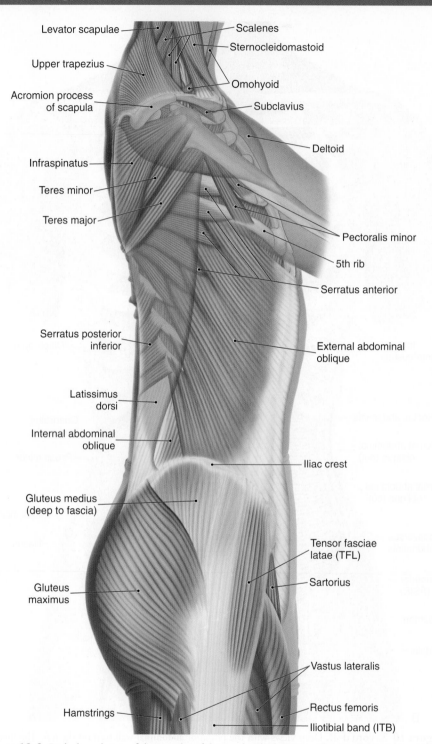

Levator scapulae

Scalenes

Sternocleidomastoid

Upper trapezius

Omohyoid

Acromion process
of scapula

Subclavius

Deltoid

Infraspinatus

Teres minor

Teres major

Pectoralis minor

5th rib

Serratus anterior

Serratus posterior
inferior

External abdominal
oblique

Latissimus
dorsi

Internal abdominal
oblique

Iliac crest

Gluteus medius
(deep to fascia)

Tensor fasciae
latae (TFL)

Sartorius

Gluteus
maximus

Vastus lateralis

Rectus femoris

Hamstrings

Iliotibial band (ITB)

Figure 10-3 Right lateral view of the muscles of the trunk. The latissimus dorsi and deltoid have been ghosted in.

Transverse Plane Cross Sections of the Trunk

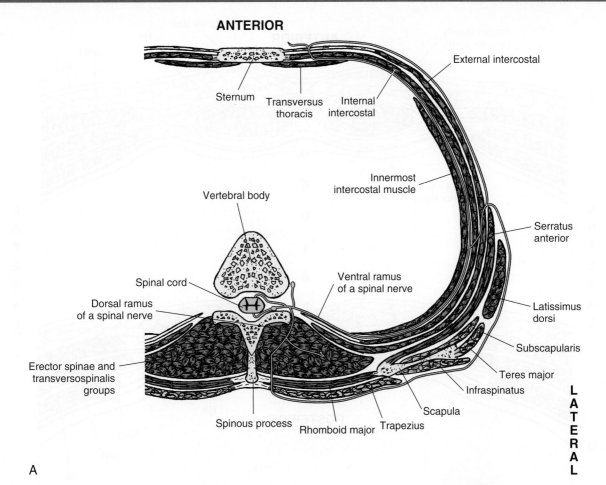

ANTERIOR

Sternum

Transversus thoracis

Internal intercostal

External intercostal

Innermost intercostal muscle

Vertebral body

Spinal cord

Dorsal ramus of a spinal nerve

Ventral ramus of a spinal nerve

Serratus anterior

Latissimus dorsi

Subscapularis

Erector spinae and transversospinalis groups

Teres major

Infraspinatus

Spinous process

Rhomboid major

Trapezius

Scapula

LATERAL

A

Vertebral body

Diaphragm (crura)

Transversus abdominis

Quadratus lumborum

External abdominal oblique

Internal abdominal oblique

Latissimus dorsi

Serratus posterior inferior

Thoracolumbar fascia

Spinous process

POSTERIOR

B

Figure 10-4 Transverse plane cross sections of the trunk. **A,** Thoracic cross section. **B,** Lumbar cross section.

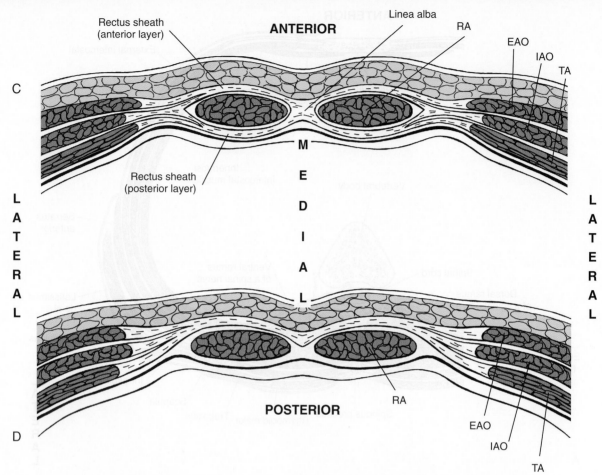

Figure 10-4, cont'd C, Cross section of anterior abdominal wall above the arcuate line. The aponeuroses of the three anterolateral abdominal wall muscles pass anterior and posterior to the rectus abdominis, ensheathing it. **D,** Cross section of anterior abdominal wall below the arcuate line. The aponeuroses of all three anterolateral abdominal wall muscles pass anterior to the rectus abdominis. *EAO,* External abdominal oblique; *IAO,* internal abdominal oblique; *RA,* rectus abdominis; *TA,* transverse abdominis.

Posterior Views of the Neck and Upper Back Region—Superficial Views

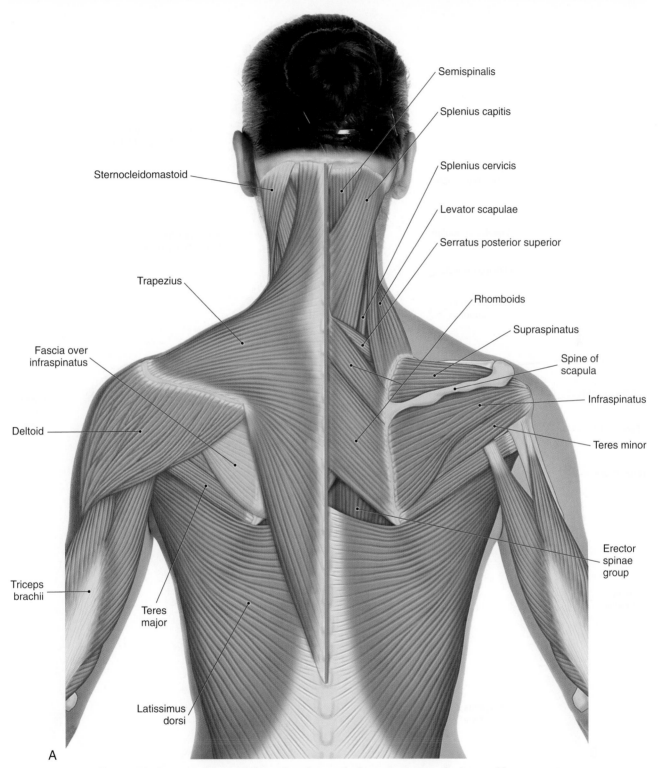

Semispinalis

Splenius capitis

Splenius cervicis

Levator scapulae

Serratus posterior superior

Rhomboids

Supraspinatus

Spine of scapula

Infraspinatus

Teres minor

Erector spinae group

Sternocleidomastoid

Trapezius

Fascia over infraspinatus

Deltoid

Triceps brachii

Teres major

Latissimus dorsi

A

Figure 10-5 Posterior views of the neck and upper back region. **A,** Superficial views. The trapezius, sternocleidomastoid, and deltoid have been removed on the right side.

Posterior Views of the Neck and Upper Back Region—Intermediate Views

10

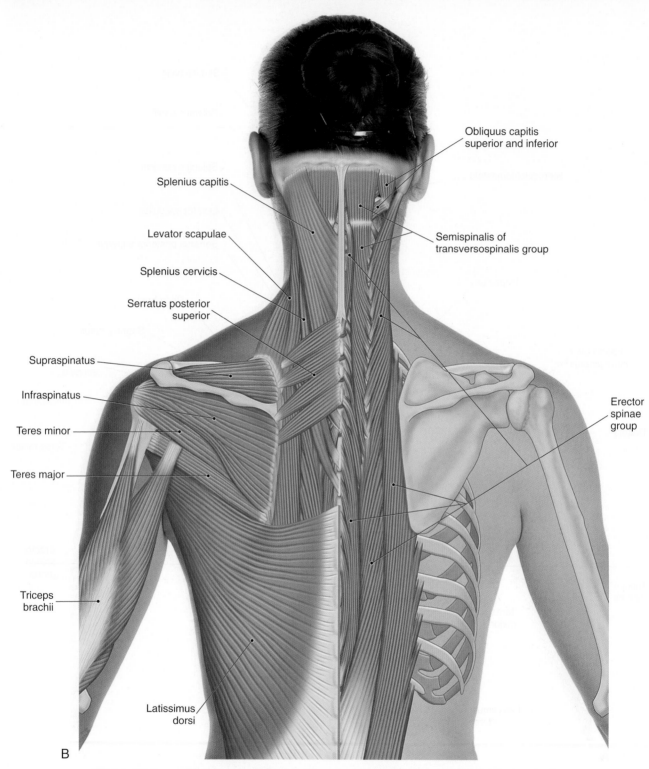

Obliquus capitis
superior and inferior

Splenius capitis

Levator scapulae

Splenius cervicis

Serratus posterior
superior

Semispinalis of
transversospinalis group

Supraspinatus

Infraspinatus

Teres minor

Teres major

Erector
spinae
group

Triceps
brachii

Latissimus
dorsi

B

Figure 10-5, cont'd B, Intermediate views. The serratus posterior superior, splenius capitis and cervicis, levator scapulae, supraspinatus, infraspinatus, teres minor and major, and triceps brachii have been removed on the right side.

Posterior Views of the Neck and Upper Back Region—Deep Views

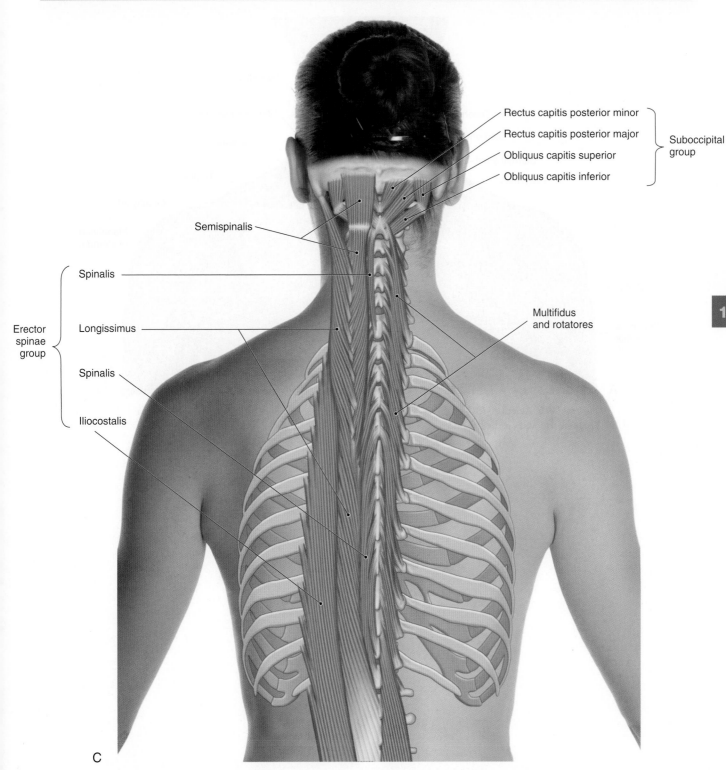

Rectus capitis posterior minor
Rectus capitis posterior major
Obliquus capitis superior
Obliquus capitis inferior
Suboccipital group

Semispinalis

Spinalis

Erector spinae group

Longissimus

Multifidus and rotatores

Spinalis

Iliocostalis

C

Figure 10-5, cont'd C, Deep views. The iliocostalis, longissimus, and spinalis of the erector spinae group and the semispinalis of the transversospinalis group have been removed on the right side.

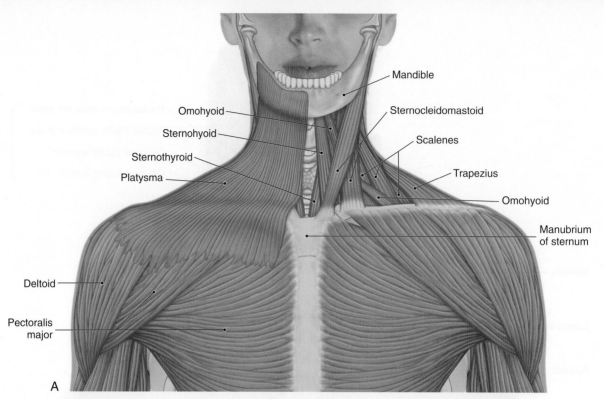

Figure 10-6 Anterior views of the neck and upper chest region. **A,** Superficial views. The platysma has been removed on the left side.

Anterior Views of the Neck and Upper Chest Region—Intermediate and Deep Views

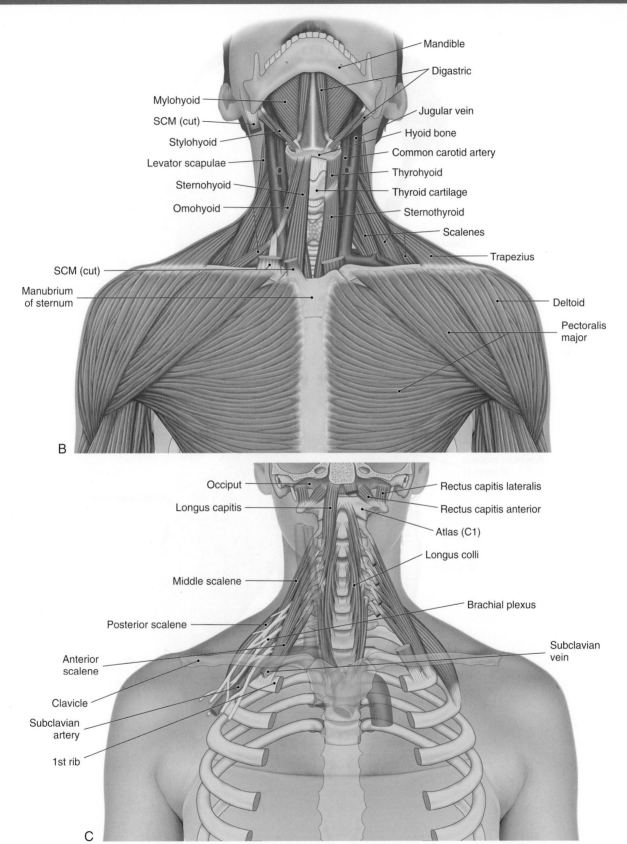

Figure 10-6, cont'd B, Intermediate view with the head extended. The sternocleidomastoid (SCM) has been cut on the right side; the SCM and omohyoid have been removed and the sternohyoid has been cut on the left side. **C,** Deep view. The anterior scalene and longus capitis, as well as the brachial plexus of the nerves and subclavian artery and vein, have been cut and/or removed on the left side. The clavicles and blood vessels have been ghosted in.

Right Lateral View of the Muscles of the Neck Region

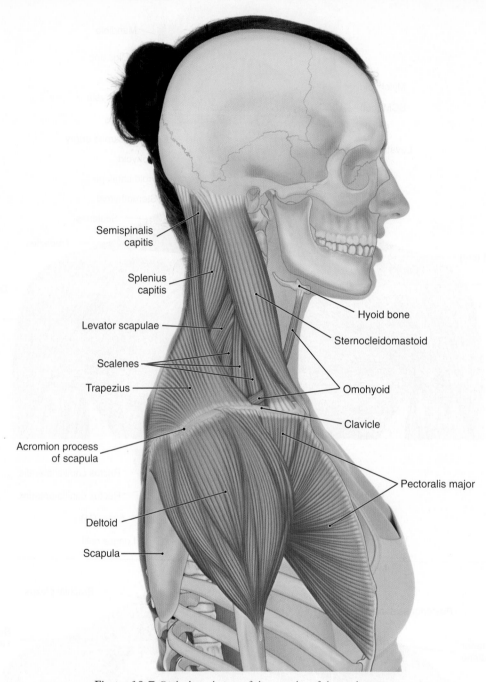

Semispinalis
capitis

Splenius
capitis

Levator scapulae

Scalenes

Trapezius

Acromion process
of scapula

Deltoid

Scapula

Hyoid bone

Sternocleidomastoid

Omohyoid

Clavicle

Pectoralis major

Figure 10-7 Right lateral view of the muscles of the neck region.

Cross-Sectional View of the Neck

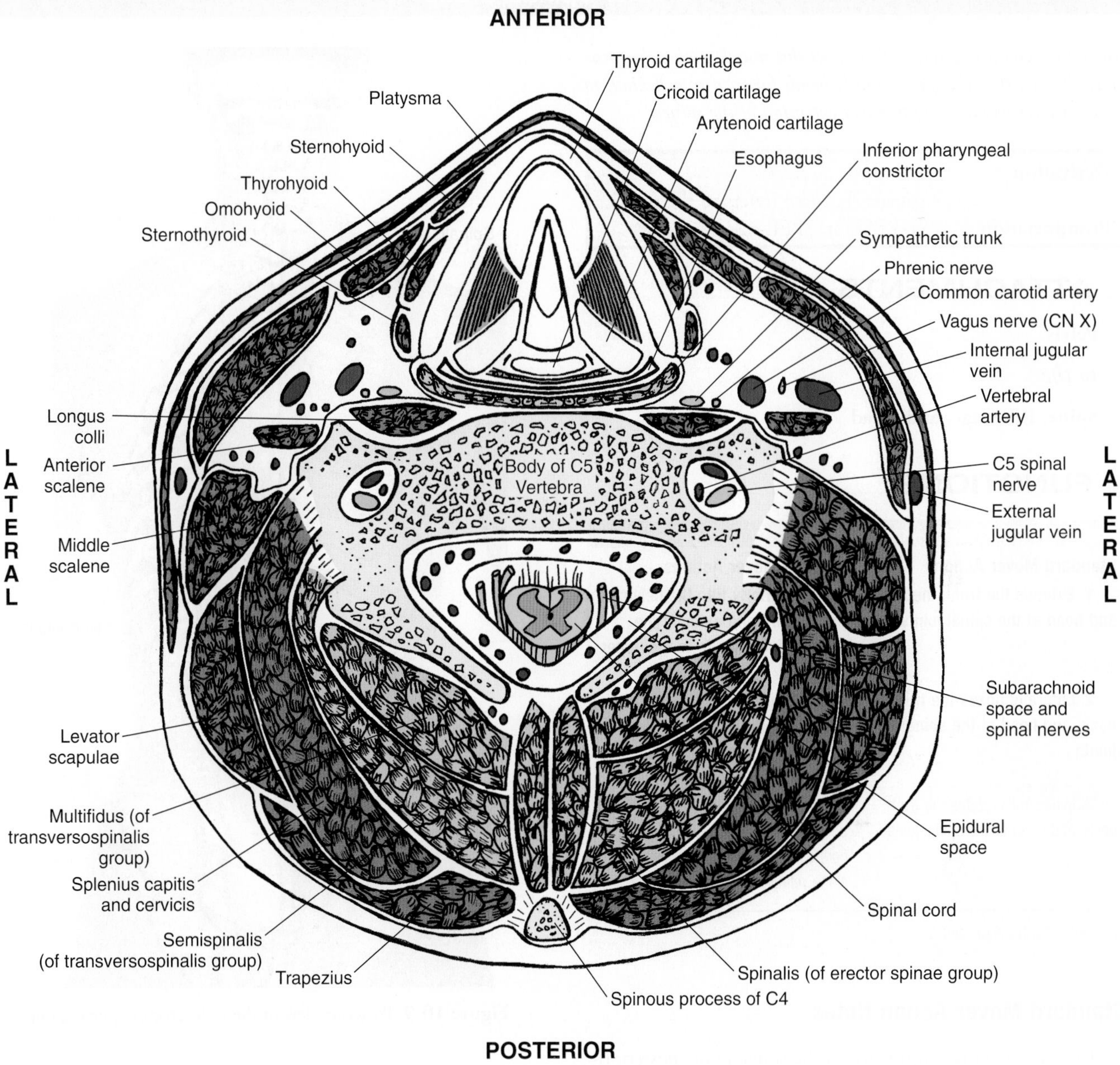

ANTERIOR

Thyroid cartilage
Platysma
Cricoid cartilage
Sternohyoid
Arytenoid cartilage
Thyrohyoid
Esophagus
Inferior pharyngeal constrictor
Omohyoid
Sternothyroid
Sympathetic trunk
Phrenic nerve
Common carotid artery
Vagus nerve (CN X)
Internal jugular vein
Longus colli
Vertebral artery
Anterior scalene
Body of C5 Vertebra
C5 spinal nerve
External jugular vein
Middle scalene

LATERAL

LATERAL

10

Levator scapulae

Subarachnoid space and spinal nerves

Multifidus (of transversospinalis group)

Epidural space

Splenius capitis and cervicis

Spinal cord

Semispinalis (of transversospinalis group)

Spinalis (of erector spinae group)

Trapezius

Spinous process of C4

POSTERIOR

Figure 10-8 Cross section of the neck at the C5 vertebral level.

FULL SPINE
Erector Spinae Group

The name, erector spinae, *tells us that this muscle makes the spine erect. (Given that the spine usually bends forward into flexion, to make it erect would be to perform extension of the spine.)*

Derivation	☐ erector: L. *to erect.*
	spinae: L. *thorn* (refers to the spine).
Pronunciation	☐ ee-REK-tor, SPEE-nee

■ ATTACHMENTS

☐ **Pelvis**

to the

☐ **Spine, Rib Cage, and Head**

■ FUNCTIONS

Concentric (Shortening) Mover Actions	
Standard Mover Actions	**Reverse Mover Actions**
☐ **1. Extends the trunk, neck, and head at the spinal joints**	☐ **1. Anteriorly tilts the pelvis at the LS joint and extends the lower spine relative to the upper spine**
☐ **2. Laterally flexes the trunk, neck, and head at the spinal joints**	☐ 2. Elevates the same-side pelvis at the LS joint and laterally flexes the lower spine relative to the upper spine
☐ 3. Ipsilaterally rotates the trunk, neck, and head at the spinal joints	☐ 3. Contralaterally rotates the pelvis at the LS joint and contralaterally rotates the lower spine relative to the upper spine

LS joint = lumbosacral joint

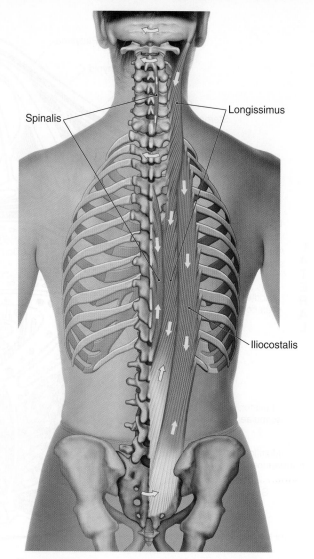

Figure 10-9 Posterior view of the right erector spinae group.

Standard Mover Action Notes

- The erector spinae group crosses the spinal joints posteriorly from the pelvis all the way to the head (with its fibers running vertically in the sagittal plane). Therefore the erector spinae group extends the trunk and the neck at the spinal joints and extends the head at the atlanto-occipital joint (AOJ). (action 1)
- The erector spinae group crosses the spinal joints laterally from the pelvis all the way to the head (with its fibers running vertically in the frontal plane). Therefore the erector spinae group laterally flexes the trunk and the neck at the spinal joints and laterally flexes the head at the AOJ. (action 2)
- The arrangement of the erector spinae group is generally such that its inferior attachment is medial and its superior attachment is more lateral (with its fibers running somewhat horizontally in the transverse plane). When the inferior attachment is fixed and the erector spinae group contracts,

it pulls this superolateral attachment posteromedially toward the midline, causing the anterior surface of the trunk and/ or the neck and/or the head to face the same side of the body on which the erector spinae group is attached. Therefore the erector spinae group ipsilaterally rotates the trunk and the neck at the spinal joints and ipsilaterally rotates the head at the AOJ. (action 3)

Reverse Mover Action Notes

- When we think of motions of the spine, we usually think of the upper spine moving relative to the fixed lower spine. However, the reverse action of moving the lower spine relative to the upper spine is also possible; these reverse actions usually occur when the client is lying down so that the lower attachment is mobile. Furthermore, if the pelvis is moved,

Erector Spinae Group—*cont'd*

because the LS joint does not allow a large degree of motion, the lumbar spine will move with the pelvis, causing the lumbar spine to move under the thoracic spine. (reverse actions 1, 2, 3)

- With the superior attachments fixed, the erector spinae group, by pulling superiorly on the posterior pelvis, anteriorly tilts the pelvis at the LS joint. (reverse action 1)
- When the erector spinae contracts and the superior attachments are fixed, it pulls superiorly on the lateral pelvis (because the fibers are running vertically), elevating the pelvis on that side at the LS joint. Elevation of one side of the pelvis causes the other side to depress. Therefore the erector spinae group ipsilaterally elevates and contralaterally depresses the pelvis. (reverse action 2)
- When the superior attachments of the erector spinae group are fixed and the erector spinae group contracts, it pulls on the inferior pelvic attachment. (Because the fibers of the erector spinae group have a slight horizontal orientation in the transverse plane, the pelvis will rotate in the transverse plane.) The posterior pelvis is pulled posterolaterally toward the side of the body on which the erector spinae group is attached, causing the anterior pelvis to face the opposite side of the body from the side of the body on which the erector spinae group is attached. Therefore the erector spinae group contralaterally rotates the pelvis at the LS joint. (reverse action 3)
- The reverse action of ipsilaterally rotating the upper spine (relative to the fixed lower spine and pelvis) is to contralaterally rotate the pelvis and lower spine (relative to the fixed upper spine). In other words, if the right-sided erector spinae group does right rotation of the upper spine, then its reverse action would be to do left rotation of the pelvis and lower spine. (reverse action 3)

Eccentric Antagonist Functions

1. Restrains/slows flexion, opposite-side lateral flexion, and contralateral rotation of the trunk, neck, and head
2. Restrains/slows posterior tilt and ipsilateral depression of the pelvis
3. Restrains/slows ipsilateral rotation of the pelvis and lower spine

Eccentric Antagonist Function Note

- The eccentric function of restraining/slowing flexion of the trunk is extremely important. The erector spinae eccentrically contracts to control our descent toward the floor every time we bend over into flexion.

Isometric Stabilization Functions

1. Stabilizes the spinal joints
2. Stabilizes the ribs at the sternocostal and costospinal joints
3. Stabilizes the sacroiliac joint

Isometric Stabilization Function Notes

- The erector spinae group can help stabilize the sacroiliac joint because the iliocostalis and longissimus attach inferiorly to the iliac crest and sacrum.

Additional Notes on Functions

1. Only the longissimus muscle of the erector spinae group attaches onto the head and can move the head at the AOJ (the capitis portion of the spinalis usually fuses with and is considered to be part of the semispinalis capitis of the transversospinalis group).
2. Only the iliocostalis and longissimus muscles of the erector spinae group attach onto the pelvis and can move the pelvis at the LS joint.

INNERVATION
□ Spinal Nerves
  □ dorsal rami of cervical, thoracic, and lumbar spinal nerves

ARTERIAL SUPPLY
□ The dorsal branches of the Posterior Intercostal and Lumbar Arteries (all branches of the Aorta)
  □ and the Thoracodorsal Artery (a branch of the Subclavian Artery)

PALPATION

1. With the client prone, place palpating hands lateral to the spinous processes of the vertebral column in the lumbar region and feel for the vertical orientation of the fibers of the erector spinae.
2. Continue palpating the erector spinae inferiorly and superiorly toward its attachments.
3. To engage the erector spinae group, ask the client to actively extend the upper part of the body (trunk, neck, and head) off the table and feel for the contraction of the erector spinae group, particularly in the lumbar and lower thoracic regions.

■ RELATIONSHIP TO OTHER STRUCTURES

□ Although much of the erector spinae group lies on either side of the spinous processes of the spine in the laminar groove (over the laminae, between the spinous processes and the transverse processes), especially in the lower back, keep in mind that this group also attaches to the ribs and attaches quite far laterally.

10

☐ The erector spinae group is deep in the back and neck. In the lumbar region, the erector spinae group is deep to the latissimus dorsi and the serratus posterior inferior. In the thoracic region the erector spinae group is deep to the trapezius, latissimus dorsi, rhomboids major and minor, serratus posterior superior, splenius capitis, and splenius cervicis. In the cervical region, the erector spinae group is deep to the trapezius, splenius capitis, splenius cervicis, and sternocleidomastoid.

☐ In the trunk, the transversospinalis muscle group, the quadratus lumborum, and the rib cage are deep to the erector spinae group. In the neck, the suboccipital muscle group is deep to the erector spinae group.

☐ The erector spinae group is located within the superficial back line and spiral line myofascial meridians.

■ MISCELLANEOUS

1. The erector spinae group can be divided into three subgroups. These three subgroups are (from lateral to medial) the iliocostalis, the longissimus, and the spinalis.

2. Generally, the following statements can be made regarding the erector spinae subgroups:
   • The iliocostalis attaches from the ilium to the ribs.
   • The longissimus is the longest of the three subgroups.
   • The spinalis attaches from spinous processes to spinous processes.

3. Of the three subgroups of the erector spinae, only the iliocostalis and longissimus attach onto the pelvis, and only the longissimus attaches onto the head. (Occasionally the spinalis capitis attaches to the head.)

4. Each of the three subgroups of the erector spinae can be further subdivided into three subgroups. They are the iliocostalis lumborum, thoracis, and cervicis; the longissimus thoracis, cervicis, and capitis; and the spinalis thoracis, cervicis, and capitis. (Note: The spinalis capitis often blends with and is therefore considered to be a part of the semispinalis capitis of the transversospinalis group.)

5. The erector spinae group is also known as the *sacrospinalis* group.

6. The term *paraspinal* musculature is also used to describe the erector spinae and the transversospinalis groups together.

Iliocostalis (of Erector Spinae Group)

The name, iliocostalis, *tells us that this muscle attaches from the ilium to the ribs.*

Derivation	☐ ilio:	L. *refers to the ilium.*
	costalis:	L. *refers to the ribs.*
Pronunciation	☐ IL-ee-o-kos-TA-lis	

■ ATTACHMENTS

☐ **ENTIRE ILIOCOSTALIS: Sacrum, Iliac Crest, and Ribs Three through Twelve**
- ☐ ILIOCOSTALIS LUMBORUM: Medial Iliac Crest and the Medial and Lateral Sacral Crests
- ☐ ILIOCOSTALIS THORACIS: Angles of Ribs Seven through Twelve
- ☐ ILIOCOSTALIS CERVICIS: Angles of Ribs Three through Six

to the

☐ **ENTIRE ILIOCOSTALIS: Ribs One through Twelve and Transverse Processes of C4-C7**
- ☐ ILIOCOSTALIS LUMBORUM: Angles of Ribs Seven through Twelve
- ☐ ILIOCOSTALIS THORACIS: Angles of Ribs One through Six and the Transverse Process of C7
- ☐ ILIOCOSTALIS CERVICIS: Transverse Processes of C4-C6

■ FUNCTIONS

Concentric (Shortening) Mover Actions	
Standard Mover Actions	**Reverse Mover Actions**
☐ **1. Extends the trunk and neck at the spinal joints**	☐ 1. Anteriorly tilts the pelvis at the LS joint and extends the lower spine relative to the upper spine
☐ **2. Laterally flexes the trunk and neck at the spinal joints**	☐ 2. Elevates the same-side pelvis at the LS joint and laterally flexes the lower spine relative to the upper spine
☐ 3. Ipsilaterally rotates the trunk and neck at the spinal joints	☐ 3. Contralaterally rotates the pelvis at the LS joint and contralaterally rotates the lower spine relative to the upper spine

LS joint = lumbosacral joint

Standard Mover Action Notes

- The iliocostalis crosses the spinal joints posteriorly from the pelvis all the way to the lower neck (with its fibers running vertically in the sagittal plane); therefore it extends the trunk and the neck at the spinal joints. (action 1)

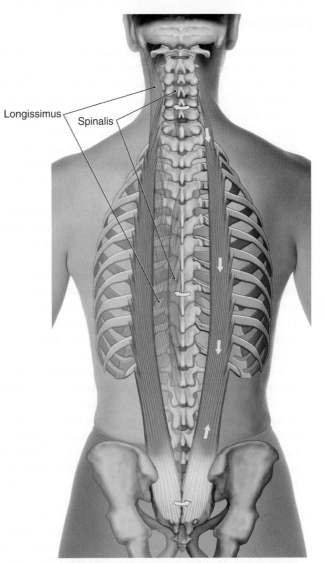

Longissimus   Spinalis

Figure 10-10 Posterior view of the iliocostalis bilaterally. The other two erector spinae muscles have been ghosted in on the left side.

- The iliocostalis crosses the spinal joints laterally from the pelvis all the way to the lower neck (with its fibers running vertically in the frontal plane); therefore it laterally flexes the trunk and the neck at the spinal joints. (action 2)
- The arrangement of the iliocostalis is generally such that its inferior attachment is medial and its superior attachment is more lateral (with its fibers running somewhat horizontally in the transverse plane). When the inferior attachment is fixed and the iliocostalis contracts, it pulls this superolateral attachment posteromedially toward the midline, causing the anterior surface of the trunk and/or the neck to face the same side of the body on which the iliocostalis is attached. Therefore the iliocostalis ipsilaterally rotates the trunk and the neck at the spinal joints. (action 3)

10

Reverse Mover Action Notes

- When we think of motions of the spine, we usually think of the upper spine moving relative to the fixed lower spine. However, the reverse action of moving the lower spine relative to the upper spine is also possible (this usually occurs when the client is lying down so the lower attachment is mobile). Further, if the pelvis is moved, because the LS joint does not allow a large degree of motion, the lumbar spine will move with the pelvis, causing the lumbar spine to move under the thoracic spine. (reverse actions 1, 2, 3)
- When the iliocostalis contracts and the superior attachments are fixed, it pulls superiorly on the posterior pelvis, anteriorly tilting the pelvis at the LS joint (in the sagittal plane). (reverse action 1)
- When the iliocostalis contracts and the superior attachments are fixed, it pulls superiorly on the lateral pelvis, elevating the pelvis on that side (in the frontal plane) at the LS joint. Elevation of one side of the pelvis causes the other side to depress. Therefore the iliocostalis ipsilaterally elevates and contralaterally depresses the pelvis. (reverse action 2)
- When the iliocostalis contracts and the superior attachments are fixed, it pulls the posterior pelvis posterolaterally toward the side of the body to which the iliocostalis is attached (note that there is a horizontal component in the transverse plane to the direction of the fibers), causing the anterior pelvis to face the opposite side of the body from the side of the body to which the iliocostalis is attached. Therefore the iliocostalis contralaterally rotates the pelvis at the LS joint. (reverse action 3)
- The reverse action of ipsilaterally rotating the upper spine (relative to the fixed lower spine and pelvis) is to contralaterally rotate the pelvis and lower spine (relative to the fixed upper spine). In other words, if the right-sided iliocostalis does right rotation of the upper spine, its reverse action would be to do left rotation of the pelvis and lower spine. (reverse action 3)

Eccentric Antagonist Functions

1. Restrains/slows flexion, opposite-side lateral flexion, and contralateral rotation of the trunk and neck
2. Restrains/slows posterior tilt and same-side depression of the pelvis
3. Restrains/slows ipsilateral rotation of the pelvis and lower spine

Eccentric Antagonist Function Note

- The eccentric function of restraining/slowing flexion of the trunk is extremely important. The iliocostalis eccentrically contracts to control our descent toward the floor every time we bend over into flexion.

Isometric Stabilization Functions

1. Stabilizes the spinal joints
2. Stabilizes the ribs at the sternocostal and costospinal joints
3. Stabilizes the sacroiliac joint

Isometric Stabilization Function Note

- Because the iliocostalis attaches inferiorly to the iliac crest and sacrum, it can help stabilize the sacroiliac joint.

Additional Note on Functions

1. Only the iliocostalis and longissimus muscles of the erector spinae group attach onto the pelvis and can move the pelvis at the LS joint.

INNERVATION
☐ Spinal Nerves
  ☐ dorsal rami of the lower cervical and the thoracic and upper lumbar spinal nerves

ARTERIAL SUPPLY
☐ The dorsal branches of the Posterior Intercostal and Lumbar Arteries (all branches of the Aorta)
  ☐ and the Thoracodorsal Artery (a branch of the Subclavian Artery)

✋ PALPATION

1. With the client prone, locate the erector spinae group in the lumbar and thoracic regions (see the Palpation section for this muscle group on page 285).
2. Once located, the iliocostalis will be the most lateral fibers of the erector spinae group.
3. Palpate the iliocostalis from the pelvis to the rib attachments.

■ RELATIONSHIP TO OTHER STRUCTURES

☐ The iliocostalis, as part of the erector spinae group, is fairly deep in the posterior trunk.
☐ The iliocostalis is deep to the latissimus dorsi, serratus posterior inferior, trapezius, rhomboids major and minor, serratus posterior superior, splenius capitis, and splenius cervicis (as well as the longissimus and semispinalis capitis in the neck).
☐ Deep to the iliocostalis are the multifidus, the quadratus lumborum, the rib cage, and the external and internal intercostal muscles.

Iliocostalis (of Erector Spinae Group)—*cont'd*

☐ The iliocostalis is the most lateral of the erector spinae muscles. It often runs far enough laterally to be deep to the scapula.

☐ The iliocostalis is located within the superficial back line and spiral line myofascial meridians.

■ MISCELLANEOUS

1. The iliocostalis is also known as the *iliocostocervicalis.*
2. The iliocostalis can be subdivided into the iliocostalis lumborum, the iliocostalis thoracis, and the iliocostalis cervicis.

3. Of the three subgroups of the erector spinae group, the iliocostalis has the most lateral attachment (onto the ribs). Keep this in mind when working on the erector spinae group. The iliocostalis often attaches lateral enough to be deep to the scapula!

10

Longissimus (of Erector Spinae Group)

The name, longissimus, *tells us that this muscle is long. It is the longest of the erector spinae subgroups.*

| **Derivation** | ☐ longissimus: L. *very long.* |
| **Pronunciation** | ☐ lon-JIS-i-mus |

■ ATTACHMENTS

☐ **ENTIRE LONGISSIMUS: Sacrum, Iliac Crest, Transverse Processes and Spinous Processes of L1-L5 and T1-T5, and the Articular Processes of C5-C7**
  ☐ LONGISSIMUS THORACIS: Medial Iliac Crest, Posterior Sacrum, and the Transverse Processes of L1-L5
  ☐ LONGISSIMUS CERVICIS: Transverse Processes of the Upper Five Thoracic Vertebrae
  ☐ LONGISSIMUS CAPITIS: Transverse Processes of the Upper Five Thoracic Vertebrae and the Articular Processes of the Lower Three Cervical Vertebrae

to the

☐ **ENTIRE LONGISSIMUS: Ribs Four through Twelve, Transverse Processes of T1-T12 and C2-C6, and the Mastoid Process of the Temporal Bone**
  ☐ LONGISSIMUS THORACIS: Transverse Processes of all the Thoracic Vertebrae and the Lower Nine Ribs (between the tubercles and the angles)
  ☐ LONGISSIMUS CERVICIS: Transverse Processes of C2-C6 (posterior tubercles)
  ☐ LONGISSIMUS CAPITIS: Mastoid Process of the Temporal Bone

■ FUNCTIONS

Concentric (Shortening) Mover Actions	
Standard Mover Actions	**Reverse Mover Actions**
☐ **1. Extends the trunk, neck, and head at the spinal joints**	☐ **1. Anteriorly tilts the pelvis at the LS joint and extends the lower spine relative to the upper spine**
☐ **2. Laterally flexes the trunk, neck, and head at the spinal joints**	☐ 2. Elevates the same-side pelvis at the LS joint and laterally flexes the lower spine relative to the upper spine
☐ 3. Ipsilaterally rotates the trunk, neck, and head at the spinal joints	☐ 3. Contralaterally rotates the pelvis at the LS joint and contralaterally rotates the lower spine relative to the upper spine

LS joint = lumbosacral joint

Standard Mover Action Notes

• The longissimus crosses the spinal joints posteriorly from the pelvis all the way to the head (with its fibers running verti-

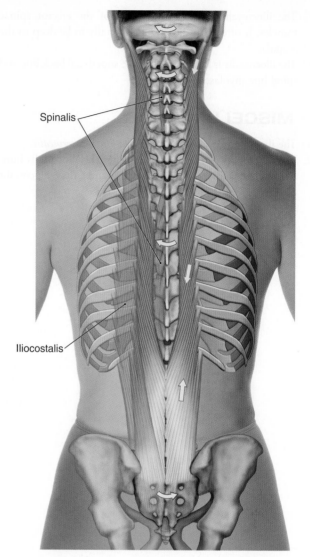

Figure 10-11 Posterior view of the longissimus bilaterally. The other two erector spinae muscles have been ghosted in on the left side.

cally in the sagittal plane). Therefore the longissimus extends the trunk and the neck at the spinal joints and extends the head at the atlanto-occipital joint (AOJ). (action 1)
• The longissimus crosses the spinal joints laterally from the pelvis all the way to the head (with its fibers running vertically in the frontal plane). Therefore the longissimus laterally flexes the trunk and the neck at the spinal joints and laterally flexes the head at the AOJ. (action 2)
• The arrangement of the longissimus is generally such that its inferior attachment is medial and its superior attachment is more lateral (with its fibers running somewhat horizontally in the transverse plane). When the inferior attachment is fixed and the longissimus contracts, it pulls this superolateral attachment posteromedially toward the midline, causing the anterior surface of the trunk and/or the neck and/or the head

Longissimus (of Erector Spinae Group)—*cont'd*

to face the same side of the body on which the longissimus is attached. Therefore the longissimus ipsilaterally rotates the trunk and the neck at the spinal joints and ipsilaterally rotates the head at the AOJ. (reverse action 3)

Reverse Mover Action Notes

- When we think of motions of the spine, we usually think of the upper spine moving relative to the fixed lower spine. However, the reverse action of moving the lower spine relative to the upper spine is also possible (this usually occurs when the client is lying down so the lower attachment is mobile). Further, if the pelvis is moved, because the LS joint does not allow a large degree of motion, the lumbar spine will move with the pelvis, causing the lumbar spine to move under (relative to) the thoracic spine. (reverse actions 1, 2, 3)
- When the longissimus contracts and the superior attachments are fixed, it pulls superiorly on the posterior pelvis, anteriorly tilting the pelvis at the LS joint. (reverse action 1)
- When the longissimus contracts and the superior attachments are fixed, it pulls superiorly on the lateral pelvis (because the fibers are running vertically), elevating the pelvis on that side at the LS joint. Elevation of one side of the pelvis causes the other side to depress. Therefore the longissimus ipsilaterally elevates and contralaterally depresses the pelvis. (reverse action 2)
- When the longissimus contracts and the superior attachments are fixed, it pulls the posterior pelvis posterolaterally toward the side of the body on which the longissimus is attached (note that there is a horizontal component to the direction of fibers), causing the anterior pelvis to face the opposite side of the body from the side of the body on which the longissimus is attached. Therefore the longissimus contralaterally rotates the pelvis at the LS joint. (reverse action 3)
- The reverse action of ipsilaterally rotating the upper spine (relative to the fixed lower spine and pelvis) is to contralaterally rotate the pelvis and lower spine (relative to the fixed upper spine). In other words, if the right-sided longissimus does right rotation of the upper spine, its reverse action would be to do left rotation of the pelvis and lower spine. (reverse action 3)

Eccentric Antagonist Functions

1. Restrains/slows flexion, opposite-side lateral flexion, and contralateral rotation of the trunk, neck, and head
2. Restrains/slows posterior tilt and same-side depression of the pelvis
3. Restrains/slows ipsilateral rotation of the pelvis and lower spine

Eccentric Antagonist Function Note

- The eccentric function of restraining/slowing flexion of the trunk is extremely important. The longissimus eccentrically

contracts to control our descent toward the floor every time we bend over into flexion.

Isometric Stabilization Functions

1. Stabilizes the spinal joints
2. Stabilizes the ribs at the sternocostal and costospinal joints
3. Stabilizes the sacroiliac joint

Isometric Stabilization Function Note

- Because longissimus attaches inferiorly to the iliac crest and sacrum, it can help stabilize the sacroiliac joint.

Additional Notes on Functions

1. Only the longissimus muscle of the erector spinae group attaches onto the head and can move the head at the AOJ (the capitis portion of the spinalis usually fuses with and is considered to be part of the semispinalis capitis of the transversospinalis group).
2. Only the iliocostalis and longissimus muscles of the erector spinae group attach onto the pelvis and can move the pelvis at the LS joint.

INNERVATION
☐ Spinal Nerves
  ☐ dorsal rami of the lower cervical and the thoracic and lumbar spinal nerves

ARTERIAL SUPPLY
☐ The dorsal branches of the Posterior Intercostal and Lumbar Arteries (all branches of the Aorta)

✋ PALPATION

1. With the client prone, locate the erector spinae group in the lumbar and thoracic regions (see the Palpation section for this muscle group on page 285).
2. Once located, palpate the longissimus between the spinalis (medially) and the iliocostalis (laterally). The longissimus will be palpable as a mass of musculature running vertically.
3. Note that the longissimus gradually courses further lateral as it ascends the trunk.

■ RELATIONSHIP TO OTHER STRUCTURES

☐ The longissimus is located between the iliocostalis (which is directly lateral to it) and the spinalis (which is directly medial to it).

10

Longissimus (of Erector Spinae Group)—*cont'd*

☐ The longissimus is deep to the latissimus dorsi, serratus posterior inferior, trapezius, rhomboids major and minor, serratus posterior superior, splenius capitis, and splenius cervicis.

☐ From the posterior perspective, the longissimus attachment onto the mastoid process of the temporal bone is deep to the mastoid process attachment of the sternocleidomastoid and the splenius capitis.

☐ Deep to the longissimus are the multifidus, rotatores, levatores costarum, intertransversarii, quadratus lumborum, the rib cage, and the external and internal intercostal muscles.

☐ The longissimus cervicis' inferior attachment is in the thoracic region, medial to the longissimus thoracis.

☐ Most of the longissimus cervicis is deep to the longissimus capitis.

☐ The longissimus capitis lies between the longissimus cervicis (which is directly lateral to it) and the splenius capitis (which is directly medial to it).

☐ The longissimus is located within the superficial back line and spiral line myofascial meridians.

■ MISCELLANEOUS

1. The longissimus can be subdivided into the longissimus thoracis, the longissimus cervicis, and the longissimus capitis.

2. The longissimus is the longest and the largest of the three subgroups of the erector spinae group.

3. Of the three subgroups of the erector spinae group, the longissimus has the most superior attachment (onto the mastoid process of the temporal bone).

4. In the lumbar region, the longissimus blends with the iliocostalis. In the thoracic region, the longissimus blends with the spinalis.

5. The longissimus thoracis also attaches into the thoracolumbar fascia.

10

Spinalis (of Erector Spinae Group)

The name, spinalis, *tells us that this muscle attaches from spinous processes to spinous processes.*

Derivation	☐ spinalis: L. *refers to spinous processes.*
Pronunciation	☐ spy-NA-lis

■ ATTACHMENTS

☐ **ENTIRE SPINALIS: Spinous Processes of T11-L2; and the Spinous Process of C7 and the Nuchal Ligament**
   ☐ SPINALIS THORACIS: Spinous Processes of T11-L2
   ☐ SPINALIS CERVICIS: Inferior Nuchal Ligament and the Spinous Process of C7
   ☐ SPINALIS CAPITIS: Usually Considered to Be the Medial Part of the Semispinalis Capitis

to the

☐ **ENTIRE SPINALIS: Spinous Processes of T4-T8; and the Spinous Process of C2**
   ☐ SPINALIS THORACIS: Spinous Processes of T4-T8
   ☐ SPINALIS CERVICIS: Spinous Process of C2
   ☐ SPINALIS CAPITIS: Usually Considered to Be the Medial Part of the Semispinalis Capitis

■ FUNCTIONS

Concentric (Shortening) Mover Actions	
Standard Mover Actions	**Reverse Mover Actions**
☐ **1. Extends the trunk and neck at the spinal joints**	☐ 1. Extends the lower spine relative to the upper spine
☐ **2. Laterally flexes the trunk and neck at the spinal joints**	☐ 2. Laterally flexes the lower spine relative to the upper spine

LS joint = lumbosacral joint

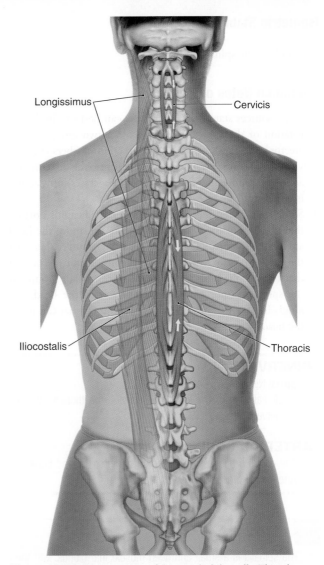

Figure 10-12 Posterior view of the spinalis bilaterally. The other two erector spinae muscles have been ghosted in on the left side.

Standard Mover Action Notes

- The spinalis crosses the spinal joints posteriorly (with its fibers running vertically in the sagittal plane). Therefore the spinalis extends the trunk and the neck at the spinal joints. (action 1)
- The spinalis crosses the spinal joints laterally (with its fibers running vertically in the frontal plane). Therefore the spinalis laterally flexes the trunk and the neck at the spinal joints. (action 2)
- Extension is the strongest action of the spinalis. Its lateral flexion ability is weak. (actions 1, 2)

Reverse Mover Action Note

- When we think of motions of the spine, we usually think of the upper spine moving relative to the fixed lower spine.

However, the reverse action of moving the lower spine relative to the fixed upper spine is also possible. These reverse actions usually occur when the client is lying down so that the inferior attachment is mobile. (reverse actions 1, 2)

Eccentric Antagonist Functions

1. Restrains/slows flexion and opposite-side lateral flexion of the trunk and neck.

Eccentric Antagonist Function Note

- The eccentric function of restraining/slowing flexion of the trunk is extremely important. The spinalis eccentrically contracts to control our descent toward the floor every time we bend over into flexion.

Spinalis (of Erector Spinae Group)—*cont'd*

Isometric Stabilization Function

1. Stabilizes the spinal joints

Additional Notes on Functions

1. Some sources state that the spinalis can perform ipsilateral rotation of the spine, as can the other two groups of the erector spinae group. Given the direction of fibers (there is virtually no horizontal component because the attachments are from spinous processes to spinous processes), this action is either unlikely or extremely weak.
2. Some sources consider the spinalis to have a capitis portion that attaches to the head and therefore can move the head at the atlanto-occipital joint (AOJ). Other sources state that the capitis portion fuses with and is considered to be part of the semispinalis capitis (of the transversospinalis group). If the spinalis is not considered to attach to the head, the longissimus is the only erector spinae muscle that can move the head at the AOJ.

INNERVATION
☐ Spinal Nerves
  ☐ dorsal rami of the lower cervical and the thoracic spinal nerves

ARTERIAL SUPPLY
☐ The dorsal branches of the Posterior Intercostal and Lumbar Arteries (all branches of the Aorta)

✋ PALPATION

1. The spinalis is a small and deep muscle that blends with the longissimus and semispinalis. It is best palpated along with the longissimus (see the Palpation section for this muscle on page 291).
2. If palpable, the spinalis will be the most medial fibers of the erector spinae. It can be very challenging to distinguish from the adjacent erector spinae and transversospinalis musculature.

■ RELATIONSHIP TO OTHER STRUCTURES

☐ The spinalis fibers are the most medial of all the fibers of the erector spinae group.
☐ The spinalis is deep to the latissimus dorsi, serratus posterior inferior, trapezius, rhomboids major and minor, serratus posterior superior, splenius capitis, and splenius cervicis.
☐ Deep to the spinalis are the multifidus, the rotatores, and the vertebrae.
☐ The spinalis is located within the superficial back line and spiral line myofascial meridians.

■ MISCELLANEOUS

1. The spinalis can be subdivided into the spinalis thoracis, the spinalis cervicis, and the spinalis capitis.
2. Of the three subgroups of the erector spinae group, the spinalis is the smallest and located the most medial.
3. The spinalis is significant in the thoracic region only.
4. The spinalis thoracis usually blends intimately with the longissimus.
5. The spinalis capitis is also known as the *biventer cervicis,* because a band of tendon cuts across it transversely, effectively dividing it into two bellies (*biventer* means two bellies).
6. Usually the spinalis capitis blends with the medial part of the semispinalis capitis (of the transversospinalis group) and is therefore usually considered to be a part of the semispinalis capitis. When the spinalis capitis is present as a distinct muscle, it is very small, and deep to the semispinalis capitis.
7. The spinalis cervicis is often absent.
8. When present, the attachment levels of the spinalis cervicis are variable. Its inferior attachment often reaches to T1-T2 and its superior attachment often reaches to C3-C4.

Transversospinalis Group

The name, transversospinalis, *tells us that this muscle group attaches from transverse processes (inferiorly) to spinous processes (superiorly).*

Derivation	☐ transverso: L. *refers to transverse processes.*
	spinalis: L. *refers to spinous processes.*
Pronunciation	☐ trans-VER-so-spy-NA-lis

■ ATTACHMENTS

☐ **Pelvis**

to the

☐ **Spine and the Head**
   ☐ Generally running from transverse process below to spinous process above

■ FUNCTIONS

Concentric (Shortening) Mover Actions	
Standard Mover Actions	**Reverse Mover Actions**
☐ **1. Extends the trunk, neck, and head at the spinal joints**	☐ **1. Anteriorly tilts the pelvis at the LS joint and extends the lower spine relative to the upper spine**
☐ **2. Laterally flexes the trunk, neck, and head at the spinal joints**	☐ 2. Elevates the same-side pelvis at the LS joint and laterally flexes the lower spine relative to the upper spine
☐ **3. Contralaterally rotates the trunk and neck at the spinal joints**	☐ 3. Ipsilaterally rotates the pelvis at the LS joint and ipsilaterally rotates the lower spine relative to the upper spine

LS joint = lumbosacral joint

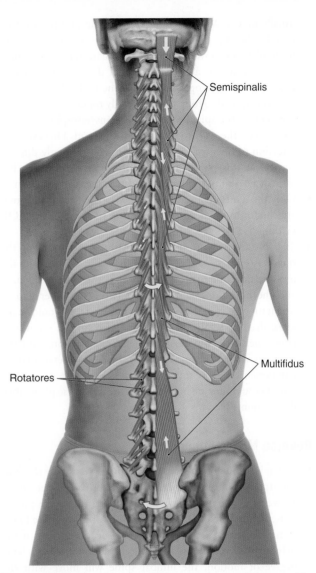

Figure 10-13 Posterior view of the transversospinalis group. The semispinalis and multifidus are seen on the right; the rotatores are seen on the left.

Standard Mover Action Notes

• The transversospinalis group crosses the spinal joints posteriorly from the pelvis all the way to the head (with its fibers running vertically in the sagittal plane). Therefore the transversospinalis group extends the trunk and the neck at the spinal joints and extends the head at the atlanto-occipital joint (AOJ). (action 1)

• Of the three muscles of the transversospinalis group, the semispinalis is best suited to create extension because its fibers are the most vertical in orientation (in the sagittal plane). The semispinalis capitis of the semispinalis muscle is the largest muscle in the posterior neck and likely the most powerful extensor of the neck and head. (action 1)

• The transversospinalis group crosses the spinal joints laterally from the pelvis all the way to the head (with its fibers running vertically in the frontal plane). Therefore the transversospinalis group laterally flexes the trunk and the neck at the spinal joints and laterally flexes the head at the AOJ. (action 2)

• The arrangement of the transversospinalis group is generally from a transverse process inferolaterally to a spinous process superomedially (with its fibers running somewhat horizontally in the transverse plane). The inferior attachment is usually more fixed (because the inferior attachment on the trunk and/or pelvis is connected to the thighs, legs, and feet, which are grounded); therefore the superior attachment

Transversospinalis Group—*cont'd*

usually moves. When the transversospinalis group contracts, it pulls the superior attachment on the spinous processes posterolaterally toward the more inferolateral transverse processes, causing the anterior surface of the body part that is moved to face the opposite side of the body. Therefore the transversospinalis group contralaterally rotates the trunk and the neck at the spinal joints. (The transversospinalis group also crosses the AOJ to attach onto the head. However, the direction of fibers of the transversospinalis is nearly directly vertical at this point. Therefore the transversospinalis has little or no ability to rotate the head at the AOJ.) (action 3)

- Only the semispinalis muscle of the transversospinalis group attaches onto the head and can move the head at the AOJ. (actions 1, 2,)
- The direction of the fibers of the three subgroups of the transversospinalis varies. The semispinalis subgroup is the most vertical, the rotatores subgroup is the most horizontal, and the multifidus subgroup is between the other two in orientation. Given these directions of fibers, it would make sense that the semispinalis is best suited for the extension/lateral flexion component of their spinal actions and the rotatores would be best suited for the contralateral rotation component of their spinal actions. (Hence the name *rotatores;* because they are horizontal in the transverse plane, they do rotation.) (actions 1, 2, 3)

Reverse Mover Action Notes

- When we think of motions of the spine, we usually think of the upper spine moving relative to the fixed lower spine. However, if the upper attachment of the transversospinalis musculature is fixed, the reverse action of moving the lower spine relative to the upper spine can occur. Further, if the pelvis is moved, because the LS joint does not allow a large degree of motion, the lumbar spine will move with the pelvis, causing the lumbar spine to move under and relative to the thoracic spine. (reverse actions 1, 2, 3)
- When the transversospinalis musculature contracts and the superior attachments are fixed, it pulls superiorly on the posterior pelvis, anteriorly tilting the pelvis at the LS joint. (reverse action 1)
- When the transversospinalis musculature contracts and the superior attachments are fixed, it pulls superiorly on the lateral pelvis, elevating the pelvis on that side (in the frontal plane) at the LS joint. Elevation of one side of the pelvis causes the other side to depress. Therefore the transversospinalis group ipsilaterally elevates and contralaterally depresses the pelvis. (reverse action 2)
- When the transversospinalis musculature contracts and the superior attachments are fixed, it pulls on the inferior pelvic attachment. Because the fibers of the transversospinalis group have a slight horizontal orientation in the transverse plane, the pelvis will rotate. When the transversospinalis group contracts, it pulls the posterior pelvis posteromedially toward the spine, causing the anterior pelvis to face the same side of the body on which the transversospinalis group is attached. Therefore the transversospinalis group ipsilaterally rotates the pelvis at the LS joint. (reverse action 3)

- The reverse action of contralaterally rotating the upper spine (relative to the fixed lower spine and pelvis) is to ipsilaterally rotate the pelvis and lower spine (relative to the fixed upper spine). In other words, if the right-sided transversospinalis group does left rotation of the upper spine, its reverse action would be to do right rotation of the pelvis and lower spine. (reverse action 3)
- Only the multifidus of the transversospinalis group attaches onto the pelvis and can move the pelvis at the LS joint. (reverse actions 1, 2, 3)

Eccentric Antagonist Functions

1. Restrains/slows flexion and opposite-side lateral flexion of the trunk, neck, and head
2. Restrains/slows ipsilateral rotation of the trunk and neck
3. Restrains/slows posterior tilt and same-side depression of the pelvis
4. Restrains/slows contralateral rotation of the pelvis and lower spine

Isometric Stabilization Functions

Stabilizes the spinal joints
Stabilizes the sacroiliac joint

Isometric Stabilization Function Notes

1. The multifidus is credited, along with the transversus abdominis, as being one of the most important muscles of core stabilization.
2. Because the multifidus attaches inferiorly to the iliac crest and sacrum, the transversospinalis group can help stabilize the sacroiliac joint. The multifidus is also the largest muscle of the low back.

INNERVATION
- ☐ Spinal Nerves
  - ☐ dorsal rami of cervical, thoracic, and lumbar spinal nerves

ARTERIAL SUPPLY
- ☐ The Occipital Artery (a branch of the External Carotid Artery) and the dorsal branches of the Posterior Intercostal and Lumbar Arteries (all branches of the Aorta)
  - ☐ and the Deep Cervical Artery (a branch of the Thyrocervical Trunk)

Transversospinalis Group—*cont'd*

 PALPATION

1. With the client prone, place palpating fingers over the laminar groove of the thoracic spine.
2. Have the client slightly extend the neck and trunk and rotate to the opposite side and feel for the contraction of the transversospinalis musculature. Palpate the transversospinalis throughout the thoracic and lumbar regions.
3. To palpate the transversospinalis of the neck, have the client supine and palpate deep to the upper trapezius between the spine and the splenius capitis.

■ RELATIONSHIP TO OTHER STRUCTURES

☐ The transversospinalis group is very deep in the back and lies in the laminar groove (over the laminae, between the spinous processes and the transverse processes) of the spine.

☐ In the trunk, the transversospinalis group is directly deep to the erector spinae group. In the neck the transversospinalis group is deep to the trapezius, the splenius capitis and the sternocleidomastoid.

☐ In the trunk, the vertebrae are directly deep to the transversospinalis group.

☐ In the neck, the suboccipitals are directly deep to the transversospinalis group.

☐ The transversospinalis group is located within the superficial back line myofascial meridian.

■ MISCELLANEOUS

1. The name, *transversospinalis,* tells us that this muscle group attaches from a transverse process *(transverso)* to a spinous process *(spinalis).* The transverse process attachment is the inferior attachment; the spinous process attachment is the superior attachment.

2. The inferior attachment of the transversospinalis group is not always precisely onto the transverse processes. Sometimes the inferior attachment is onto the mamillary or articular processes of the vertebrae.

3. The transversospinalis muscle group can be divided into three subgroups. These three subgroups are (from superficial to deep) the semispinalis, the multifidus, and the rotatores.

4. The following statements can be made regarding the transversospinalis subgroups:
   • The rotatores attach superiorly to the vertebrae one to two levels above the inferior attachment.
   • The multifidus attaches superiorly to vertebrae three to four levels above the inferior attachment.
   • The semispinalis attaches superiorly to vertebrae five or more levels above the inferior attachment.

5. Of the three subgroups of the transversospinalis, only the multifidus attaches onto the pelvis, and only the semispinalis attaches onto the head.

6. The term *paraspinal musculature* is also used to describe the erector spinae and the transversospinalis groups together.

7. The semispinalis is best developed and quite massive in the cervical region.

8. The multifidus is best developed and quite massive in the lumbar region.

10

Semispinalis (of Transversospinalis Group)

The name, semispinalis, *tells us that this muscle is associated with spinous processes.*

Derivation	□ semi: L. *half.*
	spinalis: L. *refers to spinous processes.*
Pronunciation	□ SEM-ee-spy-NA-lis

■ ATTACHMENTS

□ **ENTIRE SEMISPINALIS: Transverse Processes of C7-T10 and the Articular Processes of C4-C6**
  - □ SEMISPINALIS THORACIS: Transverse Processes of T6-T10
  - □ SEMISPINALIS CERVICIS: Transverse Processes of T1-T5
  - □ SEMISPINALIS CAPITIS: Transverse Processes of C7-T6 and the Articular Processes of C4-C6

to the

□ **ENTIRE SEMISPINALIS: Spinous Processes of C2-T4 and the Occipital Bone (Five-Six Segmental Levels Superior to the Inferior Attachment)**
  - □ SEMISPINALIS THORACIS: Spinous Processes of C6-T4
  - □ SEMISPINALIS CERVICIS: Spinous Processes of C2-C5
  - □ SEMISPINALIS CAPITIS: Occipital Bone between the Superior and Inferior Nuchal Lines

■ FUNCTIONS

Concentric (Shortening) Mover Actions	
Standard Mover Actions	**Reverse Mover Actions**
□ **1. Extends the trunk, neck, and head at the spinal joints**	□ 1. Extends the lower spine relative to the upper spine
□ **2. Laterally flexes the trunk, neck, and head at the spinal joints**	□ 2. Laterally flexes the lower spine relative to the upper spine
□ **3. Contralaterally rotates the trunk and neck at the spinal joints**	□ 3. Ipsilaterally rotates the lower spine relative to the upper spine

Standard Mover Action Notes

- The semispinalis crosses the spinal joints posteriorly from the thoracic region all the way to the head (with its fibers running vertically in the sagittal plane). Therefore the semispinalis extends the trunk and the neck at the spinal joints and extends the head at the atlanto-occipital joint (AOJ). (action 1)
- Of the three muscles of the transversospinalis group, the semispinalis is best suited to create extension because its fibers are the most vertical in orientation (in the sagittal plane). The semispinalis capitis is the largest muscle in the

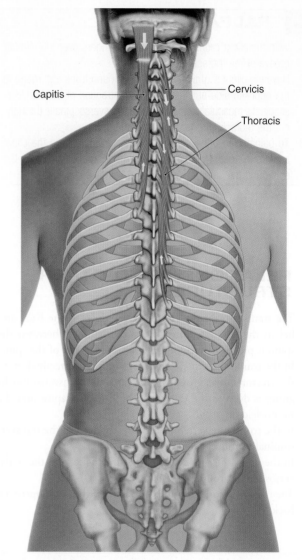

Figure 10-14 Posterior view of the semispinalis. The semispinalis thoracic and cervicis are seen on the right; the semispinalis capitis is seen on the left.

posterior neck and likely the most powerful extensor of the neck and head. (action 1)
- The semispinalis crosses the spinal joints laterally from the thoracic region all the way to the head (with its fibers running vertically in the frontal plane). Therefore the semispinalis laterally flexes the trunk and the neck at the spinal joints and laterally flexes the head at the AOJ. (action 2)
- The arrangement of the semispinalis is generally from a transverse process inferolaterally to a spinous process superomedially (with its fibers running somewhat horizontally in the transverse plane). The inferior attachment is usually more fixed (because the inferior attachment on the trunk is connected to the pelvis, thighs, legs, and feet, which are grounded); therefore the superior attachment usually moves. When the semispinalis contracts, it pulls the superior attachment on the spinous processes posterolaterally toward the

Semispinalis (of Transversospinalis Group)—*cont'd*

more inferolateral transverse processes, causing the anterior surface of the body part that is moved to face the opposite side of the body. Therefore the semispinalis contralaterally rotates the trunk and the neck at the spinal joints. (action 3)

- The semispinalis only attaches as low as T10. Therefore it only moves the thoracic spine of the trunk (not the lumbar spine). (actions 1, 2, 3)
- Only the semispinalis muscle of the transversospinalis group attaches onto the head and can move the head at the AOJ. (actions 1, 2)
- The semispinalis cannot contralaterally rotate the head at the AOJ because its fibers are perfectly vertical when they cross the AOJ. (action 3)

Reverse Mover Action Notes

- When we think of motions of the spine, we usually think of the upper spine moving relative to the fixed lower spine. However, the reverse action of moving the lower spine relative to the fixed upper spine is also possible. These reverse actions often occur when the client is lying down so that the inferior attachment is mobile. (reverse actions 1, 2, 3)
- The reverse action of contralaterally rotating the upper spine (relative to the fixed lower spine) is to ipsilaterally rotate the lower spine (relative to the fixed upper spine). In other words, if the right-sided semispinalis does left rotation of the upper spine, its reverse action would be to do right rotation of the lower spine. (reverse action 3)

Eccentric Antagonist Functions

1. Restrains/slows flexion and opposite-side lateral flexion of the trunk, neck, and head
2. Restrains/slows ipsilateral rotation of the trunk and neck
3. Restrains/slows contralateral rotation of the lower spine relative to the upper spine

Isometric Stabilization Functions

1. Stabilizes the spinal joints
2. Stabilizes the head at the AOJ

INNERVATION
- ☐ Spinal Nerves
  - ☐ dorsal rami of cervical and thoracic spinal nerves

ARTERIAL SUPPLY
- ☐ The Occipital Artery (a branch of the External Carotid Artery) and the dorsal branches of the Posterior Intercostal Arteries (branches of the Aorta)
  - ☐ and the Deep Cervical Artery (a branch of the Costocervical Trunk)

✋ PALPATION

1. With the client supine with the hand in the small of the back (to help relax the trapezius), place palpating fingers in the posteromedial neck and feel for the semispinalis capitis deep to the trapezius.
2. Continue palpating the semispinalis superiorly toward the occipital attachment between the superior and inferior nuchal lines.

■ RELATIONSHIP TO OTHER STRUCTURES

- ☐ The semispinalis thoracis is directly deep to the erector spinae group.
- ☐ The semispinalis cervicis is deep to the spinalis cervicis and the semispinalis capitis.
- ☐ In the neck, the semispinalis capitis is deep to the upper trapezius, splenius capitis, splenius cervicis, and sternocleidomastoid and superficial to the suboccipital muscles.
- ☐ The occipital attachment of the semispinalis capitis is sandwiched between the trapezius and sternocleidomastoid more superficially, and the suboccipitals deeper.
- ☐ The semispinalis is located within the superficial back line myofascial meridian.

■ MISCELLANEOUS

1. A semispinalis muscle attaches to a transverse process inferiorly and runs superiorly to attach onto the spinous process of a vertebra, five or more levels above the inferior attachment. Most commonly, a semispinalis muscle attaches six levels superior to the inferior attachment.
2. The semispinalis can be subdivided into the semispinalis thoracis, the semispinalis cervicis, and the semispinalis capitis.
3. The semispinalis capitis is the largest of the three subdivisions of the semispinalis and is the largest muscle of the neck.
4. The spinalis capitis (of the erector spinae group) usually blends with the medial part of the semispinalis capitis. Therefore the spinalis capitis is usually considered to be a part of the semispinalis capitis. (Occasionally, the spinalis capitis is a distinct muscle.)
5. When the spinalis capitis of the erector spinae group does blend with the medial portion of the semispinalis capitis, this muscle may be known as the *biventer cervicis,* because a band of tendon often cuts across it transversely, effectively dividing it into two bellies (*biventer* means two bellies), and because it is in the neck (*cervicis* means neck).
6. The inferior attachments of the semispinalis capitis are variable and often attach to the transverse process of T7 and/or to the spinous processes of C7-T1.

7. The inferior attachments of the semispinalis cervicis are variable and often attach to the transverse process of T6.

8. The greater occipital nerve, which innervates the posterior half of the scalp, pierces through the semispinalis capitis (and the upper trapezius). When the semispinalis capitis is tight, the greater occipital nerve can be compressed, causing a *tension headache* that is felt in the posterior head. (This condition is also known as *greater occipital neuralgia*.)

Multifidus (of Transversospinalis Group)

The name, multifidus, *tells us that this muscle is made up of many separate muscles that split to go to separate attachments.*

Derivation	☐ multi: L. *many.*
	fidus: L. *to split.*
Pronunciation	☐ mul-TIF-id-us

■ ATTACHMENTS

☐ **Posterior Sacrum, Posterior Superior Iliac Spine (PSIS), Posterior Sacroiliac Ligament, and L5-C4 Vertebrae**
  ☐ LUMBAR REGION: All Mamillary Processes (not transverse processes)
  ☐ THORACIC REGION: All Transverse Processes
  ☐ CERVICAL REGION: The Articular Processes of C4-C7 (not transverse processes)

to the

☐ **Spinous processes of Vertebrae Three-Four Segmental Levels Superior to the Inferior Attachment**

■ FUNCTIONS

Concentric (Shortening) Mover Actions	
Standard Mover Actions	**Reverse Mover Actions**
☐ **1. Extends the trunk and neck at the spinal joints**	☐ **1. Anteriorly tilts the pelvis at the LS joint and extends the lower spine relative to the upper spine**
☐ **2. Laterally flexes the trunk and neck at the spinal joints**	☐ 2. Elevates the same-side pelvis at the LS joint and laterally flexes the lower spine relative to the upper spine
☐ **3. Contralaterally rotates the trunk and neck at the spinal joints**	☐ 3. Ipsilaterally rotates the pelvis at the LS joint and ipsilaterally rotates the lower spine relative to the upper spine

LS joint = lumbosacral joint

Standard Mover Action Notes

- The multifidus crosses the spinal joints posteriorly from the pelvis all the way to the cervical spine (with its fibers running vertically in the sagittal plane). Therefore the multifidus extends the trunk and the neck at the spinal joints. (action 1)
- The multifidus crosses the spinal joints laterally from the pelvis all the way to the cervical spine (with its fibers running vertically in the frontal plane). Therefore the multifidus laterally flexes the trunk and the neck at the spinal joints. (action 2)

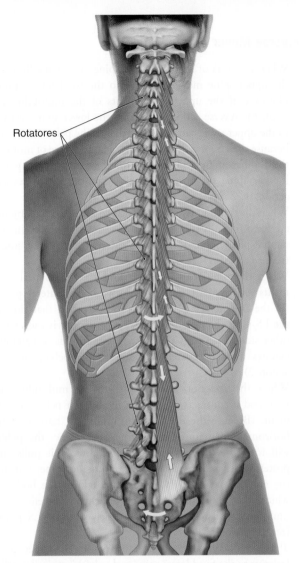

Rotatores

Figure 10-15 Posterior view of the right multifidus. The rotatores have been ghosted in on the left.

- The arrangement of the multifidus is generally from a transverse process (or mamillary process or articular process) inferolaterally to a spinous process superomedially (with its fibers running somewhat horizontally in the transverse plane). The inferior attachment is usually more fixed (because the inferior attachment on the trunk and/or pelvis is connected to the thighs, legs, and feet, which are grounded); therefore the superior attachment usually moves. When the multifidus contracts, it pulls the superior attachment on the spinous processes posterolaterally toward the more inferolateral transverse processes, causing the anterior surface of the body part that is moved to face the opposite side of the body. Therefore the multifidus contralaterally rotates the trunk and the neck at the spinal joints. (action 3)

10

Reverse Mover Action Notes

- When we think of motions of the spine, we usually think of the upper spine moving relative to the fixed lower spine. However, if the upper attachments of the multifidus are fixed, the reverse action of moving the lower spine relative to the upper spine can occur. Further, if the pelvis is moved, because the LS joint does not allow a large degree of motion, the lumbar spine will move with the pelvis, causing the lumbar spine to move under the thoracic spine. (reverse actions 1, 2, 3)

- When the multifidus contracts and the superior attachments are fixed, it pulls superiorly on the posterior pelvis (in the sagittal plane), anteriorly tilting the pelvis at the LS joint. (reverse action 1)

- When the multifidus contracts and the superior attachments are fixed, it pulls superiorly on the lateral pelvis (in the frontal plane), elevating the pelvis on that side at the LS joint. Elevation of one side of the pelvis causes the other side to depress. Therefore the multifidus ipsilaterally elevates and contralaterally depresses the pelvis. (reverse action 2)

- When the superior attachments of the multifidus are fixed and it contracts, it pulls on the inferior pelvic attachment. (Because the fibers of the multifidus have a slight horizontal orientation in the transverse plane, the pelvis will rotate.) When the multifidus contracts, it pulls the posterior pelvis posteromedially toward the spine, causing the anterior pelvis to face the same side of the body to which the multifidus group is attached. Therefore the multifidus ipsilaterally rotates the pelvis at the LS joint. (reverse action 3)

- The reverse action of contralaterally rotating the upper spine (relative to the fixed lower spine and pelvis) is to ipsilaterally rotate the pelvis and lower spine (relative to the fixed upper spine). In other words, if the right-sided multifidus does left rotation of the upper spine, its reverse action would be to do right rotation of the pelvis and lower spine. (reverse action 3)

Eccentric Antagonist Functions

1. Restrains/slows flexion, opposite-side lateral flexion, and ipsilateral rotation of the trunk and neck
2. Restrains/slows posterior tilt and same-side depression of the pelvis
3. Restrains/slows ipsilateral rotation of the pelvis and lower spine

Isometric Stabilization Functions

1. Stabilizes the spinal joints
2. Stabilizes the sacroiliac joint

Isometric Stabilization Function Notes

- The multifidus is credited, along with the transversus abdominis, as being one of the most important muscles of core stabilization.
- Because the multifidus attaches inferiorly to the iliac crest and sacrum, it can help stabilize the sacroiliac joint.

Additional Note on Functions

1. Only the multifidus of the transversospinalis group attaches onto the pelvis and can move the pelvis at the LS joint.

INNERVATION
☐ Spinal Nerves
  ☐ dorsal rami of cervical, thoracic, and lumbar spinal nerves

ARTERIAL SUPPLY
☐ The dorsal branches of the Posterior Intercostal and Lumbar Arteries (all branches of the Aorta)

👋 PALPATION

1. With the client prone, place palpating fingers just lateral to the midline of the upper sacrum.
2. Have the client extend (and perhaps slightly contralaterally rotate) the trunk, neck, and head off the table and feel for the contraction of the multifidus.
3. Continue palpating the multifidus into the lumbar and thoracic regions.

■ RELATIONSHIP TO OTHER STRUCTURES

☐ In the lumbar region, the multifidus group is directly deep to the erector spinae musculature. In the thoracic and cervical region, the multifidus group is directly deep to the semispinalis.
☐ The rotatores and vertebrae are directly deep to the multifidus group.
☐ The multifidus is located within the superficial back line myofascial meridian.

■ MISCELLANEOUS

1. The attachments for the multifidus group are from a transverse process (or mamillary process or articular process) inferiorly to a spinous process superiorly.

Multifidus (of Transversospinalis Group)—*cont'd*

2. By the usual definition, the multifidus group attaches to a spinous process three to four levels superior to its inferior attachment.
3. The multifidus group is bulkiest in the lumbosacral region and is the largest muscle in the low back.
4. Some sources describe the multifidus group as having layers that span from one to four vertebrae superior to the inferior attachment. More specifically, they describe three layers. The most superficial layer goes from a transverse process inferiorly, to spinous processes three to four levels superiorly. The

next layer goes from the same transverse process to spinous processes two to three levels superiorly. Some sources state that the deepest layer goes from the same transverse process to the spinous process of the very next vertebra superiorly. (More conventional naming of the transversospinalis group would name some of these fibers as *rotatores*.)

5. Very little erector spinae musculature overlies the multifidus in the lumbar region. However, in this region, the tendinous fibers of the erector spinae are very thick and difficult to palpate through.

Rotatores (of Transversospinalis Group)

The name, rotatores, *tells us that these muscles perform rotation.*

Derivation	☐ rotatores: L. *to turn, a muscle revolving a body part on its axis.*
Pronunciation	☐ ro-ta-TO-reez

■ ATTACHMENTS

☐ **Transverse Process (inferiorly)**

to the

☐ **Lamina (superiorly)**
　☐ One-Two Segmental Levels Superior to the Inferior Attachment

■ FUNCTIONS

Concentric (Shortening) Mover Actions	
Standard Mover Actions	**Reverse Mover Actions**
☐ **1. Contralaterally rotate the trunk and neck at the spinal joints**	☐ 1. Ipsilaterally rotate the lower spine relative to the upper spine
☐ **2. Extend the trunk and neck at the spinal joints**	☐ 2. Extend the lower spine relative to the upper spine
☐ **3. Laterally flex the trunk and neck at the spinal joints**	☐ 3. Laterally flex the lower spine relative to the upper spine

Standard Mover Action Notes

• The arrangement of the rotatores group is generally from a transverse process inferolaterally to a lamina superomedially (with its fibers running nearly horizontally in the transverse plane). The inferior attachment is usually more fixed (because the inferior attachment on the trunk is connected to the pelvis, thighs, legs, and feet, which are grounded); therefore the superior attachment usually moves. When the rotatores group contracts, it pulls the superior attachment on the lamina posterolaterally toward the more inferolateral transverse processes, causing the anterior surface of the body part that is moved to face the opposite side of the body. Therefore the rotatores group contralaterally rotates the trunk and the neck at the spinal joints. (action 1)

• Of the three muscles of the transversospinalis group, the rotatores are best suited to create rotation because their fibers are the most horizontal in orientation (in the transverse plane), hence the name *rotatores*. (action 1)

• The rotatores group crosses the spinal joints posteriorly from a transverse process inferiorly, to a lamina superiorly (with their fibers running somewhat vertically in the sagittal plane). Therefore the Rotatores extend the trunk and the neck at the spinal joints. (action 2)

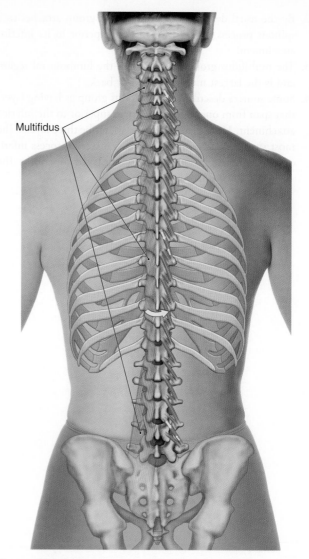

Multifidus

Figure 10-16 Posterior view of the right rotatores. The multifidus has been ghosted in on the left.

• The rotatores cross the spinal joints laterally (with their fibers running slightly vertically in the frontal plane). Therefore the multifidus laterally flexes the trunk and neck at the spinal joints. (action 3)

• Because the fiber direction of the rotatores is nearly horizontal and only slightly vertically, the rotatores are very weak at extension and lateral flexion. (actions 2, 3)

Reverse Mover Action Notes

• When we think of motions of the spine, we usually think of the upper spine moving relative to the fixed lower spine. However, if the upper attachments of the rotatores are fixed, the reverse action of moving the lower spine relative to the upper spine can occur. (reverse actions 1, 2, 3)

10

Rotatores (of Transversospinalis Group)—*cont'd*

• The reverse action of contralaterally rotating the upper spine (relative to the fixed lower spine) is to ipsilaterally rotate the lower spine (relative to the fixed upper spine). In other words, if the right-sided rotatores do left rotation of the upper spine, their reverse action would be to do right rotation of the lower spine. (reverse action 1)

Eccentric Antagonist Functions

1. Restrains/slows ipsilateral rotation, flexion, and opposite-side lateral flexion of the trunk and neck
2. Restrains/slows contralateral rotation of the lower spine relative to the upper spine

Isometric Stabilization Function

1. Stabilizes the spinal joints

Isometric Stabilization Function Note

1. Being very deep and small muscles, the rotatores are probably more important for stabilization than for movement of the spine.

INNERVATION
☐ Spinal Nerves
   ☐ dorsal rami of cervical, thoracic, and lumbar spinal nerves

ARTERIAL SUPPLY
☐ The dorsal branches of the Posterior Intercostal and Lumbar Arteries (all branches of the Aorta)

✋ PALPATION

1. With the client prone, place your palpating fingers in the client's laminar groove of the thoracic region.
2. Have the client slightly extend and rotate the trunk to the opposite side and feel for the contraction of the rotatores.
3. Note: The rotatores are very small and extremely deep muscles that are virtually impossible to palpate and discern from adjacent musculature.

■ RELATIONSHIP TO OTHER STRUCTURES

☐ The rotatores are extremely deep in the laminar groove. They are directly deep to the multifidus.
☐ Deep to the rotatores are the vertebrae.
☐ The rotatores are located within the superficial back line myofascial meridian.

■ MISCELLANEOUS

1. By the usual definition, the rotatores group attaches to a lamina one to two levels superior to its inferior attachment.
2. The rotatores are usually divided into a *brevis* component that attaches to the vertebra immediately superior and a *longus* component that skips one vertebra to attach to the vertebra two above it.
3. The rotatores can also be subdivided into three subgroups: the rotatores lumborum, rotatores thoracis, and rotatores cervicis.
4. Only the rotatores thoracis subgroup is well developed. The rotatores lumborum and rotatores cervicis are only represented by irregular muscle bundles that are similar in arrangement to the rotatores thoracis.
5. Some sources believe that the main role of the rotatores is proprioceptive by providing precise monitoring of spinal joint positions.

10

Interspinales

The name, interspinales, *tells us that these muscles are located between spinous processes of the vertebrae.*

Derivation	☐ inter:	L. *between.*
	spinales:	L. *refers to spinous processes.*
Pronunciation	☐ IN-ter-spy-NA-leez	

■ ATTACHMENTS

☐ **From a Spinous Process**

to the

☐ **Spinous Process directly superior**
   ☐ CERVICAL REGION: There are six pairs of interspinales located between T1-C2
   ☐ THORACIC REGION: There are two pairs of interspinales located between T2-T1 and T12-T11
   ☐ LUMBAR REGION: There are four pairs of interspinales located between L5-L1

■ FUNCTIONS

Concentric (Shortening) Mover Actions	
Standard Mover Actions	**Reverse Mover Actions**
☐ **1. Extend the neck and trunk at the spinal joints**	☐ 1. Extend the lower spine relative to the upper spine

Standard Mover Action Notes

- Each interspinalis muscle attaches from a spinous process of a vertebra inferiorly to the spinous process of the vertebra directly superior. Therefore the interspinales cross the vertebral joints posteriorly (with their fibers running vertically in the sagittal plane). Assuming the inferior vertebral attachment is fixed, when an interspinalis muscle contracts, it pulls the superior vertebra posteriorly and inferiorly toward the inferior vertebra, which creates extension of the superior vertebra of the neck and/or trunk at the spinal joint between them. (action 1)
- The interspinales only extend the cervical and lumbar spinal joints. (action 1)

Reverse Mover Action Notes

- When we think of motions of the spine, we usually think of the upper spine moving relative to the fixed lower spine. However, if the upper attachment of the interspinales is fixed, the reverse action of moving the lower spine relative to the upper spine can occur. This usually occurs when the client is lying down so that the lower attachment is mobile. (reverse action 1)

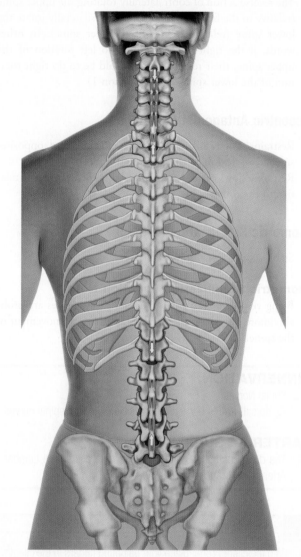

Figure 10-17 Posterior view of the right and left interspinales.

Eccentric Antagonist Functions

1. Restrains/slows flexion of the neck and trunk at the spinal joints

Isometric Stabilization Functions

1. Stabilizes the cervical and lumbar spinal joints

Isometric Stabilization Function Note

- Some sources believe that the interspinales do not have sufficient strength or leverage to actually create movement of the spine, but they may be important as fixing (stabilizing) muscles of the spine.

Interspinales—*cont'd*

Additional Notes on Functions

1. Some sources believe that the main role of the interspinales is proprioceptive by providing precise monitoring of spinal joint positions.
2. If the vertebrae are rotated away from anatomic position, the interspinales' line of pull could rotate them back toward anatomic position. In this regard, the interspinales can act as movers to rotate the spine toward anatomic position, and act as antagonists to restrain/slow rotation of the spine away from anatomic position.

INNERVATION
□ Spinal Nerves
  □ dorsal rami

ARTERIAL SUPPLY
□ The dorsal branches of the Posterior Intercostal Arteries (branches of the Aorta)

✋ PALPATION

1. With the client seated, place a palpating finger between two adjacent vertebral spinous processes in the lumbar region.
2. Have the client slightly flex the trunk and feel for the interspinales.
3. Then have the client extend the trunk back to its starting position and feel for the contraction of the interspinales.
4. The same approach can be tried in the cervical region. However, because of the thickness of the nuchal ligament, palpation of the cervical interspinales can be difficult.

■ RELATIONSHIP TO OTHER STRUCTURES

□ The interspinales are paired muscles that are located on either side of the interspinous ligaments, between the apices of spinous processes of adjacent vertebrae.
□ The interspinales are located deep to the supraspinous ligament (the nuchal ligament in the cervical region).
□ The interspinales are located within the superficial back line myofascial meridian.

■ MISCELLANEOUS

1. The interspinales are paired muscles on either side of the interspinous ligaments.
2. The interspinales are not located throughout the entire spine. They are primarily found in the cervical region (six pairs between C2 and T1) and the lumbar region (four pairs between L1 and L5). In the thoracic region, there are usually only two pairs found at T2-T1 and T12-T11.
3. The interspinales vary in location and are occasionally also found at T3-T2, L1-T12, and S1-L5.

10

Intertransversarii

The name, intertransversarii, *tells us that these muscles are located between transverse processes of the vertebrae.*

Derivation	☐ inter:	L. *between.*
	transversarii:	L. *refers to transverse processes.*
Pronunciation	☐ IN-ter-trans-ver-SA-ri-eye	

■ ATTACHMENTS

☐ **From a Transverse Process**

   to the

☐ **Transverse process directly superior**

   ☐ CERVICAL REGION: There are seven pairs of inter-transversarii muscles (anterior and posterior sets) located between C1 and T1 on each side of the body.

   ☐ THORACIC REGION: There are three intertransversarii muscles between T10 and L1 on each side of the body.

   ☐ LUMBAR REGION: There are four pairs of intertransversarii muscles (medial and lateral sets) located between L1 and L5 on each side of the body.

■ FUNCTIONS

Concentric (Shortening) Mover Actions	
Standard Mover Actions	**Reverse Mover Actions**
☐ **1. Laterally flex the neck and trunk at the spinal joints**	☐ 1. Laterally flex the lower spine relative to the upper spine

Standard Mover Action Notes

• Each intertransversarii muscle attaches from a transverse process of one vertebra and runs superiorly to attach onto the transverse process of the vertebra directly superior. Therefore it crosses the spinal joint laterally (with its fibers running vertically in the frontal plane). Assuming the inferior vertebral attachment is fixed, when an intertransversarii muscle contracts, it pulls the superior vertebra inferiorly and laterally toward the inferior vertebra, which creates lateral flexion of the superior vertebra of the neck and/or trunk at the spinal joint between them. (action 1)

• The intertransversarii only laterally flex the cervical and lumbar spinal joints. (action 1)

Reverse Mover Action Notes

• When we think of motions of the spine, we usually think of the upper spine moving relative to the fixed lower spine. However, if the upper attachment of the intertransversarii is fixed, the reverse action of moving the lower spine relative to the upper spine can occur. This usually occurs when the

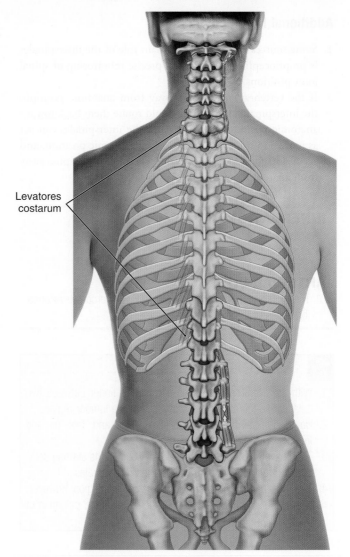

Levatores costarum

Figure 10-18 Posterior view of the right intertransversarii. The levatores costarum have been ghosted in on the left.

client is lying down so that the lower attachment is mobile. (reverse action 1)

Eccentric Antagonist Functions

1. Restrains/slows opposite-side lateral flexion of the neck and trunk at the spinal joints

Isometric Stabilization Functions

1. Stabilizes the cervical and lumbar spinal joints

Isometric Stabilization Function Note

• The intertransversarii are considered to be primarily important not as movers of the spine, but as fixing (i.e., stabilizing) postural muscles.

Intertransversarii—cont'd

Additional Note on Functions

1. If the vertebrae are rotated away from anatomic position, the intertransversarii's line of pull could rotate them back toward anatomic position. In this regard, the intertransversarii can act as movers to rotate the spine toward anatomic position, and act as antagonists to restrain/slow rotation of the spine away from anatomic position.

INNERVATION
□ Spinal Nerves
   □ dorsal and ventral rami

ARTERIAL SUPPLY
□ The dorsal branches of the Posterior Intercostal Arteries (branches of the Aorta)

✋ PALPATION

1. The intertransversarii muscles are small and very deep muscles. Palpating and distinguishing them from adjacent musculature is extremely difficult if not impossible.

■ RELATIONSHIP TO OTHER STRUCTURES

□ The thoracic and lumbar intertransversarii are located between transverse processes and are very deep. The latissimus dorsi, erector spinae, and serratus posterior inferior are all superficial to the thoracic and lumbar intertransversarii.

□ The cervical intertransversarii are located between the transverse processes and are very deep. The trapezius, splenius capitis, splenius cervicis, and semispinalis capitis are all superficial to the cervical intertransversarii.

□ The intertransversarii are located within the superficial back line myofascial meridian.

■ MISCELLANEOUS

1. The anterior cervical intertransversarii attach onto the anterior tubercles of the transverse processes of the cervical spine, and the posterior cervical intertransversarii attach onto the posterior tubercles of the transverse processes of the cervical spine. The lumbar medial intertransversarii attach to accessory and mamillary processes of the lumbar vertebrae, and the lumbar lateral intertransversarii attach to transverse processes of the lumbar vertebrae.

2. The intertransversarii between C1 (atlas) and C2 (axis) are often absent.

3. Essentially, the intertransversarii do not exist in the thoracic region. The levatores costarum and the intercostals are considered to be homologous with the two sets of intertransversarii in the thoracic region.

4. Ventral and dorsal rami of spinal nerves run between and pierce through the intertransversarii, especially in the cervical region.

5. Some sources believe that the main role of the intertransversarii is proprioceptive by providing precise monitoring of spinal joint positions.

10

NECK AND HEAD
Sternocleidomastoid (SCM)

The name, sternocleidomastoid, *tells us that this muscle attaches to the sternum, the clavicle, and the mastoid process of the temporal bone.*

Derivation	☐	sterno:	Gr. *refers to the sternum.*
		cleido:	Gr. *refers to the clavicle.*
		mastoid:	Gr. *refers to the mastoid process.*
Pronunciation	☐	STER-no-KLI-do-MAS-toyd	

■ ATTACHMENTS

☐ **STERNAL HEAD: Manubrium of the Sternum**
  ☐ the anterior superior surface
☐ **Clavicular Head: Medial Clavicle**
  ☐ the medial ⅓

to the

☐ **Mastoid Process of the Temporal Bone**
  ☐ and the lateral ½ of the superior nuchal line of the occipital bone

■ FUNCTIONS

Concentric (Shortening) Mover Actions	
Standard Mover Actions	**Reverse Mover Actions**
☐ 1. Flexes the lower neck at the spinal joints	☐ 1. Elevates the sternum and clavicle
☐ 2. Extends the upper neck and head at the spinal joints	
☐ 3. Laterally flexes the neck and head at the spinal joints	
☐ 4. Contralaterally rotates the neck and head at the spinal joints	☐ 2. Ipsilaterally rotates the trunk at the spinal joints

Standard Mover Action Notes

- The sternocleidomastoid (SCM) crosses the joints of the lower neck anteriorly (with its fibers running vertically in the sagittal plane); therefore it flexes the lower neck at the cervical spinal joints. (action 1)
- Because the SCM courses posteriorly as it ascends from the sternum/clavicle to the head, it crosses the joints of the upper neck posteriorly. Therefore, it extends the upper neck at the cervical spinal joints and extends the head at the atlanto-occipital joint (AOJ). (action 2)
- The SCM is the only muscle that can flex one region of the neck and extend another region (every other muscle either flexes or extends the neck). Exactly where the dividing line is located is determined by the degree of curvature of the client's neck. (actions 1, 2)
- The SCM crosses the spinal joints laterally (with its fibers running vertically in the frontal plane); therefore it laterally

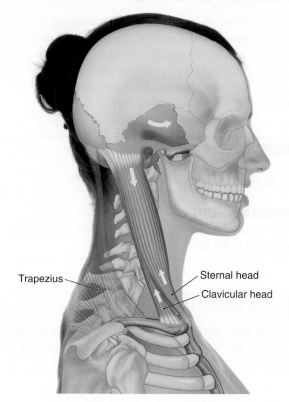

Figure 10-19 Lateral view of the right sternocleidomastoid. The trapezius has been ghosted in.

flexes the neck at the cervical spinal joints and laterally flexes the head at the AOJ. (action 3)
- The clavicular head is more active than the sternal head with lateral flexion of the neck and head. (action 3)
- The SCM wraps around the neck from the sternum/clavicle anteriorly to the cranium more posteriorly (with its fibers running somewhat horizontally in the transverse plane). When the SCM contracts, it pulls on the cranium, causing the anterior surface of the neck and/or the head to face the opposite side of the body from the side to which it is attached. Therefore the SCM contralaterally rotates the neck at the cervical spinal joints and the head at the AOJ. (action 4)
- The sternal head is more active than the clavicular head with contralateral rotation of the neck and head. (action 4)

Reverse Mover Action Notes

- If the cranial attachment of the SCM is fixed, the sternal/clavicular attachment must move. Because the SCM has its fibers running vertically from the sternum/clavicle, the sternum and the clavicle would be elevated toward the cranial attachment. Elevating the sternum and clavicle can assist in lifting the rib cage during inspiration (breathing in). Therefore the SCM is an accessory muscle of respiration. (reverse action 1)

Sternocleidomastoid (SCM)—*cont'd*

- With the cranial attachment of the SCM fixed, the sternal/clavicular attachment will be pulled in the transverse plane such that the anterior surface of the trunk will come to face the same side of the body to which the SCM is attached. Therefore the SCM can ipsilaterally rotate the trunk at the spinal joints (the reverse action of contralateral rotation of the upper spine relative to the fixed lower spine is ipsilateral rotation of the lower spine relative to the fixed upper spine). This reverse action requires the cranial attachment to be sufficiently fixed so that the weight of the trunk is moved relative to it. (reverse action 2)

Eccentric Antagonist Functions

1. Restrains/slows extension of the lower neck at the spinal joints
2. Restrains/slows flexion of the upper neck and head at the spinal joints
3. Restrains/slows opposite-side lateral flexion and ipsilateral rotation of the neck and head at the spinal joints
4. Restrains/slows depression of the sternum and clavicle
5. Restrains/slows ipsilateral rotation of the trunk

Isometric Stabilization Functions

1. Stabilizes the cervical spinal joints and the sternoclavicular joint

Isometric Stabilization Function Note

- The SCM stabilizes the entire neck, including the head at the AOJ. By attaching to the sternum and clavicle, it also helps to stabilize the sternoclavicular joint.

Additional Notes on Functions

1. Some sources state that the action of the SCM on the head at the AOJ can change from extension to flexion if the position of the head changes sufficiently, thus changing the line of pull of the SCM relative to the AOJ. This becomes more likely as a person ages and tends to posturally carry the head more anteriorly.
2. The SCM may also be able to weakly upwardly rotate the clavicle at the sternoclavicular joint.

INNERVATION
- Spinal Accessory Nerve (CN XI)
  - and C2, C3

ARTERIAL SUPPLY
- The Occipital and Posterior Auricular Arteries (branches of the External Carotid Artery)
  - and the Superior Thyroid Artery (a branch of the External Carotid Artery)

✋ PALPATION

1. Have the client supine with the neck and head rotated contralaterally.
2. Then have the client lift the head and neck up into the air and the SCM will visibly contract.
3. Palpate the SCM from attachment to attachment.

■ RELATIONSHIP TO OTHER STRUCTURES

- Except for the platysma (which is superficial to all anterior neck muscles), the SCM is superficial throughout its entire course.
- The following muscles are deep to the SCM (listed from inferior to superior): infrahyoids, scalenes, levator scapulae, digastric, and splenius capitis.
- The attachment of the SCM onto the mastoid process of the temporal bone and the superior nuchal line of the occipital bone is superficial to the splenius capitis and lateral to the trapezius.
- The SCM is located within the superficial front line and lateral line myofascial meridians.

■ MISCELLANEOUS

1. The SCM's major superior attachment is the mastoid process attachment of the temporal bone. However, it also has a thin aponeurotic attachment to the occipital bone.
2. The carotid sinus of the common carotid artery lies directly deep and medial to the SCM, midway up the neck. Given the neurologic reflex that occurs to lower blood pressure when the carotid sinus is pressed, massage to this region must be done judiciously, especially with weak and/or elderly clients.
3. The SCM and the scalenes, are often injured as a result of car accidents. This trauma is usually called *whiplash,* wherein the head and neck are forcefully thrown anteriorly and posteriorly (like a whip being lashed). When the head and the neck are thrown posteriorly, the anterior cervical musculature may be torn; or the muscle spindle reflex may occur, causing the anterior cervical musculature to spasm. When the head and the neck are thrown anteriorly, the same trauma may occur to the posterior musculature.
4. The SCM is an excellent landmark for palpating other muscles of the neck. Locate the posterior (lateral) border of the SCM and the anterior border of the upper trapezius, and then palpate in the tall narrow triangular space that is located between them; this triangular area is called the *posterior triangle of the neck.* Locating the medial border of the SCM can be used as a landmark for palpating the longus colli and longus capitis (of the prevertebral group).

10

The scalenes are a group of muscles that are found in the antero-lateral neck. There are three scalene muscles: the anterior scalene, middle scalene, and posterior scalene.

■ ATTACHMENTS

☐ As a group, the scalenes attach from superiorly on the transverse processes of the cervical spine to inferiorly on the first and second ribs.

☐ The names of the scalenes refer to their relative location with respect to each other: the anterior scalene is the most anterior of the three; the posterior scalene is the most posterior of the three; and the middle scalene is in the middle, sandwiched between the other two.

■ FUNCTIONS

☐ As a group, the scalenes flex and laterally flex the neck at the spinal joints and/or elevate the first and second ribs at the sternocostal and costospinal joints.

☐ The scalenes are considered to be the prime movers of lateral flexion of the neck at the spinal joints.

☐ By elevating the first and second ribs, the scalenes can help elevate and expand the rib cage, which expands the thoracic cavity, thereby creating more space for the lungs to expand for inspiration. Therefore the scalenes are accessory muscles of respiration.

☐ There is controversy regarding the role of the scalenes with respect to rotation of the neck. Some sources state that the scalenes perform contralateral rotation; other sources state that they perform ipsilateral rotation. Other sources state that the scalenes perform rotation without specifying whether it is contralateral or ipsilateral rotation. Still others are silent on this issue. Given the direction of fibers and the consequent line of pull, it seems likely that of all the scalenes, the anterior scalene is best suited for rotation, and that it would perform contralateral rotation of the neck at the cervical spinal joints.

■ MISCELLANEOUS

1. Of the scalenes, the middle scalene is the longest and the largest, and the posterior scalene is the shortest and the smallest.

2. When palpating the scalenes, care must be taken because the brachial plexus of nerves and the subclavian artery exit between the anterior and middle scalenes.

3. There is a fourth scalene muscle called the *scalenus minimus* that is sometimes present, unilaterally or bilaterally. When present, it is usually found posterior to the anterior scalene, attaching from the tranverse process (anterior tubercle) of C7 to the first rib (inner border) and the pleural membrane of the lung.

4. The scalenes are located within the deep front line myofascial meridian.

INNERVATION
☐ The scalenes are innervated by cervical spinal nerves (ventral rami).

ARTERIAL SUPPLY
☐ Arterial supply to the scalenes is provided by either the ascending cervical artery or the transverse cervical artery.

■ CLINICAL APPLICATIONS

☐ The scalenes, and the sternocleidomastoid, are often injured as a result of car accidents. This trauma is usually called *whiplash,* wherein the head and neck are forcefully thrown anteriorly and posteriorly (like a whip being lashed). When the head and the neck are thrown posteriorly, the anterior cervical musculature may be torn; or the muscle spindle reflex may occur, causing the anterior cervical musculature to spasm. When the head and the neck are thrown anteriorly, the same trauma may occur to the posterior musculature.

☐ The brachial plexus of nerves and the subclavian artery run between the anterior and middle scalenes. If these muscles are tight, entrapment of these nerves and/or the artery can occur. When this happens, it is called *anterior scalene syndrome,* one of the four types of *thoracic outlet syndrome.* This condition can cause sensory symptoms (e.g., tingling, pain, numbness) and/or motor symptoms (e.g., weakness and/or partial paralysis) in the upper extremity.

☐ Tight scalenes can also contribute to another type of *thoracic outlet syndrome* called *costoclavicular syndrome.* Costoclavicular syndrome is an entrapment of the brachial plexus of nerves and/or the subclavian artery and vein between the clavicle and the first rib. If the scalenes are tight, they can contribute to this condition by pulling the first rib up against the clavicle, compressing these neurovascular structures.

10

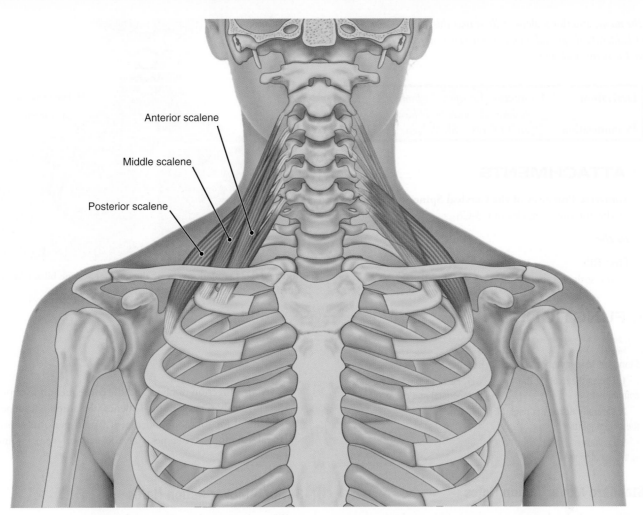

Figure 10-20 Anterior view of the scalenes. All three scalenes are seen on the right; the posterior scalene and ghosted-in middle scalene are seen on the left.

10

Anterior Scalene (of Scalene Group)

The name, anterior scalene, *tells us that this muscle has a steplike or ladderlike shape and is located anteriorly (anterior to the middle and posterior scalenes).*

Derivation	☐ anterior: L. *before, in front of.*
	scalene: L. *uneven, ladder.*
Pronunciation	☐ an-TEE-ri-or, SKAY-leen

■ ATTACHMENTS

☐ **Tranverse Processes of the Cervical Spine**
  ☐ the anterior tubercles of C3-C6

to the

☐ **First Rib**
  ☐ the scalene tubercle on the inner border

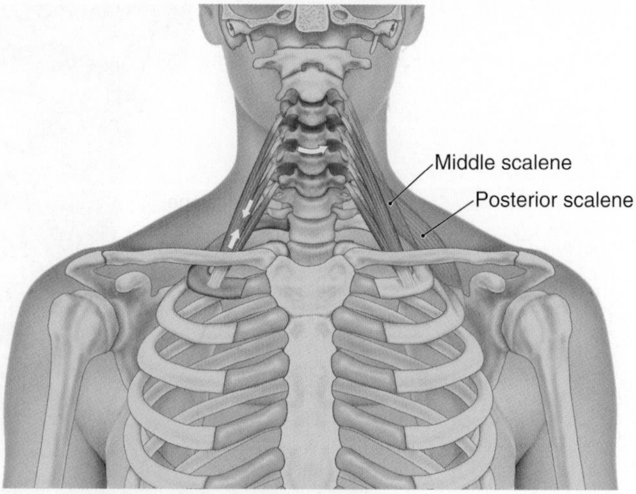

■ FUNCTIONS

Concentric (Shortening) Mover Actions	
Standard Mover Actions	**Reverse Mover Actions**
☐ 1. Flexes the neck at the spinal joints	☐ 1. Elevates the first rib at the sternocostal and costospinal joints
☐ 2. Laterally flexes the neck at the spinal joints	
☐ 3. Contralaterally rotates the neck at the spinal joints	

Standard Mover Action Notes

- The anterior scalene crosses the cervical spinal joints anteriorly (with its fibers running vertically in the sagittal plane); therefore it flexes the neck at the cervical spinal joints. (action 1)
- The anterior scalene crosses the cervical spinal joints laterally (with its fibers running vertically in the frontal plane); therefore it laterally flexes the neck at the cervical spinal joints. (action 2)
- The attachment of the anterior scalene onto the first rib is more anterior than the transverse process attachments (therefore the fibers are running slightly horizontally in the transverse plane). When the anterior scalene contracts, it pulls the transverse processes anteromedially toward the first rib, causing the anterior surface of the vertebrae to face the opposite side of the body from the side to which the anterior scalene is attached. Therefore the anterior scalene contralaterally rotates the neck at the cervical spinal joints. (action 3)
- There is controversy regarding the role of the scalene group with respect to rotation of the neck. Some sources state that the scalenes perform contralateral rotation; other sources state that they perform ipsilateral rotation. Other sources state rotation without specifying whether it is contralateral or ipsilateral rotation, and still others are silent on this issue.

Figure 10-21 Anterior view of the anterior scalene bilaterally. The other two scalenes have been ghosted in on the left side.

Given the direction of fibers and the consequent line of pull, it seems likely that of all the scalenes, the anterior scalene is best suited for rotation, and that it would perform contralateral rotation of the neck at the cervical spinal joints. (action 3)

Reverse Mover Action Notes

- When the cervical attachment of the anterior scalene is fixed, the first rib must move. Given that the fiber direction of the anterior scalene is vertical from the first rib up to the cervical vertebrae, the anterior scalene elevates the first rib at the sternocostal and the costospinal joints. (reverse action 1)
- By elevating the first rib, the anterior scalene can help elevate and expand the rib cage, which expands the thoracic cavity, thereby creating more space for the lungs to expand for inspiration. Therefore the anterior scalene is an accessory muscle of respiration. Knowing that it contracts with inspiration is important when engaging it to palpate it. (reverse action 1)

Eccentric Antagonist Functions

1. Restrains/slows extension, opposite-side lateral flexion, and ipsilateral rotation of the neck at the spinal joints
2. Restrains/slows depression of the first rib at the sternocostal and costospinal joints

Isometric Stabilization Functions

1. Stabilizes the cervical spinal joints
2. Stabilizes the first rib

Anterior Scalene (of Scalene Group)—*cont'd*

INNERVATION

☐ Cervical Spinal Nerves
  ☐ ventral rami; C4-C6

ARTERIAL SUPPLY

☐ The Ascending Cervical Artery (a branch of the Inferior Thyroid Artery)

 PALPATION

1. With the client seated or supine, place palpating fingers just superior to the clavicle and just lateral to the lateral border of the clavicular head of the sternocleidomastoid.
2. Have the client take in short, quick breaths through the nose and feel for the contraction of the anterior scalene. The middle scalene will also contract; it is located directly lateral to the anterior scalene.
3. Note: Because of the proximity of the brachial plexus and subclavian artery, palpation in this area must be done carefully.

■ RELATIONSHIP TO OTHER STRUCTURES

☐ The inferior portion of the anterior scalene is superficial, except where the clavicle and the omohyoid (and the platysma, which is superficial to all anterior neck muscles) cross in front of it.
☐ The superior portion of the anterior scalene is deep to the sternocleidomastoid.
☐ Directly posterolateral to the anterior scalene is the middle scalene.
☐ Deep to the anterior scalene are the brachial plexus of nerves, the subclavian artery, and the pleural membrane of the lung.
☐ If one looks at the relationship between the anterior scalene and the longus capitis, as well as the superior part of the longus colli, it can be seen that, except for the interruption of the attachment to the tranverse processes of the cervical spine, there is a continuous line of pull from the first rib

(the most inferior attachment of the anterior scalene) to the atlas (C1) and the head (the most superior attachments of the longus colli and longus capitis).
☐ The anterior scalene is located within the deep front line myofascial meridian.

■ MISCELLANEOUS

1. The anterior scalene is part of the scalene group, which comprises the anterior, middle, and posterior scalenes.
2. The brachial plexus of nerves and the subclavian artery run between the anterior and middle scalenes. If these muscles are tight, entrapment of these nerves and/or the artery can occur. When this happens, it is called *anterior scalene syndrome,* one of the four types of *thoracic outlet syndrome.* This condition can cause sensory symptoms (e.g., tingling, pain, numbness) and/or motor symptoms (e.g., weakness and/or partial paralysis) in the upper extremity.
3. The anterior scalene can also contribute to another type of *thoracic outlet syndrome* called *costoclavicular syndrome.* Costoclavicular syndrome is an entrapment of the brachial plexus of nerves and/or the subclavian artery and vein between the clavicle and the first rib. If the anterior scalene is tight, it can contribute to this condition by pulling the first rib up against the clavicle, compressing these neurovascular structures.
4. Very close to the superior attachment of the anterior scalene is the common carotid artery. Given the neurologic reflex that occurs to lower blood pressure when the carotid sinus of the common carotid artery is pressed, massage to this region must be done judiciously, especially with weak and/or elderly clients.
5. The scalenes, and the sternocleidomastoid, are often injured as a result of car accidents. This trauma is usually called *whiplash,* wherein the head and neck are forcefully thrown anteriorly and posteriorly (like a whip being lashed). When the head and neck are thrown posteriorly, the anterior cervical musculature may be torn; or the muscle spindle reflex may occur, causing the anterior cervical musculature to spasm. When the head and neck are thrown anteriorly, the same trauma may occur to the posterior musculature.

10

Middle Scalene (of Scalene Group)

The name, middle scalene, *tells us that this muscle has a steplike or ladderlike shape and is located in the middle of the scalene group (between the anterior and posterior scalenes).*

Derivation	☐ middle: L. *middle (between).*
	scalene: L. *uneven, ladder.*
Pronunciation	☐ MI-dil, SKAY-leen

■ ATTACHMENTS

☐ **Tranverse Processes of the Cervical Spine**
  ☐ the posterior tubercles of C2-C7

to the

☐ **First Rib**
  ☐ the superior surface

■ FUNCTIONS

Concentric (Shortening) Mover Actions	
Standard Mover Actions	**Reverse Mover Actions**
☐ 1. Flexes the neck at the spinal joints	☐ 1. Elevates the first rib at the sternocostal and costospinal joints
☐ 2. Laterally flexes the neck at the spinal joints	

Standard Mover Action Notes

• The middle scalene crosses the cervical spinal joints anteriorly (with its fibers running vertically in the sagittal plane); therefore it flexes the neck at the cervical spinal joints. (action 1)
• The middle scalene crosses the cervical spinal joints laterally (with its fibers running vertically in the frontal plane); therefore it laterally flexes the neck at the cervical spinal joints. (action 2)

Reverse Mover Action Notes

• When the cervical attachment of the middle scalene is fixed, the first rib must move. Given that the fiber direction of the middle scalene is vertical from the first rib up to the cervical vertebrae, the middle scalene elevates the first rib at the sternocostal and costospinal joints. (reverse action 1)
• By elevating the first rib, the middle scalene can help elevate and expand the rib cage, which expands the thoracic cavity, thereby creating more space for the lungs to expand for inspiration. Therefore the middle scalene is an accessory muscle of respiration. Knowing that it contracts with inspiration is important when engaging it to palpate it. (reverse action 1)

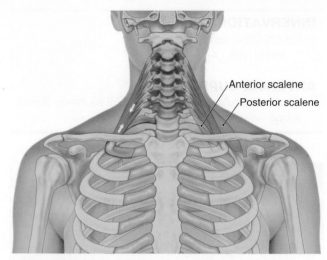

Figure 10-22 Anterior view of the middle scalene bilaterally. The other two scalenes have been ghosted in on the left side.

Eccentric Antagonist Functions

1. Restrains/slows extension and opposite-side lateral flexion of the neck at the spinal joints
2. Restrains/slows depression of the first rib at the sternocostal and costospinal joints

Isometric Stabilization Functions

1. Stabilizes the cervical spinal joints
2. Stabilizes the first rib

INNERVATION
☐ Cervical Spinal Nerves
  ☐ ventral rami; C3-C8

ARTERIAL SUPPLY
☐ The Transverse Cervical Artery (a branch of the Thyrocervical Trunk)

✋ PALPATION

1. With the client seated or supine, place palpating fingers just superior to the clavicle, in the middle of the posterior triangle of the neck (between the sternocleidomastoid and upper trapezius).
2. Have the client take in short, quick breaths through the nose and feel for the contraction of the middle scalene. The anterior and posterior scalenes will also contract. The anterior scalene is located medial to the middle scalene and the posterior scalene is located lateral to the middle scalene.
3. Note: Because of the proximity of the brachial plexus and subclavian artery, palpation in this area must be done carefully.

10

Middle Scalene (of Scalene Group)—*cont'd*

■ RELATIONSHIP TO OTHER STRUCTURES

☐ Like the anterior scalene, the inferior portion of the middle scalene is superficial, except where the clavicle and the omohyoid (and the platysma, which is superficial to all anterior neck muscles) cross in front of it.

☐ The superior portion of the middle scalene, like the anterior scalene, is deep to the sternocleidomastoid.

☐ Directly anteromedial to the middle scalene is the anterior scalene.

☐ Posterolateral to the middle scalene are the posterior scalene and the levator scapulae.

☐ The middle scalene is located within the deep front line myofascial meridian.

■ MISCELLANEOUS

1. The middle scalene is part of the scalene group, which comprises the anterior, middle, and posterior scalenes.
2. The middle scalene is the largest and the longest of the scalenes.
3. The nerve to the rhomboids (the dorsal scapula nerve) and some of the spinal nerve segments to the nerve to the serratus anterior (long thoracic nerve) pierce the middle scalene.

4. The brachial plexus of nerves and the subclavian artery run between the anterior and middle scalenes. If these muscles are tight, entrapment of these nerves and/or the artery can occur. When this happens, it is called *anterior scalene syndrome,* one of the four types of *thoracic outlet syndrome.* This condition can cause sensory symptoms (e.g., tingling, pain, numbness) and/or motor symptoms (e.g., weakness and/or partial paralysis) in the upper extremity.

5. The middle scalene can also contribute to another type of *thoracic outlet syndrome* called *costoclavicular syndrome.* Costoclavicular syndrome is an entrapment of the brachial plexus of nerves and/or the subclavian artery and vein between the clavicle and the first rib. If the middle scalene is tight, it can contribute to this condition by pulling the first rib up against the clavicle, compressing these neurovascular structures.

6. The scalenes, and the sternocleidomastoid, are often injured as a result of car accidents. This trauma is usually called *whiplash,* wherein the head and neck are forcefully thrown anteriorly and posteriorly (like a whip being lashed). When the head and neck are thrown posteriorly, the anterior cervical musculature may be torn; or the muscle spindle reflex may occur, causing the anterior cervical musculature to spasm. When the head and neck are thrown anteriorly, the same trauma may occur to the posterior musculature.

10

Posterior Scalene (of Scalene Group)

The name, posterior scalene, *tells us that this muscle has a steplike or ladderlike shape and is located posteriorly (posterior to the middle and anterior scalenes).*

Derivation	☐ posterior: L. *behind, toward the back.*
	scalene: L. *uneven, ladder.*
Pronunciation	☐ pos-TEE-ri-or, SKAY-leen

■ ATTACHMENTS

☐ **Tranverse Processes of the Cervical Spine**
  ☐ the posterior tubercles of C5-C7

to the

☐ **Second Rib**
  ☐ the external surface

■ FUNCTIONS

Concentric (Shortening) Mover Actions	
Standard Mover Actions	**Reverse Mover Actions**
☐ **1. Laterally flexes the neck at the spinal joints**	☐ **1. Elevates the second rib at the sternocostal and costospinal joints**

Standard Mover Action Notes

• The posterior scalene crosses the cervical spinal joints laterally (with its fibers running vertically in the frontal plane); therefore it laterally flexes the neck at the cervical spinal joints. Given that the posterior scalene only crosses the lower three cervical vertebrae, its action of lateral flexion would occur only at the lower neck. (action 1)

Reverse Mover Action Notes

• When the cervical attachment of the posterior scalene is fixed, the second rib must move. Given that the fiber direction of the posterior scalene is vertical from the second rib up to the cervical vertebrae, the posterior scalene elevates the second rib at the sternocostal and costospinal joints. (reverse action 1)

• By elevating the second rib, the posterior scalene can help elevate and expand the rib cage, which expands the thoracic cavity, thereby creating more space for the lungs to expand for inspiration. Therefore the posterior scalene is an accessory muscle of respiration. Knowing that it contracts with inspiration is important when engaging it to palpate it. (reverse action 1)

Eccentric Antagonist Functions

1. Restrains/slows opposite-side lateral flexion of the neck at the spinal joints and depression of the second rib at the sternocostal and costospinal joints.

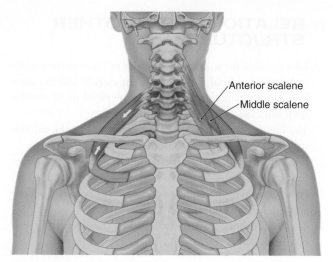

Figure 10-23 Anterior view of the posterior scalene bilaterally. The other two scalenes have been ghosted in on the left side.

Isometric Stabilization Functions

1. Stabilizes the lower cervical spinal joints
2. Stabilizes the second rib

INNERVATION
☐ Cervical Spinal Nerves
  ☐ ventral rami; C6-C8

ARTERIAL SUPPLY
☐ The Transverse Cervical Artery (a branch of the Thyrocervical Trunk)

✋ PALPATION

1. With the client seated, place palpating fingers just superior to the clavicle and just medial to the clavicular attachment of the upper trapezius.
2. Have the client take in short, quick breaths through the nose and feel for the contraction of the posterior scalene. The anterior and middle scalenes will also contract. They are located medial to the posterior scalene.

■ RELATIONSHIP TO OTHER STRUCTURES

☐ The posterior scalene is the most posterior of the three scalenes. Consequently, it is situated almost directly lateral in the inferior neck and is the most superficial from the lateral perspective.

☐ There is a small area within the *posterior triangle of the neck* (bounded by the trapezius posteriorly and the sternocleidomastoid anteriorly), in which the posterior scalene is super-

Posterior Scalene (of Scalene Group)—*cont'd*

ficial. In this space the posterior scalene is directly anterior to the upper trapezius and the levator scapulae and directly posterior to the middle scalene.

☐ To attach onto the second rib, the posterior scalene passes over (on the external side of) the first rib.

☐ The posterior scalene is located within the deep front line myofascial meridian.

■ MISCELLANEOUS

1. The posterior scalene is part of the scalene group, which comprises the anterior, middle, and posterior scalenes.

2. The posterior scalene is the smallest and the shortest of the three scalenes.

3. The scalenes, and the sternocleidomastoid, are often injured as a result of car accidents. This trauma is usually called *whiplash,* wherein the head and neck are forcefully thrown anteriorly and posteriorly (like a whip being lashed). When the head and neck are thrown posteriorly, the anterior cervical musculature may be torn; or the muscle spindle reflex may occur, causing the anterior cervical musculature to spasm. When the head and neck are thrown anteriorly, the same trauma may occur to the posterior musculature.

10

Prevertebral Group

The prevertebral group comprises four muscles that are situated deep in the anterior neck. They are called the prevertebrals because they are just in front of (before, i.e., the prefix *pre-*) the vertebral column from the anterior perspective. The four muscles of the prevertebral group are the longus colli and longus capitis of the anterior neck and head, and the two smaller rectus capitis anterior and rectus capitis lateralis, running from the atlas to the occiput.

The prevertebrals are clinically important because they function primarily to stabilize the neck and head. These muscles are commonly injured during a whiplash trauma when the neck and head are forcefully thrown back into extension. When injured or overused (for example, when doing a lot of sit-ups/crunches/curl-ups), the longus muscles often create the sensation of a sore throat, especially when swallowing. Whereas the two rectus muscles are difficult if not impossible to palpate and work, the two longus muscles can be fairly easily accessed.

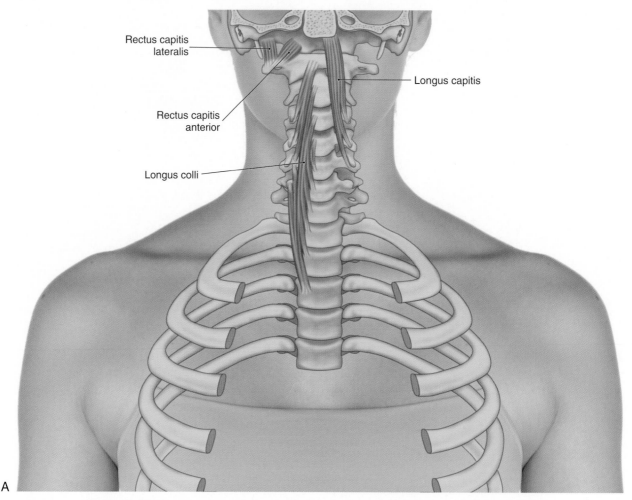

Rectus capitis lateralis

Rectus capitis anterior

Longus colli

Longus capitis

A

Figure 10-24 Anterior views of the prevertebral group. The prevertebral group is composed of the longus colli, longus capitis, rectus capitis anterior, and rectus capitis lateralis. **A,** All four prevertebral muscles are shown on the right side. The longus capitis has been removed on the left side.

Prevertebral Group—*cont'd*

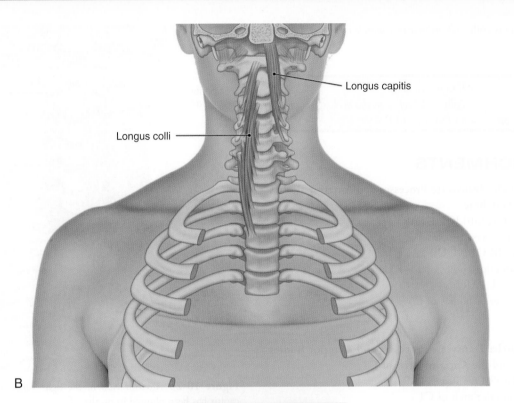

Longus capitis

Longus colli

B

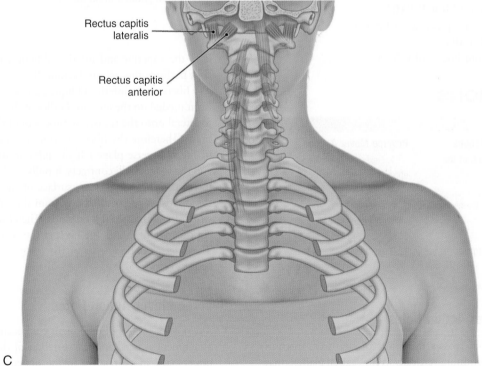

Rectus capitis lateralis

Rectus capitis anterior

C

Figure 10-24, cont'd B, the longus colli is seen on the right and the longus capitis is seen on the left. The rectus capitis anterior and rectus capitis lateralis have been ghosted in bilaterally. **C,** the rectus capitis anterior and rectus capitis lateralis are seen bilaterally. The longus colli has been ghosted in on the right and the longus capitis has been ghosted in on the left.

Longus Colli (of Prevertebral Group)

The name, longus colli, *tells us that this muscle is long and found in the neck.*

Derivation	□ longus: L. *long.*
	colli: L. *refers to the neck.*
Pronunciation	□ LONG-us, KOL-eye

■ ATTACHMENTS

□ **Entire Muscle: Transverse Processes and Anterior Bodies of C3-T3 Vertebrae**
  □ SUPERIOR OBLIQUE PART:
    □ the transverse processes of C3-C5
  □ INFERIOR OBLIQUE PART:
    □ the anterior bodies of T1-T3
  □ VERTICAL PART:
    □ the anterior bodies of C5-T3

to the

□ **Entire Muscle: Transverse Processes and Anterior Bodies of C2-C6 and the Anterior Arch of C1**
  □ SUPERIOR OBLIQUE PART:
    □ the anterior arch of C1
  □ INFERIOR OBLIQUE PART:
    □ the transverse processes of C5-C6
  □ VERTICAL PART:
    □ the anterior bodies of C2-C4

■ FUNCTIONS

Concentric (Shortening) Mover Actions	
Standard Mover Actions	**Reverse Mover Actions**
□ **1. Flexes the neck at the spinal joints**	□ 1. Flexes the lower neck and upper back relative to the upper neck
□ 2. Laterally flexes the neck at the spinal joints	□ 2. Laterally flexes the lower neck and upper back relative to the upper neck
□ 3. Contralaterally rotates the neck at the spinal joints	□ 3. Ipsilaterally rotates the lower neck and upper back relative to the upper neck

Standard Mover Action Notes

- The longus colli crosses the joints of the neck anteriorly (with its fibers running vertically in the sagittal plane); therefore it flexes the neck at the cervical spinal joints. All parts of the longus colli perform this action. (action 1)
- The longus colli is considered to be a strong flexor of the neck at the cervical spinal joints. (action 1)
- The longus colli crosses the joints of the neck laterally (with its fibers running vertically in the frontal plane); therefore it laterally flexes the neck at the cervical spinal joints. Particu-

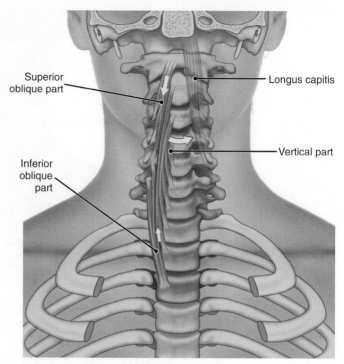

Figure 10-25 Anterior view of the right longus colli. The longus capitis has been ghosted in on the left.

larly the superior and inferior oblique parts of the longus colli perform this action. (action 2)
- The fibers of the inferior oblique part of the longus colli run from medial on the anterior bodies of the inferior vertebrae, to lateral onto the transverse processes of the superior vertebrae. (Therefore the fibers are running slightly horizontally in the transverse plane.) If the inferior attachment is fixed and the longus colli contracts, it pulls on the superior attachment, causing the anterior surface of the vertebrae to face the opposite side of the body from the side of the body to which the longus colli is attached. Therefore the longus colli contralaterally rotates the neck at the cervical spinal joints. The inferior oblique part of the longus colli performs this action. (action 3)

Reverse Mover Action Notes

- The reverse actions of the longus colli occur when the upper attachment is fixed and the vertebrae of the lower neck and upper back move relative to the upper neck. This usually occurs when the client is lying down so that the lower attachment is mobile. (reverse actions 1, 2, 3)
- The reverse action of contralaterally rotating the upper neck (relative to the fixed lower attachment) is to ipsilaterally rotate the lower spine (relative to the fixed upper attachment). In other words, if the right-sided longus colli does left rotation of the upper neck, its reverse action would be

right rotation of the lower neck and upper back (relative to the upper neck). This reverse action usually occurs when the client is lying down so that the lower attachment is mobile. (reverse action 3)

Eccentric Antagonist Functions

1. Restrains/slows extension and opposite-side lateral flexion of the neck at the spinal joints
2. Restrains/slows ipsilateral rotation of the neck at the spinal joints
3. Restrains/slows contralateral rotation of the lower neck and upper back at the spinal joints (relative to the upper attachment)

Isometric Stabilization Functions

1. Stabilizes the cervical and upper thoracic spinal joints

Isometric Stabilization Function Note

- The longus colli and other prevertebral muscles are important for fixing (stabilizing) the neck and head while talking, swallowing, coughing, and sneezing. They also fix the neck during rapid arm movements.

INNERVATION
- Cervical Spinal Nerves
  - ventral rami; C2-C6

ARTERIAL SUPPLY
- The Inferior Thyroid Artery (a branch of the Thyrocervical Trunk) and the Vertebral Artery (a branch of the Subclavian Artery)
  - and the Ascending Pharyngeal Artery (a branch of the External Carotid Artery)

✋ PALPATION

1. With the client seated or supine, place palpating fingers just medial to the medial border of the sternocleidomastoid.
2. Press gently but firmly into the client's anterior neck in a posterior and slightly medial direction, feeling for the bodies and transverse processes of the cervical spine.
3. Have the client flex the head and neck against gentle resistance and feel for the contraction of the longus colli. Discerning the longus colli from the longus capitis is difficult.
4. Note: Be careful with palpation in this region because the common carotid artery and trachea are located nearby.

■ RELATIONSHIP TO OTHER STRUCTURES

- The longus colli is deep in the anterior neck (along with the longus capitis). The longus colli is deep to the hyoid bone, the suprahyoid and infrahyoid muscles, the trachea, and the esophagus. The longus colli lies against the cervical and upper thoracic vertebral bodies.
- The longus colli is generally inferior to the longus capitis. Where they overlap, the longus colli is deep to the longus capitis.
- If one looks at the relationship between the longus colli (and the longus capitis) to the anterior scalene, it can be seen that, except for the interruption of the attachment to the transverse processes of the cervical spine, there is a continuous line of pull from the first rib (the most inferior attachment of the anterior scalene) to the atlas (C1) and the head (the most superior attachments of the longus colli and longus capitis).
- The inferior part of the longus colli (the inferior part of the inferior oblique part) lies deep to the sternum.
- The longus colli is located within the deep front line myofascial meridian.

■ MISCELLANEOUS

1. The longus colli and the longus capitis, along with the rectus capitis anterior and the rectus capitis lateralis, are often grouped together and called the *prevertebral muscles.* (From an anterior perspective, they are just before [i.e., *pre-*] the vertebral column.)
2. The longus colli has three parts: the *superior oblique part,* the *inferior oblique part,* and the *vertical part.*
3. There is a general pattern of attachments for the longus colli. The attachments of the vertical part are from anterior bodies to anterior bodies. The attachments of the inferior oblique part are from anterior bodies to transverse processes. The attachments of the superior oblique part are from transverse processes to the anterior arch of the atlas (C1). All transverse process attachments are to the anterior tubercles of the transverse processes.
4. The longus colli and longus capitis are often injured in a whiplash accident, wherein the head and neck are forcefully thrown anteriorly and posteriorly (like a whip being lashed).
5. The longus colli and longus capitis are also often aggravated when doing a lot of sit-ups/crunches/curl-ups.
6. Talking, swallowing, coughing, and sneezing can exacerbate deep anterior neck pain in people who have a tight or injured longus colli.
7. Clients with a tight longus colli and/or longus capitis often describe feeling as though they have a sore throat, especially when swallowing.

10

Longus Capitis (of Prevertebral Group)

The name, longus capitis, *tells us that this muscle is long and attaches to the head.*

Derivation	□ longus: L. *long.*
	capitis: L. *refers to the head.*
Pronunciation	□ LONG-us, KAP-i-tis

■ ATTACHMENTS

□ **Transverse Processes of the Cervical Spine**
  □ the anterior tubercles of C3-C5

to the

□ **Occiput**
  □ the inferior surface of the basilar part of the occiput (just anterior to the foramen magnum)

■ FUNCTIONS

Concentric (Shortening) Mover Actions	
Standard Mover Actions	**Reverse Mover Actions**
□ **1. Flexes the neck and head at the spinal joints**	□ 1. Flexes the lower neck relative to the head
□ 2. Laterally flexes the neck and head at the spinal joints	□ 2. Laterally flexes the lower neck relative to the head

Standard Mover Action Notes

• The longus capitis crosses the atlanto-occipital joint (AOJ) and the joints of the upper neck anteriorly (with its fibers running vertically in the sagittal plane); therefore it flexes the head at the AOJ and the upper neck at the cervical spinal joints. (action 1)
• The longus capitis crosses the AOJ and the joints of the upper neck laterally (with its fibers running vertically in the frontal plane); therefore it laterally flexes the head at the AOJ and the upper neck at the cervical spinal joints. (action 2)

Reverse Mover Action Note

• The usual action of the longus capitis is to move the upper neck and head relative to the fixed lower attachment. The reverse action of the longus capitis occurs when the upper attachment is fixed and the vertebrae of the lower neck move relative to the upper neck and head. This usually occurs when the client is lying down so that the inferior attachment is mobile. (reverse actions 1, 2)

Eccentric Antagonist Functions

1. Restrains/slows extension and opposite-side lateral flexion of the neck and head at the spinal joints

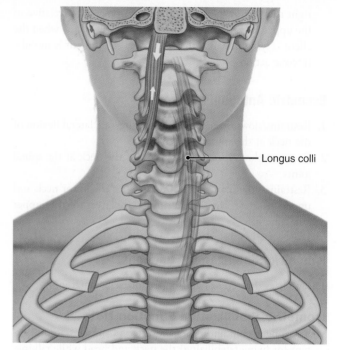

Figure 10-26 Anterior view of the right longus capitis. The longus colli has been ghosted in on the left.

Isometric Stabilization Function

1. Stabilizes the upper cervical spinal joints, including the head at the AOJ

Isometric Stabilization Function Note

• The longus capitis and other prevertebral muscles are important for fixing (stabilizing) the neck and head while talking, swallowing, coughing, and sneezing. They also fix the neck during rapid arm movements.

Additional Note on Functions

1. Some sources state that the longus capitis is capable of rotating the head and the neck at the spinal joints. Given the fiber direction of the longus capitis, it would seem likely that the line of pull would cause contralateral rotation of the head and neck.

INNERVATION
□ Cervical Spinal Nerves
  □ ventral rami; C1-C3

ARTERIAL SUPPLY
□ The Inferior Thyroid Artery (a branch of the Thyrocervical Trunk) and the Vertebral Artery (a branch of the Subclavian Artery)
  □ and the Ascending Pharyngeal Artery (a branch of the External Carotid Artery)

10

Longus Capitis (of Prevertebral Group)—*cont'd*

 PALPATION

1. With the client seated or supine, place palpating fingers just medial to the medial border of the sternocleidomastoid.
2. Press gently but firmly into the client's anterior neck in a posterior and slightly medial direction, feeling for the bodies and transverse processes of the cervical spine.
3. Have the client flex the head and neck against gentle resistance and feel for the contraction of the longus capitis. Discerning the longus capitis from the longus colli is difficult.
4. Note: Be careful with palpation in this region because the common carotid artery and trachea are located nearby.

■ RELATIONSHIP TO OTHER STRUCTURES

☐ The longus capitis is deep in the anterior neck (along with the longus colli). The longus capitis is deep to the hyoid bone, the suprahyoid muscles, the trachea, and the esophagus.

☐ The longus capitis is generally superior to the longus colli. Where they overlap, the longus colli is deep to the longus capitis. The rectus capitis anterior is also deep to the longus capitis.

☐ If one looks at the relationship between the longus capitis (and the superior part of the longus colli) and the anterior scalene, it can be seen that, except for the interruption of the attachment to the transverse processes of the cervical spine, there is a continuous line of pull from the first rib (the most inferior attachment of the anterior scalene) to the atlas (C1) and the head (the most superior attachments of the longus colli and longus capitis).

☐ The longus capitis is located within the deep front line myofascial meridian.

■ MISCELLANEOUS

1. The longus capitis and the longus colli, along with the rectus capitis anterior and the rectus capitis lateralis, are often grouped together and called the *prevertebral muscles*. (From an anterior perspective, they are just before [i.e., *pre*-] the vertebral column.)
2. The vertebral attachments of the longus capitis are variable; the longus capitis often attaches to C6.
3. The longus capitis and longus colli are often injured in a whiplash accident, wherein the head and neck are forcefully thrown anteriorly and posteriorly (like a whip being lashed).
4. The longus capitis and longus colli are also often aggravated when doing a lot of sit-ups/crunches/curl-ups.
5. Talking, swallowing, coughing, and sneezing can exacerbate deep anterior neck pain in people who have a tight or injured longus capitis.
6. Clients with a tight longus capitis and/or longus colli often describe feeling as though they have a sore throat, especially when swallowing.

10

Rectus Capitis Anterior (of Prevertebral Group)

The name, rectus capitis anterior, tells us that the fibers of this muscle run straight and attach to the head anteriorly.

Derivation	☐ rectus: L. *straight.*
	capitis: L. *refers to the head.*
	anterior: L. *before, in front of.*
Pronunciation	☐ REK-tus, KAP-i-tis, an-TEE-ri-or

■ ATTACHMENTS

☐ **The Atlas (C1)**
    ☐ the anterior surface of the base of the transverse process

to the

☐ **Occiput**
    ☐ the inferior surface of the basilar part of the occiput (just anterior to the foramen magnum)

■ FUNCTIONS

Concentric (Shortening) Mover Actions	
Standard Mover Actions	**Reverse Mover Actions**
☐ **1. Flexes the head at the AOJ**	☐ 1. Flexes the atlas relative to the head at the AOJ

AOJ = atlanto-occipital joint

Standard Mover Action Notes

• The rectus capitis anterior crosses the AOJ between the atlas (C1) and the occiput anteriorly (with its fibers running vertically in the sagittal plane); therefore it flexes the head on the atlas at the AOJ. (action 1)

Reverse Mover Action Notes

• The usual action of the rectus capitis anterior is to flex the head relative to the atlas. The reverse action would be if the head is fixed and the atlas flexes toward the head at the AOJ. This usually only happens if the client is lying supine so the lower attachment is mobile (e.g., if the client is lying supine and brings the feet up and over and behind the head. (reverse action 1)

Eccentric Antagonist Function

1. Restrains/slows extension of the AOJ

Isometric Stabilization Function

1. Stabilizes the head at the AOJ

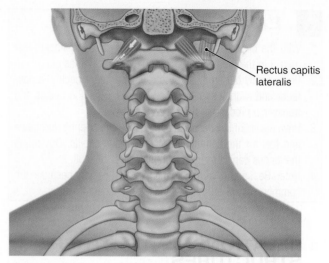

Figure 10-27 Anterior view of the rectus capitis anterior bilaterally. The rectus capitis lateralis has been ghosted in on the left.

Isometric Stabilization Function Note

• The rectus capitis anterior and other prevertebral muscles are important for fixing (stabilizing) the neck and head while talking, swallowing, coughing, and sneezing.

Additional Note on Functions

1. Some sources state that the rectus capitis anterior can ipsilaterally rotate the head at the AOJ.

INNERVATION
☐ Cervical Spinal Nerves
☐ ventral rami; C1-C2

ARTERIAL SUPPLY
☐ The Vertebral Artery (a branch of the Subclavian Artery)

✋ **PALPATION**
1. The rectus capitis anterior is located very deep and high in the anterior neck between the atlas (C1) and the occiput and is usually not palpable.

■ RELATIONSHIP TO OTHER STRUCTURES

☐ The rectus capitis anterior is very deep in the anterior neck.
☐ Directly superficial to the rectus capitis anterior is the longus capitis.
☐ The attachment of the rectus capitis anterior on the atlas (C1) is directly medial to the attachment of the rectus capitis lateralis on the atlas. From the atlas attachments, the rectus capitis anterior runs superiorly and medially to attach onto

the occiput, whereas the rectus capitis lateralis runs superiorly and slightly laterally to attach onto the occiput.

☐ The rectus capitis anterior is located within the deep front line myofascial meridian.

■ MISCELLANEOUS

1. The rectus capitis anterior and the rectus capitis lateralis, along with the longus colli and the longus capitis, are often grouped together and called the *prevertebral muscles*. (From an anterior perspective, they are just before [i.e., *pre-*] the vertebral column.)

2. In addition to the rectus capitis anterior, there is also a rectus capitis lateralis, a rectus capitis posterior major, and a rectus capitis posterior minor. These four muscles attach onto the occiput (hence, *capitis*).

3. The rectus capitis anterior is often injured in a whiplash accident.

4. Because the rectus capitis anterior contracts to stabilize the head when talking, swallowing, coughing, and sneezing, these activities can exacerbate deep anterior neck pain in people who have a tight or injured rectus capitis anterior.

Rectus Capitis Lateralis (of Prevertebral Group)

The name, rectus capitis lateralis, *tells us that the fibers of this muscle run straight and attach to the head laterally.*

Derivation	☐ rectus: L. *straight.*
	capitis: L. *refers to the head.*
	lateralis: L. *refers to the side.*
Pronunciation	☐ REK-tus, KAP-i-tis, la-ter-A-lis

■ ATTACHMENTS

☐ **The Atlas (C1)**
  ☐ the superior surface of the transverse process

to the

☐ **Occiput**
  ☐ the inferior surface of the jugular process of the occiput

■ FUNCTIONS

Concentric (Shortening) Mover Actions	
Standard Mover Actions	**Reverse Mover Actions**
☐ **1. Laterally flexes the head at the AOJ**	☐ 1. Laterally flexes the atlas relative to the head at the AOJ

AOJ = atlanto-occipital joint

Standard Mover Action Notes

• The rectus capitis lateralis crosses the AOJ between the atlas (C1) and the occiput laterally (with its fibers running vertically in the frontal plane); therefore it laterally flexes the head on the atlas at the AOJ. (action 1)

Reverse Mover Action Notes

• The usual action of the rectus capitis lateralis is to laterally flex the head relative to the atlas. The reverse action would be if the head is fixed and the atlas laterally flexes toward the head at the AOJ. This usually only happens if the client is lying down so that the lower attachment is mobile. (reverse action 1)

Eccentric Antagonist Function

1. Restrains/slows opposite-side lateral flexion at the AOJ

Isometric Stabilization Function

1. Stabilizes the head at the AOJ

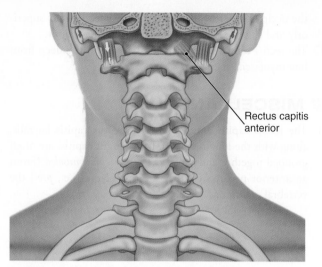

Rectus capitis anterior

Figure 10-28 Anterior view of the rectus capitis lateralis bilaterally. The rectus capitis anterior has been ghosted in on the left.

Additional Note on Functions

1. The rectus capitis lateralis and other prevertebral muscles are important for fixing (stabilizing) the neck and head when talking, swallowing, coughing, and sneezing.

INNERVATION
☐ Cervical Spinal Nerves
  ☐ ventral rami; C1-C2

ARTERIAL SUPPLY
☐ The Vertebral Artery (a branch of the Subclavian Artery) and the Occipital Artery (a branch of the External Carotid Artery)

✋ PALPATION

1. With the client seated or supine, place palpating fingers just superior to the transverse process of the atlas (the transverse process of the atlas is posterior to the ramus of the mandible, anterior to the mastoid process of the temporal bone, and inferior to the ear).
2. Palpate superiorly to the transverse processes of the atlas and a bit deeper and feel for the rectus capitis lateralis. Discerning its muscle belly from the adjacent musculature is difficult.
3. Note: The styloid process of the temporal bone is very close to this region. Care must be taken to not use too much pressure because the styloid process is a delicate structure.

■ RELATIONSHIP TO OTHER STRUCTURES

☐ The rectus capitis lateralis is deep in the anterolateral neck.
☐ The attachment of the rectus capitis lateralis on the atlas is directly lateral to the attachment of the rectus capitis ante-

Rectus Capitis Lateralis (of Prevertebral Group)—*cont'd*

rior on the atlas. From the atlas attachments, the rectus capitis lateralis runs superiorly and slightly laterally to attach onto the occiput, whereas the rectus capitis anterior runs superiorly and medially to attach onto the occiput.

☐ From a lateral perspective, the styloid process of the temporal bone is superficial to the rectus capitis lateralis.

☐ The rectus capitis lateralis may be involved with the deep front line and lateral line myofascial meridians.

■ MISCELLANEOUS

1. The rectus capitis lateralis and the rectus capitis anterior, along with the longus colli and the longus capitis, are often grouped together and called the *prevertebral muscles*. (From an anterior perspective, they are just before [i.e., *pre-*] the vertebral column.)

2. In addition to the rectus capitis lateralis, there is also a rectus capitis anterior, a rectus capitis posterior major, and a rectus capitis posterior minor. These four muscles attach onto the occiput (hence, *capitis*).

3. The rectus capitis lateralis is often injured in a whiplash accident.

4. Because the rectus capitis lateralis contracts to stabilize the head when talking, swallowing, coughing, and sneezing, these activities can exacerbate deep anterior neck pain in people who have a tight or injured rectus capitis lateralis.

5. The rectus capitis lateralis muscles are considered to be homologous to the posterior intertransversarii muscles of the spine.

10

Splenius Capitis

The name, splenius capitis, *tells us that this muscle is shaped like a bandage (a narrow rectangle) and attaches onto the head.*

Derivation	☐ splenius: Gr. *bandage.*
	capitis: L. *refers to the head.*
Pronunciation	☐ SPLEE-nee-us, KAP-i-tis

■ ATTACHMENTS

☐ **Nuchal Ligament from C3-C6 and the Spinous Processes of C7-T4**

to the

☐ **Mastoid Process of the Temporal Bone and the Occipital Bone**

☐ the lateral ⅓ of the superior nuchal line of the occiput

■ FUNCTIONS

Concentric (Shortening) Mover Actions	
Standard Mover Actions	**Reverse Mover Actions**
☐ **1. Extends the head and neck at the spinal joints**	☐ 1. Extends the upper thoracic and lower cervical spine relative to the head and upper cervical spine
☐ **2. Laterally flexes the head and neck at the spinal joints**	☐ 2. Laterally flexes the upper thoracic and lower cervical spine relative to the head and upper cervical spine
☐ **3. Ipsilaterally rotates the head and neck at the spinal joints**	☐ 3. Contralaterally rotates the upper thoracic and lower cervical spine relative to the head and upper cervical spine

Standard Mover Action Notes

- The splenius capitis crosses the atlanto-occipital joint (AOJ) and the joints of the cervical spine posteriorly (with its fibers running vertically in the sagittal plane). Therefore the splenius capitis extends the head at the AOJ and the neck at the cervical spinal joints. (action 1)
- The splenius capitis crosses the AOJ and the joints of the cervical spine laterally (with its fibers running vertically in the frontal plane). Therefore the splenius capitis laterally flexes the head at the AOJ and the neck at the cervical spinal joints. (action 2)
- The splenius capitis attaches from the nuchal ligament/spinous processes attachment and then wraps around the neck anteriorly to attach onto the cranium (with its fibers running somewhat horizontally in the transverse plane). When the splenius capitis contracts, it pulls the cranial attachment posteromedially, causing the anterior surface of the head and/or the neck to face the same side of the body

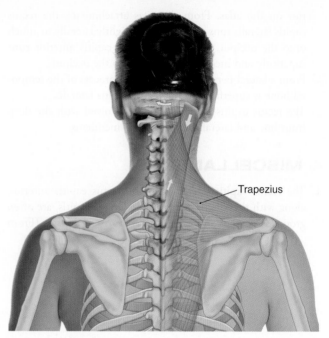

Trapezius

Figure 10-29 Posterior view of the right splenius capitis. The trapezius has been ghosted in.

to which the splenius capitis is attached. Therefore the splenius capitis ipsilaterally rotates the head at the AOJ and the neck at the cervical spinal joints. (action 3)

Reverse Mover Action Notes

- When we think of motions of the spine, we usually think of the upper spine moving relative to the fixed lower spine. However, the reverse action of moving the lower spine relative to the fixed upper spine is also possible. This usually occurs when the client is lying down so that the inferior attachment is mobile. (reverse actions 1, 2, 3)
- The reverse action of ipsilateral rotation of the head and upper spine relative to the fixed lower spine is to contralaterally rotate the lower spine relative to the fixed head and upper spine. In other words, if the right-sided splenius capitis does right rotation of the head and neck, its reverse action would be to do left rotation of the upper thoracic and lower cervical spine. (reverse action 3)

Eccentric Antagonist Functions

- Restrains/slows flexion, opposite-side lateral flexion, and contralateral rotation of the head and neck
- Restrains/slows flexion, opposite-side lateral flexion, and ipsilateral rotation of the lower spinal attachment relative to the head

Splenius Capitis—*cont'd*

Isometric Stabilization Functions

• Stabilizes the head, neck, and upper thoracic vertebrae

INNERVATION
☐ Cervical Spinal Nerves
   ☐ dorsal rami of the middle cervical spinal nerves

ARTERIAL SUPPLY
☐ The Occipital Artery (a branch of the External Carotid Artery)

✋ PALPATION

1. With the client seated, place your palpating hand in the superior aspect of the posterior triangle of the neck (the area between the sternocleidomastoid and the upper trapezius).
2. Ask the client to actively rotate the head and the neck and feel for the contraction of the same-side splenius capitis. Resistance can be added.
3. Try to continue palpating the splenius capitis toward its superior attachment deep to the sternocleidomastoid, and its inferior attachment deep to the upper trapezius.

■ RELATIONSHIP TO OTHER STRUCTURES

☐ Most of the splenius capitis is deep to the trapezius inferiorly and the sternocleidomastoid superiorly.

☐ The most inferior part of the splenius capitis is deep to the rhomboid minor and the serratus posterior superior.
☐ The attachment of the splenius capitis onto the mastoid process is deep (anterior) to the sternocleidomastoid but superficial (posterior) to the longissimus capitis.
☐ There is a small part of the splenius capitis that is superficial in the posterior triangle of the neck between the trapezius and the sternocleidomastoid.
☐ The inferior portion of the splenius cervicis lies directly inferior to the splenius capitis.
☐ The erector spinae group lies deep to the splenius capitis.
☐ The splenius capitis is located within the lateral line and spiral line myofascial meridians.

■ MISCELLANEOUS

1. The left and right splenius capitis muscles bilaterally form a V shape. Because of their V shape, the left and right splenius capitis muscles are sometimes known as the *golf tee* muscles.
2. The inferior attachment of the splenius capitis is variable and often attaches only as far inferior as the spinous process of T3.
3. The mastoid attachment of the splenius capitis is sandwiched between the attachment of the sternocleidomastoid (which is posterior to it) and the attachment of the longissimus capitis (which is anterior to it).
4. The splenius capitis and splenius cervicis often blend together. By definition, any fibers that attach superiorly onto the head are defined as splenius capitis and any fibers that attach superiorly onto the cervical spine are defined as splenius cervicis.

10

Splenius Cervicis

The name, splenius cervicis, *tells us that this muscle is shaped like a bandage (a narrow rectangle) and attaches onto the cervical spine (the neck).*

Derivation	☐ splenius: Gr. *bandage.*
	cervicis: L. *refers to the cervical spine.*
Pronunciation	☐ SPLEE-nee-us, SER-vi-sis

■ ATTACHMENTS

☐ **Spinous Processes of T3-T6**

to the

☐ **Transverse Processes of C1-C3**
  ☐ the posterior tubercles of the transverse processes

■ FUNCTIONS

Concentric (Shortening) Mover Actions	
Standard Mover Actions	**Reverse Mover Actions**
☐ 1. Extends the neck at the spinal joints	☐ 1. Extends the upper thoracic spine relative to the upper cervical spine
☐ 2. Laterally flexes the neck at the spinal joints	☐ 2. Laterally flexes the upper thoracic spine relative to the upper cervical spine
☐ 3. Ipsilaterally rotates the neck at the spinal joints	☐ 3. Contralaterally rotates the upper thoracic spine relative to the upper cervical spine

Standard Mover Action Notes

- The splenius cervicis crosses the joints of the cervical spine posteriorly (with its fibers running vertically in the sagittal plane). Therefore the splenius cervicis extends the neck at the cervical spinal joints. (action 1)
- The splenius cervicis crosses the joints of the cervical spine laterally (with its fibers running vertically in the frontal plane). Therefore the splenius cervicis laterally flexes the neck at the cervical spinal joints. (action 2)
- The splenius cervicis attaches from the spinous processes of the upper thoracic region and then wraps around the neck anteriorly to attach onto the upper cervical transverse processes (with its fibers running somewhat horizontally in the transverse plane). When the splenius cervicis contracts, it pulls the neck posteromedially, causing the anterior surface of the neck to face the same side of the body to which the splenius cervicis is attached. Therefore the splenius cervicis ipsilaterally rotates the neck at the cervical spinal joints. (action 3)

Reverse Mover Action Notes

- When we think of motions of the spine, we usually think of the upper spine moving relative to the fixed lower spine.

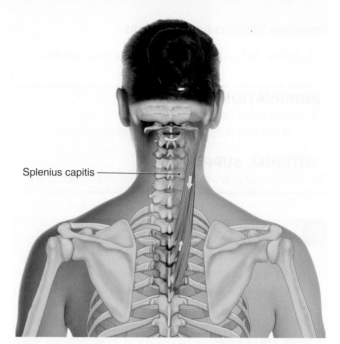

Figure 10-30 Posterior view of the right splenius cervicis. The splenius capitis has been ghosted in.

However, the reverse action of moving the lower spine relative toward the fixed upper spine is also possible. This usually occurs when the client is lying down so that the inferior attachment is mobile. (reverse actions 1, 2, 3)

- The reverse action of ipsilateral rotation of the upper spine relative to the fixed lower spine is to contralaterally rotate the lower spine relative to the fixed upper spine. In other words, if the right-sided splenius cervicis does right rotation of the neck, its reverse action would be to do left rotation of the upper thoracic spine. (reverse action 3)

Eccentric Antagonist Functions

1. Restrains/slows flexion, opposite-side lateral flexion, and contralateral rotation of the neck
2. Restrains/slows flexion, opposite-side lateral flexion, and ipsilateral rotation of the lower spinal attachment relative to the upper cervical spine

Isometric Stabilization Functions

1. Stabilizes the cervical and upper thoracic vertebrae

Additional Note on Functions

1. The splenius capitis and splenius cervicis have the same actions except that the splenius capitis moves the head and neck whereas the splenius cervicis only moves the neck (because the splenius capitis crosses the atlanto-occipital joint to attach to and move the head; the splenius cervicis does not).

Splenius capitis

10

Splenius Cervicis—*cont'd*

INNERVATION
☐ Cervical Spinal Nerves
   ☐ dorsal rami of the lower cervical spinal nerves

ARTERIAL SUPPLY
☐ The Occipital Artery (a branch of the External Carotid Artery) and the dorsal branches of the Upper Posterior Intercostal Arteries

---

✋ PALPATION

1. With the client seated, place palpating hand over the splenius cervicis between the splenius capitis and levator scapulae.
2. Ask the client to actively rotate the neck and feel for the contraction of the same-side splenius cervicis. Gentle resistance can be given.
3. Palpate as much of the splenius cervicis as possible.
4. Note: It is challenging to palpate and discern this muscle from adjacent musculature.

■ RELATIONSHIP TO OTHER STRUCTURES

☐ The splenius cervicis is deep to the trapezius, the rhomboids, and the serratus posterior superior. Toward its superior attachment, the splenius cervicis is also deep to the splenius capitis.
☐ From the posterior perspective, the cervical transverse process attachment of the splenius cervicis is superficial (posterior) to the cervical transverse process attachments of the levator scapulae and the scalenes.
☐ The inferior portion of the splenius cervicis lies directly inferior to the splenius capitis.
☐ The erector spinae musculature lies deep to the splenius cervicis.
☐ The splenius cervicis is located within the spiral line myofascial meridian.

■ MISCELLANEOUS

1. The left and right splenius cervicis muscles bilaterally form a V shape.
2. The superior attachment of the splenius cervicis is variable and often attaches only onto the transverse processes of C1-C2.

10

The suboccipitals are a group of four short muscles located deep in the posterior suboccipital region. There are four suboccipital muscles: the rectus capitis posterior major, rectus capitis posterior minor, obliquus capitis inferior, and obliquus capitis superior.

ATTACHMENTS

The names of the suboccipital muscles generally refer to their fiber direction:

☐ *Rectus* means straight. The rectus capitis posterior major and minor attach from the spinous process of C2 and the posterior tubercle of C1, respectively, and run straight up to the inferior nuchal line of the occiput.

☐ *Obliquus* means slanted. The obliquus capitis inferior and superior run in a slanted fashion. The obliquus capitis inferior slants from the spinous process of C2 to the transverse process of C1, and the obliquus capitis superior slants from the transverse process of C1 to the occiput (between the inferior and superior nuchal lines).

☐ The suboccipitals are found deep to the upper trapezius, sternocleidomastoid, splenius capitis, and semispinalis capitis (of the transversospinalis group).

FUNCTIONS

☐ The major actions of the suboccipital group are extension and anterior translation (protraction) of the head on the neck at the atlanto-occipital joint.

☐ The obliquus capitis inferior ipsilaterally rotates the atlas (C1) on the axis (C2) at the atlantoaxial joint.

☐ The suboccipital muscles are generally thought to be more important as postural stabilization muscles, providing fine control of head posture, than as movers.

☐ Some sources believe that the main role of the suboccipital group is proprioceptive by providing precise monitoring of the position of the head and upper cervical vertebrae.

MISCELLANEOUS

1. The suboccipital muscles are not the only muscles located in the suboccipital region. When tight muscles are palpated in this region, they are not always the suboccipital muscles; they can also be the superior attachments of the trapezius, splenius capitis, splenius cervicis, semispinalis capitis, or perhaps even the longissimus capitis or the sternocleidomastoid.

2. When the suboccipital musculature is chronically tight, tension headaches often occur.

3. The suboccipital muscles are located within the superficial back line myofascial meridian.

INNERVATION

☐ The four suboccipital muscles are innervated by the suboccipital nerve (dorsal ramus of C1).

ARTERIAL SUPPLY

☐ The four suboccipital muscles receive the majority of their arterial supply from the occipital artery.

10

Views of the Suboccipital Group

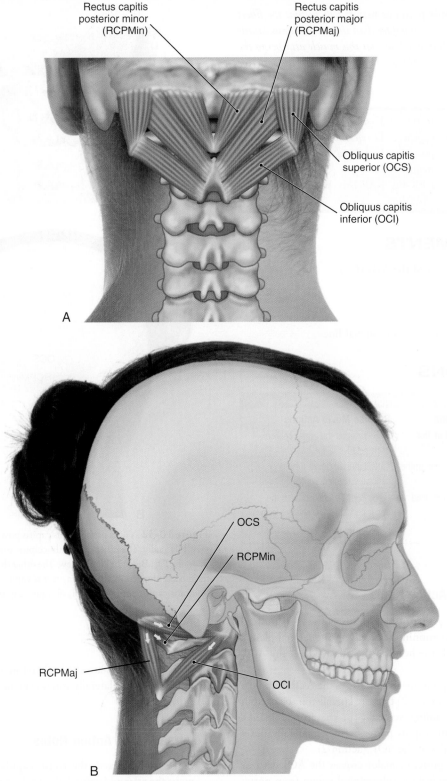

Figure 10-31 Views of the suboccipital group. **A,** Posterior view. **B,** Right lateral view. Note the anterior to posterior horizontal direction of the rectus capitis posterior minor (RCPMin) and the obliquus capitis superior (OCS). This fiber direction is ideal for anterior translation of the head at the atlanto-occipital joint.

Rectus Capitis Posterior Major (of Suboccipital Group)

The name, rectus capitis posterior major, *tells us that the fibers of this muscle run straight (straighter than the two obliquus capitis suboccipital muscles). It also tells us that this muscle attaches to the head posteriorly and is large (larger than the rectus capitis posterior minor).*

Derivation	☐ rectus: L. *straight.*
	capitis: L. *refers to the head.*
	posterior: L. *behind, toward the back.*
	major: L. *larger.*
Pronunciation	☐ REK-tus, KAP-i-tis, pos-TEE-ri-or, MAY-jor

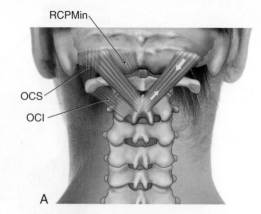

■ ATTACHMENTS

☐ **The Spinous Process of the Axis (C2)**

to the

☐ **Occiput**
　　☐ the lateral ½ of the inferior nuchal line

■ FUNCTIONS

Concentric (Shortening) Mover Actions	
Standard Mover Actions	**Reverse Mover Actions**
☐ **1. Extends the head at the AOJ**	☐ 1. Extends the upper cervical spine relative to the head
☐ 2. Laterally flexes the head at the AOJ	☐ 2. Laterally flexes the upper cervical spine relative to the head
☐ 3. Ipsilaterally rotates the head at the AOJ	☐ 3. Contralaterally rotates the upper cervical spine relative to the head

AOJ = atlanto-occipital joint

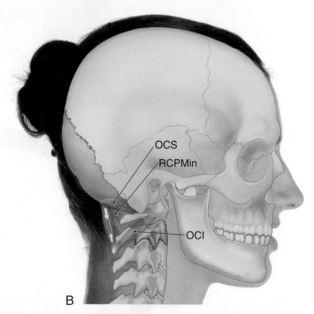

Figure 10-32 Views of the rectus capitis posterior major. **A,** Posterior view bilaterally. The other three suboccipital muscles have been ghosted in on the left. **B,** Right lateral view. The other three suboccipital muscles have been ghosted in. RCPMin, rectus capitis posterior minor; OCS, obliquus capitis superior; OCI, obliquus capitis inferior.

Standard Mover Action Notes

• The rectus capitis posterior major crosses the AOJ posteriorly (with its fibers running vertically in the sagittal plane); therefore it extends the head on the atlas (C1) at the AOJ. (action 1)

• The rectus capitis posterior major crosses the AOJ from near the midline on the axis (C2) to more laterally on the occiput (with its fibers running vertically in the frontal plane). Therefore the rectus capitis posterior major laterally flexes the head on the atlas at the AOJ. (action 2)

• The rectus capitis posterior major crosses the AOJ with its fibers wrapping around the suboccipital region from posteriorly on the axis, to more anteriorly on the occiput (with its fibers running somewhat horizontally in the transverse plane). When the rectus capitis posterior major contracts, it pulls on the occiput, causing the anterior surface of the head to face the same side of the body to which the rectus capitis

posterior major is attached. Therefore the rectus capitis posterior major ipsilaterally rotates the head on the atlas at the AOJ. (action 3)

Reverse Mover Action Notes

• If the head is fixed, the rectus capitis posterior major can move the atlas and axis relative to the head. This is only likely to occur when the client is lying down so that the inferior attachments are mobile. (reverse actions 1, 2, 3)

• The reverse action of ipsilateral rotation of the head relative to the spine is to contralaterally rotate the spine relative to the head. (reverse action 3)

Rectus Capitis Posterior Major (of Suboccipital Group)—*cont'd*

Eccentric Antagonist Functions

1. Restrains/slows flexion, opposite-side lateral flexion, and contralateral rotation of the head

Isometric Stabilization Functions

1. Stabilizes the head and atlas at the AOJ
2. Stabilizes the atlantoaxial joint

Isometric Stabilization Function Note

- The suboccipital muscles are generally thought to be more important as postural stabilization muscles, providing fine control of head posture, than as movers.

Additional Notes on Functions

1. The rectus capitis posterior major crosses the joint between the atlas and the axis (the atlantoaxial joint) in the same manner that it crosses the joint between the head and the atlas (the AOJ). Therefore the rectus capitis posterior major can perform the same actions at the atlantoaxial joint that it performs at the AOJ, except that the atlantoaxial joint does not permit lateral flexion. Therefore the rectus capitis posterior major extends and ipsilaterally rotates the atlas (C1) on the axis (C2) at the atlantoaxial joint.
2. Some sources believe that the main role of the suboccipital group is proprioceptive by providing precise monitoring of the position of the head and upper cervical vertebrae.

INNERVATION

- □ The Suboccipital Nerve
  - □ dorsal ramus of C1

ARTERIAL SUPPLY

- □ The Occipital Artery (a branch of the External Carotid Artery) and the Deep Cervical Artery (a branch of the Costocervical Trunk)
  - □ and the muscular branches of the Vertebral Artery (a branch of the Subclavian Artery)

✋ PALPATION

1. With the client supine and as relaxed as possible, place palpating fingers slightly superior and lateral to the spinous process of the axis (C2), which is the most prominent spinous process in the upper cervical region.
2. Feel for the fibers of the rectus capitis posterior major running superolaterally from the spinous process of the axis toward the occiput.

■ RELATIONSHIP TO OTHER STRUCTURES

- □ The rectus capitis posterior major, as with all the suboccipital muscles, is very deep in the suboccipital region. It is deep to the trapezius and the semispinalis capitis.
- □ Deep to the rectus capitis posterior major are the occiput, the atlas (C1), and the axis (C2).
- □ The rectus capitis posterior major lies directly lateral to the rectus capitis posterior minor.
- □ The occipital attachment of the rectus capitis posterior major is deep to the occipital attachment of the obliquus capitis superior.
- □ The rectus capitis posterior major borders the *suboccipital triangle* of the neck. The suboccipital triangle is located between the rectus capitis posterior major, the obliquus capitis inferior, and the obliquus capitis superior. The suboccipital nerve and the vertebral artery are located in the suboccipital triangle.
- □ The rectus capitis posterior major is located within the superficial back line myofascial meridian.

■ MISCELLANEOUS

1. The rectus capitis posterior major is one of four muscles that are called the *suboccipital muscles.* They are the rectus capitis posterior major, rectus capitis posterior minor, obliquus capitis inferior, and obliquus capitis superior.
2. In addition to the four suboccipital muscles, there is a rectus capitis anterior and a rectus capitis lateralis.
3. The rectus capitis posterior major and the rectus capitis posterior minor both attach to the inferior nuchal line of the occiput.

10

Rectus Capitis Posterior Minor (of Suboccipital Group)

The name, rectus capitis posterior minor, *tells us that the fibers of this muscle run straight (straighter than the two obliquus capitis suboccipital muscles). It also tells us that this muscle attaches to the head posteriorly and is small (smaller than the rectus capitis posterior major).*

Derivation	☐ rectus: L. *straight.*
	capitis: L. *refers to the head.*
	posterior: L. *behind, toward the back.*
	minor: L. *smaller.*
Pronunciation	☐ REK-tus, KAP-i-tis, pos-TEE-ri-or, MY-nor

■ ATTACHMENTS

☐ **The Posterior Tubercle of the Atlas (C1)**

to the

☐ **Occiput**
 ☐ the medial ½ of the inferior nuchal line

■ FUNCTIONS

Concentric (Shortening) Mover Actions	
Standard Mover Actions	**Reverse Mover Actions**
☐ **1. Protracts the head at the AOJ**	☐ 1. Retracts the atlas relative to the head
☐ 2. Extends the head at the AOJ	☐ 2. Extends the atlas relative to the head
☐ 3. Laterally flexes the head at the AOJ	☐ 3. Laterally flexes the atlas relative to the head
AOJ = atlanto-occipital joint	

Standard Mover Action Notes

- The rectus capitis posterior minor runs primarily horizontally from the atlas anteriorly to the occiput posteriorly (this is best appreciated when the muscle is viewed laterally). When it contracts, it pulls the occiput anteriorly toward the atlas; therefore it protracts (anteriorly translates) the head at the AOJ. (action 1)
- The rectus capitis posterior minor crosses the AOJ posteriorly (with its fibers running slightly vertically in the sagittal plane); therefore it extends the head on the atlas (C1) at the AOJ. This action is relatively weak because the muscle's fibers primarily run horizontally. (action 2)
- The rectus capitis posterior minor crosses the AOJ from near the midline on the atlas (C1) to more laterally on the occiput (with its fibers running slightly vertically in the frontal plane). Therefore it laterally flexes the head on the atlas at

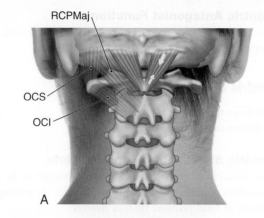

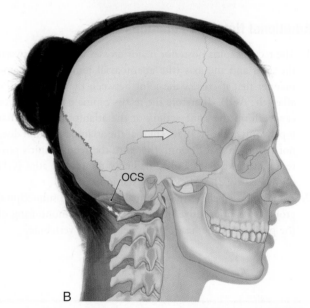

Figure 10-33 Views of the rectus capitis posterior minor. **A,** Posterior view bilaterally. The other three suboccipital muscles have been ghosted in on the left. **B,** Right lateral view. The obliquus capitis superior (OCS) has been ghosted in. OCI, obliquus capitis inferior; RCPMaj, rectus capitis posterior major.

the AOJ. This action is relatively weak because the muscle's fibers primarily run horizontally. (action 3)

Reverse Mover Action Notes

- If the head is fixed, the rectus capitis posterior minor can move the atlas relative to the head. This is only likely to occur when the client is lying down so the inferior attachment is mobile. (reverse actions 1, 2, 3)

Eccentric Antagonist Functions

1. Restrains/slows retraction, flexion, and opposite-side lateral flexion of the head

Rectus Capitis Posterior Minor (of Suboccipital Group)—*cont'd*

Isometric Stabilization Function

1. Stabilizes the head and atlas at the AOJ

Isometric Stabilization Function Notes

• The suboccipital muscles are generally thought to be more important as postural stabilization muscles, providing fine control of head posture, than as movers.

Additional Notes on Functions

1. The rectus capitis posterior minor has an attachment directly into the dura mater of the brain and spinal cord at the foramen magnum. The purpose of the dura mater attachment seems to be to protect the dura mater from folding on itself and/or getting pinched when the head protracts on the atlas at the AOJ.
2. Some sources believe that the main role of the suboccipital group is proprioceptive by providing precise monitoring of the position of the head and upper cervical vertebrae.

INNERVATION
☐ The Suboccipital Nerve
  ☐ dorsal ramus of C1

ARTERIAL SUPPLY
☐ The Occipital Artery (a branch of the External Carotid Artery) and muscular branches of the Vertebral Artery (a branch of the Subclavian Artery)
  ☐ and the Deep Cervical Artery (a branch of the Costocervical Trunk)

✋ PALPATION

1. With the client supine and as relaxed as possible, place palpating fingers just inferior to the occiput and very slightly lateral of midline, and feel for the fibers of the rectus capitis posterior minor running superiorly from the posterior tubercle of the atlas (C1) toward the occiput.

■ RELATIONSHIP TO OTHER STRUCTURES

☐ The rectus capitis posterior minor, as with all the suboccipital muscles, is very deep in the suboccipital region. It is deep to the trapezius and the semispinalis capitis.
☐ Deep to the rectus capitis posterior minor are the occiput and the atlas (C1).
☐ The rectus capitis posterior minor lies directly medial to the rectus capitis posterior major.
☐ The rectus capitis posterior minor is located within the superficial back line myofascial meridian.

■ MISCELLANEOUS

1. The rectus capitis posterior minor is one of four muscles that are called the *suboccipital muscles*. They are the rectus capitis posterior major, rectus capitis posterior minor, obliquus capitis inferior, and obliquus capitis superior.
2. In addition to the four suboccipital muscles, there is a rectus capitis anterior and a rectus capitis lateralis.
3. The rectus capitis posterior major and the rectus capitis posterior minor both attach to the inferior nuchal line of the occiput.
4. In addition to the inferior nuchal line attachment, the rectus capitis posterior minor also attaches more inferiorly onto the occiput between the inferior nuchal line and the foramen magnum. A connective tissue attachment of the rectus capitis posterior minor has been discovered that attaches directly into the dura mater. Although tightness of any of the posterior cervical musculature in the suboccipital region may cause *tension headaches,* given this dura mater attachment, tightness of the rectus capitis posterior minor may more easily precipitate a tension headache than the other muscles in the region.
5. Given its action of protraction of the head at the atlanto-occipital joint, a tight rectus capitis posterior minor can contribute to a posture of the head being held anteriorly, in other words, protracted.

10

Obliquus Capitis Inferior (of Suboccipital Group)

The name, obliquus capitis inferior, *tells us that the fibers of this muscle run obliquely (in comparison to the two rectus capitis posterior suboccipital muscles). It also tells us that this muscle attaches near the head (this is the only one of the four suboccipital muscles that does not attach directly onto the head) and is located inferiorly (inferior to the obliquus capitis superior).*

Derivation	☐ obliquus: L. *oblique.*
	capitis: L. *refers to the head.*
	inferior: L. *below.*
Pronunciation	☐ ob-LEE-kwus, KAP-i-tis,
	in-FEE-ri-or

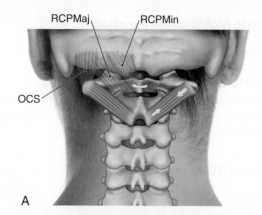

A

■ **ATTACHMENTS**

☐ **The Spinous Process of the Axis (C2)**

to the

☐ **Transverse Process of the Atlas (C1)**

■ **FUNCTIONS**

Concentric (Shortening) Mover Actions	
Standard Mover Actions	**Reverse Mover Actions**
☐ **1. Ipsilaterally rotates the atlas at the AAJ**	☐ 1. Contralaterally rotates the axis relative to the atlas

AAJ = atlantoaxial joint

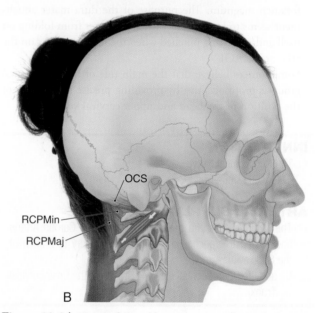

B

Figure 10-34 Views of the obliquus capitis inferior. **A,** Posterior view bilaterally. The other three suboccipital muscles have been ghosted in on the left. **B,** Right lateral view. The other three suboccipital muscles have been ghosted in. OCS, obliquus capitis superior; RCPMaj, rectus capitis posterior major; RCPMin, rectus capitis posterior minor.

Standard Mover Action Notes

- The obliquus capitis inferior attaches from the spinous process of the axis (C2) to the transverse process of the atlas (C1), with its fibers running horizontally in the transverse plane. When the obliquus capitis inferior contracts, it pulls the transverse process of the atlas toward the spinous process of the axis, causing the anterior surface of the atlas to face the same side of the body to which the obliquus capitis inferior is attached. Therefore the obliquus capitis inferior ipsilaterally rotates the atlas on the axis at the AAJ. (Note: If the head is fixed to the atlas, the head will "go along for the ride" and the head and the atlas together will rotate on the axis.) (action 1)
- Rotation of the atlas relative to the axis at the AAJ is an extremely important motion. Nearly half of the rotation of the craniocervical region occurs at the AAJ. (action 1)

Reverse Mover Action Notes

- If the head and atlas are fixed, the obliquus capitis inferior can move the axis (C2) relative to the atlas (C1). This is only likely to occur when the client is lying down so that the inferior attachment is mobile. (reverse action 1)

- The reverse action of ipsilateral rotation of the atlas at the AAJ is contralateral rotation of the axis at the AAJ. (reverse action 1)

Eccentric Antagonist Functions

1. Restrains/slows contralateral rotation of the atlas
2. Restrains/slows ipsilateral rotation of the axis

Isometric Stabilization Function

1. Stabilizes the atlas and axis at the AAJ

Obliquus Capitis Inferior (of Suboccipital Group)—*cont'd*

Isometric Stabilization Function Note

• The suboccipital muscles are generally thought to be more important as postural stabilization muscles of the head/upper cervical region than as movers. However, of the four suboccipitals, the obliquus capitis inferior is the most important as a mover, because its location affords it excellent leverage to rotate the atlas.

Additional Notes on Functions

1. The obliquus capitis inferior is the only suboccipital muscle that does not cross the atlanto-occipital joint to attach to the head. Therefore it is the only suboccipital muscle that cannot move the head at the atlanto-occipital joint. It moves the atlas (C1) at the AAJ joint.
2. Some sources believe that the main role of the suboccipital group is proprioceptive by providing precise monitoring of the position of the head and upper cervical vertebrae.

INNERVATION
☐ The Suboccipital Nerve
   ☐ dorsal ramus of C1

ARTERIAL SUPPLY
☐ The Deep Cervical Artery (a branch of the Costocervical Trunk) and the descending branch of the Occipital Artery (a branch of the External Carotid Artery)
   ☐ and the muscular branches of the Vertebral Artery (a branch of the Subclavian Artery)

✋ PALPATION

1. With the client supine and as relaxed as possible, place palpating fingers on the spinous process of the axis (C2), which is the most prominent spinous process in the upper cervical region, and feel for the fibers of the obliquus capitis inferior running laterally and slightly superiorly from the spinous process of the axis toward the transverse process of the atlas (C1).
2. Have the client gently ipsilaterally rotate the head and neck and feel for the contraction of the muscle. Resistance may be added.

■ RELATIONSHIP TO OTHER STRUCTURES

☐ The obliquus capitis inferior, as with all of the suboccipital muscles, is very deep in the suboccipital region. It is deep to the trapezius, splenius capitis, semispinalis capitis, and the sternocleidomastoid.
☐ Deep to the obliquus capitis inferior are the atlas (C1) and the axis (C2).
☐ The obliquus capitis inferior borders the *suboccipital triangle* of the neck. The suboccipital triangle is located between the rectus capitis posterior major, the obliquus capitis inferior, and the obliquus capitis superior. The suboccipital nerve and the vertebral artery are located in the suboccipital triangle.
☐ The greater occipital nerve exits from deeper in the neck directly inferior to the obliquus capitis inferior.
☐ The obliquus capitis inferior is located within the superficial back line myofascial meridian.

■ MISCELLANEOUS

1. The obliquus capitis inferior is one of four muscles that are called the *suboccipital muscles.* They are the rectus capitis posterior major, rectus capitis posterior minor, obliquus capitis inferior, and obliquus capitis superior.
2. In addition to the four suboccipital muscles, there is a rectus capitis anterior and a rectus capitis lateralis.
3. The obliquus capitis inferior and the obliquus capitis superior both attach to the transverse process of the atlas. Four other muscles also attach to the transverse process of the atlas: the levator scapulae, splenius cervicis, rectus capitis anterior, and rectus capitis lateralis.
4. The name *obliquus capitis inferior* is a misnomer in that this muscle does not attach to the head, therefore the word *capitis* should not be in the name.

10

Obliquus Capitis Superior (of Suboccipital Group)

The name, obliquus capitis superior, *tells us that the fibers of this muscle run obliquely (in comparison to the two rectus capitis posterior suboccipital muscles). It also tells us that this muscle attaches onto the head and is located superiorly (superior to the obliquus capitis inferior).*

Derivation	☐ obliquus: L. *oblique.*
	capitis: L. *refers to the head.*
	superior: L. *above.*
Pronunciation	☐ ob-LEE-kwus, KAP-i-tis,
	sue-PEE-ri-or

■ ATTACHMENTS

☐ **The Transverse Process of the Atlas (C1)**

to the

☐ **Occiput**
  ☐ between the superior and inferior nuchal lines

■ FUNCTIONS

Concentric (Shortening) Mover Actions	
Standard Mover Actions	**Reverse Mover Actions**
☐ **1. Protracts the head at the AOJ**	☐ 1. Retracts the atlas relative to the head
☐ 2. Laterally flexes the head at AOJ	☐ 2. Laterally flexes the atlas relative to the head
☐ 3. Extends the head at the AOJ	☐ 3. Extends the atlas relative to the head
☐ 4. Contralaterally rotates the head at the AOJ	☐ 4. Ipsilaterally rotates the atlas relative to the head

AOJ = atlanto-occipital joint

Standard Mover Action Notes

- The obliquus capitis superior runs primarily horizontally from the atlas anteriorly to the occiput posteriorly (this is best appreciated when the muscle is viewed laterally). When it contracts, it pulls the occiput anteriorly toward the atlas; therefore it protracts (anteriorly translates) the head on the atlas (C1) at the AOJ. (action 1)
- The obliquus capitis superior crosses the AOJ laterally (with its fibers running slightly vertically in the frontal plane); therefore it laterally flexes the head on the atlas at the AOJ. (action 2)
- The obliquus capitis superior crosses the AOJ posteriorly (with its fibers running slightly vertically in the sagittal plane); therefore it extends the head on the atlas at the AOJ. (action 3)
- When the obliquus capitis superior contracts and moves the occiput, it pulls the occipital attachment laterally toward the

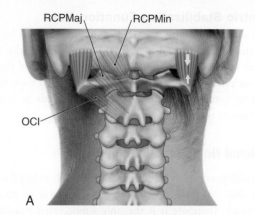

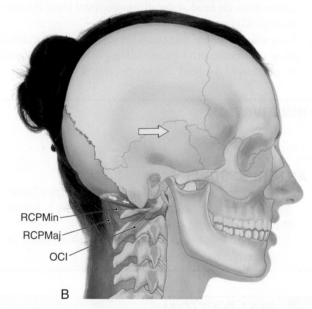

Figure 10-35 Views of the obliquus capitis superior. **A,** Posterior view bilaterally. The other three suboccipital muscles have been ghosted in on the left. **B,** Right lateral view. The other three suboccipital muscles have been ghosted in. OCI, obliquus capitis inferior; RCPMaj, rectus capitis posterior major; RCPMin, rectus capitis posterior minor.

attachment on the atlas. This causes the head to face the opposite side of the body from which the obliquus capitis superior is attached. Therefore, the obliquus capitis superior contralaterally rotates the head on the atlas at the AOJ. (action 4)

Reverse Mover Action Notes

- If the head is fixed, the obliquus capitis superior can move the atlas relative to the head. This is only likely to occur when the client is lying down so that the inferior attachment is mobile. (reverse actions 1, 2, 3, 4)
- The reverse action of contralateral rotation of the head at the AOJ is ipsilateral rotation of the atlas at the AOJ. (reverse action 4)

Obliquus Capitis Superior (of Suboccipital Group)—*cont'd*

Eccentric Antagonist Functions

1. Restrains/slows retraction, opposite-side lateral flexion, flexion, and ipsilateral rotation of the head

Isometric Stabilization Function

1. Stabilizes the head and atlas at the AOJ

Isometric Stabilization Function Note

• The suboccipital muscles are generally thought to be more important as postural stabilization muscles, providing fine control of head posture, than as movers.

Additional Note on Functions

1. Some sources believe that the main role of the suboccipital group is proprioceptive by providing precise monitoring of the position of the head and upper cervical vertebrae.

INNERVATION
☐ The Suboccipital Nerve
   ☐ dorsal ramus of C1

ARTERIAL SUPPLY
☐ The Occipital Artery (a branch of the External Carotid Artery) and the Deep Cervical Artery (a branch of the Costocervical Trunk)
   ☐ and the muscular branches of the Vertebral Artery (a branch of the Subclavian Artery)

✋ PALPATION

1. With the client supine and as relaxed as possible, place palpating fingers just inferior to the occiput, between the transverse process of the atlas (C1) and the occiput, and feel for the fibers of the obliquus capitis superior running superiorly and medially from the transverse process of the atlas toward the occiput.
2. This muscle is challenging to palpate and discern from adjacent musculature.

■ RELATIONSHIP TO OTHER STRUCTURES

☐ The obliquus capitis superior, as with all of the suboccipital muscles, is very deep in the suboccipital region. It is deep to the trapezius, the splenius capitis, the semispinalis capitis, and the sternocleidomastoid.
☐ Deep to the obliquus capitis superior are the occiput and the atlas (C1).
☐ The occipital attachment of the obliquus capitis superior is superficial to the occipital attachment of the rectus capitis posterior major.
☐ The occipital attachment of the obliquus capitis superior is slightly lateral (and partially deep) to the occipital attachment of the semispinalis capitis.
☐ The obliquus capitis superior borders the *suboccipital triangle* of the neck. The suboccipital triangle is located between the rectus capitis posterior major, the obliquus capitis inferior, and the obliquus capitis superior. The suboccipital nerve and the vertebral artery are located in the suboccipital triangle.
☐ The obliquus capitis superior is located within the superficial back line and the lateral line myofascial meridians.

■ MISCELLANEOUS

1. The obliquus capitis superior is one of four muscles that are called the *suboccipital muscles.* They are the rectus capitis posterior major, rectus capitis posterior minor, obliquus capitis inferior, and obliquus capitis superior.
2. In addition to the four suboccipital muscles, there is a rectus capitis anterior and a rectus capitis lateralis.
3. The obliquus capitis superior and the obliquus capitis inferior both attach to the transverse process of the atlas (C1). Four other muscles also attach to the transverse process of the atlas: the levator scapulae, splenius cervicis, rectus capitis anterior, and rectus capitis lateralis.
4. Given its action of protraction of the head at the atlanto-occipital joint, a tight obliquus capitis superior can contribute to a posture of the head being held anteriorly, in other words, protracted.

10

LOW BACK
Quadratus Lumborum (QL)

The name, quadratus lumborum, *tells us that this muscle is shaped somewhat like a square and is located in the lumbar (i.e., lower back) region.*

Derivation	☐ quadratus: L. *squared.*
	lumborum: L. *loin* (low back).
Pronunciation	☐ kwod-RAY-tus, lum-BOR-um

■ ATTACHMENTS

☐ **Twelfth Rib and the Transverse Processes of L1-L4**
   ☐ the medial ½ of the inferior border of the twelfth rib

to the

☐ **Posterior Iliac Crest**
   ☐ the posteromedial iliac crest and the iliolumbar ligament

■ FUNCTIONS

Concentric (Shortening) Mover Actions	
Standard Mover Actions	**Reverse Mover Actions**
☐ 1. Elevates the same-side pelvis at the LS joint and laterally flexes the lower lumbar spine relative to the upper lumbar spine	☐ 1. Laterally flexes the trunk at the spinal joints
	☐ 2. Depresses the twelfth rib at the costospinal joints
☐ 2. Anteriorly tilts the pelvis at the LS joint and extends the lower lumbar spine relative to the upper lumbar spine	☐ 3. Extends the trunk at the spinal joints

LS joint = lumbosacral joint

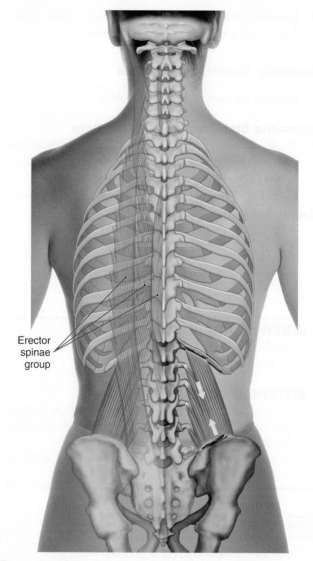

Erector spinae group

Figure 10-36 Posterior view of the quadratus lumborum (QL). The erector spinae group has been ghosted in on the left side.

Standard Mover Action Notes

• With the superior attachments fixed, the quadratus lumborum elevates the same-side (ipsilateral) pelvis at the LS joint (in the frontal plane) by pulling up on the lateral pelvis. Elevation of one side of the pelvis causes the other side to depress. Therefore the quadratus lumborum performs ipsilateral elevation and contralateral depression of the pelvis. (action 1)

• With the superior attachments fixed, the quadratus lumborum anteriorly tilts the pelvis (in the sagittal plane) at the LS joint by pulling up on the posterior pelvis. (action 2)

• When the pelvis moves, because the LS joint does not allow a large degree of motion, the lower lumbar spine will move with the pelvis, causing the lower lumbar spine to laterally flex or extend under the upper lumbar spine. (actions 1, 2)

Reverse Mover Action Notes

• The quadratus lumborum crosses the spinal joints laterally (with its fibers running vertically in the frontal plane); therefore when it contracts and the inferior pelvic attachment is fixed, it laterally flexes the trunk at the spinal joints. (reverse action 1)

• When the pelvic attachment is fixed and the quadratus lumborum contracts, it pulls the twelfth rib inferiorly toward the pelvis. Therefore the quadratus lumborum depresses the twelfth rib at the costospinal joints. (reverse action 2)

• The reverse action of the quadratus lumborum is when the upper attachment moves instead of the lower (pelvic) attach-

Quadratus Lumborum (QL)—cont'd

ment. The quadratus lumborum has two upper attachments, the lumbar spine and the twelfth rib. Therefore it is has two frontal plane reverse actions to ipsilateral (same-side) elevation of the pelvis: lateral flexion of the spine and depression of the twelfth rib. (reverse actions 1, 2)

- The quadratus lumborum crosses the spinal joints posteriorly (with its fibers running vertically in the sagittal plane); therefore when it contract and the inferior pelvis attachment is fixed, it extends the trunk at the spinal joints. (reverse action 3)

Eccentric Antagonist Functions

1. Restrains/slows same-side depression and posterior tilt of the pelvis
2. Restrains/slows flexion and opposite-side lateral flexion of the trunk
3. Restrains/slows elevation of the twelfth rib

Isometric Stabilization Functions

1. Stabilizes the pelvis, lumbar spinal joints, and the twelfth rib

Isometric Stabilization Function Note

- Stabilization of the twelfth rib is an important function of the quadratus lumborum. The quadratus lumborum's force of depression of the twelfth rib stabilizes the twelfth rib from elevating when the diaphragm contracts and pulls superiorly on it. By stabilizing the rib cage attachment of the diaphragm, the contraction of the diaphragm acts to drop its dome, thereby increasing the superior to inferior volume of the thoracic cavity for inspiration (this occurs during abdominal [belly] breathing).

Additional Note on Functions

1. According to some sources, the primary function of the lateral fibers of the quadratus lumborum is to act as a mover of the trunk and/or the pelvis, whereas the primary function of the medial fibers is to posturally stabilize the trunk.

INNERVATION
- ☐ Lumbar Plexus
  - ☐ T12, L1, L2, L3

ARTERIAL SUPPLY
- ☐ Branches of the Subcostal and Lumbar Arteries (all branches of the Aorta)
  - ☐ and the Iliolumbar Artery (a branch of the Internal Iliac Artery)

✋ PALPATION

1. With the client prone, place palpating hand superior to the iliac crest and just lateral to the erector spinae musculature.
2. Have the client elevate the pelvis on the side you are palpating and press in medially, deep to the erector spinae, feeling for the contraction of the quadratus lumborum. (Note: Elevation of the pelvis in this position involves moving the pelvis along the plane of the table, toward the head.)
3. Continue palpating the quadratus lumborum deep to the erector spinae; palpate medially toward the lumbar transverse processes, superomedially toward the twelfth rib, and inferomedially toward the iliac crest.

■ RELATIONSHIP TO OTHER STRUCTURES

- ☐ The quadratus lumborum is very deep and forms part of the posterior abdominal body wall.
- ☐ The majority of the quadratus lumborum is deep to the erector spinae. A small portion of the lateral part of the quadratus lumborum is deep to the muscles of the abdominal wall (external abdominal oblique, internal abdominal oblique, and transversus abdominis).
- ☐ Deep (anterior) to the quadratus lumborum are the abdominal viscera.
- ☐ Slightly anterior and medial to the quadratus lumborum is the psoas major.
- ☐ The quadratus lumborum is involved with the lateral line and located within the deep front line myofascial meridians.

■ MISCELLANEOUS

1. A common variation of the quadratus lumborum is to also have an attachment onto the transverse process of L5.
2. When working on the quadratus lumborum, you can position the client either prone, supine, or side lying. However, because much of it is deep (to the massive erector spinae musculature), it must be accessed with palpatory pressure from lateral to medial (i.e., come in from the side).
3. Keep in mind that the quadratus lumborum is not the only muscle in the lateral lumbar region and should not be blamed for all pain in that area. The erector spinae group is also present in the lateral lumbar region, is functionally active, and also is likely to develop tension and pain.
4. The quadratus lumborum can elevate the pelvis. Often the term *hiking up the hip* is used to describe this action. However, this term can be misleading and ambiguous. Generally when the term *hip* is used (unless the context is otherwise made very clear) it is assumed that movement of the femur at the hip joint is meant, not movement of the pelvis at the lumbosacral joint.
5. Presence of the quadratus lumborum muscles helps to cushion and protect the kidneys.

10

Anterior Abdominal Wall Muscles

The anterior abdominal wall consists of four muscles that attach from the trunk to the pelvis. These muscles are the rectus abdominis, external abdominal oblique, internal abdominal oblique, and transversus abdominis.

ATTACHMENTS

☐ The rectus abdominis is located anteromedially.
☐ The external and internal abdominal obliques and the transversus abdominis are located anterolaterally (and laterally and posterolaterally).
  ☐ The external abdominal oblique is the most superficial of the three anterolateral abdominal wall muscles.
  ☐ The internal abdominal oblique is in the middle.
  ☐ The transversus abdominis is the deepest of the three anterolateral abdominal wall muscles.
  ☐ These three anterolateral abdominal muscles attach far posterior into the low back.
☐ The rectus abdominis is enclosed within the *rectus sheath* (a sheath of muscular fascia).
☐ The midline aponeuroses of the external abdominal oblique, internal abdominal oblique, and the transversus abdominis muscles come together to form the rectus sheath (also known as the *abdominal aponeurosis*), which encloses (ensheathes) the rectus abdominis.
☐ The rectus sheath covers the entire anterior surface of the rectus abdominis. However, posteriorly it only covers the upper 2/3 of the muscle, from the superior attachment of the muscle to the *arcuate line*, located approximately halfway between the umbilicus and the pubic bone. (See cross-sectional Figures 10-4*C*, and 10-4*D*, on page 276.)
☐ The inguinal ligament is actually part of the inferior fascial attachment of the external abdominal oblique.

FUNCTIONS

☐ All four muscles of the anterior abdominal wall can compress the abdominal contents, which plays an important role in expiration and expulsion of abdominal contents (e.g., vomiting, expulsion of feces from the intestines, and expulsion of urine from the bladder).
☐ All of the muscles of the anterior abdominal wall, except for the transversus abdominis, can flex and laterally flex the trunk at the spinal joints and posteriorly tilt and elevate the same-side pelvis at the lumbosacral joint.
☐ The transversus abdominis cannot move the skeleton. Its action is compression of the abdominal contents.
☐ The external abdominal oblique of one side of the body is synergistic with the internal abdominal oblique on the opposite side of the body, with respect to rotation of the trunk at the spinal joints. Note the similarity of the direction of fibers of these muscles.

MISCELLANEOUS

1. Two other muscles, the pyramidalis and the cremaster, are also located in the anterior abdominal wall. See the Evolve website. ⊜volve
2. The anterior abdominal wall muscles are located within the superficial front line, the lateral line, and the spiral line myofascial meridians.

INNERVATION
☐ The anterior abdominal wall muscles are innervated by intercostal nerves.

ARTERIAL SUPPLY
☐ The rectus abdominis receives the majority of its arterial supply from the superior and inferior epigastric arteries. The three lateral anterior abdominal wall muscles receive the majority of their arterial supply from the posterior intercostal and subcostal arteries.

Anterior Abdominal Wall Muscles—Superficial Views

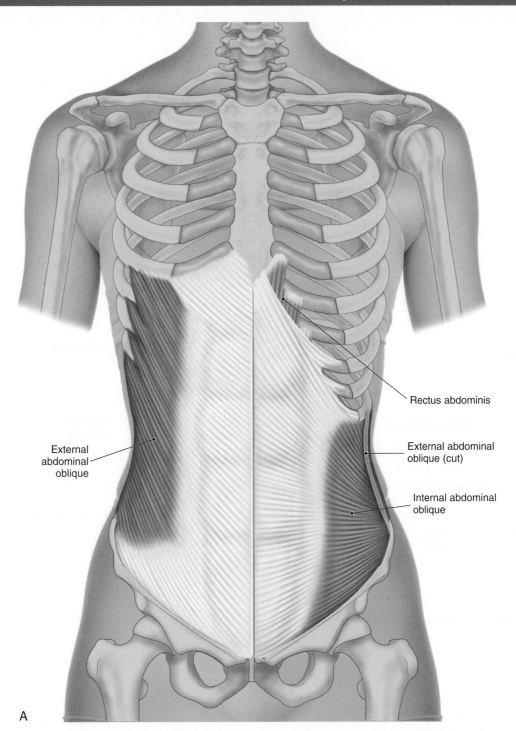

Rectus abdominis

External
abdominal
oblique

External abdominal
oblique (cut)

Internal abdominal
oblique

A

Figure 10-37 Anterior views of the four muscles of the anterior abdominal wall. **A,** Superficial views.

10

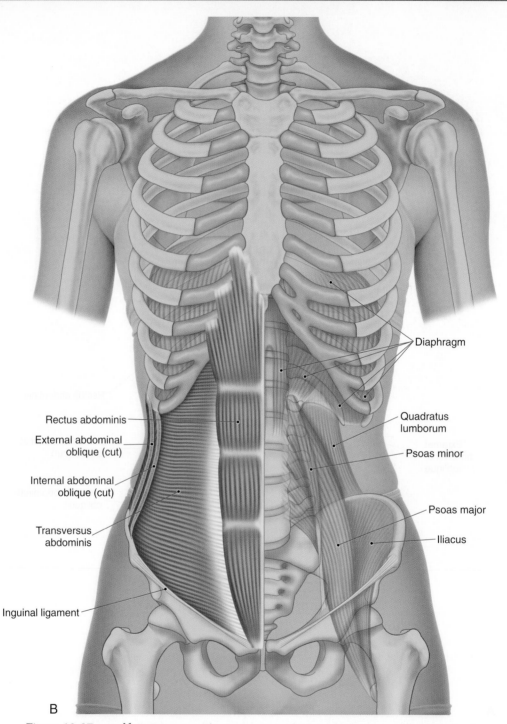

Rectus abdominis

External abdominal oblique (cut)

Internal abdominal oblique (cut)

Transversus abdominis

Inguinal ligament

Diaphragm

Quadratus lumborum

Psoas minor

Psoas major

Iliacus

B

Figure 10-37, cont'd B, Deep view. The psoas major and minor, diaphragm, and quadratus lumborum have been ghosted in on the left.

Rectus Abdominis (of Anterior Abdominal Wall)

The name, rectus abdominis, *tells us that this muscle runs straight up the abdomen.*

Derivation	☐ rectus: L. *straight.*
	abdominis: L. *refers to the abdomen.*
Pronunciation	☐ REK-tus, ab-DOM-i-nis

■ ATTACHMENTS

☐ **Pubis**

   ☐ the crest and symphysis of the pubis

to the

☐ **Xiphoid Process and the Cartilage of Ribs Five through Seven**

■ FUNCTIONS

Concentric (Shortening) Mover Actions	
Standard Mover Actions	**Reverse Mover Actions**
☐ **1. Flexes the trunk at the spinal joints**	☐ **1. Posteriorly tilts the pelvis at the LS joint and flexes the lower trunk relative to the upper trunk**
☐ **2. Laterally flexes the trunk at the spinal joints**	☐ 2. Elevates the same-side pelvis at the LS joint and laterally flexes the lower trunk relative to the upper trunk
☐ 3. Compresses the abdominopelvic cavity	☐ 3. Compresses the abdominopelvic cavity
☐ 4. Depresses the rib cage	☐ 4. Posteriorly tilts and elevates the same-side pelvis (as indicated above)

LS joint = lumbosacral joint

Standard Mover Action Notes

- The rectus abdominis crosses the spinal joints anteriorly (with its fibers running vertically in the sagittal plane) and attaches onto the pelvis. When the pelvis is fixed and the rectus abdominis contracts, it pulls the trunk toward the pelvis anteriorly. Therefore the rectus abdominis flexes the trunk at the spinal joints. (action 1)
- The rectus abdominis crosses the spinal joints slightly on the lateral side (with its fibers running vertically in the frontal plane). When the pelvis is fixed and the rectus abdominis contracts, it pulls the trunk toward the pelvis laterally. Therefore the rectus abdominis laterally flexes the trunk at the spinal joints. Because the rectus abdominis is very close to the midline, it has poor leverage for this action. (action 2)
- The rectus abdominis attaches from the trunk to the pelvis in the anterior abdominal wall (with its fibers running vertically). When both the trunk and the pelvis are fixed and the rectus abdominis contracts, it tautens in toward the abdomen

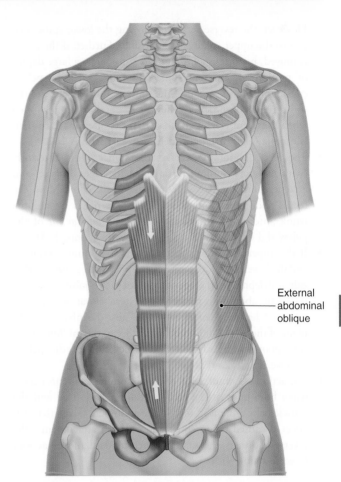

External abdominal oblique

Figure 10-38 Anterior view of the rectus abdominis bilaterally. The external abdominal oblique has been ghosted in on the left.

and exerts a compressive force on the abdominal contents. Compressing the abdominopelvic cavity also causes compression of the thoracic cavity because the abdominal contents push up against the diaphragm. Compression of the body cavities is important when expelling matter from the body, such as when breathing out, coughing, sneezing, vomiting, urinating, defecating, or giving birth. Helping to breathe out means that the rectus abdominis is an accessory muscle of respiration. (action 3)
- If the pelvic attachment of the rectus abdominis is fixed and the muscle contracts, it will pull the rib cage attachment inferiorly. Normally, this would flex the entire trunk at the spinal joints. However, if extensor muscles of the trunk fix (stabilize) the trunk and prevent it from flexing, the lower rib cage will depress. This action is important when breathing out. Therefore the rectus abdominis can act directly on the rib cage as an accessory muscle of respiration. (action 4)

Reverse Mover Action Notes

- When we think of motions of the spine, we usually think of the upper spine moving relative to the fixed lower spine.

Rectus Abdominis (of Anterior Abdominal Wall)—*cont'd*

However, the reverse action of moving the lower spine relative to the upper spine is also possible. Further, if the pelvis is moved, because the LS joint does not allow a large degree of motion, the lumbar spine will move with the pelvis, causing the lower region of the spine to move relative to the upper region of the spine. These reverse actions often happen when the client is lying down so that the inferior attachment is mobile (e.g., turning in bed). (reverse actions 1, 2, 4)

- The rectus abdominis crosses the spinal joints anteriorly (with its fibers running vertically in the sagittal plane) and attaches onto the pelvis. When the trunk is fixed and the rectus abdominis contracts, it pulls the pelvis toward the trunk anteriorly. This motion is called *posterior tilt* of the pelvis and occurs at the LS joint. (reverse actions 1, 4)
- If the upper attachment of the rectus abdominis stays fixed and the lower attachment moves, the pelvis will elevate on that side and depress on the opposite side at the LS joint. Therefore the rectus abdominis performs ipsilateral elevation and contralateral depression of the pelvis. Because the inferior attachment of the rectus abdominis is so close to the midline, it has very poor leverage for ipsilateral elevation of the pelvis. (reverse actions 2, 4)
- The action of compression of the abdominal contents occurs when both ends of the rectus abdominis are fixed and the muscle belly tautens in toward the abdomen. Given that this effect is caused by an equal pull on both attachments, the reverse action is the same as the standard mover action. (reverse action 3)

Eccentric Antagonist Functions

1. Restrains/slows extension and opposite-side lateral flexion of the trunk
2. Restrains/slows anterior tilt and same-side depression of the pelvis
3. Restrains/slows expansion of the abdominopelvic cavity
4. Restrains/slows elevation of the rib cage

Eccentric Antagonist Function Note

- The eccentric function of restraining/slowing extension of the trunk is important when returning to the floor during a curl-up exercise.

Isometric Stabilization Functions

1. Stabilizes the lumbar spinal joints
2. Stabilizes the pelvis
3. Stabilizes the rib cage

Isometric Stabilization Function Note

- Stabilization of the lumbar spinal joints and the pelvis is stabilization of the *core of the body*. Although the transversus abdominis is best known for this function, the other abdominal muscles can assist.

Additional Notes on Functions

1. Performing curl-ups (crunches, sit-ups) is an effective way to engage and strengthen the rectus abdominis. If neck discomfort occurs, reverse curl-ups can be done in which the pelvis is anteriorly tilted toward the trunk and lifted from the floor (and the lower trunk flexes up toward the upper trunk) instead of flexing the (upper) trunk toward the pelvis.

2. It is often asserted that moving the superior attachment of the rectus abdominis (such as flexing the trunk when doing a curl-up) only engages the upper compartments, and moving the inferior attachment (such as posteriorly tilting the pelvis when doing a reverse curl-up) only engages the lower compartments. However, it is not possible for the upper or lower compartments to generate tension if the entire muscle does not engage. For example, if the upper compartments were to be relaxed and the lower compartments were to engage to move the pelvis, the lower compartments would end up exerting their pull on the fibers of the upper compartments, stretching them longer, instead of exerting their pull to move the pelvis. Similarly, if the lower compartments were relaxed and the upper compartments engaged, their tension force would be dissipated pulling on (and lengthening) the relaxed lower compartment fibers. Therefore, regardless of which attachment moves, all compartments of the rectus abdominis must engage and contract.

INNERVATION
- ☐ Intercostal Nerves
  - ☐ ventral rami of T5-T12

ARTERIAL SUPPLY
- ☐ The Superior Epigastric Artery (a branch of the Internal Thoracic Artery) and the Inferior Epigastric Artery (a branch of the External Iliac Artery)
  - ☐ and the terminal branches of the Subcostal and Posterior Intercostal Arteries (all branches of the Aorta)

✋ PALPATION

1. With the client supine with a pillow placed under the knees, place palpating hands between the xiphoid process of the sternum and the adjacent ribs superiorly, and the pubis inferiorly.
2. Have the client alternate between mild flexion of the trunk (a small curl-up) and relaxation so that you can feel for the contraction of the rectus abdominis.
3. Palpate the rectus abdominis superiorly toward its rib cage attachment and inferiorly toward its pelvic attachment.

10

Rectus Abdominis (of Anterior Abdominal Wall)—*cont'd*

■ RELATIONSHIP TO OTHER STRUCTURES

☐ The rectus abdominis is superficial in the anteromedial abdomen. It is encased in the rectus sheath (also known as the abdominal aponeurosis), which is made up of the aponeuroses of the external and internal abdominal obliques and the transversus abdominis.

☐ Deep to the rectus abdominis is the peritoneum of the abdominal cavity.

☐ Lateral to the rectus abdominis are the other three muscles of the anterior abdominal wall, the external and internal abdominal obliques and the transversus abdominis.

☐ Medial to the rectus abdominis is the linea alba.

☐ The rectus abdominis is located within the superficial front line myofascial meridian.

■ MISCELLANEOUS

1. Three fibrous bands known as *tendinous inscriptions* transect the rectus abdominis muscles and divide each one of them into four sections or boxes. For this reason, the rectus abdominis muscles in a well-developed individual are often known as the *eight-pack (8-pack) muscle*. (Actually, it is more often incorrectly labeled the *six-pack [6-pack] muscle,* because six of the eight compartments are more visible.)

2. Each rectus abdominis is encased in the rectus sheath, which is made up of the aponeuroses of the other three anterior abdominal wall muscles (the external and internal abdominal obliques and the transversus abdominis). The two rectus sheaths (left and right) meet in the midline of the abdomen and form the *linea alba.*

3. The four muscles of the anterior abdominal wall are the rectus abdominis, external abdominal oblique, internal abdominal oblique, and transversus abdominis. All of these muscles compress against the abdominal contents and help create a flat abdomen.

4. When old-fashioned straight-legged sit-ups are done, the movement that occurs is not flexion of the trunk at the spinal joints but rather is anterior tilt of the pelvis at the hip joints (with the trunk moving up into the air because it is fixed to the pelvis). In this circumstance, the movers are not the abdominal wall muscles but rather the flexors of the hip joints (because anterior tilt of the pelvis at the hip joint is the reverse action of flexion of the thigh at the hip joint). The abdominal wall muscles do contract, but not as movers; they contract as fixators (i.e., stabilizers) of the pelvis, locking it to the trunk.

10

External Abdominal Oblique (of Anterior Abdominal Wall)

The name, external abdominal oblique, *tells us that this muscle is located externally in the abdomen (superficial to the internal abdominal oblique) and its fibers are oriented obliquely.*

Derivation	☐ external:	L. *outside.*
	abdominal:	L. *refers to the abdomen.*
	oblique:	L. *slanting, diagonal.*
Pronunciation	☐ EKS-turn-al, ab-DOM-in-al,	
	o-BLEEK	

■ ATTACHMENTS

☐ **Anterior Iliac Crest, Pubic Bone, and the Abdominal Aponeurosis**
  ☐ the pubic crest and tubercle

to the

☐ **Lower Eight Ribs (Ribs Five through Twelve)**
  ☐ the inferior border of the ribs

■ FUNCTIONS

Concentric (Shortening) Mover Actions	
Standard Mover Actions	**Reverse Mover Actions**
☐ **1. Flexes the trunk at the spinal joints**	☐ **1. Posteriorly tilts the pelvis at the LS joint and flexes the lower trunk relative to the upper trunk**
☐ **2. Laterally flexes the trunk at the spinal joints**	☐ 2. Elevates the same-side pelvis at the LS joint and laterally flexes the lower trunk relative to the upper trunk
☐ **3. Contralaterally rotates the trunk at the spinal joints**	☐ 3. Ipsilaterally rotates the pelvis at the LS joint and ipsilaterally rotates the lower trunk relative to the upper trunk
☐ 4. Compresses the abdominopelvic cavity	☐ 4. Compresses the abdominopelvic cavity
☐ 5. Depresses the rib cage	☐ 5. Posteriorly tilts, elevates the same-side, and ipsilaterally tilts the pelvis (as indicated above)

LS joint = lumbosacral joint

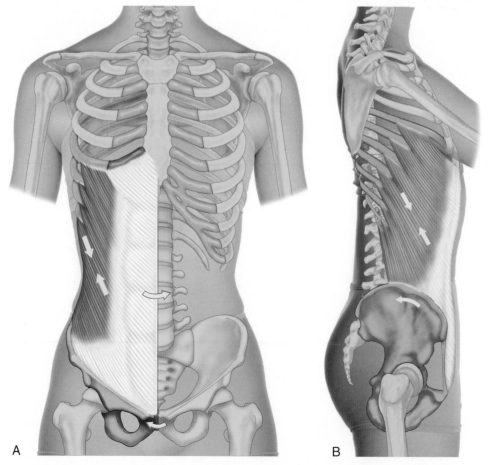

Figure 10-39 Views of the right external abdominal oblique. **A,** Anterior view. **B,** Right lateral view.

10

External Abdominal Oblique (of Anterior Abdominal Wall)—cont'd

Standard Mover Action Notes

- The external abdominal oblique crosses the spinal joints anteriorly (with its fibers running vertically in the sagittal plane) and attaches onto the pelvis. When the pelvis is fixed and the external abdominal oblique contracts, it pulls the trunk toward the pelvis anteriorly. Therefore the external abdominal oblique flexes the trunk at the spinal joints. (action 1)
- The external abdominal oblique crosses the spinal joints laterally (with its fibers running vertically in the frontal plane). When the pelvis is fixed and the external abdominal oblique contracts, it pulls the trunk toward the pelvis laterally. Therefore the external abdominal oblique laterally flexes the trunk at the spinal joints. (action 2)
- The external abdominal oblique wraps around the trunk (with its fibers running somewhat horizontally in the transverse plane). When the pelvis is fixed and the external abdominal oblique contracts, it pulls on the trunk, causing the anterior surface of the trunk to face the opposite side of the body from the side of the body to which it is attached. Therefore the external abdominal oblique contralaterally rotates the trunk at the spinal joints. (action 3)
- The external and internal abdominal obliques are the prime movers of rotation of the trunk at the spinal joints. (action 3)
- The external abdominal oblique attaches from the trunk to the pelvis in the abdominal wall (with its fibers running somewhat vertically). When both the trunk and the pelvis are fixed and the external abdominal oblique contracts, it exerts a compressive force on the abdomen. Compressing the abdominopelvic cavity also causes compression of the thoracic cavity because the abdominal contents push up against the diaphragm. Compression of the body cavities is important when expelling matter from the body, such as when breathing out, coughing, sneezing, vomiting, urinating, defecating, or giving birth. Helping to breathe out means that the external abdominal oblique is an accessory muscle of respiration. (action 4)
- If the pelvic attachment of the external abdominal oblique is fixed and it contracts, it will pull the rib cage attachment inferiorly. Normally, this would flex and/or laterally flex the entire trunk at the spinal joints. However, if extensor and opposite-side lateral flexor muscles of the trunk fix (stabilize) the trunk and prevent it from moving, the lower eight ribs will depress. This action is important when breathing out. Therefore the external abdominal oblique can act directly on the rib cage as an accessory muscle of respiration. (action 5)

Reverse Mover Action Notes

- When we think of motions of the spine, we usually think of the upper spine moving relative to the fixed lower spine.

However, the reverse action of moving the lower spine relative to the upper spine is also possible. Further, if the pelvis is moved, because the LS joint does not allow a large degree of motion, the lumbar spine will move with the pelvis, causing the lower region of the spine to move relative to the upper region of the spine. These reverse actions often happen when the client is lying down so that the inferior attachment is mobile (e.g., turning in bed). (reverse actions 1, 2, 3, 5)

- The external abdominal oblique crosses the spinal joints anteriorly (with its fibers running vertically in the sagittal plane) and attaches onto the pelvis. When the trunk is fixed and the external abdominal oblique contracts, it pulls the pelvis toward the trunk anteriorly. This motion is called *posterior tilt* of the pelvis and occurs at the LS joint. (reverse actions 1, 5)
- When the superior attachments of the external abdominal oblique are fixed and it contracts, it pulls the lateral pelvis superiorly toward the rib cage. Therefore the external abdominal oblique elevates the pelvis on that side at the LS joint. Elevation of one side of the pelvis causes the other side to depress. Therefore the external abdominal oblique performs ipsilateral elevation and contralateral depression of the pelvis. (reverse actions 2, 5)
- When the superior attachments of the external abdominal oblique are fixed and it contracts, it pulls on the inferior attachment, the pelvis, causing the anterior surface of the pelvis to face the same side of the body to which the external abdominal oblique is attached (because the fibers of the external abdominal oblique have a horizontal orientation in the transverse plane). Therefore the external abdominal oblique ipsilaterally rotates the pelvis at the LS joint. (reverse action 3)
- The reverse action of contralaterally rotating the upper spine (relative to the fixed lower spine and pelvis) is to ipsilaterally rotate the pelvis and lower spine (relative to the fixed upper spine). In other words, if the right-sided external abdominal oblique does left rotation of the upper spine, its reverse action would be to do right rotation of the pelvis at the LS joint and to do right rotation of the lower spine relative to the upper spine. (reverse actions 3, 5)
- The action of compression of the abdominal contents occurs when both ends of the external abdominal oblique are fixed and the muscle belly tautens in toward the abdomen. Given that this effect is caused by an equal pull on both attachments, the reverse action is the same as the standard mover action. (reverse action 4)

Eccentric Antagonist Functions

1. Restrains/slows extension and opposite-side lateral flexion of the trunk
2. Restrains/slows anterior tilt and same-side depression of the pelvis

10

External Abdominal Oblique (of Anterior Abdominal Wall)—cont'd

3. Restrains/slows ipsilateral rotation of the upper trunk and contralateral rotation of the pelvis and lower trunk
4. Restrains/slows expansion of the abdominopelvic cavity
5. Restrains/slows elevation of the rib cage

Eccentric Antagonist Function Note

• The eccentric function of restraining/slowing extension of the trunk is important when returning to the floor during a curl-up exercise.

Isometric Stabilization Functions

1. Stabilizes the lumbar spinal joints
2. Stabilizes the pelvis
3. Stabilizes the rib cage

Isometric Stabilization Function Note

• Stabilization of the lumbar spinal joints and the pelvis is stabilization of the *core of the body*. Although the transversus abdominis is best known for this function, the other abdominal muscles can assist.

Additional Notes on Functions

1. It is very interesting to compare exactly how the four abdominal oblique muscles are synergistic and/or antagonistic to each other. For example, the right external abdominal oblique and left internal abdominal oblique are synergistic with regard to flexion in the sagittal plane, antagonistic with regard to lateral flexions in the frontal plane, and synergistic with regard to left rotation in the transverse plane. Hence, two muscles may be both synergistic and antagonistic to each other. This exemplifies the idea that whenever we look to determine whether two muscles are synergistic or antagonistic to each other, we need to do so relative to a specific joint action within one plane.
2. With regard to flexion, all four abdominal obliques are synergistic to each other.
3. With regard to lateral flexion of the trunk at the spinal joints, the external and internal abdominal obliques on the same side are synergistic to each other.
4. The external abdominal oblique is a contralateral rotator of the trunk at the spinal joints, and the internal abdominal oblique is an ipsilateral rotator of the trunk at the spinal joints; hence with regard to trunk rotation (i.e., transverse plane actions), they are antagonistic to each other. However, the external abdominal oblique on one side of the body is synergistic with the internal abdominal oblique on the opposite side of the body during trunk rotation. Similarly, the external abdominal oblique is an ipsilateral rotator of the pelvis at the LS joint, and the internal abdominal oblique is a contralateral rotator of the pelvis at the LS joint; hence with regard to pelvic rotation (i.e., transverse plane actions),

they are antagonistic to each other. However, the external abdominal oblique on one side of the body is synergistic with the internal abdominal oblique on the opposite side of the body during pelvic rotation. Note the similarity of the direction of their fibers.

5. Performing curl-ups (crunches, sit-ups) is an effective way to engage and strengthen the external abdominal obliques, especially if rotation is added to the flexion (some repetitions rotated to the right and some repetitions rotated to the left). If neck discomfort occurs, reverse curl-ups can be done in which the pelvis is anteriorly tilted toward the trunk and lifted from the floor (and the lower trunk flexes up toward the upper trunk) instead of flexing the (upper) trunk toward the pelvis. The pelvis can also be rotated as it is lifted to better engage the external abdominal obliques.

INNERVATION

☐ Intercostal Nerves
  ☐ ventral rami of T7-T12

ARTERIAL SUPPLY

☐ The Subcostal and Posterior Intercostal Arteries (all branches of the Aorta) and the Deep Circumflex Iliac Artery (a branch of the External Iliac Artery)
  ☐ and the Inferior Epigastric Artery (a branch of the External Iliac Artery)

✋ PALPATION

1. With the client supine with a pillow placed under the knees, place palpating hands on the anterolateral abdomen between the iliac crest and the lower ribs.
2. Ask the client to rotate the trunk at the spinal joints to the opposite side (along with slight flexion of the trunk) and feel for the contraction of the external abdominal oblique.
3. Continue palpating the external abdominal oblique superolaterally toward the rib attachments and inferomedially toward the iliac crest and the abdominal aponeurosis.

■ RELATIONSHIP TO OTHER STRUCTURES

☐ The external abdominal oblique is located lateral to the rectus abdominis.
☐ The external abdominal oblique is the most superficial of the three layers of the anterolateral abdominal wall. Directly deep to the external abdominal oblique is the internal abdominal oblique, and deep to that is the transversus abdominis.
☐ The external abdominal oblique interdigitates with the serratus anterior (at ribs five through nine) along the antero-

External Abdominal Oblique (of Anterior Abdominal Wall)—*cont'd*

lateral body wall. The external abdominal oblique's fibers also meet fibers of the latissimus dorsi (at approximately a perpendicular angle at ribs ten through twelve) along the posterolateral body wall.

☐ Keep in mind that the external abdominal oblique is located not only in the anterior abdominal wall but also in the lateral abdominal wall; it reaches all the way to the posterior abdominal wall, where it interdigitates with the latissimus dorsi at ribs ten through twelve.

☐ The external abdominal oblique is located within the lateral line and spiral line and involved with the superficial front line myofascial meridians.

■ MISCELLANEOUS

1. If you were to put your hand into a coat pocket, your fingers would be pointing along the direction of the fibers of the external abdominal oblique on that side. For this reason, the external abdominal obliques are sometimes called the *pocket muscles.*

2. The aponeurosis of the external abdominal oblique, between the anterior superior iliac spine and the pubic tubercle, forms the inguinal ligament.

3. The abdominal aponeurosis is actually the midline aponeurosis of the three anterolateral abdominal wall muscles (external and internal abdominal obliques and the transversus abdominis). The abdominal aponeurosis is also known as the rectus sheath because it envelops/ensheathes the rectus abdominis.

10

Internal Abdominal Oblique (of Anterior Abdominal Wall)

The name, internal abdominal oblique, *tells us that this muscle is located internally in the abdomen (deep to the external abdominal oblique) and its fibers are oriented obliquely.*

Derivation	☐ internal: L. *inside.*
	abdominal: L. *refers to the abdomen.*
	oblique: L. *slanting, diagonal.*
Pronunciation	☐ in-TURN-al, ab-DOM-in-al,
	o-BLEEK

■ ATTACHMENTS

☐ **Inguinal Ligament, Iliac Crest, and the Thoracolumbar Fascia**

  ☐ the lateral ⅔ of the inguinal ligament

to the

☐ **Lower Three Ribs (Ten through Twelve) and the Abdominal Aponeurosis**

■ FUNCTIONS

Concentric (Shortening) Mover Actions

Standard Mover Actions	Reverse Mover Actions
☐ 1. Flexes the trunk at the spinal joints	☐ 1. Posteriorly tilts the pelvis at the LS joint and flexes the lower trunk relative to the upper trunk
☐ 2. Laterally flexes the trunk at the spinal joints	☐ 2. Elevates the same-side pelvis at the LS joint and laterally flexes the lower trunk relative to the upper trunk
☐ 3. Ipsilaterally rotates the trunk at the spinal joints	☐ 3. Contralaterally rotates the pelvis at the LS joint and contralaterally rotates the lower trunk relative to the upper trunk
☐ 4. Compresses the abdominopelvic cavity	☐ 4. Compresses the abdominopelvic cavity
☐ 5. Depresses the rib cage	☐ 5. Posteriorly tilts, elevates the same-side, and contralaterally rotates the pelvis (as indicated above)

LS joint = lumbosacral joint

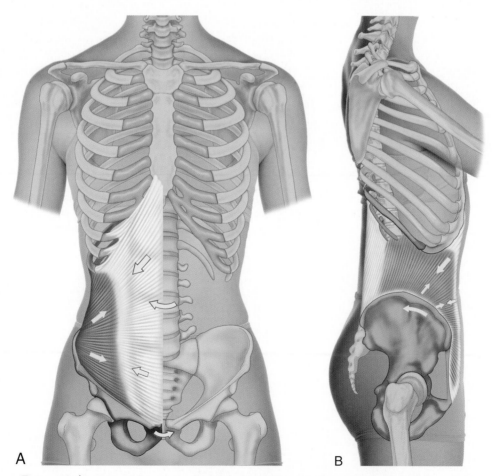

Figure 10-40 Views of the right internal abdominal oblique. **A,** Anterior view. **B,** Right lateral view.

10

Internal Abdominal Oblique (of Anterior Abdominal Wall)—*cont'd*

Standard Mover Action Notes

- The internal abdominal oblique crosses the spinal joints anteriorly (with its fibers running vertically in the sagittal plane) and attaches onto the pelvis. When the pelvis is fixed and the internal abdominal oblique contracts, it pulls the trunk toward the pelvis anteriorly. Therefore the internal abdominal oblique flexes the trunk at the spinal joints. (action 1)

- The internal abdominal oblique crosses the spinal joints laterally (with its fibers running vertically in the frontal plane). When the pelvis is fixed and the internal abdominal oblique contracts, it pulls the trunk toward the pelvis laterally. Therefore the internal abdominal oblique laterally flexes the trunk at the spinal joints. (action 2)

- The internal abdominal oblique wraps around the trunk (with its fibers running somewhat horizontally in the transverse plane). When the pelvis is fixed and the internal abdominal oblique contracts, it pulls on the trunk, causing the anterior surface of the trunk to face the same side of the body to which it is attached. Therefore the internal abdominal oblique ipsilaterally rotates the trunk at the spinal joints. (action 3)

- The external and internal abdominal obliques are the prime movers of rotation of the trunk at the spinal joints. (action 3)

- The internal abdominal oblique attaches from the trunk to the pelvis in the anterior abdominal wall (with its fibers running somewhat vertically). When both the trunk and the pelvis are fixed and the internal abdominal oblique contracts, it exerts a compressive force on the abdomen. Compressing the abdominopelvic cavity also causes compression of the thoracic cavity because the abdominal contents push up against the diaphragm. Compression of the body cavities is important when expelling matter from the body, such as when breathing out, coughing, sneezing, vomiting, urinating, defecating, or giving birth. Helping to breathe out means that the internal abdominal oblique is an accessory muscle of respiration. (action 4)

- If the pelvic attachment of the internal abdominal oblique is fixed and it contracts, it will pull the rib cage attachment inferiorly. Normally, this would flex and/or laterally flex the entire trunk at the spinal joints. However, if extensor and opposite-side lateral flexor muscles of the trunk fix (stabilize) the trunk and prevent it from moving, the lower ribs will depress. This action is important when breathing out. Therefore the internal abdominal oblique can act directly on the rib cage as an accessory muscle of respiration. (action 5)

Reverse Mover Action Notes

- When we think of motions of the spine, we usually think of the upper spine moving relative to the fixed lower spine. However, the reverse action of moving the lower spine relative to the upper spine is also possible. Further, if the pelvis is moved, because the LS joint does not allow a large degree of motion, the lumbar spine will move with the pelvis, causing the lower region of the spine to move relative to the upper region of the spine. These reverse actions often happen when the client is lying down so that the inferior attachment is mobile (e.g., turning in bed). (reverse actions 1, 2, 3, 5)

- The internal abdominal oblique crosses the spinal joints anteriorly (with its fibers running vertically in the sagittal plane) and attaches onto the pelvis. When the trunk is fixed and the internal abdominal oblique contracts, it pulls the pelvis toward the trunk anteriorly. This motion is called *posterior tilt* of the pelvis and occurs at the LS joint. (reverse actions 1, 5)

- When the superior attachments of the internal abdominal oblique are fixed and it contracts, it pulls the lateral pelvis superiorly toward the rib cage. Therefore the internal abdominal oblique elevates the pelvis on that side at the LS joint. Elevation of one side of the pelvis causes the other side to depress. Therefore the internal abdominal oblique performs ipsilateral elevation and contralateral depression of the pelvis. (reverse actions 2, 5)

- When the superior attachments of the internal abdominal oblique are fixed and it contracts, it pulls on the inferior attachment, the pelvis, causing the anterior surface of the pelvis to face the opposite side of the body from the side of the body on which the internal abdominal oblique is attached (because the fibers of the internal abdominal oblique have a horizontal orientation in the transverse plane). Therefore the internal abdominal oblique contralaterally rotates the pelvis at the LS joint. (reverse action 3)

- The reverse action of ipsilaterally rotating the upper spine (relative to the fixed lower spine and pelvis) is to contralaterally rotate the pelvis and lower spine (relative to the fixed upper spine). In other words, if the right-sided internal abdominal oblique does right rotation of the upper spine, its reverse action would be to do left rotation of the pelvis at the LS joint and to do left rotation of the lower spine relative to the upper spine. (reverse actions 3, 5)

- The action of compression of the abdominal contents occurs when both ends of the internal abdominal oblique are fixed and the muscle belly tautens in toward the abdomen. Given that this effect is caused by an equal pull on both attachments, the reverse action is the same as the standard mover action. (reverse action 4)

Eccentric Antagonist Functions

1. Restrains/slows extension and opposite-side lateral flexion of the trunk
2. Restrains/slows anterior tilt and same-side depression of the pelvis
3. Restrains/slows contralateral rotation of the trunk and ipsilateral rotation of the pelvis and lower trunk

Internal Abdominal Oblique (of Anterior Abdominal Wall)—*cont'd*

4. Restrains/slows expansion of the abdominopelvic cavity
5. Restrains/slows elevation of the rib cage

Eccentric Antagonist Function Note

- The eccentric function of restraining/slowing extension of the trunk is important when returning to the floor during a curl-up exercise.

Isometric Stabilization Functions

1. Stabilizes the spinal joints
2. Stabilizes the pelvis
3. Stabilizes the rib cage

Isometric Stabilization Function Notes

- Stabilization of the lumbar spinal joints and the pelvis is stabilization of the *core of the body*. Although the transversus abdominis is best known for this function, the other abdominal muscles can assist.

Additional Notes on Functions

1. It is very interesting to compare exactly how the four abdominal oblique muscles are synergistic and/or antagonistic to each other. For example, the right internal abdominal oblique and right external abdominal oblique are synergistic with regard to flexion in the sagittal plane, synergistic with regard to right lateral flexion in the frontal plane, and antagonistic with regard to rotations in the transverse plane. Hence, two muscles may be both synergistic and antagonistic to each other. This exemplifies the idea that whenever we look to determine whether two muscles are synergistic or antagonistic to each other, we need to do so relative to a specific joint action within one plane.
2. With regard to flexion, all four abdominal obliques are synergistic to each other.
3. With regard to lateral flexion of the trunk at the spinal joints, the external and internal abdominal obliques on the same side are synergistic to each other.
4. The internal abdominal oblique is an ipsilateral rotator of the trunk at the spinal joints, and the external abdominal oblique is a contralateral rotator of the trunk at the spinal joints; hence with regard to trunk rotation (i.e., transverse plane actions), they are antagonistic to each other. However, the internal abdominal oblique on one side of the body is synergistic with the external abdominal oblique on the opposite side of the body during trunk rotation. Similarly, the internal abdominal oblique is a contralateral rotator of the pelvis at the LS joint, and the external abdominal oblique is an ipsilateral rotator of the pelvis at the LS joint; hence with regard to pelvic rotation (i.e., transverse plane actions), they are antagonistic to each other. However, the internal abdominal oblique on one side of the body is synergistic with the external abdominal oblique on the opposite side of

the body during pelvic rotation. Note the similarity of the direction of their fibers.
5. Performing curl-ups (crunches, sit-ups) is an effective way to engage and strengthen the internal abdominal obliques, especially if rotation is added to the flexion (some repetitions rotated to the right and some repetitions rotated to the left). If neck discomfort occurs, reverse curl-ups can be done in which the pelvis is anteriorly tilted toward the trunk and lifted from the floor (and the lower trunk flexes up toward the upper trunk) instead of flexing the (upper) trunk toward the pelvis. The pelvis can also be rotated as it is lifted to better engage the internal abdominal obliques.

INNERVATION
- [ ] Intercostal Nerves
  - [ ] ventral rami of T7-L1

ARTERIAL SUPPLY
- [ ] The Subcostal and Posterior Intercostal Arteries (all branches of the Aorta) and the Deep Circumflex Iliac Artery (a branch of the External Iliac Artery)
  - [ ] and the Inferior Epigastric Artery (a branch of the External Iliac Artery)

✋ PALPATION

1. With the client supine with a pillow placed under the knees, place palpating hands on the anterolateral abdomen between the iliac crest and the lower ribs.
2. Ask the client to actively rotate the trunk at the spinal joints to the same side (along with slight flexion of the trunk) and feel for the contraction of the internal abdominal oblique.
3. Continue palpating the internal abdominal oblique superiorly and inferiorly toward its attachments.
4. Note: Discerning the contraction of the internal abdominal oblique from the contraction of the external abdominal oblique can be challenging if the client has not developed these muscles.

■ RELATIONSHIP TO OTHER STRUCTURES

- [ ] The internal abdominal oblique is located lateral to the rectus abdominis.
- [ ] The internal abdominal oblique is the middle muscle of the three anterolateral abdominal wall muscles. It is deep to the external abdominal oblique and superficial to the transversus abdominis.
- [ ] Keep in mind that the internal abdominal oblique is located not only in the anterior abdominal wall but also in the lateral abdominal wall and posterior abdominal wall. It attaches

10

Internal Abdominal Oblique (of Anterior Abdominal Wall)—*cont'd*

posteriorly into the thoracolumbar fascia (just lateral to the erector spinae), and via the thoracolumbar fascia, attaches into the transverse processes of the lumbar spine.

☐ The internal abdominal oblique is located within the lateral line and spiral line and involved with the superficial front line myofascial meridians.

■ MISCELLANEOUS

1. If you were to put your hand into a coat pocket, your fingers would be pointing along the direction of the fibers of the external abdominal oblique on that side. The fibers of the internal abdominal oblique are exactly 90 degrees opposite (i.e., perpendicular) to those of the external abdominal oblique.

2. The midline aponeuroses of the external abdominal oblique, the internal abdominal oblique, and the transversus abdominis form the rectus sheath that envelops/ensheathes the rectus abdominis. Part of the internal abdominal oblique's midline aponeurosis actually splits and wraps around the rectus abdominis both superficially and deep. (This occurs superior to the arcuate line, which is located approximately halfway between the umbilicus and the pubic bone. See cross-sectional Figures 10-4, *C,* and 10-4, *D,* on page 276.)

Transversus Abdominis (of Anterior Abdominal Wall)

The name, transversus abdominis, *tells us that this muscle runs transversely across the abdomen.*

Derivation	☐ transversus: L. *running transversely.*
	abdominis: L. *refers to the abdomen.*
Pronunciation	☐ trans-VER-sus, ab-DOM-i-nis

■ ATTACHMENTS

☐ **Inguinal Ligament, Iliac Crest, Thoracolumbar Fascia, and the Lower Costal Cartilages**
  ☐ the lateral ⅔ of the inguinal ligament; the lower six costal cartilages (of ribs seven through twelve)

  to the

☐ **Abdominal Aponeurosis**

■ FUNCTIONS

Concentric (Shortening) Mover Actions	
Standard Mover Actions	**Reverse Mover Actions**
☐ **1. Compresses abdominopelvic cavity**	☐ 1. Compresses abdominopelvic cavity

Standard Mover Action Notes

• The transversus abdominis attaches from the thoracolumbar fascia posteriorly, to the linea alba anteriorly, and from the lower ribs superiorly, to the iliac crest and inguinal ligament inferiorly (with its fibers running horizontally). The transversus abdominis does not cause skeletal movement. Instead, the two transversus abdominis muscles bilaterally act like a sphincter muscle, pulling in and compressing the abdominopelvic cavity. Compressing the abdominopelvic cavity also causes compression of the thoracic cavity because the abdominal contents push up against the diaphragm. Compression of the body cavities is important when expelling matter from the body, such as when breathing out, coughing, sneezing, vomiting, urinating, defecating, or giving birth. Helping to breathe out means that the transversus abdominis is an accessory muscle of respiration. (action 1)

Reverse Mover Action Notes

• The action of compression of the abdominal contents occurs when both ends of the transversus abdominis are fixed and

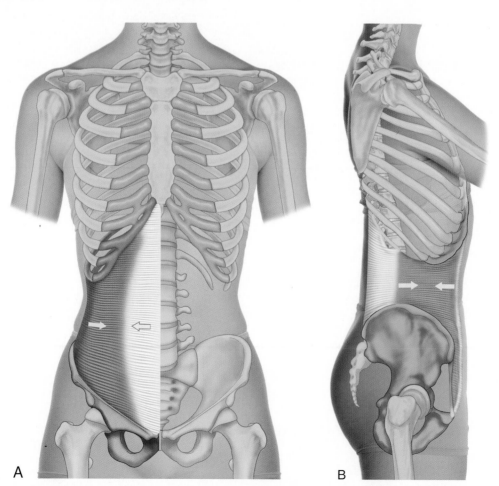

Figure 10-41 Views of the right transversus abdominis. **A,** Anterior view. **B,** Right lateral view.

Transversus Abdominis (of Anterior Abdominal Wall)—*cont'd*

the muscle belly tautens in toward the abdomen. Given that this effect is caused by an equal pull on both attachments, the reverse action is the same as the standard action. (reverse action 1)

Eccentric Antagonist Function

1. Restrains/slows expansion of the abdominopelvic cavity

Isometric Stabilization Functions

1. Stabilizes the lumbar spinal joints
2. Stabilizes the pelvis
3. Stabilizes the lower ribs

Isometric Stabilization Function Notes

- The transversus abdominis, along with the multifidus, is credited as being one of the most important muscles for core stabilization of the body.
- The transversus abdominis can also tighten and stabilize the linea alba. This can help increase the efficiency of the actions of the external and internal abdominal obliques because they attach via the abdominal aponeurosis into the linea alba.

Additional Note on Functions

1. Because the fibers of the transversus abdominis run horizontally in the transverse plane, it would seem that this muscle is ideally suited to create rotation of the trunk at the spinal joints; however, this action seems to be negligible at best. For rotation to occur, its anterior attachment (abdominal aponeurosis) would have to stay fixed, so that it could pull on its spinal attachment (theoretically causing the spinous processes to rotate to that side, which rotates the anterior surfaces of the vertebral bodies to the opposite side, creating contralateral rotation of the trunk). However, fixing the anterior attachment (abdominal aponeurosis) cannot be done by the contralateral transversus abdominis because it would then also pull on the same vertebrae from the opposite side, fighting the ability of the other transversus abdominis to rotate the vertebrae. (Note: The same problem would occur if the contralateral external abdominal oblique were to contract to stabilize the abdominal aponeurosis. Therefore, for rotation to occur, the abdominal aponeurosis would have to be stabilized by the contralateral internal abdominal oblique.)

INNERVATION

- ☐ Intercostal Nerves
  - ☐ ventral rami of T7-L1

ARTERIAL SUPPLY

- ☐ The Subcostal and Posterior Intercostal Arteries (all branches of the Aorta) and the Deep Circumflex Iliac Artery (a branch of the External Iliac Artery)
- ☐ and the Inferior Epigastric Artery (a branch of the External Iliac Artery)

✋ PALPATION

1. With the client supine with a pillow placed under the knees, place palpating hands on the anterolateral abdomen between the iliac crest and the lower ribs.
2. Have the client forcefully exhale and feel for the contraction of the transversus abdominis.
3. The external and internal abdominal obliques will likely engage with this action as well. Discerning the contraction of the transversus abdominis from these other muscles will be extremely challenging.

■ RELATIONSHIP TO OTHER STRUCTURES

- ☐ The transversus abdominis is lateral to the rectus abdominis.
- ☐ The transversus abdominis is the deepest of the three anterolateral abdominal wall muscles. It is directly deep to the internal abdominal oblique.
- ☐ Deep to the transversus abdominis is the peritoneum of the abdominal cavity.
- ☐ Keep in mind that the transversus abdominis is located not only in the anterior abdominal wall but also in the lateral abdominal wall and the posterior abdominal wall. It attaches posteriorly into the thoracolumbar fascia (just lateral to the erector spinae), and via the thoracolumbar fascia, attaches into the transverse processes of the lumbar spine.
- ☐ The transversus abdominis is involved with the superficial front line, lateral line, and spiral line myofascial meridians.

■ MISCELLANEOUS

1. The transversus abdominis contributes (along with the external and internal abdominal obliques) to the rectus sheath, which encloses/ensheathes the rectus abdominis.
2. The upper fibers of the transversus abdominis are contiguous and blend with the diaphragm and the transversus thoracis (another muscle that runs transversely in the trunk).
3. The transversus abdominis is sometimes called the *corset* muscle because it wraps around the abdomen like a corset and, like a corset, it functions to hold in the abdomen.

10

Psoas Minor

The name, psoas minor, *tells us that this muscle is located in the loin (low back) area and is small (smaller than the psoas major).*

Derivation	☐ psoas: Gr. *loin (low back)*.
	minor: L. *smaller.*
Pronunciation	☐ SO-as, MY-nor

■ ATTACHMENTS

☐ **Anterolateral Bodies of T12 and L1**
  ☐ and the disc between T12 and L1

to the

☐ **Pubis**
  ☐ the pectineal line of the pubis and the iliopectineal eminence (of the ilium and the pubis)

■ FUNCTIONS

Concentric (Shortening) Mover Actions	
Standard Mover Actions	**Reverse Mover Actions**
☐ 1. Flexes the trunk at the spinal joints	☐ 1. Posteriorly tilts the pelvis at the LS joint and flexes the lower trunk relative to the upper trunk
☐ 2. Laterally flexes the trunk at the spinal joints	☐ 2. Elevates the same-side pelvis at the LS joint and laterally flexes the lower trunk relative to the upper trunk
LS joint = lumbosacral joint	

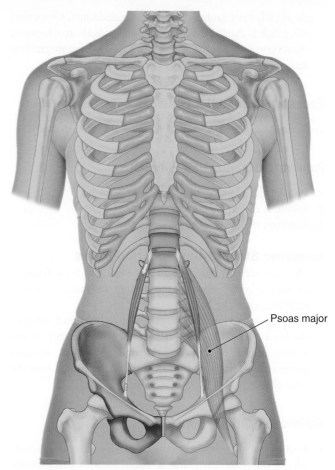

Psoas major

Figure 10-42 Anterior view of the psoas minor bilaterally. The psoas major has been ghosted in on the left.

Standard Mover Action Notes

- The psoas minor crosses the vertebral column anteriorly (with its fibers running vertically in the sagittal plane) and attaches onto the pelvis. When the pelvis is fixed and the psoas minor contracts, the trunk flexes at the spinal joints toward the pelvis. (action 1)
- The psoas minor crosses the spinal joints slightly on the lateral side (with its fibers running vertically in the frontal plane). When the pelvis is fixed and the psoas minor contracts, it pulls the trunk toward the pelvis laterally. Therefore the psoas minor laterally flexes the trunk at the spinal joints. However, because the psoas minor is very close to the midline, it has poor leverage for this action. (action 2)

Reverse Mover Action Notes

- When we think of motions of the spine, we usually think of the upper spine moving relative to the fixed lower spine. However, the reverse action of moving the lower spine relative to the upper spine is also possible (this usually occurs when the client is lying down so that the inferior attachment is mobile). Further, if the pelvis is moved, because the LS joint does not allow a large degree of motion, the lumbar spine will move with the pelvis, causing the lower spine to move relative to the upper spine. (reverse actions 1, 2)
- The psoas minor crosses the vertebral column anteriorly (with its fibers running vertically in the sagittal plane) and attaches onto the pelvis. When the trunk is fixed and the psoas minor contracts, it pulls the pelvis anteriorly and superiorly toward the spine. This motion is called *posterior tilt* of the pelvis and occurs at the LS joint. (reverse action 1)
- If the upper attachment of the psoas minor stays fixed and the lower attachment moves, the pelvis will elevate on that side and depress on the opposite side. Therefore the psoas minor ipsilaterally elevates and contralaterally depresses the pelvis at the LS joint. (reverse action 2)
- Because the inferior attachment of the psoas minor is so close to the midline, it has very poor leverage for ipsilateral elevation of the pelvis. (reverse action 2)

10

Psoas Minor—*cont'd*

Eccentric Antagonist Functions

1. Restrains/slows extension and opposite-side lateral flexion of the trunk
2. Restrains/slows anterior tilt and same-side depression of the pelvis

Isometric Stabilization Functions

1. Stabilizes the lumbar spinal joints
2. Stabilizes the pelvis

Additional Note on Functions

1. The psoas minor is fairly weak and usually not considered to be a very important muscle.

INNERVATION
□ L1 Spinal Nerve
  □ a branch from L1

ARTERIAL SUPPLY
□ Lumbar Arteries (branches of the Descending Aorta)
  □ and the Arteria Lumbalis Ima of the Median Sacral Artery (a branch of the Aorta), the lumbar branch of the Iliolumbar Artery (a branch of the Internal Iliac Artery), and the Common Iliac Artery (a branch of the Aorta)

✋ PALPATION

1. With the client supine, place your palpating fingers on the anterior abdomen, halfway between the umbilicus and anterior superior iliac spine (ASIS), just lateral to the rectus abdominis.
2. First locate the psoas major (see the Palpation section for this muscle on page 478).
3. Now palpate for the psoas minor lying on the psoas major. Do not engage the psoas minor because it will cause the more superficial abdominal wall muscles to contract and block your palpation.
4. If the psoas minor is tight, it may be possible to feel and distinguish it from the psoas major.

■ RELATIONSHIP TO OTHER STRUCTURES

□ The psoas minor is deep in the abdomen and lies directly anterior to the psoas major.
□ Anterior (superficial) to the psoas minor are the abdominal viscera.
□ The psoas minor is located within the deep front line myofascial meridian.

■ MISCELLANEOUS

1. The psoas minor is absent in about 40% of the population.
2. The iliopectineal eminence (of the ilium and pubis) is also known as the *iliopubic eminence.*
3. A condition called *psoas minor syndrome* has been reported wherein the psoas minor in teenagers has not kept up with the growth of the trunk and pelvis and consequently is pulled taut and becomes painful.

10

Muscles of the Rib Cage Joints

CHAPTER **OUTLINE**

CHAPTER **OVERVIEW**

The muscles addressed in this chapter are the muscles whose principal function is usually considered to be movement of the rib cage (at the sternocostal and costospinal joints). Other muscles in the body can also move the ribs, but they are placed in different chapters because their primary function is usually considered to be at another joint. These muscles are covered in Chapters 4, 5, and 10.

Overview of Structure

☐ Structurally, muscles that move the rib cage attach to the rib cage. The other attachment of these muscles is usually considered to be either superior or inferior to the rib attachment for elevation or depression motions, respectively. These muscles may be located anteriorly, posteriorly, and/or laterally.

Overview of Function

The following general rules regarding actions can be stated for the functional groups of muscles of the rib cage:

☐ If a muscle attaches to the rib cage and its other attachment is superior to the rib cage attachment, it can elevate the ribs to which it is attached at the sternocostal and costospinal joints.

☐ If a muscle attaches to the rib cage and its other attachment is inferior to the rib cage attachment, it can depress the ribs to which it is attached at the sternocostal and costospinal joints.

☐ As a rule, muscles that elevate ribs contract with inspiration and muscles that depress ribs contract with expiration.

☐ One notable exception to this rule is when muscles that depress the lower ribs contract to stabilize the lower rib cage attachment of the diaphragm so that when the diaphragm contracts, it can better depress its dome (central tendon) toward the rib cage attachment for abdominal (belly) breathing.

Posterior Views of the Muscles of the Trunk—Superficial and Intermediate Views

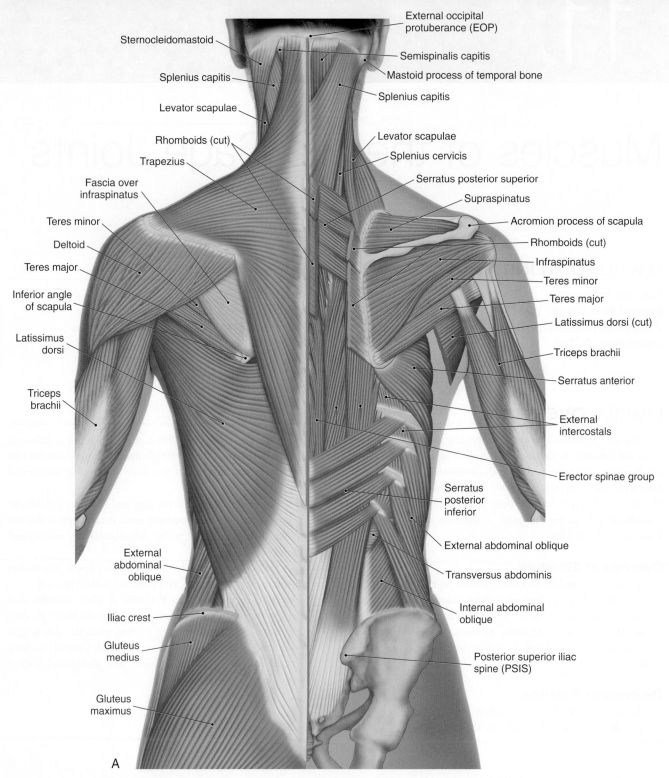

Figure 11-1 Posterior views of the muscles of the trunk. **A,** Superficial view on the left and an intermediate view on the right.

Posterior Views of the Muscles of the Trunk—Deep Views

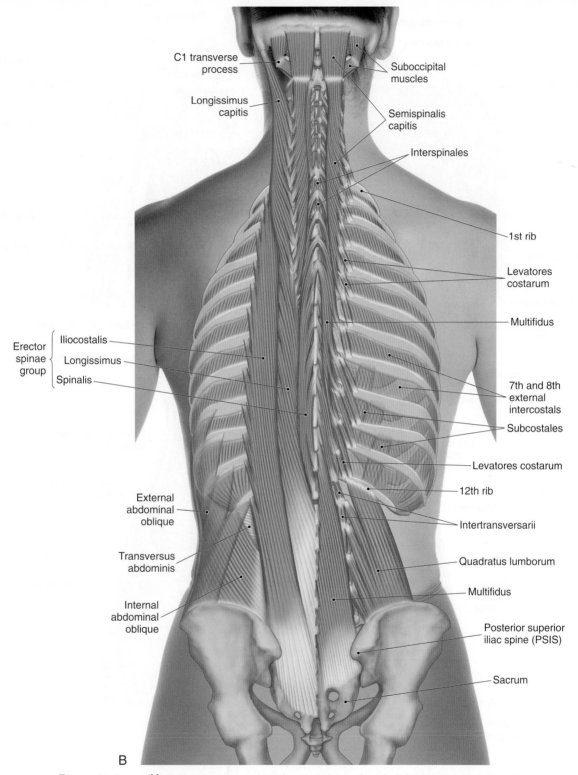

C1 transverse process

Suboccipital muscles

Longissimus capitis

Semispinalis capitis

Interspinales

1st rib

Levatores costarum

Multifidus

Erector spinae group

Iliocostalis

Longissimus

Spinalis

7th and 8th external intercostals

Subcostales

Levatores costarum

12th rib

External abdominal oblique

Intertransversarii

Transversus abdominis

Quadratus lumborum

Multifidus

Internal abdominal oblique

Posterior superior iliac spine (PSIS)

Sacrum

B

Figure 11-1, cont'd B, Two deep views; the right side is deeper than the left. The external abdominal oblique has been ghosted in on the left side. The intercostals have been ghosted in on the right side between ribs eight and twelve to show the subcostales.

Anterior Views of the Muscles of the Trunk—Superficial and Intermediate Views

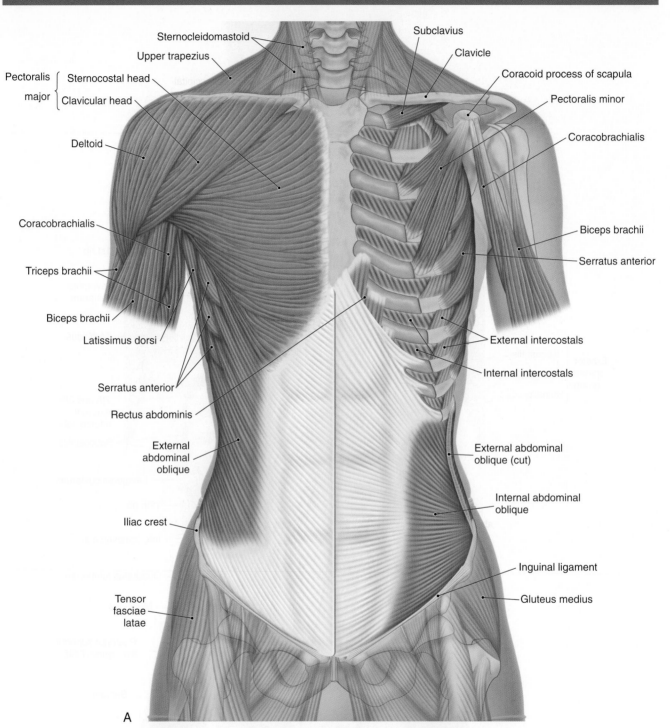

Figure 11-2 Anterior views of the muscles of the trunk. **A,** Superficial view on the right and an intermediate view on the left. The muscles of the neck and thigh have been ghosted in.

Anterior Views of the Muscles of the Trunk—Deep Views

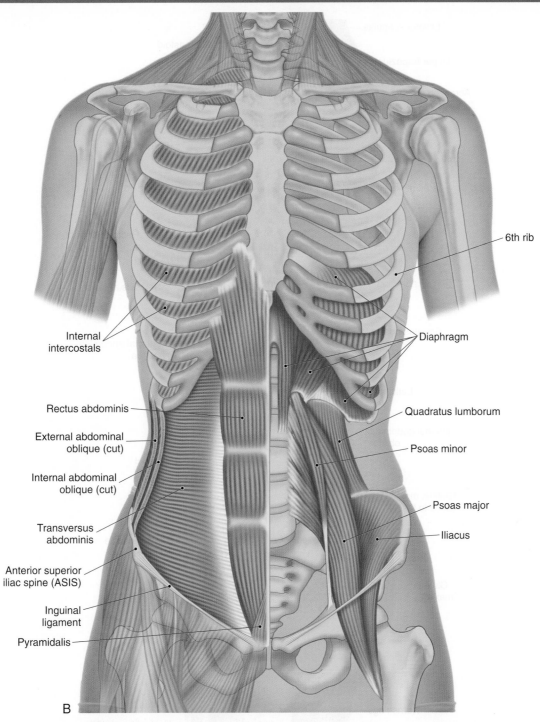

6th rib

Internal
intercostals

Diaphragm

Rectus abdominis

Quadratus lumborum

External abdominal
oblique (cut)

Psoas minor

Internal abdominal
oblique (cut)

Psoas major

Transversus
abdominis

Iliacus

Anterior superior
iliac spine (ASIS)

Inguinal
ligament

Pyramidalis

B

Figure 11-2, cont'd B, Deep views with the posterior abdominal wall seen on the left. The muscles of the neck, arm, and thigh have been ghosted in.

Right Lateral View of the Muscles of the Trunk—Superficial View

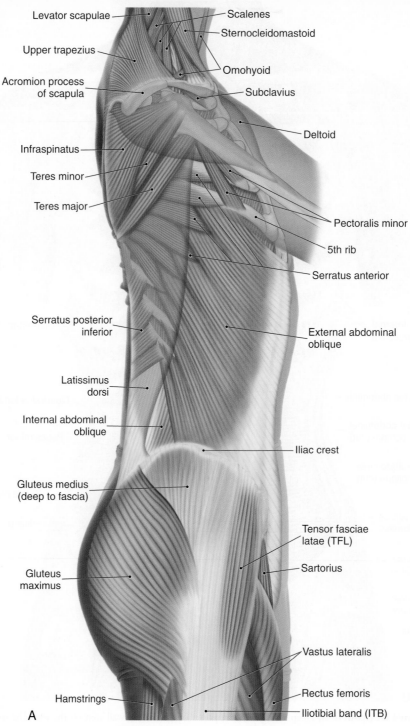

Figure 11-3 Right lateral view of the muscles of the trunk. **A,** Superficial view. The latissimus dorsi and deltoid have been ghosted in.

Right Lateral View of the Muscles of the Trunk—Deep View

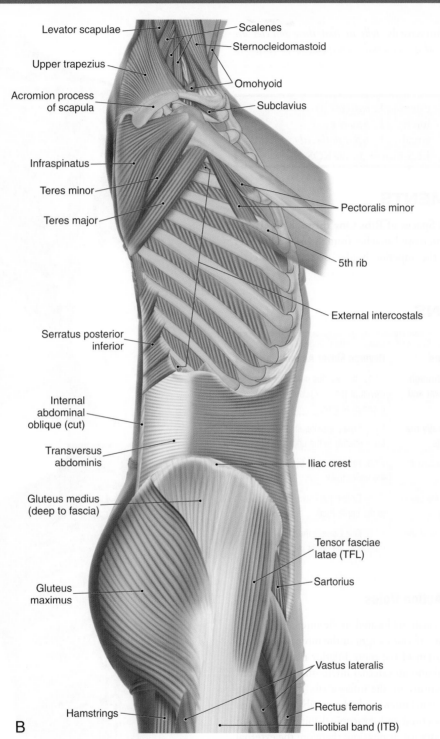

Levator scapulae

Scalenes

Sternocleidomastoid

Upper trapezius

Omohyoid

Acromion process
of scapula

Subclavius

Infraspinatus

Teres minor

Teres major

Pectoralis minor

5th rib

External intercostals

Serratus posterior
inferior

Internal
abdominal
oblique (cut)

Transversus
abdominis

Iliac crest

Gluteus medius
(deep to fascia)

Tensor fasciae
latae (TFL)

Sartorius

Gluteus
maximus

Vastus lateralis

Rectus femoris

Hamstrings

Iliotibial band (ITB)

B

Figure 11-3, cont'd B, Deep view.

External Intercostals

The name, external intercostals, *tells us that these muscles are located between ribs and are external (superficial to the internal intercostals).*

Derivation	☐ external: L. *outside.*
	inter: L. *between.*
	costals: L. *refers to the ribs.*
Pronunciation	☐ EKS-turn-al, in-ter-KOS-tals

■ ATTACHMENTS

☐ **In the Intercostal Spaces of Ribs One through Twelve**
  ☐ Each external intercostal attaches from the inferior border of one rib to the superior border of the rib directly inferior.

■ FUNCTIONS

Concentric (Shortening) Mover Actions	
Standard Mover Actions	**Reverse Mover Actions**
☐ **1. Elevate ribs two through twelve at the sternocostal and costospinal joints**	☐ 1. Depress ribs one through eleven at the sternocostal and costospinal joints
☐ **2. Rotate contralaterally the trunk at the spinal joints**	☐ 2. Rotate ipsilaterally the lower trunk relative to the upper trunk
☐ 3. Flex the trunk at the spinal joints	☐ 3. Flex the lower trunk relative to the upper trunk
☐ 4. Extend the trunk at the spinal joints	☐ 4. Extend the lower trunk relative to the upper trunk
☐ 5. Flex laterally the trunk at the spinal joints	☐ 5. Flex laterally the lower trunk relative to the upper trunk

Standard Mover Action Notes

- The external intercostals are located in the intercostal spaces and attach from the inferior margin of the more superior rib to the superior margin of the more inferior rib. When the superior rib is fixed and an external intercostal muscle contracts, it pulls superiorly on the inferior rib, thus elevating it. Therefore the external intercostals elevate ribs two through twelve at the sternocostal and costospinal joints. Elevation of the ribs is necessary for inspiration; therefore the external intercostals are respiratory muscles. (action 1)

- The external intercostals have the same fiber direction as the external abdominal oblique on the same side of the body; therefore they have the same actions of the trunk, namely, contralateral rotation, flexion, and lateral flexion. (actions 2, 3, 5)

- The anterior external intercostal fibers can do flexion. The posterior fibers can do extension. All fibers, but especially the most lateral ones, can do lateral flexion. (actions 3, 4, 5)

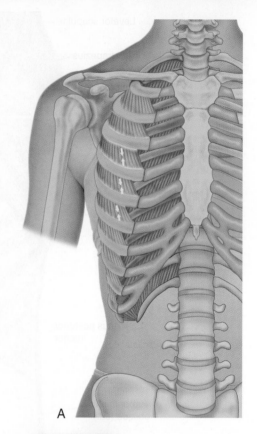

A

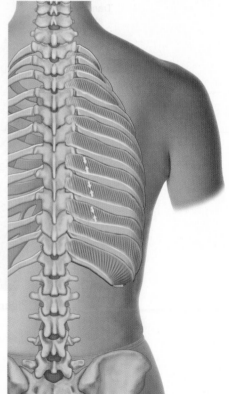

B

Figure 11-4 Views of the right external intercostals. **A,** Anterior view. **B,** Posterior view.

External Intercostals—cont'd

Reverse Mover Action Notes

- The external intercostals are located in the intercostal spaces and attach from the inferior margin of the more superior rib to the superior margin of the more inferior rib. If the lower rib is fixed and an external intercostal muscle contracts, it pulls inferiorly on the superior rib, thus depressing it. Therefore the external intercostals depress ribs one through eleven at the sternocostal and costospinal joints. Depression of the ribs is necessary for expiration; therefore the external intercostals are respiratory muscles. (reverse action 1)
- The standard mover action occurs when the upper trunk moves toward the lower trunk. The reverse mover action occurs if the superior attachments are fixed and the inferior attachments move so that the lower trunk moves toward the upper trunk. This usually occurs when the client is lying down so that the lower trunk is mobile. It should be noted that the reverse action of flexion is flexion, the reverse action of extension is extension, and the reverse action of lateral flexion is lateral flexion. The only difference is that the lower trunk moves toward the upper trunk instead of vice versa. However, the reverse action of contralateral rotation of the upper trunk is ipsilateral rotation of the lower trunk. (reverse actions 2, 3, 4, 5)

Eccentric Antagonist Functions

1. Restrains/slows depression of ribs two through twelve and elevation of ribs one through eleven
2. Restrains/slows ipsilateral rotation of the upper trunk and contralateral rotation of the lower trunk
3. Restrains/slows flexion, extension, and opposite-side lateral flexion of the trunk at the spinal joints

Isometric Stabilization Functions

1. Stabilizes the ribs
2. Stabilizes the spinal joints

Isometric Stabilization Function Note

- The external intercostals (and internal intercostals) are also involved in fixation (i.e., stabilization) of the rib cage during other movements of the body.

Additional Note on Actions

1. Given the location of the external intercostals, it is clear that they are involved in respiration. However, there is controversy regarding whether they elevate or depress the ribs during respiration. Generally, it is stated that they act during inspiration by elevating ribs; however, this is not known for certain. Given that the external intercostals are located in eleven intercostal spaces, and that these eleven intercostal spaces are located in the anterior, lateral, and posterior trunk, it is likely that different parts of this muscle group are active in different parts of the respiratory cycle. Some sources state that the upper and more lateral external intercostals are especially active with inspiration.

INNERVATION
- ☐ Intercostal Nerves

ARTERIAL SUPPLY
- ☐ Anterior Intercostal Arteries (branches of the Internal Thoracic Artery) and the Posterior Intercostal Arteries (branches of the Aorta)
  - ☐ and the branches of the Costocervical Trunk (a branch of the Subclavian Artery) and the Superior Thoracic Artery (a branch of the Axillary Artery)

✋ PALPATION

1. With the client supine, locate the hard surfaces of two adjacent ribs and place palpating fingers into the intercostal space between them.
2. Feel for the external intercostal muscle. Distinguishing between the external and internal intercostals is extremely difficult.
3. Palpate the external intercostals in other regions of the rib cage wherever possible.

■ RELATIONSHIP TO OTHER STRUCTURES

- ☐ The external intercostals are located in the intercostal spaces between ribs one through twelve. Therefore they are deep to all muscles that overlie the rib cage. Note that the external intercostals are not located between the costal cartilages of the ribs.
- ☐ The external intercostals are directly superficial to the internal intercostals.
- ☐ The external intercostals are located within the lateral line myofascial meridian.

■ MISCELLANEOUS

1. The fibers of the external intercostals are oriented in the same direction as the fibers of the same-side external abdominal oblique. For this reason, the external intercostals between the ribs appear to be extensions of the external abdominal oblique of the abdomen.
2. The external intercostals are thicker than the internal intercostals.

3. Regardless of the controversy over the exact actions of the external intercostals, it is clear that they are involved in respiration. Therefore the external intercostals (and the internal intercostals) should be addressed in any client who has a respiratory condition. Further, athletes may also greatly benefit from having these muscles worked on because of the great demand for respiration during exercise.

4. The intercostal muscles are the meat that is eaten when one eats ribs or spare ribs.

Internal Intercostals

The name, internal intercostals, *tells us that these muscles are located between ribs and are internal (deep to the external intercostals).*

Derivation	☐ internal: L. *inside.*
	inter: L. *between.*
	costals: L. *refers to the ribs.*
Pronunciation	☐ IN-turn-al, in-ter-KOS-tals

■ ATTACHMENTS

☐ **In the Intercostal Spaces of Ribs One through Twelve**
  ☐ Each internal intercostal attaches from the superior border of one rib and its costal cartilage to the inferior border of the rib and its costal cartilage that is directly superior.

■ FUNCTIONS

Concentric (Shortening) Mover Actions	
Standard Mover Actions	**Reverse Mover Actions**
☐ **1. Depress ribs one through eleven at the sternocostal and costospinal joints**	☐ 1. Elevate ribs two through twelve at the sternocostal and costospinal joints
☐ **2. Rotate ipsilaterally the trunk at the spinal joints**	☐ 2. Rotate contralaterally the lower trunk relative to the upper trunk
☐ 3. Flex the trunk at the spinal joints	☐ 3. Flex the lower trunk relative to the upper trunk
☐ 4. Extend the trunk at the spinal joints	☐ 4. Extend the lower trunk relative to the upper trunk
☐ 5. Flex laterally the trunk at the spinal joints	☐ 5. Flex laterally the lower trunk relative to the upper trunk

Standard Mover Action Notes

- The internal intercostals are located in the intercostal spaces and attach from the inferior margin of the more superior rib to the superior margin of the more inferior rib. If the lower rib is fixed and an internal intercostal muscle contracts, it pulls inferiorly on the superior rib, thus depressing it. Therefore the internal intercostals depress ribs one through eleven at the sternocostal and costospinal joints. Depression of the ribs is necessary for expiration; therefore the internal intercostals are respiratory muscles. (action 1)
- The internal intercostals have the same fiber direction as the internal abdominal oblique on the same side of the body; therefore they have the same actions of the trunk at the spinal joints, namely, ipsilateral rotation, flexion, and lateral flexion. (actions 2, 3, 5)
- The anterior internal intercostal fibers can do flexion. The posterior fibers can do extension. All fibers, but especially the most lateral ones, can do lateral flexion. (actions 3, 4, 5)

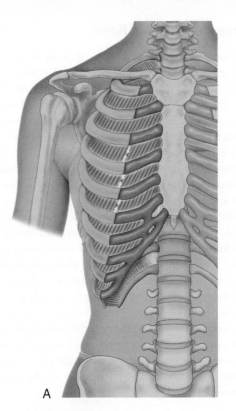

A

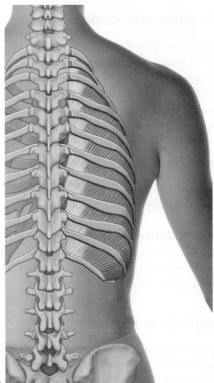

B

Figure 11-5 Views of the right internal intercostals. **A,** Anterior view. **B,** Posterior view.

Internal Intercostals—*cont'd*

Reverse Mover Action Notes

- The internal intercostals are located in the intercostal spaces and attach from the inferior margin of the more superior rib to the superior margin of the more inferior rib. When the superior rib is fixed and an internal intercostal muscle contracts, it pulls superiorly on the inferior rib, thus elevating it. Therefore the internal intercostals elevate ribs two through twelve at the sternocostal and costospinal joints. Elevation of the ribs is necessary for inspiration; therefore the internal intercostals are respiratory muscles. (reverse action 1)
- The standard mover action occurs when the upper trunk moves toward the lower trunk. The reverse mover action occurs if the superior attachments are fixed and the inferior attachments move so that the lower trunk moves toward the upper trunk. This usually occurs when the client is lying down so that the lower trunk is mobile. It should be noted that the reverse action of flexion is flexion, the reverse action of extension is extension, and the reverse action of lateral flexion is lateral flexion. The only difference is that the lower trunk moves toward the upper trunk instead of vice versa. However, the reverse action of ipsilateral rotation of the upper trunk is contralateral rotation of the lower trunk. (reverse actions 2, 3, 4, 5)

Eccentric Antagonist Functions

1. Restrains/slows elevation of ribs one through eleven and depression of ribs two through twelve
2. Restrains/slows contralateral rotation of the upper trunk and ipsilateral rotation of the lower trunk
3. Restrains/slows flexion, extension, and opposite-side lateral flexion of the trunk at the spinal joints

Isometric Stabilization Functions

1. Stabilizes the ribs
2. Stabilizes the spinal joints

Isometric Stabilization Function Note

- The internal intercostals (and external intercostals) are also involved in fixation (i.e., stabilization) of the rib cage during other movements of the body.

Additional Note on Functions

1. Given the location of the internal intercostals, it is clear that they are involved in respiration. However, there is controversy regarding whether they elevate or depress the ribs during respiration. Generally, it is stated that they act during expiration by depressing ribs; however, this is not known for certain. Given that the internal intercostals are located in eleven intercostal spaces, and that these eleven intercostal spaces are located in the anterior, lateral, and posterior

trunk, it is likely that different parts of this muscle group are active in different parts of the respiratory cycle. Some sources state that the fibers located between the costal cartilages (interchondral fibers) are especially active with inspiration and that the fibers located between the bones of the ribs themselves (interosseus fibers) are especially active with expiration.

INNERVATION
- Intercostal Nerves

ARTERIAL SUPPLY
- Anterior Intercostal Arteries (branches of the Internal Thoracic Artery) and the Posterior Intercostal Arteries (branches of the Aorta)
  - and the branches of the Costocervical Trunk (a branch of the Subclavian Artery) and the Superior Thoracic Artery (a branch of the Axillary Artery)

PALPATION

1. The internal intercostals are deep to the external intercostals, except between the costal cartilages where there are no external intercostals. The internal intercostals may be palpated superficially in the intercostal spaces between costal cartilages, or they may be palpated deep to the external intercostals. Discerning between the external and internal intercostals is extremely difficult.

■ RELATIONSHIP TO OTHER STRUCTURES

- The internal intercostals are located in the intercostal spaces between ribs one through twelve. Therefore they are deep to all muscles that overlie the rib cage. They are directly deep to the external intercostals, except in the intercostal spaces between the costal cartilages where no external intercostals muscles are located.
- The internal intercostals are superficial to the innermost intercostals, the subcostales, and the pleural membrane of the lung.
- The internal intercostals are located within the lateral line myofascial meridian.

■ MISCELLANEOUS

1. Anteriorly the internal intercostals are located in the spaces between the costal cartilages. (The external intercostals are not.)

Internal Intercostals—cont'd

2. Posteriorly, the muscle fibers of the internal intercostals only reach as far as the angle of the ribs. However, the internal intercostals attach into the internal intercostal membrane, which reaches farther medially to attach into the spine.

3. The fibers of the internal intercostals are oriented in the same direction as the fibers of the same-side internal abdominal oblique. For this reason, the internal intercostals between the ribs appear to be extensions of the internal abdominal oblique of the abdomen.

4. The internal intercostals are generally thinner than the external intercostals. The thickest region of the internal intercostals is between the costal cartilages.

5. Regardless of the controversy over the exact actions of the internal intercostals, it is clear that they are involved in respiration. Therefore the internal intercostals (and the external intercostals) should be addressed in any client who has a respiratory condition. Further, athletes may also greatly benefit from having these muscles worked on because of the great demand for respiration during exercise.

6. There is another layer of muscles called the *innermost intercostals* or *intercostals intimi,* which is located directly deep to the internal intercostals and has an identical direction of fibers to the internal intercostals. This third layer of intercostal musculature, which had always been considered to be the deeper layer of the internal intercostals, is now considered by many sources to be a distinct muscle layer.

7. The intercostal muscles are the meat that is eaten when one eats ribs or spare ribs.

Transversus Thoracis

The name, transversus thoracis, *tells us that this muscle runs transversely across the thoracic region.*

Derivation	☐ transversus: L. *running transversely.*
	thoracis: Gr. *refers to the thorax (chest).*
Pronunciation	☐ trans-VER-sus, thor-AS-is

■ ATTACHMENTS

☐ **Internal Surfaces of the Sternum, the Xiphoid Process, and the Adjacent Costal Cartilages**
   ☐ the inferior ⅔ of the sternum, and the costal cartilages of ribs four through seven

to the

☐ **Internal Surface of Costal Cartilages Two through Six**

■ FUNCTIONS

Concentric (Shortening) Mover Actions	
Standard Mover Actions	**Reverse Mover Actions**
☐ **1. Depresses ribs two through six at the sternocostal and costospinal joints**	☐ 1. Elevates the sternum

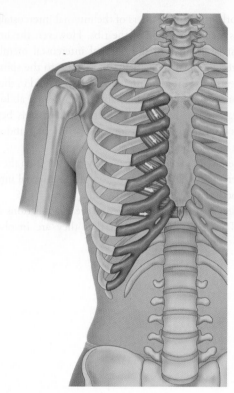

Figure 11-6 Anterior view of the right transversus thoracis.

Standard Mover Action Notes

• The transversus thoracis has its fibers running somewhat vertically, attaching from the sternum and the xiphoid process inferiorly, to the costal cartilages of ribs two through six superiorly. When the transversus thoracis contracts, it pulls the second through sixth costal cartilages inferiorly toward the sternum and xiphoid process. Therefore the transversus thoracis depresses costal cartilages two through six and thereby depresses ribs two through six at the sternocostal and costospinal joints. This action is necessary for expiration. (action 1)
• The primary role of the transversus thoracis is as a respiratory muscle. By depressing the costal cartilages, and therefore ribs two through six, the volume of the rib cage decreases for expiration.

Reverse Mover Action Notes

• The reverse action is moving the sternum toward the ribs and may occur in conjunction with lifting the trunk such as when extending and straightening the thoracic spine. Elevation of the sternum may also be involved in inspiration when breathing. (reverse action 1)

Eccentric Antagonist Functions

1. Restrains/slows elevation of ribs two through six
2. Restrains/slows depression of the sternum

Isometric Stabilization Functions

1. Stabilizes the rib cage and sternum

Additional Note on Functions

1. Muscles that depress (or elevate) the ribs are usually oriented vertically. The lower fibers of the transversus thoracis are oriented nearly perfectly horizontally, yet they can depress the ribs to which they attach because they cross inferior to the axis of motion for these ribs at the sternocostal joint.

INNERVATION
☐ Intercostal Nerves

ARTERIAL SUPPLY
☐ The Anterior Intercostal Arteries (branches of the Internal Thoracic Artery)

Transversus Thoracis—*cont'd*

 PALPATION

- The transversus thoracis is deep to the rib cage itself and essentially not discernable when palpated. A small portion of it may be palpable just lateral to the xiphoid process of the sternum, or some pressure may translate through to it if applied with your palpating fingers in the medial intercostal spaces between ribs two through six, just lateral to the sternum.

■ RELATIONSHIP TO OTHER STRUCTURES

- The transversus thoracis is deep to the rib cage and all the musculature that overlies the anterior thoracic region, as well as the intercostal muscles.

- The transversus thoracis is superficial to the pleural membrane of the lungs.
- The transversus thoracis is located within the deep front line myofascial meridian.

■ MISCELLANEOUS

1. The superior fibers of the transversus thoracis run primarily vertically, but the inferior fibers run horizontally (i.e., transversely).
2. The transversus thoracis is also known as the *sternocostalis* or as the *triangularis sternae*.
3. The transversus thoracis is internal (i.e., it is located within the thoracic cavity).
4. The inferior fibers of the transversus thoracis are contiguous with the superior fibers of the transversus abdominis, another deep trunk muscle that runs transversely.
5. The attachments of the transversus thoracis vary.

11

Diaphragm

The name, diaphragm, *tells us that this muscle is a partition.*

Derivation	☐ diaphragm: Gr. *partition.*
Pronunciation	☐ DI-a-fram

■ ATTACHMENTS

☐ **ENTIRE MUSCLE: Internal Surfaces of the Rib Cage and Sternum, and the Spine**
  ☐ COSTAL PART: Internal Surface of the Lower Six Ribs (Ribs Seven through Twelve) and their Costal Cartilages
  ☐ STERNAL PART: Internal Surface of the Xiphoid Process of the Sternum

☐ **LUMBAR PART: L1-L3**
  ☐ The lumbar attachments consist of two aponeuroses, called the *medial* and *lateral arcuate ligaments,* and two tendons, called the *right* and *left crura.*

to the

☐ **Central Tendon (Dome) of the Diaphragm**

■ FUNCTIONS

Concentric (Shortening) Mover Actions	
Standard Mover Actions	**Reverse Mover Actions**
☐ 1. Increases the volume of (expands) the thoracic cavity via abdominal breathing	☐ 1. Increases the volume of (expands) the thoracic cavity via thoracic breathing

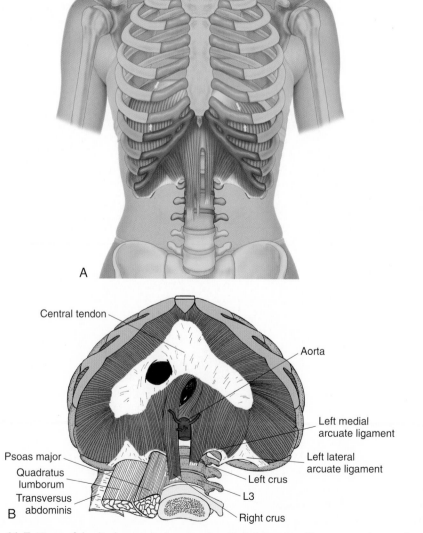

Figure 11-7 Views of the diaphragm. **A,** Anterior view. **B,** Inferior view. The psoas major, quadratus lumborum, and transversus abdominis are shown on the right side.

Diaphragm—*cont'd*

Standard Mover Action Notes

- If the bony peripheral attachments are fixed and the diaphragm contracts, the pull is on the central tendon, which causes it (i.e., the top of the dome) to drop down against the abdominal viscera. This increases the superior-inferior dimension of the thoracic cavity to allow the lungs to inflate and expand for inspiration. (action 1)
- The diaphragm is the prime mover of inspiration. (action 1)
- The diaphragm is unusual in that one of its attachments is located 360 degrees around the lower rib cage, and the other attachment is the center of the muscle itself, its dome, a region of fibrous tissue known as the central tendon (in reality a broad flat aponeurosis). Similar to any skeletal muscle, either attachment can be fixed with the other attachment mobile. Typically, the rib cage attachment is more fixed; therefore the central dome tends to move first. When this occurs, the central dome drops down, thereby increasing the superior to inferior height of the thoracic cavity, allowing for the lungs to fill with air. When this occurs, because the dome compresses into the abdominopelvic cavity, its contents are pushed out anteriorly and the belly is seen to rise. This is known as *belly breathing* or *abdominal breathing*. (action 1)

Reverse Mover Action Notes

- As the diaphragm continues to contract, the pressure caused by the resistance of the abdominal viscera prohibits the central dome from dropping any farther and the dome now becomes less able to move (i.e., more fixed). The pull exerted by the contraction of the fibers of the diaphragm now pull peripherally on the rib cage, elevating the lower ribs outward laterally and causing the anterior rib cage and sternum to push anteriorly. This further increases the volume of the thoracic cavity to allow the lungs to inflate and expand for inspiration. (reverse action 1)
- The reverse action of the diaphragm (reverse to abdominal breathing) could be considered to occur when the central dome can drop no farther because there is too much resistance from the compressed abdominal contents. At this point, the rib cage is now more mobile and is pulled upward toward the central dome. This causes the ribs to lift outward, thereby increasing the medial to lateral dimension and anterior to posterior dimension of the thoracic cavity, allowing the lungs to fill further with air for inspiration. When this occurs, the rib cage is seen to expand. This is known as *chest breathing* or *thoracic breathing*. Both aspects of diaphragm contraction (abdominal and thoracic breathing) occur when breathing in deeply. (reverse action 1)
- Keep in mind that the diaphragm only elevates the lower half (six ribs) of the rib cage. Other *accessory* muscles of respiration such as the scalenes and intercostals contract to elevate the upper half of the rib cage. (reverse action 1)

Eccentric Antagonist Function

1. Restrains/slows compression of the thoracic cavity

Isometric Stabilization Function

1. Stabilizes the trunk, including the joints of the lower rib cage and the thoracic and lumbar spinal joints

Isometric Stabilization Function Note

- When the lungs inflate with air, the thoracic cavity becomes more rigid. Further, because when it contracts, the diaphragm drops down against the abdominopelvic cavity, the abdominopelvic cavity is also compressed, becoming more rigid. The result is that core stability is increased, including the thoracic and lumbar spinal joints. Increasing the stability of the core increases the efficiency with which muscles that attach from the core to the extremities can move the extremities because their proximal attachment is held so stable. This is the reason why people intuitively take in and hold a deep breath when performing a joint action that requires great strength.

Additional Notes on Functions

1. The diaphragm is the primary muscle of respiration but is by no means the only one. The exact pattern of a client's breathing is usually determined by the precise coordination of the diaphragm with the many accessory muscles of respiration. Among respiratory muscles, the diaphragm is the only one that must contract for quiet relaxed breathing. Many other (accessory) muscles of inspiration can also contract when more forceful inspiration is needed. No muscle contraction is necessary for quiet relaxed expiration; when the diaphragm relaxes, its elastic recoil is sufficient to press up against the lungs and expel air. When forceful expiration is needed, many accessory muscles of expiration can be engaged.
2. The diaphragm is essentially shaped like a dome. This dome is somewhat asymmetric, with the anterior aspect of it being higher than the posterior aspect. Its attachments peripherally onto the posterior rib cage and the lumbar vertebrae are its lowest points. The attachments peripherally onto the anterior rib cage and the xiphoid process of the sternum are somewhat higher. From these peripheral attachments, the fibers essentially run vertically and toward the center of the body to converge together into the central tendon (dome) of the diaphragm. Thus the diaphragm attaches into itself centrally at the central tendon.

   When the diaphragm contracts, the volume of the thoracic cavity can increase in two ways. If the peripheral rib cage attachment is fixed and the central tendon drops toward the rib cage, the superior to inferior diameter of the thoracic cavity increases. This aspect of the diaphragm's contraction is usually called *abdominal breathing* or *belly breathing* because the abdominal contents are pushed outward and the

11

11

belly is seen to rise. If the central tendon is fixed and the rib cage attachment lifts outward and upward toward the central tendon, the side-to-side and front-to-back diameter of the thoracic cavity increases. This aspect of the diaphragm's contraction is usually called *thoracic breathing* or *chest breathing* because the rib cage is seen to expand. Either way, when the thoracic cavity increases in volume, the lungs can inflate and expand for inspiration.

Usually, the central tendon is the more mobile attachment and moves first until the resistance of the abdominal viscera stops it, and then the rib cage attachment moves. Which attachment moves first and to what degree will vary from person to person and be based on the relative resistance to motion of the central tendon and rib cage. If the client is overweight or wearing very tight clothing, there is greater resistance to belly breathing. If the client has tight chest muscles or degenerative joint disease (osteoarthritis) of the joints of the rib cage, there is more resistance to chest breathing.

3. Movement of the rib cage attachments laterally outward and upward is usually described as *bucket handle motion* because like a bucket handle that is fixed in two places and lifts in the center, the ribs are fixed at the sternum and spine and lift in the center (laterally) between these two attachments. The movement of the sternum that occurs is often described as a *pump handle motion* because it lifts out and up anteriorly, similar to how a pump handle moves.

INNERVATION
- The Phrenic Nerve
  - C3-C5

ARTERIAL SUPPLY
- Branches of the Aorta and the Internal Thoracic Artery (a branch of the Subclavian Artery)
  - the Superior and Inferior Phrenic Arteries (both branches of the Aorta) and the Musculophrenic and Pericardiacophrenic Arteries (both branches of the Internal Thoracic Artery)

✋ PALPATION

1. With the client supine with a pillow placed under the knees, place palpating fingers on the inferior margin of the anterior rib cage.
2. Have the client take in a deep breath and then slowly exhale.
3. As the client exhales, curl your fingertips under (inferior and then deep to) the rib cage and feel for the diaphragm, palpating gently, yet firmly, as deep as possible against the internal surface of the ribs.

■ RELATIONSHIP TO OTHER STRUCTURES

- The diaphragm separates the thoracic cavity from the abdominal cavity.
- The heart and lungs sit (superiorly) on the diaphragm. The liver and stomach are located (inferiorly) under the diaphragm.
- The medial and lateral arcuate ligaments of the diaphragm actually attach across the psoas major and the quadratus lumborum muscles, respectively.
- The diaphragm is located within the deep front line myofascial meridian.

■ MISCELLANEOUS

1. The diaphragm is a partition between the thoracic cavity and the abdominal (i.e., abdominopelvic) cavity. The term *diaphragm* means partition.
2. The medial arcuate ligament of the diaphragm surrounds the psoas major and runs from the body of L2 to the transverse process of L1. The lateral arcuate ligament of the diaphragm surrounds the quadratus lumborum and runs from the transverse process of L1 to the twelfth rib.
3. The central tendon of the diaphragm is a thin but strong aponeurosis located near the center of the muscle (at its dome). It is flattened somewhat at its center because the heart sits on it there. Each side of the dome is sometimes referred to as a *cupola*.
4. The dome of the diaphragm is higher on the right than the left because the liver pushes up on the right side. With maximal expiration, the dome is located at approximately the level of the fourth costal cartilage on the right (approximately the level of the right nipple) and the fifth costal cartilage on the left. With maximal inspiration, the dome drops as much as 4 inches (10 cm). The diaphragm is higher when a person lies down; and if lying on the side, the side of the diaphragm against the bed is higher than the other side.
5. The two crura (singular: crus) of the diaphragm are not symmetric. The right crus is broader and attaches farther inferiorly than the left crus.
6. The costal fibers of the diaphragm interdigitate with the transversus abdominis.
7. There are a number of openings in the diaphragm to allow passage of structures between the thoracic and abdominal cavities. The largest openings are for the esophagus, the aorta, and the inferior vena cava.
8. The diaphragm is unusual in that it is under both conscious control and unconscious control. More specifically, con-

Diaphragm—cont'd

traction of the diaphragm is under constant unconscious regulation by the brainstem. However, we routinely override this brainstem control whenever we choose to sing, talk, sigh, hold our breath, or otherwise consciously change our breathing pattern.

9. The innervation to the diaphragm is provided by the phrenic nerve, composed of spinal nerves C3, C4, and C5. *(C3, 4, 5 keeps the diaphragm alive!)*

10. A *hiatal hernia* is when part of the stomach herniates (ruptures) through the diaphragm into the thoracic cavity.

Serratus Posterior Superior

The name, serratus posterior superior, *tells us that this muscle has a serrated appearance and is posterior and superior in location (posterior to the serratus anterior and superior to the serratus posterior inferior).*

Derivation	☐ serratus: L. *a notching.*
	superior: L. *above.*
	posterior: L. *behind, toward the back.*
Pronunciation	☐ ser-A-tus, pos-TEE-ri-or,
	sue-PEE-ri-or

■ ATTACHMENTS

☐ **Spinous Processes of C7-T3**
  ☐ and the lower nuchal ligament

to

☐ **Ribs Two through Five**
  ☐ the superior borders and the external surfaces

■ FUNCTIONS

Concentric (Shortening) Mover Actions	
Standard Mover Actions	**Reverse Mover Actions**
☐ **1. Elevates ribs two through five at the sternocostal and costospinal joints**	☐ 1. Contralaterally rotates C7-T3 at the spinal joints

Standard Mover Action Notes

- The serratus posterior superior attaches from ribs two through five inferiorly, to the vertebral column superiorly (with its fibers running somewhat vertically). When the serratus posterior superior contracts, it pulls the ribs superiorly toward the vertebral attachment. Therefore the serratus posterior superior elevates ribs two through five at the sternocostal and costospinal joints. (action 1)
- Elevation of ribs is important for respiration. By elevating upper ribs, the thoracic cavity expands, which creates more space for the lungs to fill with air. Therefore the serratus posterior superior is a muscle of inspiration. (action 1)

Reverse Mover Action Notes

- If the rib cage attachment of the serratus posterior superior is fixed, the vertebral attachment could be pulled toward the ribs. This would result in the spinous processes of C7-T3 being pulled toward the rib attachments, which would result in the anterior surface of the vertebrae rotating to the opposite side. Therefore the serratus posterior superior can contralaterally rotate the trunk (specifically C7-T3) at the spinal joints. Given how thin this muscle is, this action would be very weak. (reverse action 1)

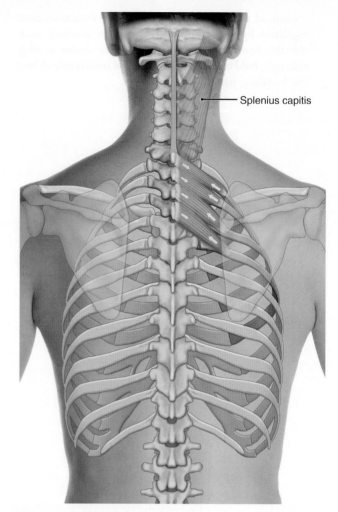

Splenius capitis

Figure 11-8 Posterior view of the right serratus posterior superior. The splenius capitis has been ghosted in.

Eccentric Antagonist Functions

1. Restrains/slows depression of ribs two through five
2. Restrains/slows ipsilateral rotation of C7-T3

Isometric Stabilization Functions

1. Stabilizes the upper ribs
2. Stabilizes upper thoracic spinal joints

INNERVATION
☐ Intercostal Nerves
  ☐ intercostal nerves two through five

ARTERIAL SUPPLY
☐ The dorsal branches of the Posterior Intercostal Arteries (branches of the Aorta)

Serratus Posterior Superior—*cont'd*

✋ PALPATION

1. With the client prone, place palpating hand in the region of the upper rhomboids.
2. Have the client take in a moderately deep breath and feel for the contraction of the serratus posterior superior.
3. Note: It is very challenging to discern the serratus posterior superior from the overlying rhomboids.

■ RELATIONSHIP TO OTHER STRUCTURES

☐ The serratus posterior superior is directly deep to the rhomboids.

☐ The serratus posterior superior is directly superficial to the erector spinae musculature and the lower portions of the splenius capitis and the splenius cervicis.

☐ The serratus posterior superior is involved with the spiral line myofascial meridian.

■ MISCELLANEOUS

1. The serrated appearance of the serratus posterior superior comes from attaching onto separate ribs, which creates the notched look of a serrated knife.
2. The serratus posterior superior is a thin, quadrilateral-shaped muscle.
3. The serratus posterior superior is variable with regard to its attachments. Its most common variation is that its spinal attachment is only C7-T2 instead of C7-T3.

11

Serratus Posterior Inferior

The name, serratus posterior inferior, *tells us that this muscle has a serrated appearance and is posterior and inferior in location (posterior to the serratus anterior and inferior to the serratus posterior superior).*

Derivation	☐ serratus: L. *a notching*
	inferior: L. *below.*
	posterior: L. *behind, toward the back.*
Pronunciation	☐ ser-A-tus, pos-TEE-ri-or,
	in-FEE-ri-or

■ ATTACHMENTS

☐ **Spinous Processes of T11-L2**

   to

☐ **Ribs Nine through Twelve**
   ☐ the inferior borders and the external surfaces

■ FUNCTIONS

Concentric (Shortening) Mover Actions	
Standard Mover Actions	**Reverse Mover Actions**
☐ **1. Depresses ribs nine through twelve at the sternocostal and costospinal joints**	☐ 1. Contralaterally rotates T11-L2 at the spinal joints

Standard Mover Action Notes

- The serratus posterior inferior attaches from ribs nine through twelve superiorly, to the vertebral column inferiorly (with its fibers running somewhat vertically). When the serratus posterior inferior contracts, it pulls the ribs inferiorly toward the vertebral attachment. Therefore the serratus posterior inferior depresses ribs nine through twelve at the sternocostal and costospinal joints. (action 1)

- The action of depressing ribs nine through twelve is considered to be important for respiration. Theoretically, the fact that the serratus posterior inferior depresses ribs nine through twelve would seem to indicate that this muscle is a muscle of expiration. However, its main function regarding the lower ribs is not to be a mover and actually move the lower ribs into depression, but rather to fix (stabilize) the lower ribs in place so that they do not elevate when the diaphragm contracts and exerts an upward pull on them. In this manner, if the lower rib cage attachments of the diaphragm are fixed, the dome of the diaphragm drops down more efficiently, thus increasing the superior to inferior size of the thoracic cavity for the lungs to expand and fill with air. Therefore the serratus posterior inferior is a muscle of inspiration (primarily as a fixator [i.e., stabilizer]). It must be noted that there is some controversy regarding the role of the serratus posterior inferior with regard to respiration. Some sources state that it is

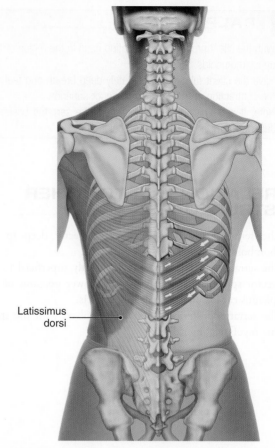

Latissimus
dorsi

Figure 11-9 Posterior view of the serratus posterior inferior bilaterally. The latissimus dorsi has been ghosted in on the left side.

not involved with respiration at all. Other sources list it as a muscle of expiration rather than inspiration. However, looking at its biomechanical role of fixing the lower ribs against the pull of the diaphragm clearly places the serratus posterior inferior as a muscle of inspiration. (action 1)

Reverse Mover Action Notes

- If the rib cage attachment of the serratus posterior inferior is fixed, the vertebral attachment could be pulled toward the ribs. This would result in the spinous processes of T11-L2 being pulled toward the rib attachments, which would result in the anterior surface of the vertebrae rotating to the opposite side. Therefore the serratus posterior inferior can contralaterally rotate the trunk (specifically T12-L2) at the spinal joints. Given how thin this muscle is, this action would be very weak. (reverse action 1)

Eccentric Antagonist Functions

1. Restrains/slows elevation of ribs nine through twelve
2. Restrains/slows ipsilateral rotation of T12-L2

Serratus Posterior Inferior—*cont'd*

Isometric Stabilization Functions

1. Stabilizes the lower ribs
2. Stabilizes thoracolumbar spinal joints

Isometric Stabilization Function Note

• Stabilization of the lower ribs is an important function of the serratus posterior inferior. Its force of depression of the lower ribs stabilizes them from elevating when the diaphragm contracts and pulls superiorly on them. By stabilizing the rib cage attachment of the diaphragm, the contraction of the diaphragm acts to drop its dome, thereby increasing the superior to inferior volume of the thoracic cavity for inspiration (this occurs during abdominal [belly] breathing). (See second Standard Mover Action Note above.)

Additional Note on Functions

1. Theoretically, if the upper two slips of the serratus posterior inferior pull on ribs nine and ten, and if these ribs are fixed to vertebrae T9 and T10, the serratus posterior inferior could ipsilaterally rotate T9 and T10 at the spinal joints (via their rib attachments).

INNERVATION
☐ Subcostal Nerve and Intercostal Nerves
   ☐ intercostal nerves nine through eleven

ARTERIAL SUPPLY
☐ The dorsal branches of the Posterior Intercostal Arteries (branches of the Aorta)

🖐 PALPATION

1. With the client prone, place palpating hand in the upper lumbar region.
2. Have the client take in a moderately deep breath and feel for the contraction of the serratus posterior inferior.
3. Note: It is very challenging to discern the serratus posterior inferior from the overlying latissimus dorsi.

■ RELATIONSHIP TO OTHER STRUCTURES

☐ The serratus posterior inferior is directly deep to the latissimus dorsi.
☐ Directly deep to the serratus posterior inferior is the erector spinae group.
☐ The serratus posterior inferior may be involved with the superficial front arm line and superficial back line myofascial meridians.

■ MISCELLANEOUS

1. The serrated appearance of the serratus posterior inferior comes from attaching onto separate ribs, which creates the notched look of a serrated knife.
2. The serratus posterior inferior is a thin, quadrilateral-shaped muscle.
3. The serratus posterior inferior is variable with regard to its spinal and costal (rib) attachments.

11

The name, levatores costarum, *tells us that these muscles elevate the ribs.*

Derivation	☐ levator: L. *lifter.*
	costarum: L. *refers to the ribs.*
Pronunciation	☐ le-va-TO-rez, (singular: le-VAY-tor),
	kos-TAR-um

■ ATTACHMENTS

☐ **Transverse Processes of C7-T11**
  ☐ the tips of the transverse processes

to

☐ **Ribs One through Twelve (inferiorly)**
  ☐ the external surfaces of the ribs, between the tubercle and the angle

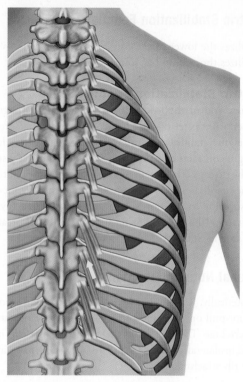

Figure 11-10 Posterior view of the right levatores costarum.

■ FUNCTIONS

Concentric (Shortening) Mover Actions	
Standard Mover Actions	**Reverse Mover Actions**
☐ **1. Elevate the ribs at the sternocostal and costospinal joints**	☐ 1. Laterally flex, extend, and contralaterally rotate the trunk at the spinal joints

Standard Mover Action Notes

- The levatores costarum attach from superiorly on a vertebral transverse process to inferiorly onto a rib (with their fibers running vertically). When the vertebral attachment is fixed and the levatores costarum contract, they pull the costal attachments (i.e., the ribs) superiorly toward the vertebral attachment. Therefore the levatores costarum elevate the ribs at the sternocostal and costospinal joints. (action 1)
- As elevators of the ribs, the levatores costarum can help increase the volume of the thoracic cavity, and therefore increase the volume of the lungs. Hence, they are muscles of inspiration (accessory muscles of respiration). (action 1)

Reverse Mover Action Notes

- When the rib attachment of the levatores costarum is fixed and the levatores costarum contract, they pull the vertebral attachment toward the rib attachment. Because the levatores costarum cross the spinal joints posteriorly (with their fibers running somewhat vertically in the sagittal plane), they extend the trunk at the spinal joints. Because the levatores costarum cross the spinal joints laterally (with their fibers running somewhat vertically in the frontal plane), they laterally flex the trunk at the spinal joints. Because the levatores costarum run somewhat horizontally (in the transverse

plane) they pull the vertebral attachment posterolaterally toward the rib attachment. This causes the anterior surface of the trunk to face the opposite side of the body from the side on which the levatores costarum are attached. Therefore the levatores costarum contralaterally rotate the trunk at the spinal joints. (reverse action 1)
- The levatores costarum's reverse action of lateral flexion, extension, and contralateral rotation of the trunk can only occur in the thoracic spine. These actions would not be very strong. (reverse action 1)

Eccentric Antagonist Functions

1. Restrains/slows depression of the ribs
2. Restrains/slows opposite-side lateral flexion, flexion, and ipsilateral rotation of the thoracic vertebrae

Isometric Stabilization Functions

1. Stabilizes the sternocostal and costospinal joints
2. Stabilizes the thoracic spinal joints

Isometric Stabilization Function Note

- Some sources state that the primary function of the levatores costarum is to stabilize the spinal joints and ribs.

Levatores Costarum—*cont'd*

Additional Note on Functions

1. The levatores costarum, although small, have excellent leverage to move the ribs. A small upward movement of a rib close to the vertebral attachment results in a large motion laterally.

INNERVATION
□ Spinal Nerves
    □ dorsal rami

ARTERIAL SUPPLY
□ The dorsal branches of the Posterior Intercostal Arteries (branches of the Aorta)

✋ PALPATION

1. With the client prone, place palpating fingers on the erector spinae musculature over the angles of the ribs. Have the client slowly and deeply breathe in and out. Try to feel for the contraction of the levatores costarum.
2. The levatores costarum are small and very deep muscles. Palpating and discerning them from the adjacent musculature is extremely difficult if not impossible.

■ RELATIONSHIP TO OTHER STRUCTURES

□ The levatores costarum are deep to the trapezius, latissimus dorsi, serratus posterior superior, serratus posterior inferior, and the erector spinae muscles.
□ Deep to the levatores costarum are the intercostal muscles.
□ The levatores costarum are located within the superficial back line myofascial meridian.

■ MISCELLANEOUS

1. The levatores costarum attach from a transverse process of a vertebra and orient inferiorly and laterally to attach onto the rib directly inferior to the vertebral attachment. However, the levatores costarum that attach to vertebrae T8-T10 have a second slip of tissue that also attaches to the second rib below that vertebral attachment (i.e., ribs ten through twelve). When this occurs, the two parts of the levatores costarum are called the *levatores costarum breves* and the *levatores costarum longi*.
2. The levatores costarum are considered to be homologous to the intertransversarii of the cervical and lumber regions.

11

Subcostales

The name, subcostales, *tells us that these muscles are "under" (i.e., deep to) the ribs.*

Derivation	☐ sub: L. *under.*
	costales: L. *refers to the ribs.*
Pronunciation	☐ sub-kos-TAL-eez

■ ATTACHMENTS

☐ **Ribs Ten through Twelve**
  ☐ the internal surface of the ribs, near the angle

to

☐ **Ribs Eight through Ten**
  ☐ the internal surfaces of the ribs, near the angle

■ FUNCTIONS

Concentric (Shortening) Mover Actions	
Standard Mover Actions	**Reverse Mover Actions**
☐ **1. Depress ribs eight through ten at the sternocostal and costospinal joints**	☐ 1. Elevate ribs ten through twelve at the sternocostal and costospinal joints

Standard Mover Action Note

- The subcostales attach from the internal surface of a rib and run superiorly (with their fibers running vertically), skipping one rib to attach onto the internal surface of a more superior rib. When the subcostales contract, they pull the more superior rib inferiorly toward the more inferior rib. Therefore the subcostales depress ribs eight through ten at the sternocostal and costospinal joints. This action assists forceful expiration by decreasing the size of the thoracic cavity; hence the subcostales are respiratory muscles. (action 1)

Reverse Mover Action Note

- If the upper ribs' (eight through ten) attachments of the subcostales are fixed, the subcostales would elevate the lower ribs (ten through twelve) instead of depressing the upper ribs. Elevating ribs is usually considered important for inspiration because lifting ribs increases the volume of the thoracic cavity, thereby allowing the lungs to fill with air. (reverse action 1)

Eccentric Antagonist Function

1. Restrains/slows elevation of ribs eight through ten or depression of ribs ten through twelve

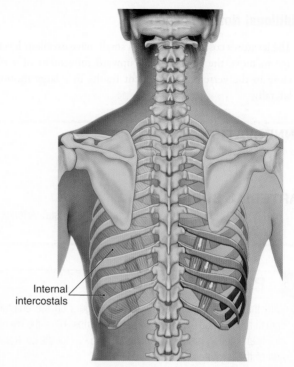

Internal intercostals

Figure 11-11 Posterior view of the subcostales bilaterally. The internal intercostals have been ghosted in on the left side.

Isometric Stabilization Function

1. Stabilizes the lower five ribs

Isometric Stabilization Function Note

1. The subcostales' primary function might be to stabilize ribs eight through ten by stopping them from elevating. This could help to stabilize the rib cage attachment of the diaphragm so that the diaphragm could more efficiently pull its dome (central tendon) down, increasing the superior to inferior volume of the thoracic cavity and therefore the lungs. This function would make the subcostales important as muscles of inspiration.

INNERVATION
☐ Intercostal Nerves
  ☐ eight through eleven

ARTERIAL SUPPLY
☐ The dorsal branches of the Posterior Intercostal Arteries (branches of the Aorta)

11

Subcostales—*cont'd*

PALPATION

☐ The subcostales are deep to the rib cage itself and are essentially not palpable. If pressure were to translate through to them, it would have to be applied with palpating fingers just lateral to the erector spinae's lateral border, in the intercostal spaces between ribs eight through twelve.

■ RELATIONSHIP TO OTHER STRUCTURES

☐ The subcostales are deep to the rib cage and all the musculature overlying the rib cage in the lower posterior thoracic region, as well as the external and internal intercostal muscles and the intercostal neurovascular bundle.

☐ The subcostales are superficial to the pleural membrane of the lungs.

☐ The subcostales are located within the superficial back line myofascial meridian.

■ MISCELLANEOUS

1. The subcostales are variable in their presentation. They are usually well developed only in the lower thoracic region. Most often, there are three subcostales muscles running from rib eight to rib ten, rib nine to rib eleven, and rib ten to rib twelve (as presented earlier in the Attachment section and shown in the individual illustration).

11

Muscles of the Temporomandibular Joints

CHAPTER OUTLINE

CHAPTER OVERVIEW

The muscles addressed in this chapter are the muscles whose principal function is usually considered to be movement of the mandible at the temporomandibular joints (TMJs). Some of these muscles are involved at other joints of the body. Principally, the muscles of the hyoid group are also involved in motions of the neck at the spinal joints.

Overview of Structure
☐ Mastication is the act of chewing. Therefore the muscles of mastication are those that attach to and are involved in movement of the mandible at the TMJs.
☐ There are four major muscles of mastication: the temporalis, masseter, lateral pterygoid, and medial pterygoid.
☐ The eight muscles of the hyoid group are also involved in mastication and are therefore covered in this chapter. The

hyoid group is comprised of four suprahyoid muscles and four infrahyoid muscles.
☐ The major muscles of mastication are located in the head. The temporalis and masseter are superficial and the two pterygoids are deeper. The lesser muscles of mastication are the muscles of the hyoid group and are located in the anterior neck.

Overview of Function
The following general rules regarding actions can be stated for the functional groups of muscles of mastication at the TMJs:
☐ If a muscle attaches to the mandible and its other attachment is superior to the mandibular attachment, it can elevate the mandible at the TMJs.

Review the muscles and bones from this chapter on the enclosed CD!

□ If a muscle attaches to the mandible and its other attachment is inferior to the mandibular attachment, it can depress the mandible at the TMJs.

□ If a muscle attaches to the mandible and its other attachment is anterior to the mandibular attachment, it can protract the mandible at the TMJs.

□ If a muscle attaches to the mandible and its other attachment is posterior to the mandibular attachment, it can retract the mandible at the TMJs.

□ If a muscle attaches to the mandible and its other attachment is medial to the mandibular attachment, it can contralaterally deviate (do opposite side deviation of) the mandible at the TMJs.

□ Reverse actions of the major muscles of mastication are unlikely because they would require movement of the entire head toward a fixed mandible (at the TMJs).

□ Reverse actions of the suprahyoid muscles of the hyoid group occur when the mandible is fixed and the hyoid bone is moved superiorly toward the mandible.

INNERVATION

□ The major muscles of mastication are innervated by the trigeminal nerve (CN V).

□ The hyoid muscles are innervated by the following nerves: the trigeminal nerve (CN V), the facial nerve (CN VII), the hypoglossal nerve (CN XII), and nerves from the cervical plexus.

ARTERIAL SUPPLY

□ The major muscles of mastication receive the majority of their arterial supply from the maxillary artery.

□ The infrahyoid muscles receive their arterial supply from the superior thyroid artery. Arterial supply to the suprahyoid muscles is varied.

Superficial Right Lateral View of the Muscles of the Head

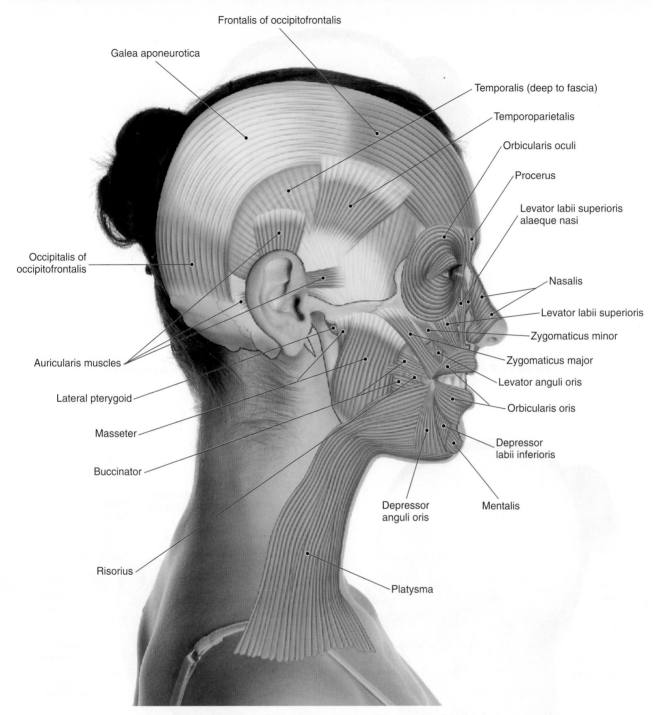

Figure 12-1 Superficial right lateral view of the muscles of the head.

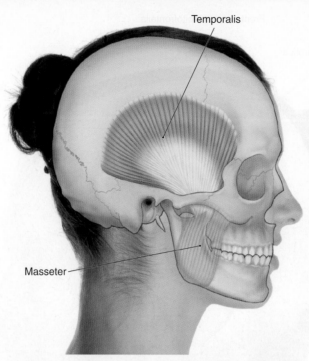

Figure 12-2 Right lateral view of the temporalis and masseter. The masseter has been ghosted in.

12

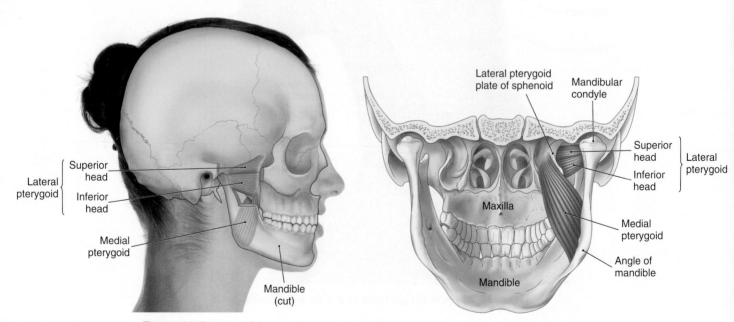

Figure 12-3 Views of the right lateral and medial pterygoids. **A,** Lateral view with the mandible partially cut away. **B,** Posterior view of the lateral and medial pterygoids with the cranial bones cut away.

Anterior Views of the Neck and Upper Chest Region

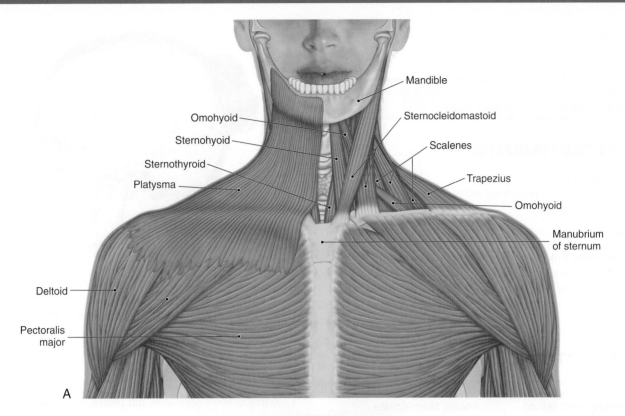

Mandible
Omohyoid
Sternocleidomastoid
Sternohyoid
Scalenes
Sternothyroid
Trapezius
Platysma
Omohyoid
Manubrium of sternum
Deltoid
Pectoralis major

A

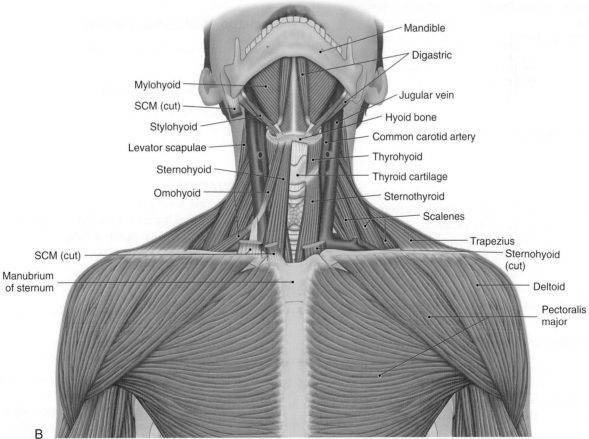

Mandible
Digastric
Mylohyoid
Jugular vein
SCM (cut)
Hyoid bone
Stylohyoid
Common carotid artery
Levator scapulae
Thyrohyoid
Sternohyoid
Thyroid cartilage
Omohyoid
Sternothyroid
Scalenes
Trapezius
SCM (cut)
Sternohyoid (cut)
Manubrium of sternum
Deltoid
Pectoralis major

B

Figure 12-4 Anterior views of the neck and upper chest region. **A,** Superficial views; the platysma has been removed on the left side. **B,** Intermediate views with the head extended. The sternocleidomastoid has been cut on the right side; the sternocleidomastoid and omohyoid have been removed and the sternohyoid has been cut on the left side.

Temporalis

The name, temporalis, *tells us that this muscle attaches onto the temporal bone.*

Derivation	☐ temporalis: L. *refers to the temple.*
Pronunciation	☐ tem-po-RA-lis

■ ATTACHMENTS

☐ **Temporal Fossa**
  ☐ the entire temporal fossa except the portion on the zygomatic bone

to the

☐ **Coronoid Process and the Ramus of the Mandible**
  ☐ the anterior border, apex, posterior border, and internal surface of the coronoid process of the mandible, as well as the anterior border of the ramus of the mandible

■ FUNCTIONS

CONCENTRIC (SHORTENING) MOVER ACTIONS	
Standard Mover Actions	**Reverse Mover Actions**
☐ **1. Elevates the mandible at the TMJs**	☐ 1. Moves the temporal bone inferiorly toward the mandible
☐ 2. Retracts the mandible at the TMJs	☐ 2. Moves the temporal bone anteriorly toward the mandible

TMJs = temporomandibular joints

Standard Mover Action Notes

- The anterior fibers of the temporalis are oriented vertically from the cranium superiorly, to the mandible inferiorly. When the temporalis contracts, it pulls the mandible superiorly toward the cranium. Therefore the temporalis elevates the mandible at the TMJs. (action 1)
- The posterior fibers of the temporalis are oriented horizontally from the cranium posteriorly, to the mandible anteriorly. When the temporalis contracts, it pulls the mandible posteriorly toward the cranium. Therefore the temporalis retracts the mandible at the TMJs. (action 2)

Reverse Mover Action Notes

- Reverse actions of moving the temporal bone toward the mandible require the mandible to be fixed and the temporal bone and entire cranium to move toward the fixed mandible at the TMJs. These reverse actions do not commonly occur. When they do occur, they would be opposite in direction to the standard mover actions. Therefore, the cranium would be pulled inferiorly and anteriorly. (reverse actions 1, 2)

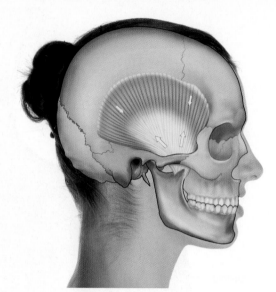

Figure 12-5 Lateral view of the right temporalis. The masseter has been ghosted in.

Eccentric Antagonist Functions

1. Restrains/slows depression and protraction of the mandible

Isometric Stabilization Function

1. Stabilizes the mandible at the TMJs

Additional Note on Functions

1. Some sources state that the temporalis also contributes to side-to-side grinding by doing ipsilateral deviation of the mandible at the TMJs.

INNERVATION
☐ The Trigeminal Nerve (CN V)
  ☐ deep temporal branches of the anterior trunk of the mandibular division of the trigeminal nerve

ARTERIAL SUPPLY
☐ The Maxillary and Superficial Temporal Arteries (branches of the External Carotid Artery)

🖐 PALPATION

1. With the client supine, place palpating fingers over the temporal fossa.
2. Have the client alternately clench and relax the teeth and feel for the contraction and relaxation of the temporalis. In this manner the majority of the temporalis superior to the zygomatic arch can be easily palpated.

■ RELATIONSHIP TO OTHER STRUCTURES

☐ The superior portion of the temporalis is superficial (except for the auriculares anterior and superior, which are superficial to it). The inferior portion of the temporalis runs deep to the zygomatic arch. Inferior to the zygomatic arch, the temporalis is deep to the masseter.

☐ Deep to the superior portion of the temporalis are the cranial bones (frontal, parietal, temporal, and sphenoid).

☐ Deep to the inferior portion of the temporalis are the lateral pterygoid, the superficial head of the medial pterygoid, and a small part of the buccinator.

☐ The temporalis is involved with the deep front line myofascial meridian.

■ MISCELLANEOUS

1. The temporalis muscle is deep to thick fibrous fascia called the *temporalis fascia*.
2. The more superficial fibers of the temporalis actually attach into the temporal fascia.
3. A tight temporalis may be involved with tension headaches and with dysfunction of the temporomandibular joint *(TMJ syndrome)*.
4. The temporal fossa is a fossa (depression) that overlies not only the temporal bone but also the frontal, parietal, zygomatic, and sphenoid bones.
5. The superficial temporal artery is superficial to the temporalis muscle, and its pulse can be palpated.
6. The temporal fossa is much deeper in carnivores, allowing for a much thicker and stronger temporalis muscle. This contributes to the strength of a carnivore's bite.

12

Masseter

The name, masseter, *tells us that this muscle is involved with chewing.*

Derivation	□ masseter: Gr. *chewer*.
Pronunciation	□ MA-sa-ter

■ ATTACHMENTS

□ **Inferior Margins of Both the Zygomatic Bone and the Zygomatic Arch of the Temporal Bone**
  □ SUPERFICIAL LAYER: the inferior margins of the zygomatic bone and the zygomatic arch
  □ DEEP LAYER: the inferior margin and the deep surface of the zygomatic arch

to the

□ **Angle, Ramus, and Coronoid Process of the Mandible**
  □ SUPERFICIAL LAYER: the angle and the inferior ½ of the external surface of the ramus of the mandible
  □ DEEP LAYER: the external surface of the coronoid process, and the superior ½ of the external surface of the ramus of the mandible

■ FUNCTIONS

CONCENTRIC (SHORTENING) MOVER ACTIONS	
Standard Mover Actions	**Reverse Mover Actions**
□ **1. Elevates the mandible at the TMJs**	□ 1. Moves the cranium inferiorly toward the mandible
□ 2. Protracts the mandible at the TMJs	□ 2. Moves the cranium posteriorly toward the mandible
□ 3. Retracts the mandible at the TMJs	□ 3. Moves the cranium anteriorly toward the mandible

TMJs = temporomandibular joints

Standard Mover Action Notes

- The fibers of the masseter are oriented vertically from the zygomatic bone and zygomatic arch of the temporal bone superiorly, to the mandible inferiorly. When the masseter contracts, it pulls the mandible superiorly toward the zygomatic bone and arch. Therefore the masseter elevates the mandible at the TMJs. (action 1)
- The masseter is the prime mover of elevation of the mandible at the TMJs. (action 1)
- The superficial layer of the masseter is somewhat oriented in a horizontal fashion from the zygomatic bone anteriorly, to the mandible posteriorly. When the superficial layer of the masseter contracts, it pulls the mandible anteriorly toward the zygomatic bone. Therefore the masseter protracts the mandible at the TMJs. (action 2)

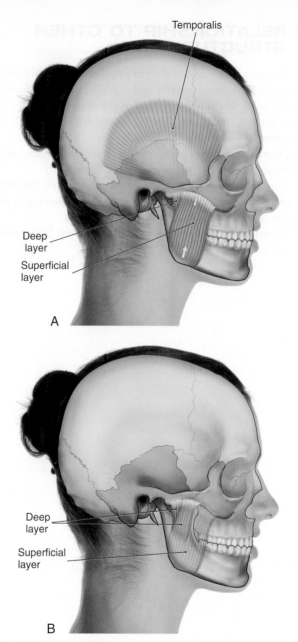

Figure 12-6 Lateral views of the right masseter. **A,** The temporalis has been ghosted in. **B,** The superficial head of the masseter has been ghosted in.

- The deep layer of the masseter is somewhat oriented in a horizontal fashion from the zygomatic arch of the temporal bone posteriorly, to the mandible anteriorly. When the deep layer of the masseter contracts, it pulls the mandible posteriorly toward the zygomatic arch. Therefore the masseter retracts the mandible at the TMJs. (Note: Keep in mind that retraction can only occur if the mandible is first protracted. When the mandible is first protracted, the horizontal orientation of the fibers of the deep layer of the masseter increases.) (action 3)

12

Masseter—*cont'd*

Reverse Mover Action Note

1. Reverse actions of moving the cranium (temporal and zygomatic bones) toward the mandible require the mandible to be fixed and the entire cranium to move toward the fixed mandible at the TMJs. These reverse actions do not commonly occur. (reverse actions 1, 2, 3)

Eccentric Antagonist Function

1. Restrains/slows depression, retraction, and protraction of the mandible

Isometric Stabilization Function

1. Stabilizes the mandible at the TMJs

Additional Note on Function

1. Some sources state that the masseter can also ipsilaterally deviate the mandible, contributing to side-to-side grinding.

INNERVATION
- ☐ The Trigeminal Nerve (CN V)
  - ☐ anterior trunk of the mandibular division of the trigeminal nerve

ARTERIAL SUPPLY
- ☐ The Maxillary Artery (a branch of the External Carotid Artery)
  - ☐ and the Transverse Facial Artery (a branch of the Superficial Temporal Artery)

✋ PALPATION

1. With the client supine, place palpating fingers between the zygomatic arch and the angle of the mandible.
2. Have the client alternately clench the teeth and relax and feel for contraction and relaxation of the masseter. When the masseter contracts, the muscle may visibly bulge out.

■ RELATIONSHIP TO OTHER STRUCTURES

- ☐ The masseter is superficial in the cheek except for the platysma, the risorius, and the zygomaticus major (muscles of facial expression).
- ☐ The large parotid gland and parotid duct are superficial to the masseter.
- ☐ Deep to the masseter are the temporalis, part of the buccinator, and the ramus of the mandible.
- ☐ The masseter is involved with the deep front line myofascial meridian.

■ MISCELLANEOUS

1. The masseter is usually divided into two layers: a *superficial layer* and a *deep layer*.
2. Some sources further subdivide the deep layer of the masseter into two layers and therefore state that overall, the masseter has three layers: a *superficial layer*, a *middle layer*, and a *deep layer*.
3. The superficial layer of the masseter is the largest.
4. The masseter and medial pterygoid form a sling that supports the mandible. The masseter is superficial to the mandible; the medial pterygoid is deep to it.
5. The masseter may be involved with dysfunction of the temporomandibular joint *(TMJ syndrome)*.
6. Proportional to its size, the masseter is stated by many sources to be the strongest muscle in the human body.

12

Lateral Pterygoid

The name, lateral pterygoid, *tells us that this muscle attaches to the sphenoid bone (the pterygoid process) and is lateral (lateral to the medial pterygoid muscle).*

Derivation	☐ lateral: L. *side.*
	pterygoid: Gr. *wing shaped.*
Pronunciation	☐ LAT-er-al, TER-i-goyd

■ ATTACHMENTS

☐ **Entire Muscle: Sphenoid Bone**
  ☐ SUPERIOR HEAD: the greater wing of the sphenoid
  ☐ INFERIOR HEAD: the lateral surface of the lateral pterygoid plate of the pterygoid process of the sphenoid

  to the

☐ **Mandible and the Temporomandibular Joint (TMJ)**
  ☐ SUPERIOR HEAD: the capsule and articular disc of the TMJ
  ☐ INFERIOR HEAD: the neck of the mandible

■ FUNCTIONS

CONCENTRIC (SHORTENING) MOVER ACTIONS	
Standard Mover Actions	**Reverse Mover Actions**
☐ **1. Protracts the mandible at the TMJs**	☐ 1. Moves the cranium posteriorly toward the mandible
☐ **2. Contralaterally deviates the mandible at the TMJs**	☐ 2. Moves the cranium laterally (ipsilateral deviation) toward the mandible

TMJs = temporomandibular joints

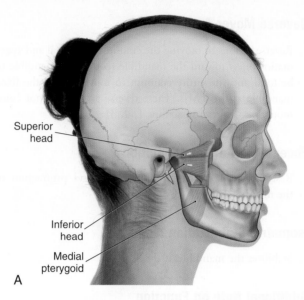

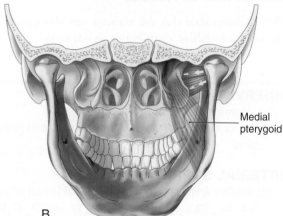

Figure 12-7 Views of the right lateral pterygoid with the medial pterygoid ghosted in. **A,** Lateral view with the mandible partially cut away. **B,** Posterior view with the cranial bones cut away.

Standard Mover Action Notes

• The lateral pterygoid attaches from the sphenoid anteriorly, to the mandible posteriorly (with its fibers running horizontally). When the lateral pterygoid contracts, it pulls the mandible anteriorly toward the sphenoid. Therefore the lateral pterygoid protracts the mandible at the TMJs. (action 1)

• The lateral pterygoid attaches from the sphenoid medially, to the mandible laterally (with its fibers running horizontally). When the lateral pterygoid contracts, it pulls the mandible medially toward the sphenoid. By pulling one side of the mandible toward the sphenoid, the entire mandible is pulled toward the opposite side of the body. This movement is called *lateral deviation of the mandible.* Because the lateral pterygoid on one side of the body pulls the mandible toward the opposite side of the body, this action is called *contralateral deviation of the mandible,* and it occurs at the TMJs. (action 2)

• Lateral deviation of the mandible at the TMJs is important for grinding and chewing food. (action 2)

Reverse Mover Action Notes

• Reverse actions of moving the sphenoid bone toward the mandible require the mandible to be fixed and the sphenoid bone and entire cranium to move toward the fixed mandible at the TMJs. These reverse actions do not commonly occur. (reverse actions 1, 2)

Eccentric Antagonist Function

1. Restrains/slows retraction and ipsilateral deviation of the mandible

Lateral Pterygoid—cont'd

Isometric Stabilization Function

1. Stabilizes the mandible at the TMJs

Additional Notes on Functions

1. As protraction of the mandible occurs with opening the jaw, the articular disc of the TMJ must also protract to stay in proper alignment between the mandibular condyle and the mandibular fossa of the temporal bone. Given its attachment into the articular disc, the lateral pterygoid guides this movement of the articular disc.
2. Some sources report that the inferior belly of the lateral pterygoid can also depress the mandible at the TMJs. Given that its mandibular attachment is higher than the sphenoid attachment, this seems likely.
3. Some sources state that the superior belly of the lateral pterygoid can elevate the mandible at the TMJs. Given that its mandibular attachment is lower than the sphenoid attachment, this seems likely.

INNERVATION
- ☐ The Trigeminal Nerve (CN V)
  - ☐ lateral pterygoid nerve from the anterior trunk of the mandibular division of the trigeminal nerve

ARTERIAL SUPPLY
- ☐ The Maxillary Artery (a branch of the External Carotid Artery)

✋ PALPATION

1. With the client seated or supine, wearing a finger cot or glove, place palpating fingers along the external surfaces of the upper teeth until you reach the back molars.
2. Press posteriorly and superiorly (it may feel like your finger is in a little pocket; this is where peanut butter often gets stuck!), and then medially against the inside wall of the mouth and laterally against the condyle of the mandible.
3. Have the client protract the mandible and feel for the contraction of the lateral pterygoid.

■ RELATIONSHIP TO OTHER STRUCTURES

- ☐ Of the two pterygoid muscles, the lateral pterygoid is named *lateral* because its attachment onto the pterygoid process of the sphenoid bone is more lateral than the attachment of the medial pterygoid onto the pterygoid process of the sphenoid bone. Regarding the gross location of the bellies of these two muscles, the lateral pterygoid is generally lateral and superior in location relative to the medial pterygoid.
- ☐ The majority of the lateral pterygoid is deep to the zygomatic arch of the temporal bone and the coronoid process of the mandible. The lateral pterygoid is also deep to the masseter muscle and the inferior tendon of the temporalis.
- ☐ The superior part of the deep head of the medial pterygoid is deep to the lateral pterygoid.
- ☐ The lateral pterygoid may be involved with the deep front line myofascial meridian.

■ MISCELLANEOUS

1. The lateral pterygoid is sometimes known as the *external pterygoid.*
2. Both the lateral pterygoid and the medial pterygoid attach onto the lateral pterygoid plate of the pterygoid process of the sphenoid bone. The two pterygoids are so named because the lateral pterygoid attaches onto the lateral surface of the lateral pterygoid plate and the medial pterygoid attaches onto the medial surface of the lateral pterygoid plate.
3. The lateral pterygoid functions to protract the mandible and the articular disc of the temporomandibular joint (TMJ). It is important that the mandible and disc protract together when the jaw is opened. Therefore if the contraction of the lateral pterygoid is not precisely coordinated with the other muscles that move the mandible, the articular disc may become jammed between the two bones of the joint and dysfunction of the TMJ *(TMJ syndrome)* may occur.
4. Although all four major muscles of mastication (temporalis, masseter, and the lateral and medial pterygoids) may be involved in *TMJ syndrome,* given the attachments of the lateral pterygoid directly into the capsule and articular disc of the TMJ, it is clear that hypertonicity of a lateral pterygoid could excessively pull on the soft tissue structures of the TMJ and therefore cause dysfunction of the TMJ *(TMJ syndrome).*

12

Medial Pterygoid

The name, medial pterygoid, *tells us that this muscle attaches to the sphenoid bone (the pterygoid process) and is medial (medial to the lateral pterygoid muscle).*

Derivation	☐ medial: L. *toward the middle.*
	pterygoid: Gr. *wing shaped.*
Pronunciation	☐ MEE-dee-al, TER-i-goyd

■ ATTACHMENTS

☐ **Entire Muscle: Sphenoid Bone**
  ☐ DEEP HEAD: the medial surface of the lateral pterygoid plate of the pterygoid process of the sphenoid, the palatine bone, and the tuberosity of the maxilla
  ☐ SUPERFICIAL HEAD: the palatine bone and the maxilla

  to the

☐ **Internal Surface of the Mandible**
  ☐ at the angle and the inferior border of the ramus of the mandible

12

■ FUNCTIONS

CONCENTRIC (SHORTENING) MOVER ACTIONS	
Standard Mover Actions	**Reverse Mover Actions**
☐ **1. Elevates the mandible at the TMJs**	☐ 1. Moves the cranium inferiorly toward the mandible
☐ **2. Protracts the mandible at the TMJs**	☐ 2. Moves the cranium posteriorly toward the mandible
☐ **3. Contralaterally deviates the mandible at the TMJs**	☐ 3. Moves the cranium laterally (ipsilateral deviation) toward the mandible

TMJs = temporomandibular joints

Standard Mover Action Notes

• The fibers of the medial pterygoid are oriented vertically from the sphenoid superiorly, to the mandible inferiorly. When the medial pterygoid contracts, it pulls the mandible superiorly toward the sphenoid. Therefore the medial pterygoid elevates the mandible at the TMJs. (action 1)

• The medial pterygoid attaches from the sphenoid anteriorly, to the mandible posteriorly, (with its fibers running somewhat horizontally). When the medial pterygoid contracts, it pulls the mandible anteriorly toward the sphenoid. Therefore the medial pterygoid protracts the mandible at the TMJs. (action 2)

• The medial pterygoid attaches from the sphenoid medially, to the mandible laterally (with its fibers running somewhat

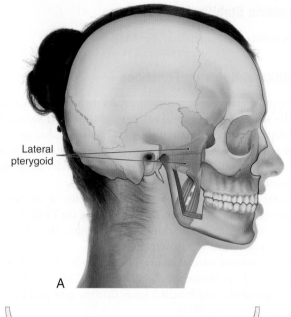

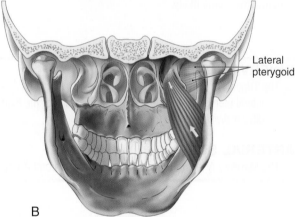

Figure 12-8 Views of the right medial pterygoid with the lateral pterygoid ghosted in. **A,** Lateral view with the mandible partially cut away. **B,** Posterior view with the cranial bones cut away.

horizontally). When the medial pterygoid contracts, it pulls the mandible medially toward the sphenoid. By pulling one side of the mandible toward the sphenoid, the entire mandible is pulled toward the opposite side of the body. This movement is called *lateral deviation of the mandible.* Because the medial pterygoid on one side of the body pulls the mandible toward the opposite side of the body, this action is called *contralateral deviation of the mandible,* and it occurs at the TMJs. (action 3)

• Lateral deviation of the mandible at the TMJs is important for grinding and chewing food. (action 3)

Reverse Mover Action Notes

• Reverse actions of moving the sphenoid bone toward the mandible require the mandible to be fixed and the sphenoid

Medial Pterygoid—*cont'd*

bone and entire cranium to move toward the fixed mandible at the TMJs. These reverse actions do not commonly occur. (reverse actions 1, 2, 3)

Eccentric Antagonist Function

1. Restrains/slows depression, retraction, and ipsilateral deviation of the mandible

Isometric Stabilization Function

1. Stabilizes the mandible at the TMJs

Additional Note on Functions

1. The medial pterygoid and masseter are oriented very similarly, attaching inferiorly to the inferior angle of the mandible and running superiorly to the other attachment. Therefore they both elevate the mandible at the TMJs.

INNERVATION
- ☐ The Trigeminal Nerve (CN V)
  - ☐ medial pterygoid nerve from the mandibular division of the trigeminal nerve

ARTERIAL SUPPLY
- ☐ The Maxillary Artery (a branch of the External Carotid Artery)

🖐 PALPATION

1. With the client seated or supine, place palpating fingers on the angle of the mandible and then hook them under onto the internal surface of the mandible.
2. Have the client clench the teeth and feel for the contraction of the medial pterygoid.
3. To palpate from inside the mouth, wearing a finger cot or glove, place palpating finger along the internal surfaces of the lower teeth until you reach the back molars.
4. Press posterolaterally against the inside wall of the mouth, have the client protract the mandible, and feel for the contraction of the medial pterygoid.

■ RELATIONSHIP TO OTHER STRUCTURES

- ☐ Of the two pterygoid muscles, the medial pterygoid is named *medial* because its attachment onto the pterygoid process of the sphenoid bone is more medial than the attachment of the lateral pterygoid onto the pterygoid process of the sphenoid bone. Regarding the gross location of the bellies of these two muscles, the medial pterygoid is generally medial and inferior in location relative to the lateral pterygoid.
- ☐ The medial pterygoid is deep to the coronoid process, the ramus, and the angle of the mandible (and the zygomatic arch as well). The medial pterygoid is also deep to the masseter and the inferior tendon of the temporalis.
- ☐ From the lateral perspective, the majority of the medial pterygoid is deep to the lateral pterygoid.
- ☐ From the posterolateral perspective, the internal wall of the mouth is deep to the medial pterygoid.
- ☐ A number of small muscles of the palate and the pharynx lie close to the medial attachment of the medial pterygoid.
- ☐ The medial pterygoid is involved with the deep front line myofascial meridian.

■ MISCELLANEOUS

1. The medial pterygoid is sometimes known as the *internal pterygoid.*
2. The medial pterygoid is a fairly thick, quadrilateral (square) muscle.
3. The medial pterygoid is usually divided into a *deep head* and a *superficial head.*
4. The deep head of the medial pterygoid is the larger of the two heads.
5. The direction of fibers of the medial pterygoid is essentially identical to the direction of the fibers of the masseter; in fact, these two muscles occupy the same position. The difference is that the masseter is external (superficial) to the mandible, and the medial pterygoid is internal (deep) to the mandible.
6. The masseter and medial pterygoid form a sling that supports the mandible.
7. Both the medial pterygoid and the lateral pterygoid attach onto the lateral pterygoid plate of the pterygoid process of the sphenoid bone. The two pterygoids are so named because the medial pterygoid attaches onto the medial surface of the lateral pterygoid plate, and the lateral pterygoid attaches onto the lateral surface of the lateral pterygoid plate.
8. A tight medial pterygoid may be involved with dysfunction of the TMJ *(TMJ syndrome).*

12

Hyoid Group

The hyoids are a group of eight muscles that are superficial in the anterior neck. They are subdivided into two groups of four, as follows:

- The infrahyoids: sternohyoid, sternothyroid, thyrohyoid, omohyoid
- The suprahyoids: digastric, mylohyoid, geniohyoid, stylohyoid

■ ATTACHMENTS

☐ All the hyoid muscles (except the sternothyroid) attach onto the hyoid bone.

☐ The infrahyoids are located inferior to the hyoid bone.

☐ The suprahyoids are located superior to the hyoid bone.

■ ACTIONS

☐ The hyoids are involved with movement of the mandible at the temporomandibular joints (TMJs). Most of the suprahyoids attach directly to the mandible and can depress it. The infrahyoids are also involved because they must stabilize the hyoid bone so that the suprahyoids' contraction acts to depress the mandible. In this manner, all hyoid muscles can act synergistically to depress the mandible at the TMJs, hence they are placed in this chapter as muscles of mastication.

☐ The suprahyoids and infrahyoids may act synergistically to stabilize the hyoid bone as a stable base of attachment for movements of the tongue. Therefore the hyoid muscles are important in chewing, swallowing, and speech.

☐ As a group, because the hyoids cross the cervical spinal joints anteriorly with their fibers running vertically, they can all act synergistically to assist with flexion of the neck at the spinal joints. For this to occur, the hyoid bone and the mandible must be fixed (stabilized).

☐ The infrahyoids depress the hyoid bone; the suprahyoids elevate the hyoid bone. In this manner, the infrahyoids and the suprahyoids may be considered to be antagonistic to each other.

■ MISCELLANEOUS

1. The carotid sinus of the common carotid artery lies directly deep and lateral to the hyoid muscles midway up the neck. Given the neurologic reflex that occurs to lower blood pressure when the carotid sinus is pressed, massage to this region must be done judiciously, especially with weak and/or elderly clients.

2. The hyoid muscles are located within the deep front line myofascial meridian.

INNERVATION

☐ The hyoid muscles are innervated by the following nerves: the trigeminal nerve (CN V), the facial nerve (CN VII), the hypoglossal nerve (CN XII), and nerves from the cervical plexus.

ARTERIAL SUPPLY

☐ The infrahyoid muscles receive their arterial supply from the superior thyroid artery. Arterial supply to the suprahyoid muscles is varied.

Hyoid Group—*cont'd*

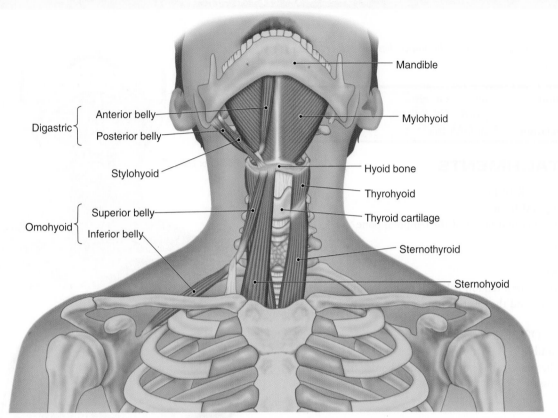

Figure 12-9 Anterior view of the hyoid muscle group. The sternohyoid, omohyoid, stylohyoid, and digastric have been removed on the left. The geniohyoid is deep to the mylohyoid and not seen.

SUPRAHYOIDS
Digastric (of Hyoid Group)

The name, digastric, *tells us that this muscle has two bellies (gaster means belly).*

Derivation	☐ di:	Gr. *two.*
	gastric:	Gr. *belly.*
Pronunciation	☐ di-GAS-trik	

■ ATTACHMENTS

☐ POSTERIOR BELLY:
  ☐ **Temporal Bone**
    ☐ the mastoid notch of the temporal bone

to the

  ☐ **Hyoid**
    ☐ the central tendon is bound to the hyoid bone at the body and the greater cornu

☐ ANTERIOR BELLY:
  ☐ **Mandible**
    ☐ the inner surface of the inferior border (the digastric fossa)

to the

  ☐ **Hyoid**
    ☐ the central tendon is bound to the hyoid bone at the body and the greater cornu

■ FUNCTIONS

CONCENTRIC (SHORTENING) MOVER ACTIONS	
Standard Mover Actions	**Reverse Mover Actions**
☐ **1. Depresses the mandible at the TMJs**	☐ **1. Elevates the hyoid bone**
☐ 2. Retracts the mandible at the TMJs	
☐ **3. Flexes the head and neck at the spinal joints**	
☐ 4. Extends the head at the AOJ	

TMJs = temporomandibular joints; AOJ = atlanto-occipital joint

Standard Mover Action Notes

- The anterior belly of the digastric attaches superiorly and anteriorly to the mandible and inferiorly and posteriorly to the hyoid bone. If the hyoid bone is fixed, the digastric pulls the mandible inferiorly and posteriorly toward the hyoid bone. Therefore it depresses and retracts the mandible at the TMJs. (actions 1, 2)
- The digastric is considered to be the prime mover of depression of the mandible at the TMJs. (action 1)

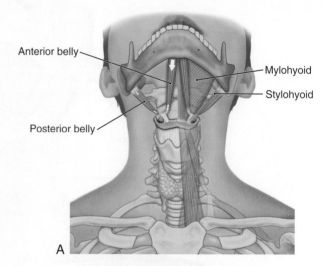

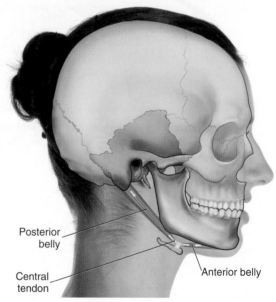

Figure 12-10 Views of the digastric. **A,** Anterior view of the digastric bilaterally with other hyoid muscles ghosted in on the client's left side. **B,** Right lateral view.

- If the anterior belly of the digastric pulls inferiorly on the mandible, and elevators of the mandible contract to fix the mandible to the cranium, then when the digastric contracts, it pulls the entire head and neck forward into flexion at the spinal joints. (action 3)
- When the hyoid bone and mandible are fixed and the posterior belly of the digastric contracts, it pulls the temporal bone toward the hyoid bone. Because its line of pull is posterior to the AOJ, it extends the head at the AOJ. (action 4)
- Even though one belly of the digastric may be primarily responsible for a certain action (as indicated in the above notes), its line of pull to create this action will not be effi-

Digastric (of Hyoid Group)—*cont'd*

client unless the other belly also contracts to stabilize the hyoid bone. (actions 1, 2, 3, 4)

Reverse Mover Action Note

- The digastric is unusual in that it has two bellies. The anterior belly attaches inferiorly to the hyoid bone and superiorly to the mandible; the posterior belly attaches inferiorly to the hyoid bone and superiorly to the temporal bone. When the mandible and temporal bone are fixed (stabilized) and the digastric contracts, it pulls the hyoid bone superiorly. Movements of the hyoid bone are important in chewing, swallowing, and speech. (reverse action 1)

Eccentric Antagonist Functions

1. Restrains/slows elevation and protraction of the mandible
2. Restrains/slows depression of the hyoid bone
3. Restrains/slows extension of the head and neck
4. Restrains/slows flexion of the head

Isometric Stabilization Functions

1. Stabilizes the TMJs
2. Stabilizes the hyoid bone
3. Stabilizes the head and neck

Additional Notes on Functions

1. The digastric can also protract and retract the hyoid bone. The anterior belly of the digastric can protract the hyoid (i.e., draw the hyoid anteriorly), and the posterior belly of the digastric can retract the hyoid (i.e., draw the hyoid posteriorly).
2. All hyoid muscles are important in moving and/or fixing (stabilizing) the hyoid bone. These functions are necessary for chewing, swallowing, and speech.
3. All hyoid muscles can assist with flexion of the neck at the spinal joints.

INNERVATION

- The Trigeminal Nerve (CN V) and the Facial Nerve (CN VII)
  - anterior belly: mylohyoid branch of the inferior alveolar nerve of posterior trunk of the mandibular division of the trigeminal nerve (CN V)
  - posterior belly: facial nerve (CN VII)

ARTERIAL SUPPLY

- The Occipital, Posterior Auricular, and Facial Arteries (branches of the External Carotid Artery)

✋ PALPATION

1. With the client supine, place palpating hand between the sternocleidomastoid and the ramus of the mandible.
2. Ask the client to depress the mandible against gentle resistance and feel for the contraction of the digastric. It will be a pencil-thin muscle running horizontally.
3. Palpate as much of the digastric as possible. Note: Discerning the posterior belly of the digastric from the stylohyoid can be challenging.

■ RELATIONSHIP TO OTHER STRUCTURES

- The digastric runs an unusual course. The posterior belly attaches to the mastoid notch of the temporal bone (deep to the sternocleidomastoid). It then runs anteriorly and slightly inferiorly toward the hyoid bone. Near the hyoid bone, the digastric becomes tendinous (the central tendon). However, the digastric does not attach directly to the hyoid bone, but rather its central tendon is attached to the hyoid by a fibrous sling of tissue. From there, the anterior belly runs superiorly and anteriorly to the inner surface of the mandible.
- Except for the occipital attachment of the sternocleidomastoid and the platysma (which is superficial to all anterior neck muscles), the digastric is superficial for its entire course in the lateral and anterior neck. The submandibular salivary gland may also be superficial to the digastric.
- The posterior belly of the digastric runs inferior to, and parallel to, the stylohyoid.
- The central tendon of the digastric perforates the attachment of the stylohyoid onto the hyoid bone.
- Deep to the posterior belly of the digastric is the transverse process of the atlas (C1).
- The digastric is located within the deep front line myofascial meridian.

■ MISCELLANEOUS

1. The digastric is one of the four suprahyoid muscles. The four suprahyoid muscles are the digastric, mylohyoid, geniohyoid, and stylohyoid.
2. The external carotid artery lies inferior and deep to the anterior belly of the digastric. Massage to this region must be done judiciously.
3. The digastric is unusual in that it has two separate bellies: a posterior belly and an anterior belly.
4. The digastric's two bellies are separated by its *central tendon* (also known as the *intermediate tendon*). Like the omohyoid (an infrahyoid muscle), the central tendon of the digastric is tethered (attached) to bone by a fibrous sling of tissue.

12

Mylohyoid (of Hyoid Group)

The name, mylohyoid, *tells us that this muscle attaches to the hyoid bone.* Mylo, *referring to the molar teeth, tells us that this muscle also attaches close to the molar teeth.*

Derivation	☐ mylo: Gr. *mill (refers to the molar teeth).*
	hyoid: Gr. *refers to the hyoid bone.*
Pronunciation	☐ MY-lo-HI-oyd

■ ATTACHMENTS

☐ **Inner Surface of the Mandible**
  ☐ the mylohyoid line of the mandible (from the symphysis menti to the molars)

  to the

☐ **Hyoid**
  ☐ the anterior surface of the body of the hyoid

■ FUNCTIONS

CONCENTRIC (SHORTENING) MOVER ACTIONS	
Standard Mover Actions	**Reverse Mover Actions**
☐ 1. Depresses the mandible at the TMJs	☐ 1. Elevates the hyoid bone
☐ 2. Flexes the head and neck at the spinal joints	

TMJs = temporomandibular joints

Standard Mover Action Notes

- The mylohyoid attaches from the mandible superiorly, to the hyoid bone inferiorly (with its fibers running somewhat vertically). When the hyoid bone is fixed and the mylohyoid contracts, it pulls the mandible inferiorly toward the hyoid bone. Therefore the mylohyoid depresses the mandible at the TMJs. (action 1)
- If the mylohyoid pulls inferiorly on the mandible, and elevators of the mandible contract to fix the mandible to the cranium, then when the mylohyoid contracts, it pulls the entire head and neck forward into flexion at the spinal joints. (action 2)

Reverse Mover Action Note

- The mylohyoid attaches from the mandible superiorly, to the hyoid bone inferiorly (with its fibers running vertically). When the mandible is fixed and the mylohyoid contracts, it pulls the hyoid bone superiorly toward the mandible. Therefore the mylohyoid elevates the hyoid bone. Movements of the hyoid bone are important in chewing, swallowing, and speech. (reverse action 1)

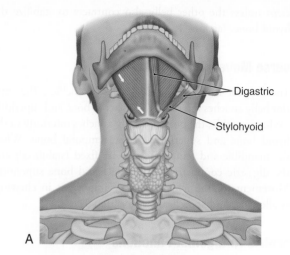

A

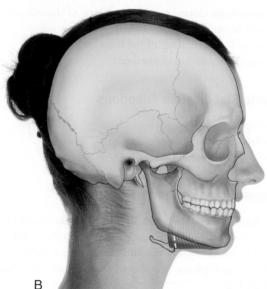

B

Figure 12-11 Views of the mylohyoid. **A,** Anterior view of the mylohyoid bilaterally with the digastric and stylohyoid shown on the client's left side. **B,** Right lateral view.

Eccentric Antagonist Functions

1. Restrains/slows elevation of the mandible
2. Restrains/slows extension of the head and neck
3. Restrains/slows depression of the hyoid bone

Isometric Stabilization Functions

1. Stabilizes the mandible at the TMJs
2. Stabilizes the hyoid bone
3. Stabilizes the head and neck

Additional Notes on Functions

1. Another function of the mylohyoid is to elevate the floor of the mouth during the first stage of swallowing.

12

Mylohyoid (of Hyoid Group)—*cont'd*

2. All hyoid muscles are important in moving and/or fixing (stabilizing) the hyoid bone. These functions are necessary for chewing, swallowing, and speech.
3. All hyoid muscles can assist with flexion of the neck at the spinal joints.

INNERVATION
☐ The Trigeminal Nerve (CN V)
  ☐ the mylohyoid branch of the inferior alveolar nerve of the posterior trunk of the mandibular division of the trigeminal nerve (CN V)

ARTERIAL SUPPLY
☐ The Inferior Alveolar Artery (a branch of the Maxillary Artery)

✋ PALPATION

1. With the client supine, place palpating fingers under the chin.
2. Ask the client to depress the mandible against resistance or push the tip of the tongue against the roof of the mouth and feel for the contraction of the mylohyoid.

◼ RELATIONSHIP TO OTHER STRUCTURES

☐ The mylohyoid is a broad, flat muscle that forms the muscular floor of the oral cavity.
☐ Superior to the mylohyoid is the geniohyoid.
☐ Inferior to the mylohyoid is the anterior belly of the digastric.
☐ From the perspective of the underside of the mandible, the mylohyoid is superficial except for the anterior belly of the digastric and the platysma.
☐ The mylohyoid is located within the deep front line myofascial meridian.

◼ MISCELLANEOUS

1. The mylohyoid is one of the four suprahyoid muscles. The four suprahyoid muscles are the digastric, mylohyoid, geniohyoid, and stylohyoid.
2. The fibers from the left and right mylohyoid muscles meet each other in the midline and form a median fibrous raphe. (A *raphe* is a seam of tissue formed by the union of the halves of a part.)

12

Geniohyoid (of Hyoid Group)

The name, geniohyoid, *tells us that this muscle attaches to the hyoid bone.* Genio, *referring to the chin, tells us that this muscle also attaches to the mandible.*

Derivation	☐ genio: Gr. *chin.*
	hyoid: Gr. *refers to the hyoid bone.*
Pronunciation	☐ JEE-nee-o-HI-oyd

■ ATTACHMENTS

☐ **Inner Surface of the Mandible**
   ☐ the inferior mental spine of the mandible

   to the

☐ **Hyoid**
   ☐ the anterior surface of the body of the hyoid

■ FUNCTIONS

CONCENTRIC (SHORTENING) MOVER ACTIONS	
Standard Mover Actions	**Reverse Mover Actions**
☐ 1. Depresses the mandible at the TMJs	☐ 1. Elevates the hyoid bone
☐ 2. Flexes the head and neck at the spinal joints	

TMJs = temporomandibular joints

Standard Mover Action Notes

- The geniohyoid attaches from the mandible superiorly, to the hyoid bone inferiorly (with its fibers running somewhat vertically). When the hyoid bone is fixed and the geniohyoid contracts, it pulls the mandible inferiorly toward the hyoid bone. Therefore the geniohyoid depresses the mandible at the TMJs. (action 1)
- If the geniohyoid pulls inferiorly on the mandible, and elevators of the mandible contract to fix the mandible to the cranium, then when the geniohyoid contracts, it pulls the entire head and neck forward into flexion at the spinal joints. (action 2)

Reverse Mover Action Note

- The geniohyoid attaches from the mandible superiorly, to the hyoid bone inferiorly (with its fibers running vertically). When the mandible is fixed and the geniohyoid contracts, it pulls the hyoid bone superiorly toward the mandible. Therefore the geniohyoid elevates the hyoid bone. Movements of the hyoid bone are important in chewing, swallowing, and speech. (reverse action 1)

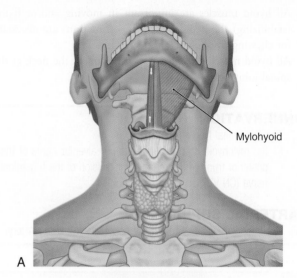

A

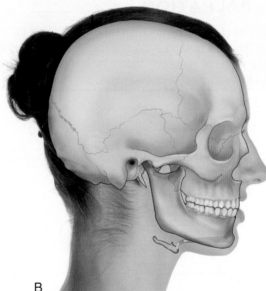

B

Figure 12-12 Views of the geniohyoid. **A,** Anterior view of the geniohyoid bilaterally with the mylohyoid ghosted in on the client's left side. **B,** Right lateral view.

Eccentric Antagonist Functions

1. Restrains/slows elevation of the mandible
2. Restrains/slows extension of the head and neck
3. Restrains/slows depression of the hyoid bone

Isometric Stabilization Functions

1. Stabilizes the mandible at the TMJs
2. Stabilizes the hyoid bone
3. Stabilizes the head and neck

Mylohyoid

Geniohyoid (of Hyoid Group)—*cont'd*

Additional Notes on Functions

1. Another action of the geniohyoid is to protract the hyoid bone (draw the hyoid bone anteriorly).
2. All hyoid muscles are important in moving and/or fixing (i.e., stabilizing) the hyoid bone. These functions are necessary for chewing, swallowing, and speech.
3. All hyoid muscles can assist with flexion of the neck at the spinal joints.

INNERVATION
- The Hypoglossal Nerve (CN XII)
  - a branch of C1 through the hypoglossal nerve

ARTERIAL SUPPLY
- The Lingual Artery (a branch of the External Carotid Artery)

PALPATION

1. With the client supine, place palpating fingers on the underside of the chin in the midline.
2. Ask the client to depress the mandible against gentle resistance or push the tip of the tongue against the roof of the mouth and feel for the contraction of the geniohyoid. Note: It is difficult to discern the geniohyoid from the more superficial mylohyoid.

■ RELATIONSHIP TO OTHER STRUCTURES

- The two geniohyoid muscles are two pencil-thin muscles that lie next to each other in the midline, sandwiched between the mylohyoid and the genioglossus muscles. The mylohyoids are inferior to the geniohyoids; the genioglossus muscles (muscles that move the tongue) (ⓔvolve see the Evolve website) are superior to the geniohyoids.
- From the perspective of the underside of the mandible, the geniohyoid is deep to the mylohyoid, the anterior belly of the digastric, and the platysma muscles.
- The geniohyoid is located within the deep front line myofascial meridian.

■ MISCELLANEOUS

1. The geniohyoid is one of the four suprahyoid muscles. The four suprahyoid muscles are the digastric, mylohyoid, geniohyoid, and stylohyoid.
2. The left and right geniohyoid muscles occasionally blend together.
3. The inferior mental spines are bony landmarks of the mandible that are on the internal (posterior) side, directly behind the symphysis menti (the midline of the mandible).

12

Stylohyoid (of Hyoid Group)

The name, stylohyoid, *tells us that this muscle attaches from the styloid process (of the temporal bone) to the hyoid bone.*

Derivation	☐ stylo: Gr. *refers to the styloid process.*
	hyoid: Gr. *refers to the hyoid bone.*
Pronunciation	☐ STI-lo-HI-oyd

■ ATTACHMENTS

☐ **Styloid Process of the Temporal Bone**
  ☐ the posterior surface

to the

☐ **Hyoid**
  ☐ at the junction of the body and the greater cornu of the hyoid bone

■ FUNCTIONS

CONCENTRIC (SHORTENING) MOVER ACTIONS	
Standard Mover Actions	**Reverse Mover Actions**
☐ 1. Elevates the hyoid bone	☐ 1. Extends the head at the AOJ

AOJ = atlanto-occipital joint

Standard Mover Action Note

• The stylohyoid attaches from the temporal bone superiorly, to the hyoid bone inferiorly (with its fibers running vertically). When the stylohyoid contracts, it pulls the hyoid bone superiorly toward the temporal bone. Therefore the stylohyoid elevates the hyoid. Movements of the hyoid bone are important in chewing, swallowing, and speech. (action 1)

Reverse Mover Action Note

• When the hyoid bone is fixed and the stylohyoid contracts, it pulls the temporal bone and entire cranium toward the hyoid bone. Because its line of pull is posterior to the AOJ, it extends the head at the AOJ. (reverse action 1)

Eccentric Antagonist Functions

1. Restrains/slows depression of the hyoid bone
2. Restrains/slows flexion of the head

Isometric Stabilization Functions

1. Stabilizes the hyoid bone
2. Stabilizes the head at the AOJ

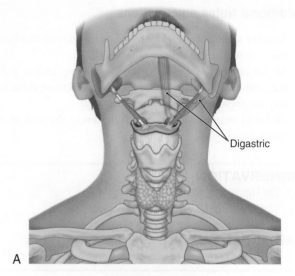

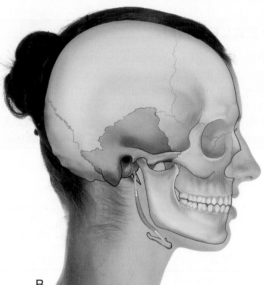

Figure 12-13 Views of the stylohyoid. **A,** Anterior view of the stylohyoid bilaterally with the digastric ghosted in on the client's left side. **B,** Right lateral view.

Additional Notes on Functions

1. The stylohyoid can also retract the hyoid bone.
2. All hyoid muscles are important in moving and/or fixing (stabilizing) the hyoid bone. These functions are necessary for chewing, swallowing, and speech.
3. All hyoid muscles can assist with flexion of the neck at the spinal joints. The stylohyoid assists by stabilizing the hyoid bone.

Stylohyoid (of Hyoid Group)—*cont'd*

INNERVATION
- ☐ The Facial Nerve (CN VII)
  - ☐ the stylohyoid branch

ARTERIAL SUPPLY
- ☐ The Occipital, Posterior Auricular, and Facial Arteries (branches of the External Carotid Artery)

 PALPATION

1. With the client supine, place palpating fingers between the sternocleidomastoid and the posterior ramus of the mandible (i.e., over the styloid process of the temporal bone). Keep your pressure light to moderate because the styloid process of the temporal bone is a delicate structure.
2. Ask the client to swallow and feel for the stylohyoid to contract.
3. Palpate as much of the stylohyoid as possible. It is a pencil-thin muscle located next to the digastric. Note: Discerning the stylohyoid from the posterior belly of the digastric can be challenging.

■ RELATIONSHIP TO OTHER STRUCTURES

☐ The stylohyoid is superior to, and runs parallel to, the posterior belly of the digastric.

☐ Except for the platysma, which is superficial to all anterior neck muscles (and the submandibular salivary gland), the stylohyoid is superficial in the superolateral neck.

☐ The attachment of the stylohyoid onto the hyoid bone is the same location where the digastric attaches (via its fibrous sling attachment that holds the central tendon of the digastric to the hyoid bone).

☐ The attachment of the stylohyoid onto the hyoid bone is perforated by the central tendon of the digastric.

☐ Deep to the stylohyoid is the transverse process of the atlas (C1).

☐ The stylohyoid is located within the deep front line myofascial meridian.

■ MISCELLANEOUS

1. The stylohyoid is one of the four suprahyoid muscles. The four suprahyoid muscles are the digastric, mylohyoid, geniohyoid, and stylohyoid.
2. The external carotid artery lies inferior and deep to the stylohyoid. Massage to this region must be done judiciously.
3. There are two other small muscles that attach to the styloid process of the temporal bone: the styloglossus and the stylopharyngeus (ⓔvolve see the Evolve website).

12

INFRAHYOIDS
Sternohyoid (of Hyoid Group)

The name, sternohyoid, *tells us that this muscle attaches from the sternum to the hyoid bone.*

Derivation	□ sterno: L. *refers to the sternum.*
	hyoid: Gr. *refers to the hyoid.*
Pronunciation	□ STER-no-HI-oyd

■ ATTACHMENTS

□ **Sternum**
  □ the posterior surface of both the manubrium of the sternum and the medial clavicle

to the

□ **Hyoid**
  □ the inferior surface of the body of the hyoid

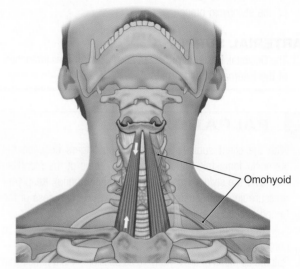

Figure 12-14 Anterior view of the sternohyoid bilaterally. The omohyoid has been ghosted in on the client's left side.

Omohyoid

■ FUNCTIONS

12

CONCENTRIC (SHORTENING) MOVER ACTIONS	
Standard Mover Actions	**Reverse Mover Actions**
□ 1. Depresses the hyoid bone	□ 1. Elevates the sternum
□ 2. Flexes the neck and head at the spinal joints	

Standard Mover Action Notes

- The sternohyoid attaches from the hyoid bone superiorly, to the sternum inferiorly (with its fibers running vertically). When the sternohyoid contracts, it pulls the hyoid bone inferiorly toward the sternum. Therefore the sternohyoid depresses the hyoid bone. Movements of the hyoid bone are important in chewing, swallowing, and speech. (action 1)
- If the inferior attachment of the sternohyoid stays fixed and the hyoid bone is pulled inferiorly, and the suprahyoids contract to fix the hyoid bone to the mandible, and elevators of the mandible contract to fix the mandible to the cranium, the sternohyoid can assist in flexing the neck and head at the spinal joints. This makes sense given that it crosses the cervical vertebrae anteriorly with a vertical direction to its fibers. (action 2)

Reverse Mover Action Note

- If the hyoid bone is fixed and the sternohyoid contracts, its pull would be exerted on its inferior attachment, the sternum, thereby pulling it superiorly. Given how small the sternohyoid is and how much resistance there is to the sternum lifting (the rib cage would have to move with it), this reverse action would not be very powerful. However, it may play a role in

lifting the rib cage when breathing in. In this manner, the sternohyoid may be considered to be an accessory muscle of breathing. (reverse action 1)

Eccentric Antagonist Functions

1. Restrains/slows elevation of the hyoid
2. Restrains/slows extension of the neck and head
3. Restrains/slows depression of the sternum

Isometric Stabilization Functions

1. Stabilizes the hyoid bone
2. Stabilizes the sternum
3. Stabilizes the temporomandibular joints (TMJs)
4. Stabilizes the neck

Isometric Function Note

- The sternohyoid can indirectly assist stabilization of the TMJs by stabilizing the hyoid bone when the suprahyoid muscles contract. With the hyoid stabilized, the suprahyoids can exert their pull on the mandible, thereby stabilizing the TMJs.

Additional Notes on Functions

1. If the sternohyoid stabilizes the hyoid bone, and the suprahyoid muscles contract, they will act to depress the mandible at the temporomandibular joints (TMJs). Therefore, via its stabilization of the hyoid, the sternohyoid can assist in

Sternohyoid (of Hyoid Group)—*cont'd*

depressing the mandible. In this manner, all infrahyoid muscles and all suprahyoid muscles can assist in depressing the mandible at the TMJs.

2. All hyoid muscles are important in moving and/or fixing (stabilizing) the hyoid bone. These functions are necessary for chewing, swallowing, and speech.

3. All hyoid muscles can assist with flexion of the neck at the spinal joints.

INNERVATION
☐ The Cervical Plexus
  ☐ ansa cervicalis (C1, C3)

ARTERIAL SUPPLY
☐ The Superior Thyroid Artery (a branch of the External Carotid Artery)

✋ PALPATION

1. With the client supine, place palpating fingers superior to the manubrium of the sternum and slightly lateral to midline. Make sure that you stay medial to the sternocleidomastoid.
2. Gently resist the client from depressing the mandible and feel for the contraction of the sternohyoid.
3. Palpate the sternohyoid superiorly toward the hyoid bone (using delicate pressure over the thyroid gland that is superficial in the anterior lower neck).

■ RELATIONSHIP TO OTHER STRUCTURES

☐ Nearly the entire sternohyoid is superficial in the anterior neck (except for the platysma, which is superficial to all anterior neck muscles). However, the inferior belly of the sternohyoid is deep to the sternocleidomastoid
☐ The inferior attachment of the sternohyoid is deep to the sternum and clavicle.
☐ The inferior portion of the sternohyoid lies directly medial to the sternocleidomastoid. The superior portion of the sternohyoid lies medial to the omohyoid.
☐ The sternohyoid lies anterior to, and just lateral to, the midline of the trachea.
☐ Deep to the sternohyoid are the sternothyroid and thyrohyoid.
☐ The sternohyoid is located within the deep front line myofascial meridian.

■ MISCELLANEOUS

1. The sternohyoid is one of the four infrahyoid muscles. The four infrahyoid muscles are the sternohyoid, sternothyroid, thyrohyoid, and omohyoid.
2. The carotid sinus of the common carotid artery lies slightly lateral to the sternohyoid (between the sternohyoid and the sternocleidomastoid, midway up the neck). Given the neurologic reflex that occurs to lower blood pressure when the carotid sinus is pressed, massage to this region must be done judiciously, especially with weak and/or elderly clients.

12

Sternothyroid (of Hyoid Group)

The name, sternothyroid, *tells us that this muscle attaches from the sternum to the thyroid cartilage.*

Derivation	☐ sterno: L. *refers to the sternum.*
	thyroid: Gr. *refers to the thyroid*
	cartilage.
Pronunciation	☐ STER-no-THI-royd

■ ATTACHMENTS

☐ **Sternum**
  ☐ the posterior surface of both the manubrium of the sternum and the cartilage of the first rib

to the

☐ **Thyroid Cartilage**
  ☐ the lamina of the thyroid cartilage

■ FUNCTIONS

CONCENTRIC (SHORTENING) MOVER ACTIONS	
Standard Mover Actions	**Reverse Mover Actions**
☐ 1. Depresses the thyroid cartilage	☐ 1. Elevates the sternum
☐ 2. Flexes the neck and head at the spinal joints	

Standard Mover Action Notes

• The sternothyroid attaches from the thyroid cartilage superiorly, to the sternum inferiorly (with its fibers running vertically). When the sternothyroid contracts, it pulls the thyroid cartilage inferiorly toward the sternum. Therefore the sternothyroid depresses the thyroid cartilage. Movements of the thyroid cartilage are important in chewing, swallowing, and speech. (action 1)

• If the inferior attachment of the sternothyroid stays fixed and the thyroid cartilage is pulled inferiorly, and the thyrohyoid contracts to fix the thyroid cartilage to the hyoid bone, and the suprahyoids contract to fix the hyoid bone to the mandible, and elevators of the mandible contract to fix the mandible to the cranium, then the sternothyroid can assist in flexing the neck and head at the spinal joints. This makes sense given that it crosses the cervical vertebrae anteriorly with a vertical direction to its fibers. Although this sounds complicated, it effectively requires only that the hyoid group contract simultaneously with elevators of the mandible. (action 2)

Reverse Mover Action Note

• If the thyroid cartilage is fixed and the sternothyroid contracts, its pull would be exerted on its inferior attachment,

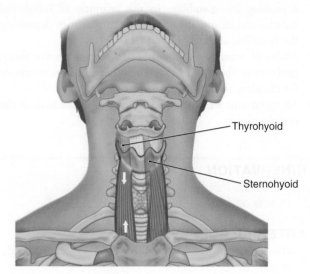

Figure 12-15 Anterior view of the sternothyroid bilaterally. The sternohyoid and thyrohyoid have been ghosted in.

Thyrohyoid

Sternohyoid

the sternum, thereby pulling it superiorly. Given how small the sternothyroid is and how much resistance there is to the sternum lifting (the rib cage would have to move with it), this reverse action would not be very powerful. However, it may play a role when the rib cage has to be lifted when breathing in. In this manner, the sternothyroid may be considered to be an accessory muscle of breathing. (reverse action 1)

Eccentric Antagonist Functions

1. Restrains/slows elevation of the thyroid cartilage
2. Restrains/slows extension of the neck and head
3. Restrains/slows depression of the sternum

Isometric Stabilization Functions

1. Stabilizes the thyroid cartilage
2. Stabilizes the hyoid bone
3. Stabilizes the sternum
4. Stabilizes the temporomandibular joints (TMJs)
5. Stabilizes the neck

Isometric Function Notes

• The sternothyroid can play a role in stabilizing the hyoid bone by stabilizing the thyroid cartilage when the thyrohyoid contracts. This allows the contraction force of the thyrohyoid to be exerted on the hyoid bone.

• The sternothyroid can indirectly assist stabilization of the TMJs by stabilizing the thyroid cartilage and hyoid bone when the suprahyoid muscles contract. With the hyoid stabilized, the suprahyoids can exert their pull on the mandible, thereby stabilizing the TMJs.

12

Sternothyroid (of Hyoid Group)—*cont'd*

Additional Notes on Functions

1. If the sternothyroid stabilizes the thyroid cartilage and hyoid bone, and the suprahyoid muscles contract, they will act to depress the mandible at the temporomandibular joints (TMJs). Therefore, via its stabilization of the hyoid, the sternothyroid can assist in depressing the mandible. In this manner, all infrahyoid muscles and all suprahyoid muscles can assist in depressing the mandible at the TMJs.
2. All hyoid muscles are important in moving and/or fixing (stabilizing) the hyoid bone. These functions are necessary for chewing, swallowing, and speech.
3. All hyoid muscles can assist with flexion of the neck at the spinal joints.

INNERVATION
- ☐ The Cervical Plexus
  - ☐ ansa cervicalis (C1, C3)

ARTERIAL SUPPLY
- ☐ The Superior Thyroid Artery (a branch of the External Carotid Artery)

PALPATION

- ☐ The sternothyroid is best palpated along with the sternohyoid (see the Palpation section for this muscle on page 417). Keep in mind that the sternothyroid does not extend superiorly beyond the thyroid cartilage, as does the sternohyoid.

■ RELATIONSHIP TO OTHER STRUCTURES

- ☐ Most of the sternothyroid lies directly deep to the sternohyoid and the omohyoid. However, part of the sternothyroid is superficial (except for the platysma, which is superficial to all anterior neck muscles) just above the sternum.
- ☐ The sternothyroid lies anterior to, and just lateral to, the midline of the trachea.
- ☐ Deep to the sternothyroid is the trachea.
- ☐ The inferior attachment of the sternothyroid is deep to the sternum and first rib.
- ☐ The sternothyroid is located within the deep front line myofascial meridian.

■ MISCELLANEOUS

1. The sternothyroid is one of the four infrahyoid muscles. The four infrahyoid muscles are the sternohyoid, sternothyroid, thyrohyoid, and omohyoid.
2. The sternothyroid is the only hyoid muscle that does not attach onto the hyoid bone.
3. The carotid sinus of the common carotid artery lies slightly lateral to the sternothyroid (between the sternothyroid and the sternocleidomastoid, midway up the neck). Given the neurologic reflex that occurs to lower blood pressure when the carotid sinus is pressed, massage to this region must be done judiciously, especially with weak and/or elderly clients.

12

Thyrohyoid (of Hyoid Group)

The name, thyrohyoid, *tells us that this muscle attaches from the thyroid cartilage to the hyoid bone.*

Derivation	☐ thyro: Gr. *refers to the thyroid cartilage.*
	hyoid: Gr. *refers to the hyoid bone.*
Pronunciation	☐ THI-ro-HI-oyd

■ ATTACHMENTS

☐ **Thyroid Cartilage**
  ☐ the lamina of the thyroid cartilage

to the

☐ **Hyoid**
  ☐ the inferior surface of the greater cornu of the hyoid

■ FUNCTIONS

CONCENTRIC (SHORTENING) MOVER ACTIONS	
Standard Mover Actions	**Reverse Mover Actions**
☐ 1. Depresses the hyoid bone	☐ 1. Elevates the thyroid cartilage
☐ 2. Flexes the neck and head at the spinal joints	

Standard Mover Action Notes

- The thyrohyoid attaches from the hyoid bone superiorly, to the thyroid cartilage inferiorly (with its fibers running vertically). When the thyroid cartilage is fixed (stabilized) and the thyrohyoid contracts, it pulls the hyoid bone inferiorly toward the thyroid cartilage. Therefore the thyrohyoid depresses the hyoid bone. Movements of the hyoid bone are important in chewing, swallowing, and speech. (action 1)
- If the thyroid cartilage attachment of the thyrohyoid stays fixed and the hyoid bone is pulled inferiorly, and the suprahyoids contract to fix the hyoid bone to the mandible, and elevators of the mandible contract to fix the mandible to the cranium, then the thyrohyoid can assist in flexing the neck and head at the spinal joints. This makes sense given that it crosses the cervical vertebrae anteriorly with a vertical direction to its fibers. (action 2)

Reverse Mover Action Note

- The thyrohyoid attaches from the thyroid cartilage inferiorly, to the hyoid bone superiorly (with its fibers running vertically). When the hyoid bone is fixed (stabilized) and the thyrohyoid contracts, it pulls the thyroid cartilage superiorly toward the hyoid bone. Therefore the thyrohyoid elevates the thyroid cartilage. Movements of the thyroid cartilage are important in chewing, swallowing, and speech. (reverse action 1)

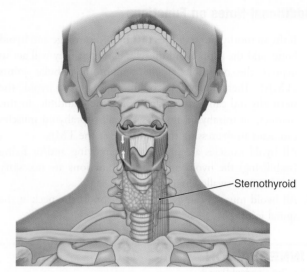

Figure 12-16 Anterior view of the thyrohyoid bilaterally. The sternothyroid has been ghosted in on the client's left side.

Eccentric Antagonist Functions

1. Restrains/slows elevation of the hyoid
2. Restrains/slows depression of the thyroid cartilage
3. Restrains/slows extension of the neck and head

Isometric Stabilization Functions

1. Stabilizes the hyoid bone and thyroid cartilage
2. Stabilizes the temporomandibular joints (TMJs)
3. Stabilizes the neck

Isometric Function Note

- The thyrohyoid can indirectly assist stabilization of the TMJs by stabilizing the hyoid bone when the suprahyoid muscles contract. With the hyoid stabilized, the suprahyoids can exert their pull on the mandible, thereby stabilizing the TMJs.

Additional Notes on Functions

1. If the thyrohyoid stabilizes the hyoid bone, and the suprahyoid muscles contract, they will act to depress the mandible at the temporomandibular joints (TMJs). Therefore, via its stabilization of the hyoid, the thyrohyoid can assist in depressing the mandible. In this manner, all infrahyoid muscles and all suprahyoid muscles can assist in depressing the mandible at the TMJs.
2. All hyoid muscles are important in moving and/or fixing (stabilizing) the hyoid bone. These functions are necessary for chewing, swallowing, and speech.
3. All hyoid muscles can assist with flexion of the neck at the spinal joints.

12

Thyrohyoid (of Hyoid Group)—*cont'd*

INNERVATION
- ☐ The Hypoglossal Nerve (CN XII)
  - ☐ a branch of C1 through the hypoglossal nerve

ARTERIAL SUPPLY
- ☐ The Superior Thyroid Artery (a branch of the External Carotid Artery)

 PALPATION

- ☐ The thyrohyoid is best palpated along with the sternohyoid (see the Palpation section for this muscle on page 417). Keep in mind that the thyrohyoid does not extend inferiorly beyond the thyroid cartilage, as does the sternohyoid.

■ RELATIONSHIP TO OTHER STRUCTURES

- ☐ The inferior part of the thyrohyoid lies directly deep to the sternohyoid and omohyoid. However, its superior part is superficial (except for the platysma, which is superficial to all anterior neck muscles).
- ☐ The thyrohyoid lies anterior to, and lateral to, the midline of the thyroid cartilage. It is inferior to the hyoid bone.
- ☐ Deep to the thyrohyoid is the thyroid cartilage.
- ☐ The thyrohyoid is located within the deep front line myofascial meridian.

■ MISCELLANEOUS

1. The thyrohyoid is one of the four infrahyoid muscles. The four infrahyoid muscles are the sternohyoid, sternothyroid, thyrohyoid, and omohyoid.
2. The carotid sinus of the common carotid artery lies directly lateral to the thyrohyoid (between the thyrohyoid and the sternocleidomastoid, superior in the neck). Given the neurologic reflex that occurs to lower blood pressure when the carotid sinus is pressed, massage to this region must be done judiciously, especially with weak and/or elderly clients.
3. The thyrohyoid can be considered to be an upward continuation of the sternothyroid muscle.

12

Omohyoid (of Hyoid Group)

The name, omohyoid, *tells us that this muscle attaches from the scapula (*omo *means shoulder, referring to the scapula) to the hyoid bone.*

Derivation	☐ omo: Gr. *shoulder.*
	hyoid: Gr. *refers to the hyoid bone.*
Pronunciation	☐ O-mo-HI-oyd

■ ATTACHMENTS

☐ INFERIOR BELLY:
  ☐ **Scapula**
    ☐ the superior border

to the

  ☐ **Clavicle**
    ☐ the central tendon is bound to the clavicle

☐ SUPERIOR BELLY:
  ☐ **Clavicle**
    ☐ the central tendon is bound to the clavicle

to the

  ☐ **Hyoid**
    ☐ the inferior surface of the body of the hyoid

■ FUNCTIONS

CONCENTRIC (SHORTENING) MOVER ACTIONS	
Standard Mover Actions	**Reverse Mover Actions**
☐ **1. Depresses the hyoid bone**	☐ 1. Elevates the scapula at the scapulocostal joint
☐ **2. Flexes the neck and head at the spinal joints**	

Standard Mover Action Notes

• The omohyoid attaches from the hyoid bone superiorly, to the clavicle inferiorly (with a continuation of its fibers to the scapula). Therefore its fibers run vertically. When the scapula and the clavicle are fixed (stabilized) and the omohyoid contracts, it pulls the hyoid bone inferiorly toward the clavicle. Therefore the omohyoid depresses the hyoid bone. Movements of the hyoid bone are important in chewing, swallowing, and speech. (action 1)

• If the inferior attachment of the omohyoid stays fixed and the hyoid bone is pulled inferiorly, and the suprahyoids contract to fix the hyoid bone to the mandible, and elevators of the mandible contract to fix the mandible to the cranium, then the omohyoid can assist in flexing the neck and head at the spinal joints. This makes sense given that it crosses the cervical vertebrae anteriorly with a vertical direction to its fibers. (action 2)

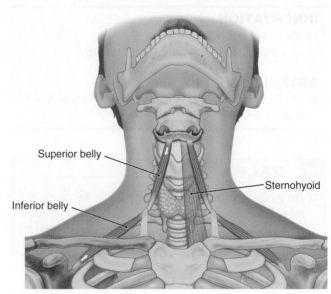

Figure 12-17 Anterior view of the omohyoid. The sternohyoid has been ghosted in on the client's left side.

Reverse Mover Action Note

• The omohyoid attaches from the hyoid bone superiorly, to the scapula inferiorly. When the hyoid bone is fixed (stabilized) and the omohyoid contracts, it pulls the scapula superiorly toward the hyoid bone. Therefore the omohyoid elevates the scapula at the scapulocostal joint. (reverse action 1)

Eccentric Antagonist Functions

1. Restrains/slows elevation of the hyoid
2. Restrains/slows depression of the scapula
3. Restrains/slows extension of the neck and head

Isometric Stabilization Functions

1. Stabilizes the hyoid bone
2. Stabilizes the scapula
3. Stabilizes the clavicle
4. Stabilizes the temporomandibular joints (TMJs)

Isometric Function Note

• The omohyoid can indirectly assist stabilization of the TMJs by stabilizing the hyoid bone when the suprahyoid muscles contract. With the hyoid stabilized, the suprahyoids can exert their pull on the mandible, thereby stabilizing the TMJs.

Additional Notes on Functions

1. If the omohyoid stabilizes the hyoid bone, and the suprahyoid muscles contract, they will act to depress the mandible

Omohyoid (of Hyoid Group)—*cont'd*

at the temporomandibular joints (TMJs). Therefore, via its stabilization of the hyoid, the omohyoid can assist in depressing the mandible. In this manner, all infrahyoid muscles and all suprahyoid muscles can assist in depressing the mandible at the TMJs.

2. All hyoid muscles are important in moving and/or fixing (stabilizing) the hyoid bone. These functions are necessary for chewing, swallowing, and speech.

3. All hyoid muscles can assist with flexion of the neck at the spinal joints.

4. Even though the omohyoid has two bellies that could theoretically contract separately, its line of pull to create an action will not be efficient unless both bellies contract together.

INNERVATION
□ The Cervical Plexus
  □ ansa cervicalis (C1-C3)

ARTERIAL SUPPLY
□ The Superior Thyroid Artery (a branch of the External Carotid Artery) and the Transverse Cervical Artery (a branch of the Thyrocervical Trunk)

✋ PALPATION

1. With the client supine, place palpating hand lateral to the sternocleidomastoid, just superior to the clavicle, and feel for the fibers of the omohyoid running nearly horizontally. Make sure you are not palpating the scalenes, which are deep to the omohyoid (and have fibers running more vertically).
2. To engage the omohyoid, ask the client to depress the mandible against mild resistance and feel for its contraction.
3. Palpate as much of the omohyoid as possible.

■ RELATIONSHIP TO OTHER STRUCTURES

□ The omohyoid runs an unusual course. The inferior belly of the omohyoid attaches onto the superior border of the scapula, just superior to the supraspinatus (near the scapular notch). From the scapula, the omohyoid runs anteriorly and slightly superiorly toward the clavicle, deep to the trapezius and superficial to the scalenes. Near the medial end of the clavicle, the omohyoid becomes tendinous (the central tendon). However, it does not attach directly to the clavicle, but rather its central tendon is attached to the clavicle by a fibrous sling of tissue. At this point, the omohyoid is deep to the sternocleidomastoid and superficial to the sternothyroid. Its superior belly then runs superiorly and attaches to the hyoid bone, just lateral to the sternohyoid.

□ Except for the platysma, the omohyoid is superficial in two locations: (1) slightly inferior to the hyoid bone and superior to the sternocleidomastoid in the anterior neck and (2) between the sternocleidomastoid and the trapezius in the inferolateral neck (within the *posterior triangle of the neck*).

□ The omohyoid is located within the deep front line myofascial meridian.

■ MISCELLANEOUS

1. The omohyoid is one of the four infrahyoid muscles. The four infrahyoid muscles are the sternohyoid, sternothyroid, thyrohyoid, and omohyoid.

2. The carotid sinus of the common carotid artery lies slightly lateral to the omohyoid (between the omohyoid and the sternocleidomastoid, midway up the neck). Given the neurologic reflex that occurs to lower blood pressure when the carotid sinus is pressed, massage to this region must be done judiciously, especially with weak and/or elderly clients.

3. The omohyoid is unusual in that it has two separate bellies: a superior belly and an inferior belly.

4. The omohyoid's two bellies are separated by its *central tendon* (also known as the *intermediate tendon*). Like the digastric (a suprahyoid muscle), the omohyoid's central tendon is tethered (i.e., attached) to bone by a fibrous sling of tissue.

12

Muscles of Facial Expression

CHAPTER **OUTLINE**

CHAPTER **OVERVIEW**

The muscles of facial expression can be subdivided into four groups, as shown above in the Chapter Outline.

Overview of Structure

☐ Some sources do not include the muscles of the scalp in the muscles of facial expression. Although they are the least active with facial expression, they can be considered to be involved; this is especially true of the occipitofrontalis.

☐ The platysma of the neck is included here as a muscle of fascial expression of the mouth. Some sources treat this muscle as a neck muscle because it is primarily located in the neck, or as a muscle of mastication because it can move the mandible at the temporomandibular joints (TMJs).

☐ The levator labii superioris alaeque nasi is a facial expression muscle of both the nose and the mouth.

☐ The orbicularis oris encircles the mouth. All other muscles of the mouth radiate out from the mouth like spokes of a wheel.

☐ The modiolus is a fibromuscular condensation approximately ¼ inch (0.5 cm) lateral to the angle of the mouth. Six muscles of the mouth attach into the modiolus: the zygomaticus major, levator anguli oris, risorius, depressor anguli oris, buccinator, and orbicularis oris.

Overview of Function

☐ All the facial muscles move the fascia and/or skin of the face and scalp. Therefore they all contribute to facial expressions, which are important for displaying emotions. Although there is certainly some universality of facial expressions expressing emotions, there can be variations from one culture to another. Further, many of these muscles may act in concert with others to add to the spectrum of facial expressions displayed. Some sources state that there are more than 1,800 separate facial expressions that can be created with combinations of the muscles of facial expression.

Review the muscles and bones from this chapter on the enclosed CD!

☐ The levator labii superioris alaeque nasi, levator labii superioris, levator anguli oris, and zygomaticus minor and major all elevate the upper lip.

☐ The zygomaticus minor, zygomaticus major, risorius, depressor anguli oris, depressor labii inferioris, and platysma all draw the lip(s) and/or the angle (corner) of the mouth laterally.

☐ The depressor anguli oris, depressor labii inferioris, mentalis, and platysma all depress the lower lip.

☐ Most muscles of facial expression are also functionally important for dilating or constricting (opening or closing) the apertures (openings) of the face (mouth, nostrils, eyes, and ears); this is functionally important to our physiology by allowing or blocking the intake of food, air, light, and sound.

☐ Long-standing contraction of a facial expression muscle creates wrinkles in the skin of the face that run perpendicular to the direction of fibers of the underlying muscle. Botox injections eliminate/remove these wrinkles because Botox paralyzes the muscle, preventing it from contracting. Because the muscle is paralyzed, Botox also decreases the ability to contract the muscle and create facial expressions to convey emotion.

INNERVATION

☐ The facial muscles (except the levator palpebrae superioris) are innervated by the facial nerve (CN VII).

ARTERIAL SUPPLY

☐ Most muscles of facial expression receive the majority of their arterial supply from the facial artery.

13

Superficial Right Lateral View of the Muscles of the Head

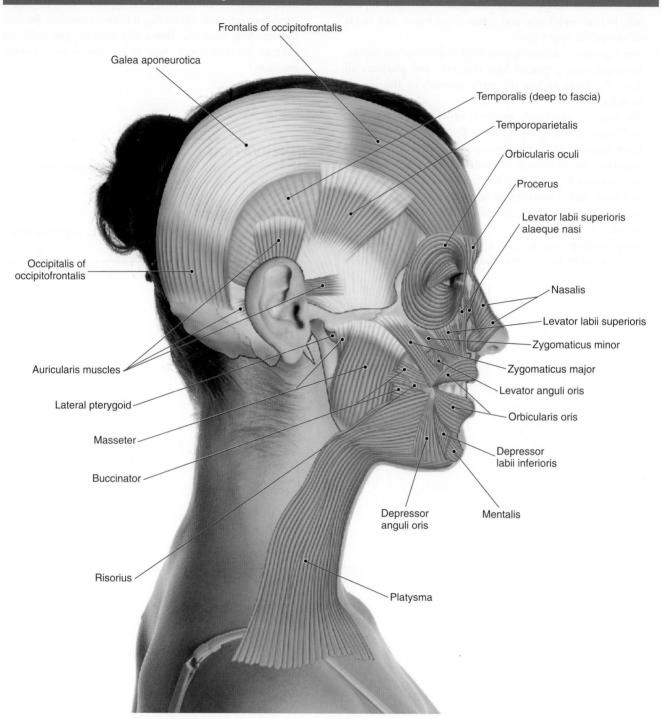

Figure 13-1 Superficial right lateral view of the muscles of the head.

13

Anterior Views of the Muscles of the Head

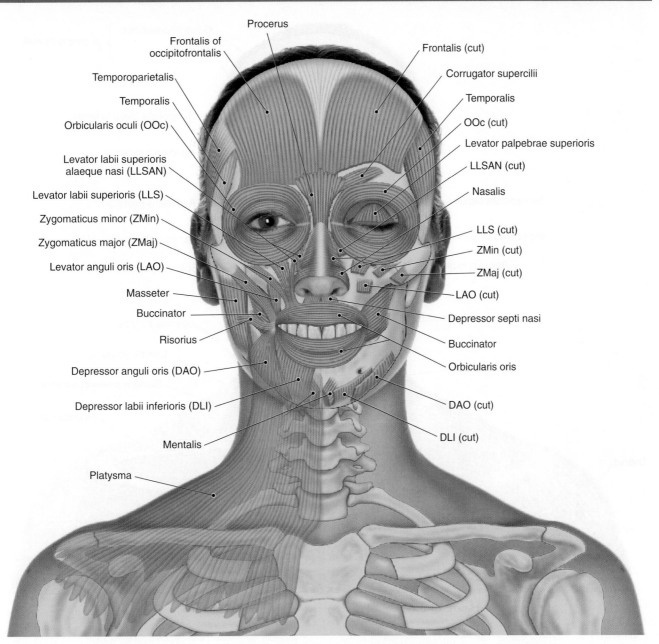

Procerus

Frontalis of occipitofrontalis

Temporoparietalis

Temporalis

Orbicularis oculi (OOc)

Levator labii superioris alaeque nasi (LLSAN)

Levator labii superioris (LLS)

Zygomaticus minor (ZMin)

Zygomaticus major (ZMaj)

Levator anguli oris (LAO)

Masseter

Buccinator

Risorius

Depressor anguli oris (DAO)

Depressor labii inferioris (DLI)

Mentalis

Platysma

Frontalis (cut)

Corrugator supercilii

Temporalis

OOc (cut)

Levator palpebrae superioris

LLSAN (cut)

Nasalis

LLS (cut)

ZMin (cut)

ZMaj (cut)

LAO (cut)

Depressor septi nasi

Buccinator

Orbicularis oris

DAO (cut)

DLI (cut)

Figure 13-2 Superficial and anterior views of the muscles of the head. The platysma has been ghosted in. Note: Acronyms used on the person's left side are defined on the right side.

Posterior View of the Muscles of the Head

13

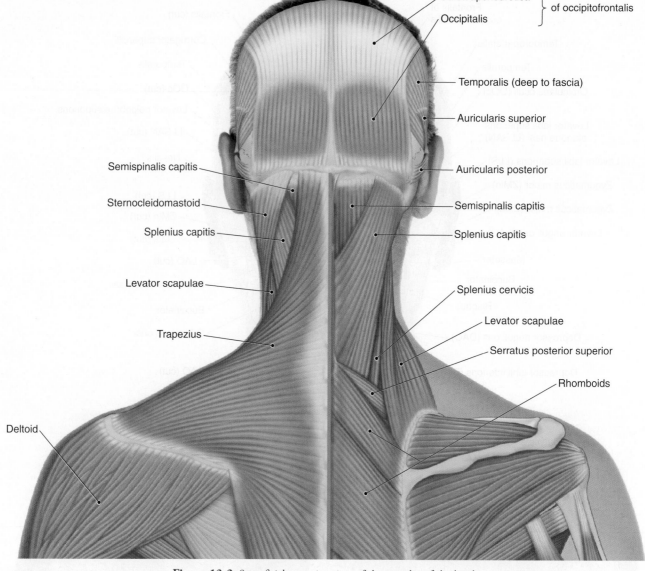

Galea aponeurotica ⎱ of occipitofrontalis
Occipitalis ⎰

Temporalis (deep to fascia)

Auricularis superior

Semispinalis capitis

Sternocleidomastoid

Splenius capitis

Levator scapulae

Trapezius

Deltoid

Auricularis posterior

Semispinalis capitis

Splenius capitis

Splenius cervicis

Levator scapulae

Serratus posterior superior

Rhomboids

Figure 13-3 Superficial posterior view of the muscles of the head.

Facial Landmarks

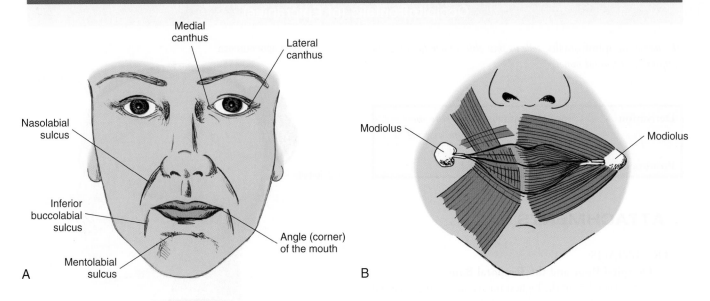

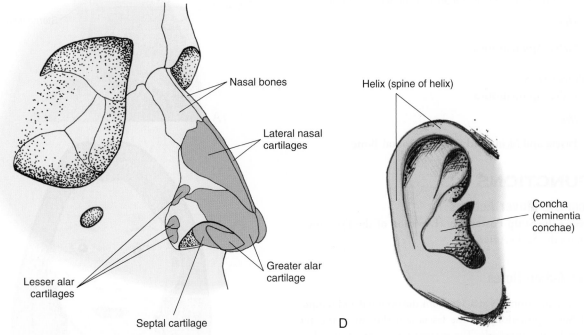

Figure 13-4 Facial landmarks. **A** and **B,** Anterior views of the face. **C,** Anterolateral view of the nose. **D,** Lateral view of the right ear.

SCALP

Occipitofrontalis (of Epicranius)

The name, occipitofrontalis, *tells us that this muscle lies over the occipital and frontal bones.*

Derivation	□ occipitofrontalis: L. *refers to the occiput and the frontal bone.*
Pronunciation	□ ok-SIP-i-to-fron-TA-lis

■ ATTACHMENTS

□ OCCIPITALIS:
- □ **Occipital Bone and the Temporal Bone**
  - □ the lateral ⅔ of the highest nuchal line of the occipital bone and the mastoid area of the temporal bone

to the

- □ **Galea Aponeurotica**

□ FRONTALIS:
- □ **Galea Aponeurotica**

to the

- □ **Fascia and Skin overlying the Frontal Bone**

■ FUNCTIONS

Concentric Mover Actions
1. **Draws the Scalp Posteriorly (Elevation of the Eyebrow)**
2. Draws the Scalp Anteriorly

Mover Action Notes

1. The occipitofrontalis attaches from the occipital and temporal bones posteriorly, to the fascia and skin overlying the frontal bone anteriorly. The posterior attachment, which is bone, is more fixed than the anterior attachment, which is soft tissue. Therefore when the posterior attachment is fixed, and the occipitofrontalis contracts, it pulls the anterior attachment toward the posterior attachment. When this occurs, the entire scalp moves posteriorly. This pulls on the fascia and skin located superior to the eye, causing the eyebrow to elevate and the skin of the forehead to wrinkle. (action 1)

2. The frontalis belly of the occipitofrontalis attaches from the fascia and skin overlying the frontal bone to the galea aponeurotica posteriorly. When the anterior attachment is fixed and the frontalis contracts, it pulls the posterior attachment (the galea aponeurotica) toward the anterior attachment. Therefore the scalp is drawn anteriorly. When this occurs, the skin of the forehead may also wrinkle. (action 2)

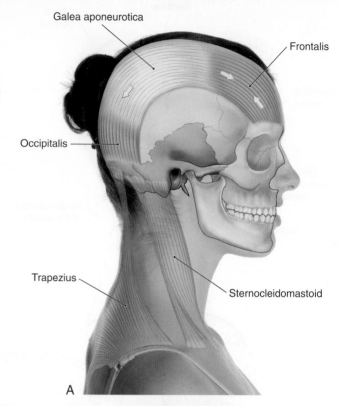

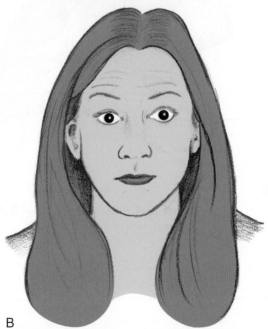

Figure 13-5 The occipitofrontalis. **A,** Lateral view of the right occipitofrontalis. The trapezius and sternocleidomastoid have been ghosted in. **B,** Expression of elevating the eyebrows created by the bilateral contraction of the occipitofrontalis.

Occipitofrontalis (of Epicranius)—*cont'd*

INNERVATION

☐ The Facial Nerve (CN VII)
☐ occipitalis: posterior auricular branch of the facial nerve
☐ frontalis: temporal branches of the facial nerve

ARTERIAL SUPPLY

☐ Occipitalis: the Occipital and Posterior Auricular Arteries (branches of the External Carotid Artery)
☐ Frontalis: supraorbital and supratrochlear branches of the Ophthalmic Artery (a branch of the Internal Carotid Artery)

✋ PALPATION

1. With the client prone or supine, place palpating hand over the occipital bone and feel for the occipitalis, over the parietal bone and feel for the galea aponeurotica, and over the frontal bone and feel for the frontalis.
2. Ask the client to wrinkle the skin of the forehead, and feel for the contraction of the muscle.

■ RELATIONSHIP TO OTHER STRUCTURES

☐ The occipitalis is directly superior to the most superficial muscles of the neck that attach into the superior nuchal line and the mastoid process, namely, the trapezius and the sternocleidomastoid.
☐ The frontalis is superior to and even blends into the procerus, the corrugator supercilii, and the orbicularis oculi.
☐ Lateral to the frontalis and the galea aponeurotica is the temporoparietalis, and deep to that, the temporalis.

☐ The occipitofrontalis is located within the superficial back line myofascial meridian.

■ MISCELLANEOUS

1. The occipitofrontalis attaches into the galea aponeurotica; the temporoparietalis also attaches into the galea aponeurotica. The occipitofrontalis and the temporoparietalis together are known as the *epicranius*. (Note: The galea aponeurotica is also known as the *epicranial aponeurosis*.)
2. The occipitofrontalis can be considered to be two separate muscles: the *occipitalis* and the *frontalis*.
3. Elevation of the eyebrows often accompanies glancing upward. Elevation of the eyebrows is associated with the expressions of surprise, shock, horror, fright, or recognition.
4. The occipitofrontalis is located within the scalp. The scalp consists of five layers: the skin, subcutaneous tissue, the epicranius and its aponeurosis (the galea aponeurotica), loose connective tissue, and the pericranium. Of these layers, the skin, the subcutaneous tissue, and the galea aponeurotica are firmly connected to each other.
5. The left and right frontalis muscles blend into each other in the midline of the head. The left and right occipitalis muscles usually have a gap between them that is filled in with an extension of the galea aponeurotica.
6. The occipitofrontalis is often ignored or only worked lightly during bodywork. It is a muscle like any other in the body, and moderate or even deeper work may be done to benefit the client. Because tension headaches often involve the occipitofrontalis, this muscle should be evaluated in any client complaining of headaches, especially tension headaches.

13

Temporoparietalis (of Epicranius)

The name, temporoparietalis, *tells us that this muscle lies over the temporal and parietal bones.*

Derivation	☐ temporoparietalis: L. *refers to the temporal and parietal bones.*
Pronunciation	☐ TEM-po-ro-pa-RI-i-TAL-is

■ ATTACHMENTS

☐ **Fascia Superior to the Ear**

to the

☐ **Lateral Border of the Galea Aponeurotica**

■ FUNCTIONS

Concentric Mover Actions

1. **Elevates the Ear**
2. Tightens the Scalp

Mover Action Notes

- The temporoparietalis attaches from the fascia superior to the ear inferiorly, to the galea aponeurotica superiorly (with its fibers running vertically). When the temporoparietalis contracts, it pulls the fascia that is superior to the ear superiorly toward the galea aponeurotica, which causes the ear to elevate. (action 1)
- Because the fibers of the temporoparietalis attach into the galea aponeurotica, when the temporoparietalis contracts it exerts a pull on the galea aponeurotica, which causes the scalp to tighten. (action 2)

INNERVATION
☐ The Facial Nerve (CN VII)
  ☐ temporal branch

ARTERIAL SUPPLY
☐ The Superficial Temporal and Posterior Auricular Arteries (branches of the External Carotid Artery)

 PALPATION

1. With the client prone or supine, place palpating hand 1 to 2 inches (2.5 to 5 cm) superior and slightly anterior to the ear.
2. Have the client contract the temporoparietalis to elevate the ear (if able to) and feel for the contraction of the temporoparietalis. Be sure that you are superior enough so that you are on the temporoparietalis and not on the auricularis superior, which can also elevate the ear.

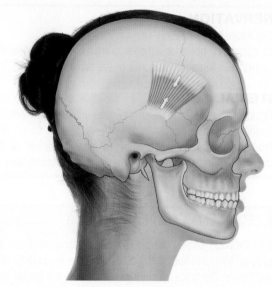

Figure 13-6 Lateral view of the right temporoparietalis.

■ RELATIONSHIP TO OTHER STRUCTURES

☐ The temporoparietalis is superficial and lies between the frontalis and the auricularis anterior and auricularis superior.
☐ The temporoparietalis is involved with the deep front line myofascial meridian.

■ MISCELLANEOUS

1. The temporoparietalis attaches into the galea aponeurotica; the occipitofrontalis also attaches into the galea aponeurotica. The occipitofrontalis and the temporoparietalis together are known as the *epicranius*. (Note: The galea aponeurotica is also known as the *epicranial aponeurosis*.)
2. The temporoparietalis is located within the scalp. The scalp consists of five layers: the skin, subcutaneous tissue, the epicranius and its aponeurosis (the galea aponeurotica), loose connective tissue, and the pericranium. Of these layers, the skin, the subcutaneous tissue, and the galea aponeurotica are firmly connected to each other.
3. The degree of development of the temporoparietalis varies. In some individuals, it is very thin; in others, it is nonexistent.
4. In addition to the galea aponeurotica, the temporoparietalis often attaches directly into the belly of the frontalis muscle.

13

Auricularis Group

There are three auricularis muscles: the auricular anterior, auricular superior, and auricularis posterior.

The name, auricularis, tells us that these muscles are involved with the ear. Anterior, superior, and posterior tell us their location relative to the ear.

Derivation	☐ auricularis: L. *ear.*
	anterior: L. *before, in front of.*
	superior: L. *upper, higher than.*
	posterior: L. *behind, toward the back.*
Pronunciation	☐ aw-RIK-u-la-ris, an-TEE-ri-or, sue-PEE-ri-or, pos-TEE-ri-or

■ ATTACHMENTS

☐ AURICULARIS ANTERIOR:
  ☐ **Galea Aponeurotica**
    ☐ the lateral margin

to the

  ☐ **Anterior Ear**
    ☐ the spine of the helix

☐ AURICULARIS SUPERIOR:
  ☐ **Galea Aponeurotica**
    ☐ the lateral margin

to the

  ☐ **Superior Ear**
    ☐ the superior aspect of the cranial surface

☐ AURICULARIS POSTERIOR:
  ☐ **Temporal Bone**
    ☐ the mastoid area of the temporal bone

to the

  ☐ **Posterior Ear**
    ☐ the ponticulus of the eminentia conchae

■ FUNCTIONS

Concentric Mover Actions

1. **Draws the Ear Anteriorly (auricularis anterior)**
2. **Elevates the Ear (auricularis superior)**
3. **Draws the Ear Posteriorly (auricularis posterior)**
4. Tightens and moves the scalp (auricularis anterior and superior)

Mover Action Notes

- The auricularis anterior attaches from the ear posteriorly, to the galea aponeurotica anteriorly (with its fibers running

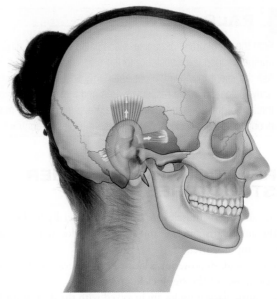

Figure 13-7 Lateral view of the right auricularis muscles.

horizontally). When the auricularis anterior contracts, it pulls the ear toward the more anterior attachment. Therefore the auricularis anterior draws the ear anteriorly. (action 1)

- The auricularis superior attaches from the ear inferiorly, to the galea aponeurotica superiorly (with its fibers running vertically). When the auricularis superior contracts, it pulls the ear toward the more superior attachment; therefore the auricularis superior elevates the ear. (Note: The auricularis anterior also has a slight vertical orientation to its fibers; therefore it can also help elevate the ear.) (action 2)
- The auricularis posterior attaches from the ear anteriorly, to the temporal bone posteriorly (with its fibers running horizontally). When the auricularis posterior contracts, it pulls the ear toward the more posterior attachment. Therefore the auricularis posterior draws the ear posteriorly. (action 3)
- If the auricular (ear) attachment is more fixed, the auricularis anterior and superior could pull on the galea aponeurotica, thereby tightening and moving the scalp. (action 4)

INNERVATION
☐ The Facial Nerve (CN VII)
    ☐ Auricularis anterior and superior: temporal branches
    ☐ Auricularis posterior: posterior auricular branch

ARTERIAL SUPPLY
☐ The Superficial Temporal and Posterior Auricular Arteries (branches of the External Carotid Artery)

PALPATION

1. With the client prone or supine. place palpating fingers directly anterior, superior, or posterior to the ear.
2. Ask the client to move the ear anteriorly, posteriorly, or superiorly, palpating in the respective area and feeling for the contraction of the corresponding muscle. Keep in mind that many people cannot consciously "will" these muscles to contract.

■ RELATIONSHIP TO OTHER STRUCTURES

☐ The auricularis muscles are located superficially in the scalp.
☐ The auricularis anterior and superior are located inferior to the temporoparietalis.
☐ The auricularis posterior is located just superior to the cranial attachment of the sternocleidomastoid.
☐ The auricularis muscles are involved with the deep front line myofascial meridian.

■ MISCELLANEOUS

1. The auricularis anterior is the smallest of the three auricularis muscles; the auricularis superior is the largest.
2. One, two, or all three of the auricularis muscles are nonfunctional in many people.
3. The spine of the helix is the cartilage in the helix of the ear.
4. The eminentia conchae is the cartilage in the concha of the ear, which forms an eminence on the cranial surface of the ear. The ponticulus of the eminentia conchae is a ridge found on the eminentia conchae that is the attachment site for the auricularis posterior muscle.
5. Although the auricularis muscles in humans are poorly formed and often nonfunctional, the analogous muscles in dogs (and many other animals) are highly developed. This is clear when one sees how a dog can direct its ears toward the location from which a sound originates.

EYE
Orbicularis Oculi

The name, orbicularis oculi, *tells us that this muscle encircles the eye.*

Derivation	☐ orbicularis: L. *a small circle.*
	oculi: L. *refers to the eye.*
Pronunciation	☐ or-BIK-you-la-ris, OK-you-lie

■ ATTACHMENTS

☐ **Medial Side of the Eye**
    ☐ ORBITAL PART: the nasal part of the frontal bone, the frontal process of the maxilla, and the medial palpebral ligament
    ☐ PALPEBRAL PART: the medial palpebral ligament
    ☐ LACRIMAL PART: the lacrimal bone

to the

☐ **Medial Side of the Eye (returns to the same attachment, encircling the eye)**
    ☐ ORBITAL PART: returns to the same attachment (these fibers encircle the eye)
    ☐ PALPEBRAL PART: the lateral palpebral ligament (these fibers run through the connective tissue of the eyelids)
    ☐ LACRIMAL PART: the medial palpebral raphe (these fibers are deeper in the eye socket)

■ FUNCTIONS

Concentric Mover Actions
1. **Closes and Squints the Eye (orbital part)**
2. Depresses the Upper Eyelid (palpebral part)
3. Elevates the Lower Eyelid (palpebral part)
4. Retraction of the Lower Eyelid (lacrimal part)
5. Assists in Tear Transport and Drainage (lacrimal part)

Mover Action Notes

• The fiber direction of the orbital part of the orbicularis oculi is circular around the eye. When the orbital part of the orbicularis oculi contracts, it acts as a circular sphincter muscle that closes in around the eye, not only forcing the two eyelids together but also closing in the tissue above and below the eye. This is often termed *forceful closure of the eye,* or more commonly, *squinting.* (Note: To understand how a circular sphincter muscle works, the following reasoning applies: if a linear muscle shortens, its length decreases. When that same linear muscle is arranged in a circular fashion and shortens, the length of the line you have to make the circle decreases and therefore the size of the circle lessens, which can close in on whatever structure is being surrounded by it.) (action 1)

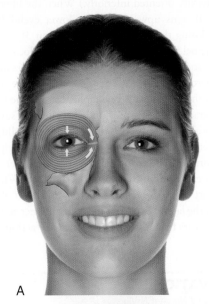

A

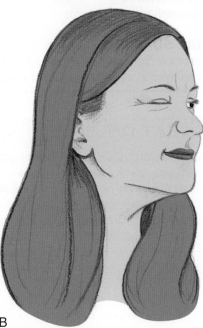

B

Figure 13-8 The orbicularis oculi. **A,** Anterior view of the right orbicularis oculi. **B,** Anterolateral view of the expression created by the contraction of the right orbicularis oculi.

• The palpebral part of the orbicularis oculi has fibers that are arranged in an arc like fashion in the upper eyelid. (The direction of the fibers is a horizontal arc with the convexity oriented superiorly.) When the fibers contract, the arc flattens down and the upper eyelid is depressed, gently closing the eye from above. (action 2)
• The palpebral part of the orbicularis oculi has fibers that are arranged in an upside-down, arc like fashion in the lower

eyelid. (The direction of the fibers is a horizontal arc with the convexity oriented inferiorly.) When the fibers contract, the arc flattens upward and the lower eyelid is elevated, gently closing the eye from below. (action 3)

- The lacrimal part of the orbicularis oculi is located deeper in the eye socket (with its fibers running horizontally from anterior to posterior). When the lacrimal part contracts, it pulls on the medial palpebral raphe, causing the lower eyelid to be retracted, and thereby pulled against the surface of the eye (this also prevents eversion of the lower eyelid). Holding the lower eyelid against the surface of the eye helps to direct (transport) tear fluid toward the medial corner of the eye where it can be drained into the lacrimal sac. When the lacrimal part of the orbicularis oculi contracts, it also exerts a pulls on the lacrimal sac that dilates it and increases its ability to drain tears from the surface of the eye. (actions 4, 5)

INNERVATION

☐ The Facial Nerve (CN VII)
  ☐ temporal and zygomatic branches

ARTERIAL SUPPLY

☐ The Branches of the Facial Artery and Superficial Temporal Artery (both branches of the External Carotid Artery)

 PALPATION

1. To palpate the orbital part, with the client supine, place palpating fingers inferior, lateral, or superior to the eye.
2. Ask the client to forcefully close the eye and feel for the contraction of the orbicularis oculi.
3. To palpate the palpebral part, place palpating fingers gently on the upper and lower eyelids.
4. Ask the client to gently close the eye and feel for its contraction.

■ RELATIONSHIP TO OTHER STRUCTURES

☐ The orbicularis oculi is superficial and encircles the eye. The orbicularis oculi is inferior to the frontalis and the corrugator supercilii and superior to the levator labii superioris alaeque nasi, levator labii superioris, zygomaticus minor, and zygomaticus major. It is lateral to the procerus and nasalis and medial to the temporoparietalis and the temporalis.

☐ Some fibers of the levator palpebrae superioris pierce through the palpebral part of the orbicularis oculi to attach into the skin of the upper eyelid.

☐ The orbicularis oculi is involved with the deep front line myofascial meridian.

■ MISCELLANEOUS

1. The palpebral part of the orbicularis oculi is under both conscious and unconscious control and may contract reflexly to close the eye (for protection and as part of blinking).
2. Superiorly, the orbital part of the orbicularis oculi blends in with fibers of the frontalis and the corrugator supercilii. Inferiorly, the orbital part of the orbicularis oculi blends in with fibers of the zygomaticus minor, levator labii superioris, and levator labii superioris alaeque nasi.
3. Some fibers of the orbital part may blend into the skin, deep to the eyebrow, creating the *depressor supercilii* muscle.
4. If the entire orbicularis oculi contracts, the eye will close forcefully (i.e., the eyelids and the surrounding tissue close in around the eye) and the skin of the eyelids and surrounding area (forehead, temple, and cheek) will be drawn medially toward the attachment at the medial eye. This action creates a facial expression in which the amount of light entering the eye decreases and wrinkles radiating out from the lateral eye form; these wrinkles are called *crow's-feet*.
5. The medial and lateral palpebral raphes are where the tissue from the upper and lower eyelids come together at the corners (canthi) of the eye. The medial and lateral palpebral ligaments are small ligaments located directly next to the raphes in the corners of the eye. (A raphe is a seam of tissue formed by the union of the halves of a part.)
6. When the tissue located superior to the eye is pulled down around the eye by the contraction of the orbicularis oculi, it helps shield the eye from bright sunlight. The corrugator supercilii and the procerus can also assist with this function of shielding the eye from bright sunlight.
7. Given that the lacrimal part of the orbicularis oculi helps drain tears from the surface of the eye into the lacrimal sac, weakness or flaccid paralysis of the lacrimal part of the orbicularis oculi results in excessive spilling of tears over the lower eyelid (i.e., crying).

Levator Palpebrae Superioris

The name, levator palpebrae superioris, tells us that this muscle elevates the upper eyelid.

Derivation	☐ levator: L. *lifter.*
	palpebrae: L. *eyelid.*
	superioris: L. *upper.*
Pronunciation	☐ LE-vay-tor, pal-PEE-bree, su-PEE-ri-OR-is

■ ATTACHMENTS

☐ **Sphenoid Bone**
    ☐ the anterior surface of the lesser wing of the sphenoid

to the

☐ **Upper Eyelid**
    ☐ the fascia and skin of the upper eyelid

■ FUNCTIONS

Concentric Mover Action

1. Elevates the Upper Eyelid

Mover Action Note

• The levator palpebrae superioris attaches from the sphenoid bone superiorly, to the upper eyelid inferiorly. When the levator palpebrae superioris contracts, it pulls the upper eyelid

superiorly toward the sphenoid bone. Therefore the levator palpebrae superioris elevates the upper eyelid (action 1).

INNERVATION

☐ The Oculomotor Nerve (CN III)

ARTERIAL SUPPLY

☐ The Ophthalmic Artery (a branch of the Internal Carotid Artery)

✋ PALPATION

1. With the client supine, have the client close the eye.
2. Gently place your palpating finger on the client's upper eyelid. Then ask the client to open the eye and feel for the contraction of the levator palpebrae superioris.

■ RELATIONSHIP TO OTHER STRUCTURES

☐ The levator palpebrae superioris begins in the orbital socket, deep to the orbicularis oculi. Some of its fibers pierce through the orbicularis oculi to attach into the skin of the eyelid, superficial to the orbicularis oculi.
☐ The levator palpebrae superioris is superior to, and somewhat conjoined to, the superior rectus muscle of the eye.
☐ The levator palpebrae superioris is involved with the deep front line myofascial meridian.

13

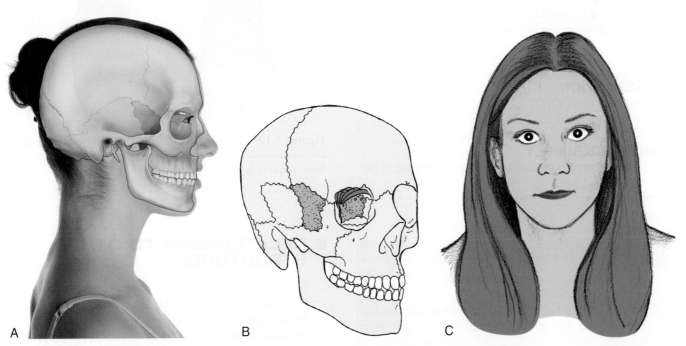

Figure 13-9 The levator palpebrae superioris. **A,** Lateral view of the right levator palpebrae superioris. **B,** Anterolateral view of the right levator palpebrae superioris. **C,** Anterior view of the expression created by the bilateral contraction of the levator palpebrae superioris.

Corrugator Supercilii

The name, corrugator supercilii, *tells us that this muscle wrinkles the skin of the eyebrow.*

Derivation	☐ corrugator: L. *to wrinkle together.*
	supercilii: L. *refers to the eyebrow.*
Pronunciation	☐ KOR-u-gay-tor, su-per-SIL-i-eye

■ ATTACHMENTS

☐ **Inferior Frontal Bone**
  ☐ the medial end of the superciliary arch of the frontal bone

to the

☐ **Fascia and Skin Deep to the Eyebrow**

■ FUNCTIONS

Concentric Mover Action

1. Draws the Eyebrow Inferomedially

Mover Action Note

- The corrugator supercilii attaches to the region of the frontal bone next to the nasal bone. From there, its fibers run superiorly and laterally to attach into the skin deep to the eyebrow. Because the frontal bone attachment is more fixed, when the corrugator supercilii contracts, it pulls the skin deep to the eyebrow inferomedially toward the frontal bone attachment (toward the other eyebrow). When both corrugator supercilii muscles contract, both eyebrows are pulled inferomedially toward each other. (action 1)

INNERVATION
☐ The Facial Nerve (CN VII)
  ☐ temporal branch

ARTERIAL SUPPLY
☐ The Supratrochlear and Supraorbital Arteries (branches of the Ophthalmic Artery)

🖐 **PALPATION**

1. With the client supine, place palpating fingers over the middle to medial portion of the eyebrow.
2. Ask the client to frown, drawing the eyebrow medially and inferiorly, and feel for the contraction of the corrugator supercilii.
3. Continue palpating the corrugator supercilii inferomedially toward its frontal bone attachment.

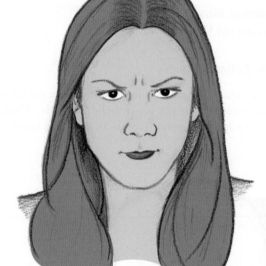

A

B

Figure 13-10 The corrugator supercilii. **A,** Anterior view of the right corrugator supercilii. **B,** Anterior view of the expression created by the bilateral contraction of the corrugator supercilii.

■ RELATIONSHIP TO OTHER STRUCTURES

☐ The corrugator supercilii is lateral to the procerus.
☐ The corrugator supercilii is deep to the frontalis.
☐ The corrugator supercilii lies toward the superior end of the orbicularis oculi. Where these two muscles overlap, the corrugator supercilii is deep to the orbicularis oculi.
☐ The corrugator supercilii is involved with the deep front line and superficial back line myofascial meridians.

13

Corrugator Supercilii—*cont'd*

■ MISCELLANEOUS

1. Some fibers of the corrugator supercilii blend in with fibers of the frontalis and the orbicularis oculi.
2. The action of drawing the eyebrows inferiorly and medially is involved in frowning. It is also useful in shielding the eyes from bright sunlight. (Note: The orbicularis oculi and the procerus can also assist with this function of shielding the eyes from bright sunlight.)
3. When the corrugator supercilii contracts, it causes vertical wrinkles superior and medial to the eyes.

NOSE
Procerus

The name, procerus, tells us that this muscle helps create the expression of superiority of a nobleman or prince.

Derivation	☐ procerus: L. *a chief noble, prince.*
Pronunciation	☐ pro-SAIR-rus

■ ATTACHMENTS

☐ **Fascia and Skin over the Nasal Bone**

> *to the*

☐ **Fascia and Skin Medial to the Eyebrow**

■ FUNCTIONS

Concentric Mover Actions
1. **Wrinkles the Skin of the Nose Upward**
2. **Draws Down the Medial Eyebrow**

Mover Action Notes

- The procerus attaches from the fascia and skin over the nose to the fascia and skin medial to the eyebrow (with its fibers running vertically). When the superior attachment is fixed and the procerus contracts, it pulls the fascia and skin of the nose superiorly, which causes the skin of the nose to wrinkle. (action 1)
- The procerus attaches from the fascia and skin over the nose to the fascia and skin medial to the eyebrow (with its fibers running vertically). When the inferior attachment is fixed and the procerus contracts, it pulls the medial eyebrow inferiorly (downward) toward the nose. Therefore the procerus draws down the medial eyebrow (this also causes the skin over the nose to wrinkle). (action 2)

INNERVATION
☐ The Facial Nerve (CN VII)
  ☐ superior buccal branches

ARTERIAL SUPPLY
The Facial Artery (a branch of the External Carotid Artery)

🖐 PALPATION

1. With the client supine, place palpating fingers directly superior to the bridge of the nose.
2. Ask the client to wrinkle the nose upward and/or draw the medial eyebrows down with a look of disdain as in frowning, and feel for the contraction of the procerus.
3. Palpate the entire procerus.

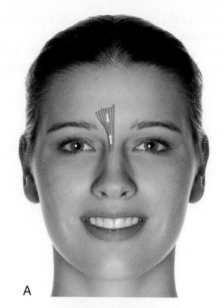

A

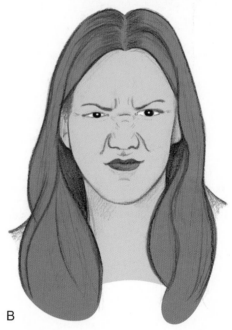

B

Figure 13-11 The procerus. **A,** Anterior view of the right procerus. **B,** Anterior view of the expression created by the bilateral contraction of the procerus.

■ RELATIONSHIP TO OTHER STRUCTURES

☐ The procerus is located superior to the nasalis, inferior to the frontalis, and medial to the corrugator supercilii and the orbicularis oculi.
☐ The procerus is involved with the deep front line and superficial back line myofascial meridians.

■ MISCELLANEOUS

1. The procerus often blends with the frontalis superiorly and the nasalis inferiorly.
2. The action of wrinkling the skin of the nose and/or drawing down the medial eyebrows can create the look of frowning or disdain that a person may make to convey an air of superiority (hence the name *procerus*, meaning chief noble or prince).
3. Bringing the medial eyebrows down is part of the facial expression of frowning, but it also helps shield the eyes from bright sunlight. (Note: The orbicularis oculi and the corrugator supercilii can also assist with this function of shielding the eyes from bright sunlight.)

Nasalis

The name, nasalis, tells us that this muscle is involved with the nose.

Derivation	☐ nasalis: L. *nose.*
Pronunciation	☐ nay-SA-lis

■ ATTACHMENTS

☐ **Maxilla**
  ☐ ALAR PART: the maxilla, lateral to the lower part of the nose
  ☐ TRANSVERSE PART: the maxilla, lateral to the upper part of the nose

to the

☐ **Cartilage of the Nose and the Opposite-Side Nasalis Muscle**
  ☐ ALAR PART: the alar cartilage of the nose
  ☐ TRANSVERSE PART: the opposite-side nasalis over the upper cartilage of the nose

■ FUNCTIONS

Concentric Mover Actions
1. **Flares the Nostril**
2. **Constricts the Nostril**

Mover Action Notes

• The alar part of the nasalis pulls directly on the lower part of the alar cartilage of the nose from the maxillary attachment, which is more lateral (the fibers are running somewhat horizontally). Therefore the lower part of the nose is pulled laterally, flaring the nostril and increasing the aperture for breathing. (action 1)

• The transverse part of each nasalis attaches into the opposite-side nasalis over the upper cartilage of the nose. When the nasalis contracts, it pulls the common midline attachment at the upper part of the nose down and in. This results in a constriction of the nose, which narrows the airway when breathing. (action 2)

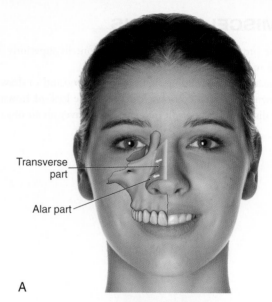

Transverse part

Alar part

A

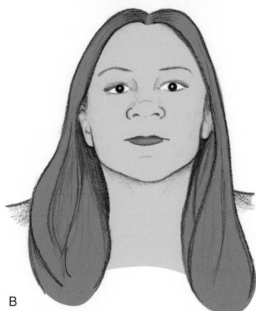

B

Figure 13-12 The nasalis. **A,** Anterior view of the right nasalis. **B,** Anterior view of the expression created by the bilateral contraction of the alar part of the nasalis.

INNERVATION
☐ The Facial Nerve (CN VII)
  ☐ superior buccal branches

ARTERIAL SUPPLY
☐ The Facial Artery (a branch of the External Carotid Artery)

✋ PALPATION

1. With the client supine, place palpating fingers over the cartilage of the nose, as well as the skin just lateral to the cartilage of the nose.
2. Have the client flare the nostrils as if taking in a deep breath and feel for the contraction of the lower alar part of the nasalis. Then have the client constrict the nostrils and palpate the upper transverse part of the nasalis.

Nasalis—*cont'd*

■ RELATIONSHIP TO OTHER STRUCTURES

☐ The nasalis is inferior to the procerus, medial to the levator labii superioris alaeque nasi, superior to the orbicularis oris, and superolateral to the depressor septi nasi.

☐ The nasalis is involved with the deep front line and superficial back line myofascial meridians.

■ MISCELLANEOUS

1. The alar part of the nasalis is sometimes called the *dilatator naris*. The transverse part of the nasalis is sometimes called the *compressor naris*.

2. The maxillary attachments of the transverse and alar parts of the nasalis often partially blend together.

3. Superiorly, the nasalis often blends in with the procerus.

4. The muscle directly inferomedial to the nasalis, the depressor septi nasi, is sometimes considered to be a part of the alar portion *(dilatator nasi)* of the nasalis.

5. The action of flaring the nostrils to increase the aperture for breathing in is important for deep inspiration. This action can also be associated with facial expressions during emotional states.

13

Depressor Septi Nasi

The name, depressor septi nasi, *tells us that this muscle depresses the nasal septum. (The septum is the midline cartilage of the nose.)*

Derivation	□ depressor: L. *depressor.*
	septi: L. *refers to the nasal septum.*
	nasi: L. *refers to the nose.*
Pronunciation	□ dee-PRES-or, SEP-ti, NAY-zi

■ ATTACHMENTS

□ **Maxilla**
  □ the incisive fossa of the maxilla

to the

□ **Cartilage of the Nose**
  □ the septum and the alar cartilage of the nose

■ FUNCTIONS

Concentric Mover Action
1. **Constricts the Nostril**

Mover Action Note

• The depressor septi nasi attaches from the maxilla inferiorly, to the cartilage of the nose superiorly (with its fibers running vertically). Given that the maxillary attachment is fixed, when the depressor septi nasi contracts, it pulls the cartilage of the nose inferiorly toward the maxilla. More specifically, the septum of the nose will be depressed and the alar cartilage will be depressed and pulled medially. These actions cause the nostril to constrict, which narrows the airway when breathing. (action 1)

INNERVATION
□ The Facial Nerve (CN VII)
  □ superior buccal branches

ARTERIAL SUPPLY
□ The Facial Artery (a branch of the External Carotid Artery)

🖐 PALPATION

1. With the client supine, place palpating fingers directly inferior to the nose.
2. Ask the client to try to pull the middle of the nose down toward the mouth and/or to constrict the nostrils and feel for the contraction of the depressor septi nasi.

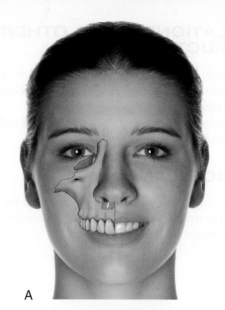

A

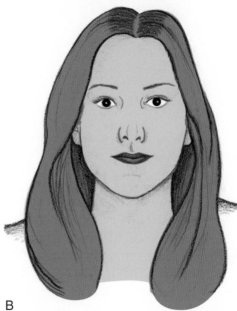

B

Figure 13-13 The depressor septi nasi. **A,** Anterior view of the right depressor septi nasi. **B,** Anterior view of the expression created by the bilateral contraction of the depressor septi nasi.

■ RELATIONSHIP TO OTHER STRUCTURES

□ The depressor septi nasi is superior to the orbicularis oris, and where they overlap, the depressor septi nasi is deep to the orbicularis oris.
□ The depressor septi nasi is inferior and medial to the nasalis (alar part).
□ The depressor septi nasi is involved with the deep front line myofascial meridian.

Depressor Septi Nasi—*cont'd*

■ MISCELLANEOUS

1. The depressor septi nasi is sometimes simply known as the *depressor septi*.

2. The depressor septi nasi is sometimes considered to be a part of the alar portion of the nasalis.

3. The action of constricting the nostrils can be associated with facial expressions during emotional states.

MOUTH
Levator Labii Superioris Alaeque Nasi

The name, levator labii superioris alaeque nasi, *tells us that this muscle elevates the upper lip and is involved with the ala (cartilage of the nostril of the nose).*

Derivation	☐ levator:	L. *lifter.*
	labii:	L. *refers to the lip.*
	superioris:	L. *upper.*
	alaeque:	L. *refers to the ala* (alar cartilage).
	nasi:	L. *refers to the nose.*
Pronunciation	☐ le-VAY-tor, LAY-be-eye, soo-PEE-ri-o-ris, a-LEE-kwe, NAY-si	

■ ATTACHMENTS

☐ **Maxilla**
   ☐ the frontal process of the maxilla near the nasal bone

to the

☐ **Upper Lip and the Nose**
   ☐ LATERAL SLIP: the muscular substance of the lateral part of the upper lip
   ☐ MEDIAL SLIP: the alar cartilage and the fascia and skin of the nose

■ FUNCTIONS

Concentric Mover Actions
1. **Elevates the Upper Lip**
2. **Flares the Nostril**
3. Everts the Upper Lip

Mover Action Notes

- The lateral slip of the levator labii superioris alaeque nasi attaches from the upper lip inferiorly and has a bony attachment near the eye superiorly (with its fibers running vertically). Because the superior attachment is into bone, it is more fixed than the other soft tissue attachment. When the levator labii superioris alaeque nasi contracts, it pulls the upper lip superiorly toward the other attachment. Therefore the levator labii superioris alaeque nasi elevates the upper lip. (action 1)

- The medial slip of the levator labii superioris alaeque nasi attaches from the alar cartilage and the fascia and skin of the nose medially, to attach onto the maxilla laterally (with its fibers running somewhat horizontally). Because the lateral attachment is into bone, it is more fixed than the other soft tissue attachment. When the levator labii superioris alaeque nasi contracts, it pulls the skin and alar cartilage of the nose toward the other attachment. Therefore the cartilage of the

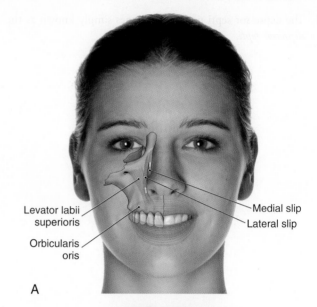

Levator labii superioris
Orbicularis oris
Medial slip
Lateral slip

A

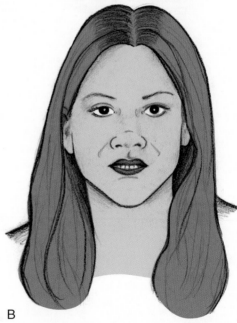

B

Figure 13-14 The levator labii superioris alaeque nasi (LLSAN). **A,** Anterior view of the right LLSAN. The levator labii superioris and the orbicularis oris have been ghosted in. **B,** Anterior view of the expression created by the bilateral contraction of the LLSAN.

nose is pulled laterally, flaring the nostril and increasing the aperture for breathing. (action 2)

- When the inferior attachment of the lateral slip of the levator labii superioris alaeque nasi is pulled superiorly toward the superior attachment, the lower margin of the upper lip is not only pulled superiorly, it is also pulled away from the mouth, curling the upper lip. This curling or pulling away

Levator Labii Superioris Alaeque Nasi—*cont'd*

of the upper lip from the face is called *eversion of the upper lip.* (action 3)

INNERVATION
□ The Facial Nerve (CN VII)
   □ buccal branches

ARTERIAL SUPPLY
□ The Infraorbital Artery (a branch of the Maxillary Artery)

✋ PALPATION

1. With the client supine, place palpating fingers just lateral to the nose.
2. Ask the client to flare the nostrils and/or elevate the upper lip to show you the upper teeth, and feel for the contraction of the levator labii superioris alaeque nasi. Try to distinguish it from the nasalis medially and the levator labii superioris laterally.

■ RELATIONSHIP TO OTHER STRUCTURES

□ The levator labii superioris alaeque nasi is located lateral to the nasalis and medial (and somewhat superficial) to the levator labii superioris. The levator labii superioris alaeque nasi is also medial to the zygomaticus minor.
□ The levator labii superioris alaeque nasi is medial and inferior to the orbicularis oculi.
□ The levator labii superioris alaeque nasi is superior to the orbicularis oris.
□ The levator labii superioris alaeque nasi is involved with the deep front line myofascial meridian.

■ MISCELLANEOUS

1. Some sources consider the levator labii superioris alaeque nasi muscle to be the *angular head* of the levator labii superioris.
2. The three main elevators of the upper lip are the levator labii superioris alaeque nasi, the levator labii superioris, and the zygomaticus minor. These three muscles were once considered to be three individual heads (named *angularis, infraorbitalis,* and *zygomaticus,* respectively) of the *musculus quadratus labii superioris.*
3. The levator labii superioris alaeque nasi blends into the levator labii superioris and the orbicularis oris.
4. In addition to increasing the aperture for breathing, flaring the nostrils can also be part of the look of anger.
5. Contraction of the lateral slip of the levator labii superioris alaeque nasi alone will elevate the upper lip, as in showing someone your upper teeth. This action, along with the contraction of other facial muscles, can contribute to the facial expression of a smile or express smugness, contempt, or disdain.

13

Levator Labii Superioris

The name, levator labii superioris, *tells us that this muscle elevates the upper lip.*

Derivation	☐ levator:	L. *lifter.*
	labii:	L. *refers to the lip.*
	superioris:	L. *upper.*
Pronunciation	☐ le-VAY-tor, LAY-be-eye,	
	soo-PEE-ri-O-ris	

■ ATTACHMENTS

☐ **Maxilla**
  ☐ at the inferior orbital margin of the maxilla

to the

☐ **Upper Lip**
  ☐ the muscular substance of the upper lip

■ FUNCTIONS

Concentric Mover Actions
1. **Elevates the Upper Lip**
2. Everts the Upper Lip

Mover Action Notes

• The levator labii superioris attaches from the upper lip inferiorly, to attach onto the maxilla superiorly (with its fibers running vertically). The superior attachment is into bone and is therefore more fixed than the other attachment, which is into soft tissue. When the levator labii superioris contracts, it pulls the upper lip superiorly toward the maxilla. Therefore the levator labii superioris elevates the upper lip. (action 1)

• When the inferior attachment of the levator labii superioris is pulled superiorly toward the superior attachment, the lower margin of the upper lip is not only pulled superiorly, it is also pulled away from the mouth, curling the upper lip. This curling or pulling away of the upper lip from the face is called *eversion of the upper lip.* (action 2)

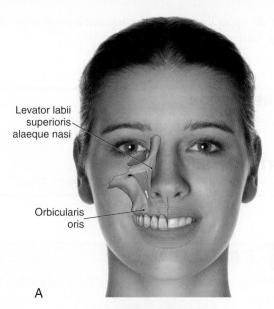

Levator labii
superioris
alaeque nasi

Orbicularis
oris

A

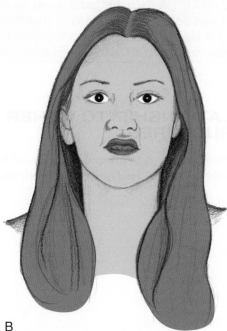

B

Figure 13-15 The levator labii superioris (LLS). **A,** Anterior view of the right LLS. The levator labii superioris alaeque nasi and the orbicularis oris have been ghosted in. **B,** Anterior view of the expression created by the bilateral contraction of the levator labii superioris.

INNERVATION
☐ The Facial Nerve (CN VII)
  ☐ buccal branches

ARTERIAL SUPPLY
☐ The Facial Artery (a branch of the External Carotid Artery)

🖐 PALPATION

1. With the client supine, place palpating fingers just superior to the upper lip approximately ½ to 1 inch (1-2 cm) medial to the corner of the mouth.
2. Ask the client to elevate the upper lip to show you the upper gums and feel for the contraction of the levator labii superioris. Try to distinguish it from the levator labii superioris alaeque nasi medially and the zygomaticus minor laterally.

13

Levator Labii Superioris—*cont'd*

■ RELATIONSHIP TO OTHER STRUCTURES

☐ The levator labii superioris is between the levator labii superioris alaeque nasi (medially) and the zygomaticus minor (laterally).

☐ The levator labii superioris is inferior to the orbicularis oculi; where they overlap, the levator labii superioris is deep to the orbicularis oculi.

☐ The levator labii superioris is superior to the orbicularis oris. When the levator labii superioris meets the orbicularis oris, the fibers of the levator labii superioris run deep to and blend into the orbicularis oris.

☐ The levator labii superioris is involved with the deep front line myofascial meridian.

■ MISCELLANEOUS

1. Some sources consider the levator labii superioris alaeque nasi muscle to be the *angular head* of the levator labii superioris.

2. The three main elevators of the upper lip are the levator labii superioris alaeque nasi, the levator labii superioris, and the zygomaticus minor. These three muscles were once considered to be three individual heads (named *angularis, infraorbitalis,* and *zygomaticus,* respectively) of the *musculus quadratus labii superioris.*

3. The levator labii superioris blends in with the levator labii superioris alaeque nasi and the orbicularis oris.

4. Contraction of the levator labii superioris alone will elevate the upper lip, as in showing someone your upper teeth. This action, along with the contraction of other facial muscles, can contribute to the facial expression of a smile or express smugness, contempt, or disdain.

13

The name, zygomaticus minor, tells us that this muscle attaches to the zygomatic bone and is small (smaller than the zygomaticus major).

Derivation	☐ zygomaticus: Gr. *refers to the zygomatic bone.*
	minor: L. *smaller.*
Pronunciation	☐ ZI-go-MAT-ik-us, MY-nor

■ ATTACHMENTS

☐ **Zygomatic Bone**
   ☐ near the zygomaticomaxillary suture

to the

☐ **Upper Lip**
   ☐ the muscular substance of the upper lip

■ FUNCTIONS

Concentric Mover Actions
1. Elevates the Upper Lip
2. Everts the Upper Lip

Mover Action Notes

- The zygomaticus minor attaches from the upper lip inferiorly, to the zygomatic bone superiorly (with its fibers running vertically). The maxillary attachment is into bone and is therefore more fixed than the other attachment, which is into soft tissue. When the zygomaticus minor contracts, it pulls the upper lip superiorly toward the zygomatic bone. Therefore the zygomaticus minor elevates the upper lip. (action 1)
- When the inferior attachment of the zygomaticus minor is pulled superiorly toward the superior attachment, the lower margin of the upper lip is not only pulled superiorly, it is also pulled away from the mouth, curling the upper lip. This curling or pulling away of the upper lip from the face is called *eversion of the upper lip.* (action 2)

INNERVATION
☐ The Facial Nerve (CN VII)
   ☐ buccal branches

ARTERIAL SUPPLY
☐ The Facial Artery (a branch of the External Carotid Artery)

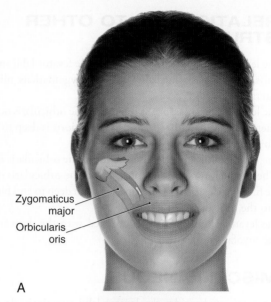

Zygomaticus major
Orbicularis oris

A

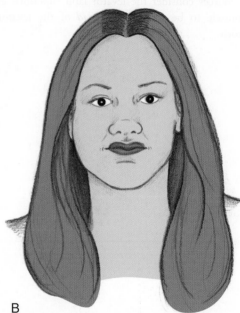

B

Figure 13-16 The zygomaticus minor. **A,** Anterior view of the right zygomaticus minor. The zygomaticus major and the orbicularis oris have been ghosted in. **B,** Anterior view of the expression created by the bilateral contraction of the zygomaticus minor.

✋ PALPATION

1. With the client supine, place palpating fingers just superior to the upper lip, approximately ½ to 1 inch (1-2 cm) medial to the angle of the mouth.
2. Have the client elevate the upper lip to show you the upper teeth and feel for the contraction of the zygomaticus minor. Try to distinguish it from the levator labii superioris and levator labii superioris alaeque nasi medially and the zygomaticus major laterally.

RELATIONSHIP TO OTHER STRUCTURES

☐ The zygomaticus minor is lateral to the levator labii superioris alaeque nasi and the levator labii superioris, and medial to the zygomaticus major.

☐ The zygomaticus minor is superior to the orbicularis oris and inferior to the orbicularis oculi.

☐ The zygomaticus minor is superficial to the levator anguli oris.

☐ The zygomaticus minor is involved with the deep front line myofascial meridian.

MISCELLANEOUS

1. The zygomaticus minor blends with the levator labii superioris.

2. The three main elevators of the upper lip are the levator labii superioris alaeque nasi, the levator labii superioris, and the zygomaticus minor. These three muscles were once considered to be three individual heads (named *angularis, infraorbitalis,* and *zygomaticus,* respectively) of the *musculus quadratus labii superioris.*

3. Contraction of the zygomaticus minor alone will elevate the upper lip, as in showing someone your upper teeth. This action, along with the contraction of other facial muscles, can contribute to the facial expression of a smile or express smugness, contempt, or disdain.

4. Contraction of the zygomaticus minor also increases the nasolabial sulcus.

13

Zygomaticus Major

The name, zygomaticus major, tells us that this muscle attaches to the zygomatic bone and is large (larger than the zygomaticus minor).

Derivation	☐ zygomaticus: Gr. *refers to the* *zygomatic bone.*
	major: L. *larger.*
Pronunciation	☐ ZI-go-MAT-ik-us, MAY-jor

■ ATTACHMENTS

☐ **Zygomatic Bone**
  ☐ near the zygomaticotemporal suture

  to the

☐ **Angle of the Mouth**
  ☐ the modiolus, just lateral to the angle of the mouth

■ FUNCTIONS

Concentric Mover Actions
1. **Elevates the Angle of the Mouth**
2. Draws Laterally the Angle of the Mouth

Mover Action Notes

• The zygomaticus major attaches from the zygomatic bone superiorly, to the angle (corner) of the mouth inferiorly (with its fibers running vertically). The zygomatic attachment is into bone and is therefore more fixed than the other attachment, which is into soft tissue. When the zygomaticus major contracts, it pulls the angle of the mouth superiorly toward the zygomatic bone. Therefore the zygomaticus major elevates the angle of the mouth. (action 1)

• The zygomaticus major attaches from the zygomatic bone laterally, to the angle (corner) of the mouth medially (with its fibers running somewhat horizontally). The zygomatic attachment is into bone and is therefore more fixed than the other attachment, which is into soft tissue. When the zygomaticus major contracts, it pulls the angle of the mouth toward the zygomatic bone. Therefore the zygomaticus major draws laterally the angle of the mouth. (action 2)

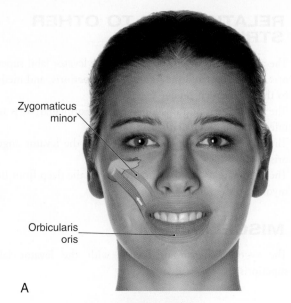

Zygomaticus minor

Orbicularis oris

A

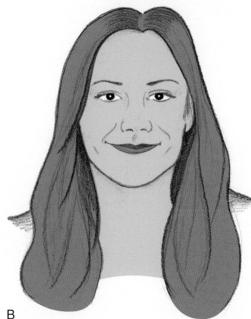

B

Figure 13-17 The zygomaticus major. **A,** Anterior view of the right zygomaticus major. The zygomaticus minor and the orbicularis oris have been ghosted in. **B,** Anterior view of the expression created by the bilateral contraction of the zygomaticus major.

INNERVATION
☐ The Facial Nerve (CN VII)
  ☐ buccal branches

ARTERIAL SUPPLY
☐ The Facial Artery (a branch of the External Carotid Artery)

✋ PALPATION

1. With the client supine, place palpating fingers superior and lateral to the angle of the mouth.
2. Have the client smile by drawing the angle of the mouth both superiorly and laterally and feel for the contraction of the belly of the zygomaticus major.

■ RELATIONSHIP TO OTHER STRUCTURES

☐ The zygomaticus major is lateral to the zygomaticus minor.

☐ The zygomaticus major is superior to the risorius and the orbicularis oris.

☐ The zygomaticus major is superficial to the buccinator and the masseter.

☐ The zygomaticus major is involved with the deep front line myofascial meridian.

■ MISCELLANEOUS

1. The zygomaticus major blends in with the levator anguli oris and the orbicularis oris.

2. The action of elevating the angle of the mouth and drawing it laterally contributes to smiling and laughing.

3. Contraction of the zygomaticus major also increases the nasolabial sulcus.

4. Six muscles attach into the modiolus: the zygomaticus major, levator anguli oris, risorius, depressor anguli oris, buccinator, and orbicularis oris.

5. The modiolus is a fibromuscular condensation approximately ¼ inch (0.5 cm) lateral to the angle of the mouth (see page 429).

Levator Anguli Oris

The name, levator anguli oris, *tells us that this muscle elevates the angle of the mouth.*

Derivation	☐ levator: L. *lifter.*
	anguli: L. *refers to the angle.*
	oris: L. *mouth.*
Pronunciation	☐ le-VAY-tor, ANG-you-lie, O-ris

■ ATTACHMENTS

☐ **Maxilla**
   ☐ the canine fossa of the maxilla (just inferior to the infra-orbital foramen)

to the

☐ **Angle of the Mouth**
   ☐ the modiolus, just lateral to the angle of the mouth

■ FUNCTIONS

Concentric Mover Action
1. Elevates the Angle of the Mouth

Mover Action Note

- The levator anguli oris attaches from the maxilla superiorly, to the tissue at the angle (corner) of the mouth inferiorly (with its fibers running vertically). The maxillary attachment is into bone and is therefore more fixed than the other attachment, which is into soft tissue. When the levator anguli oris contracts, it pulls the angle of the mouth superiorly toward the maxilla. Therefore the levator anguli oris elevates the angle of the mouth. (action 1)

INNERVATION
☐ The Facial Nerve (CN VII)
   ☐ buccal branches

ARTERIAL SUPPLY
☐ The Facial Artery (a branch of the External Carotid Artery)

✋ PALPATION

1. With the client supine, place palpating fingers just superior to the angle (corner) of the mouth.
2. Have the client elevate the angle of the mouth straight superiorly, attempting to show you the canine tooth, and feel for the contraction of the belly of the levator anguli oris. Try to distinguish it from the levator labii superioris, the zygomaticus major, and the zygomaticus minor.

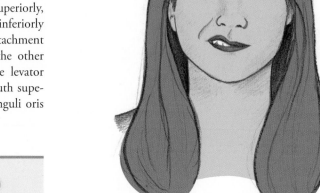

Orbicularis oris

A

B

Figure 13-18 The right levator anguli oris. **A,** Anterior view. The orbicularis oris has been ghosted in. **B,** Anterior view of the expression created by the contraction of the levator anguli oris.

■ RELATIONSHIP TO OTHER STRUCTURES

☐ Where they overlap, the levator anguli oris is deep to the levator labii superioris, the zygomaticus minor, and the zygomaticus major. The levator anguli oris is superficial between the zygomaticus minor and the zygomaticus major.

Levator Anguli Oris—*cont'd*

☐ The inferior attachment of the levator anguli oris is superficial to the buccinator.

☐ The levator anguli oris is superior to the orbicularis oris and inferior to the orbicularis oculi.

☐ The levator anguli oris is involved with the deep front line myofascial meridian.

■ MISCELLANEOUS

1. The levator anguli oris is also known as the *caninus* (kay-NI-nus). This name is given because the contraction of the levator anguli oris can result in the teeth, especially the canine tooth, becoming visible.

2. At the attachment near the angle of the mouth (the modiolus), fibers of the levator anguli oris blend in with the orbicularis oris, the zygomaticus major, and the depressor anguli oris.

3. Although the action of the levator anguli oris may contribute to a smile, its action alone (unilaterally or bilaterally) can manifest a sneer. Bilateral contraction of this muscle can also reproduce the typical *Dracula* expression wherein the canine teeth are exposed.

4. Contraction of the levator anguli oris also increases the nasolabial sulcus.

5. Six muscles attach into the modiolus: the zygomaticus major, the levator anguli oris, the risorius, the depressor anguli oris, the buccinator, and the orbicularis oris.

6. The modiolus is a fibromuscular condensation approximately ¼ inch (0.5 cm) lateral to the angle of the mouth (see page 429).

13

Risorius

The name, risorius, *tells us that this muscle is involved with laughing.*

Derivation	☐ risorius: L. *laughing*.
Pronunciation	☐ ri-SO-ri-us

■ ATTACHMENTS

☐ **Fascia and Skin Superficial to the Masseter**

  to the

☐ **Angle of the Mouth**
  ☐ the modiolus, just lateral to the angle of the mouth

■ FUNCTIONS

Concentric Mover Action
1. Draws Laterally the Angle of the Mouth

Mover Action Note

- The risorius attaches from the fascia and skin superficial to the masseter laterally, to the angle (corner) of the mouth medially (with its fibers running somewhat horizontally). If the lateral attachment is the more fixed attachment and the risorius contracts, it pulls the angle of the mouth laterally. Therefore the risorius draws laterally the angle of the mouth. (action 1)

INNERVATION
☐ The Facial Nerve (CN VII)
  ☐ buccal branches

ARTERIAL SUPPLY
☐ The Facial Artery (a branch of the External Carotid Artery)

✋ **PALPATION**

1. With the client supine, place palpating fingers directly lateral to the angle of the mouth.
2. Ask the client to draw the angle (corner) of the mouth directly lateral and feel for the contraction of the belly of the risorius. Be sure that you are not palpating too superiorly onto the zygomaticus major, which can also help draw the angle of the mouth laterally.

■ RELATIONSHIP TO OTHER STRUCTURES

☐ The risorius is inferior to the zygomaticus major and lateral to the orbicularis oris.

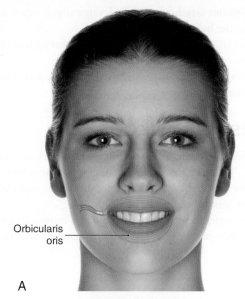

Orbicularis
  oris

A

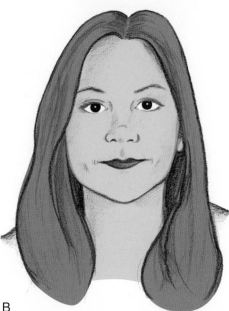

B

Figure 13-19 The risorius. **A,** Anterior view of the right risorius. The orbicularis oris has been ghosted in. **B,** Anterior view of the expression created by the bilateral contraction of the risorius.

☐ The risorius is superior to the depressor anguli oris and the platysma. Where these muscles overlap, the risorius is superficial.
☐ The risorius is superficial to the buccinator.
☐ The risorius is involved with the deep front line myofascial meridian.

■ MISCELLANEOUS

1. The lateral attachment of the risorius varies greatly in its presentation.

Risorius—*cont'd*

2. The medial attachment of the risorius also varies, often attaching approximately ¼ inch (0.5 cm) inferior to the angle of the mouth.
3. Drawing the angle of the mouth laterally is involved with grinning, smiling, and laughing.
4. Six muscles attach into the modiolus: the zygomaticus major, levator anguli oris, risorius, depressor anguli oris, buccinator, and orbicularis oris.

5. The modiolus is a fibromuscular condensation approximately ¼ inch (0.5 cm) lateral to the angle of the mouth (see page 429).

13

Depressor Anguli Oris

The name, depressor anguli oris, *tells us that this muscle depresses the angle of the mouth.*

Derivation	☐ depressor: L. *depressor.*
	anguli: L. *refers to the angle.*
	oris: L. *mouth.*
Pronunciation	☐ dee-PRES-or, ANG-you-lie, O-ris

■ ATTACHMENTS

☐ **Mandible**
    ☐ the oblique line of the mandible, inferior to the mental foramen

to the

☐ **Angle of the Mouth**
    ☐ the modiolus, just lateral to the angle of the mouth

■ FUNCTIONS

Concentric Mover Actions
1. Depresses the Angle of the Mouth
2. Draws Laterally the Angle of the Mouth

Mover Action Notes

- The depressor anguli oris attaches from the mandible inferiorly, to the tissue at the angle (corner) of the mouth superiorly (with its fibers running vertically). The mandibular attachment is into bone and is therefore more fixed than the other attachment, which is into soft tissue. When the depressor anguli oris contracts, it pulls the angle of the mouth inferiorly toward the mandible. Therefore the depressor anguli oris depresses the angle of the mouth. (action 1)
- The depressor anguli oris attaches from the mandible laterally, into the angle (corner) of the mouth medially (with its fibers running somewhat horizontally). The mandibular attachment is into bone and is therefore more fixed than the other attachment, which is into soft tissue. When the depressor anguli oris contracts, it pulls the angle of the mouth laterally toward the mandible. Therefore the depressor anguli oris draws laterally the angle of the mouth. (action 2)

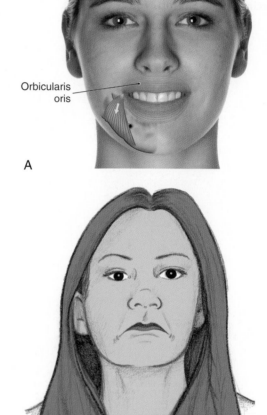

Orbicularis oris

A

B

Figure 13-20 The depressor anguli oris. **A,** Anterior view of the right depressor anguli oris. The orbicularis oris has been ghosted in. **B,** Anterior view of the expression created by the bilateral contraction of the depressor anguli oris.

INNERVATION
☐ The Facial Nerve (CN VII)
    ☐ mandibular branch

ARTERIAL SUPPLY
☐ The Facial Artery (a branch of the External Carotid Artery)

 PALPATION

1. With the client supine, place palpating fingers slightly lateral and inferior to the angle of the mouth.
2. Have the client draw the angle of the mouth inferiorly (and perhaps pull the angle of the mouth slightly laterally) and feel for the contraction of the belly of the depressor anguli oris. It may be difficult to precisely discern this muscle from the nearby depressor labii inferioris.

Depressor Anguli Oris—*cont'd*

■ RELATIONSHIP TO OTHER STRUCTURES

☐ The depressor anguli oris is lateral to the depressor labii inferioris. Where these two muscles overlap, the depressor anguli oris is superficial to the depressor labii inferioris.

☐ The depressor anguli oris is inferior to the orbicularis oris and the risorius.

☐ The depressor anguli oris is superior to the platysma.

☐ The depressor anguli oris is involved with the deep front line myofascial meridian.

■ MISCELLANEOUS

1. The depressor anguli oris blends into the platysma.
2. Occasionally, some fibers of the depressor anguli oris blend into the opposite-side depressor anguli oris and/or the same-side levator anguli oris.

3. Both the depressor anguli oris and the depressor labii inferioris arise from the oblique line of the mandible. On the oblique line, the depressor anguli oris attaches more laterally than the depressor labii inferioris.
4. The actions of the depressor anguli oris contribute to the facial expression of sadness or uncertainty.
5. Six muscles attach into the modiolus: the zygomaticus major, levator anguli oris, risorius, depressor anguli oris, buccinator, and orbicularis oris.
6. The modiolus is a fibromuscular condensation approximately ¼ inch (0.5 cm) lateral to the angle of the mouth (see page 429).

13

Depressor Labii Inferioris

The name, depressor labii inferioris, *tells us that this muscle depresses the lower lip.*

Derivation	☐ depressor: L. *depressor.*
	labii: L. *refers to the lip.*
	inferioris: L. *lower.*
Pronunciation	☐ dee-PRES-or, LAY-be-eye,
	in-FEE-ri-O-ris

■ ATTACHMENTS

☐ **Mandible**
  ☐ the oblique line of the mandible, between the symphysis menti and the mental foramen

to the

☐ **Lower Lip**
  ☐ the midline of the lower lip

■ FUNCTIONS

Concentric Mover Actions
1. **Depresses the Lower Lip**
2. Draws Laterally the Lower Lip
3. Everts the Lower Lip

Mover Action Notes

- The depressor labii inferioris attaches from the mandible inferiorly, into the lower lip superiorly (with its fibers running vertically). The mandibular attachment is into bone and is therefore more fixed than the other attachment, which is into soft tissue. When the depressor labii inferioris contracts, it pulls the lower lip inferiorly toward the mandible. Therefore the depressor labii inferioris depresses the lower lip. (action 1)
- The depressor labii inferioris attaches from the mandible laterally, into the lower lip medially (with its fibers running somewhat horizontally). The mandibular attachment is into bone and is therefore more fixed than the other attachment, which is into soft tissue. When the depressor labii inferioris contracts, it pulls the lower lip laterally toward the mandible. Therefore the depressor labii inferioris draws laterally the lower lip. (action 2)
- When the superior attachment of the depressor labii inferioris is pulled inferiorly toward the mandible, the lower margin of the lower lip is not only pulled inferiorly, it is also pulled away from the mouth, curling the lower lip. This curling or pulling away of the lower lip from the face is called *eversion of the lower lip.* (action 3)

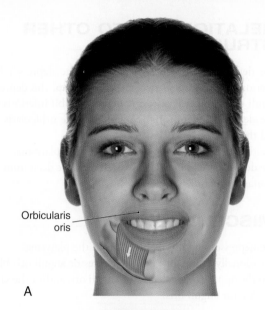

Orbicularis oris

A

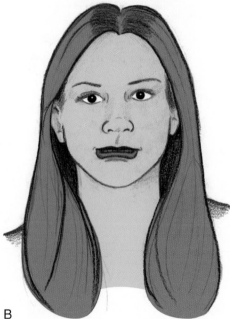

B

Figure 13-21 The depressor labii inferioris. **A,** Anterior view of the right depressor labii inferioris. The orbicularis oris has been ghosted in. **B,** Anterior view of the expression created by the bilateral contraction of the depressor labii inferioris.

INNERVATION
☐ The Facial Nerve (CN VII)
  ☐ mandibular branch

ARTERIAL SUPPLY
☐ The Facial Artery (a branch of the External Carotid Artery)

Depressor Labii Inferioris—*cont'd*

 PALPATION

1. With the client supine, place palpating fingers inferior to the lower lip, slightly lateral from the center.
2. Have the client draw the lower lip inferiorly and slightly laterally and feel for the contraction of the depressor labii inferioris. It may be difficult to precisely discern the depressor labii inferioris from the nearby mentalis and the depressor anguli oris.

■ RELATIONSHIP TO OTHER STRUCTURES

☐ The depressor labii inferioris is lateral to the mentalis. Where these two muscles overlap, the depressor labii inferioris is superficial.

☐ The depressor labii inferioris is medial to the depressor anguli oris. Where these two muscles overlap, the depressor labii inferioris is deeper.

☐ The depressor labii inferioris is inferior to the orbicularis oris and superior to the platysma.

☐ The depressor labii inferioris is involved with the deep front line myofascial meridian.

■ MISCELLANEOUS

1. The depressor labii inferioris blends with the opposite side depressor labii inferioris and the orbicularis oris at the lip. Inferiorly, the depressor labii inferioris blends with the platysma.
2. Both the depressor labii inferioris and the depressor anguli oris arise from the oblique line of the mandible. On the oblique line, the depressor labii inferioris attaches more medially than the depressor anguli oris.
3. The actions of the depressor labii inferioris can contribute to the facial expressions of sorrow, doubt, and irony.

13

Mentalis

The name, mentalis, *tells us that this muscle is related to the chin.*

Derivation	☐ mentalis: L. *the chin.*
Pronunciation	☐ men-TA-lis

■ ATTACHMENTS

☐ **Mandible**
   ☐ the incisive fossa of the mandible

to the

☐ **Fascia and Skin of the Chin**

■ FUNCTIONS

Concentric Mover Actions
1. **Elevates the Lower Lip**
2. **Everts and Protracts the Lower Lip**
3. Wrinkles the Skin of the Chin

Mover Action Notes

- The mentalis attaches from the mandible superiorly and attaches into the fascia and skin of the chin inferiorly (with its fibers running vertically). The mandibular attachment is into bone and is therefore more fixed than the other attachment, which is into soft tissue. When the mentalis contracts, it pulls the fascia and skin of the chin superiorly toward the mandible. When this occurs, the skin of the chin is pulled into the lower lip, pushing the lower lip superiorly. Therefore the mentalis elevates the lower lip. (action 1)
- When the mentalis pulls superiorly on the fascia and skin of the chin, the lower lip is elevated. As the mentalis continues to contract, the upper margin of the lower lip is forced away from the mouth anteriorly. This action is called *eversion of the lower lip*. As the mentalis continues to contract, the entire lower lip is forced away from the mouth. This action is called *protraction* (or *protrusion*) *of the lower lip*. Therefore the mentalis everts and protracts the lower lip. (action 2)
- When the mentalis contracts and pulls superiorly on the fascia and skin of the chin, the skin of the chin is wrinkled. (action 3)

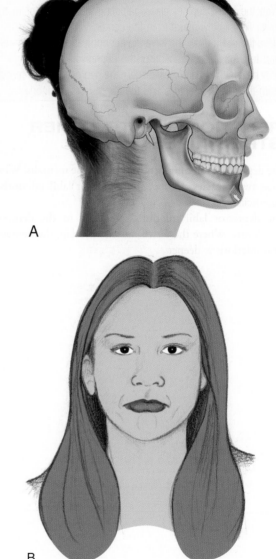

A

B

Figure 13-22 The mentalis. **A,** Right lateral view. **B,** Anterior view of the expression created by the bilateral contraction of the mentalis.

INNERVATION
☐ The Facial Nerve (CN VII)
   ☐ mandibular branch

ARTERIAL SUPPLY
☐ The Facial Artery (a branch of the External Carotid Artery)

✋ PALPATION

1. With the client supine, place palpating fingers inferior to the midline of the lower lip, just slightly lateral from the center. Be sure that you are inferior to the orbicularis oris and medial to the depressor labii inferioris.
2. Have the client stick out the lower lip as if pouting and feel for the contraction of the mentalis.

Mentalis—*cont'd*

■ RELATIONSHIP TO OTHER STRUCTURES

☐ The mentalis is medial to the depressor labii inferioris. Where these two muscles overlap, the mentalis is deeper. The mentalis is also medial to the depressor anguli oris.

☐ The mentalis is inferior to the orbicularis oris and superior to the platysma.

☐ The mentalis is involved with the deep front line myofascial meridian.

■ MISCELLANEOUS

1. The actions of the mentalis are involved in manifesting the facial expressions of doubt, pouting, or disdain.
2. Elevating, everting, and protracting the lower lip are also useful when drinking.
3. When the mentalis contracts, it also raises the mentolabial sulcus.

13

Buccinator

The name, buccinator, *tells us that this muscle is found in the cheek region.*

Derivation	☐ buccinator: L. *trumpeter, refers to the cheek.*
Pronunciation	☐ BUK-sin-A-tor

■ ATTACHMENTS

☐ **Maxilla and the Mandible**
  ☐ the external surfaces of the alveolar processes of the mandible and the maxilla (opposite the molars), and the pterygomandibular raphe

  to the

☐ **Lips**
  ☐ deeper into the musculature of the lips and the modiolus, just lateral to the angle of the mouth

■ FUNCTIONS

Concentric Mover Action
1. Compresses the Cheek against the teeth

Mover Action Note

• Posteriorly, the fibers of the buccinator arise from the maxilla and the mandible (and the pterygomandibular raphe between them). From there, the buccinator fibers travel anteriorly through the tissue of the cheek (running horizontally) to attach into the lips. The posterior attachments are into bone and are therefore more fixed than the anterior attachment, which is into soft tissue. When the buccinator contracts, the tissue of the cheek and the lips is pulled posteriorly and compressed against the teeth. (action 1)

INNERVATION
☐ The Facial Nerve (CN VII)
  ☐ buccal branches

ARTERIAL SUPPLY
☐ The Maxillary and Facial Arteries (branches of the External Carotid Artery)

✋ PALPATION

1. With the client supine, place palpating fingers on the cheek, anterior (medial) to the ramus of the mandible.
2. Have the client take in a breath, purse the lips, and press the lips against the teeth as if expelling air to play the trumpet, and feel for the contraction of the buccinator.

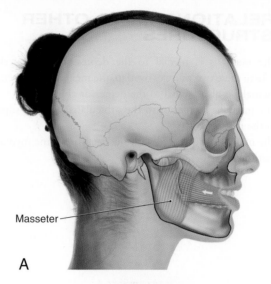

Masseter

A

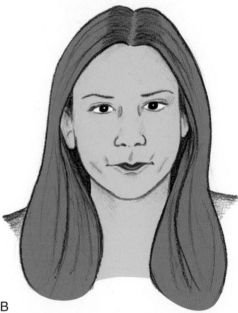

B

Figure 13-23 The buccinator. **A,** Right lateral view. **B,** Anterior view of the expression created by the bilateral contraction of the buccinator.

■ RELATIONSHIP TO OTHER STRUCTURES

☐ The anterior (medial) part of the buccinator is superficial and located in the tissue of the cheek. The posterior (lateral) part of the buccinator is deeper and located posterior (deep) to the ramus of the mandible.
☐ The anterior (medial) part of the buccinator is deep to the levator anguli oris, zygomaticus major, risorius, and depressor anguli oris.
☐ Deep to the buccinator is the mucosa of the cheek.
☐ The buccinator is involved with the deep front line myofascial meridian.

13

Buccinator—*cont'd*

■ MISCELLANEOUS

1. The buccinator has three posterior parts that all converge into the anterior attachment. These three parts come from the maxilla, the mandible, and the pterygomandibular raphe.

2. The buccinator's central posterior attachment is into the pterygomandibular raphe. (A raphe is a seam of tissue formed by the union of the halves of a part.) Essentially, the pterygomandibular raphe is composed of fibrous connective tissue that bridges the pterygoid process of the sphenoid bone to the mandible, hence, its name.

3. The pterygomandibular raphe is located deep near the sphenoid bone, posterior to the maxilla. More specifically, the pterygomandibular raphe runs from the hamulus of the medial pterygoid plate of the sphenoid bone to the posterior end of the mylohyoid line of the mandible. (The pterygomandibular raphe also serves as an attachment site for the superior pharyngeal constrictor muscle (Ⓔvolve See Evolve website). The pterygomandibular raphe can be thought of as the intersection of the buccinator and the superior pharyngeal constrictor muscle.)

4. The parotid duct pierces through the buccinator to enter the mouth.

5. The action of compressing the cheeks against the teeth by the two buccinators working bilaterally is important for forcefully expelling air from the mouth. If one is forcefully expelling air through tightly closed lips, it is the buccinator that expels the air and keeps the cheeks from distending.

6. The buccinator is the muscle that contracts when a musician blows air into a brass or woodwind instrument. In fact, the Latin word for trumpeter is *buccinator.*

7. The buccinators are also important with whistling, blowing up a balloon, and with helping to keep food from lingering in the vestibule of the mouth (between the teeth and the cheeks).

8. The buccinators are the muscles responsible for the expression made (puckering the cheeks) when a person eats something sour, such as biting into a lemon.

9. Six muscles attach into the modiolus: the zygomaticus major, levator anguli oris, risorius, depressor anguli oris, buccinator, and orbicularis oris.

10. The modiolus is a fibromuscular condensation approximately ¼ inch (0.5 cm) lateral to the angle of the mouth (see page 429).

13

Orbicularis Oris

The name, orbicularis oris, *tells us that this muscle encircles the mouth.*

Derivation	☐ orbicularis: L. *a small circle.*
	oris: L. *mouth.*
Pronunciation	☐ or-BIK-you-LA-ris, O-ris

■ ATTACHMENTS

☐ **Orbicularis oris is a muscle that, in its entirety, surrounds the mouth.**

☐ In more detail, there are four parts to the orbicularis oris: two on the left (upper and lower) and two on the right (upper and lower). Therefore there is one part in each of the four quadrants. Each of these four parts of the orbicularis oris anchors to the modiolus on that side. From there, the fibers traverse through the tissue of the upper or the lower lips. At the midline, the fibers on each side interlace with each other, thereby attaching into each other.

■ FUNCTIONS

Concentric Mover Actions
1. **Closes the Mouth**
2. **Protracts the Lips**

Mover Action Notes

• The fiber direction of the orbicularis oris is circular around the mouth. When the orbicularis oris contracts, it acts like a circular sphincter muscle that closes in around the mouth, forcing the two lips together. (Note: To understand how a circular sphincter muscle works, the following reasoning applies: If a linear muscle shortens, its length decreases. When that same linear muscle is arranged in a circular fashion and shortens, the length of the line you have to make the circle decreases and therefore the size of the circle lessens, which can close in on whatever structure is being surrounded by it.) (action 1)

• After closure of the mouth occurs, if the orbicularis oris continues to contract, the lips are pushed against each other harder and push out anteriorly. This action is called *protraction* (or *protrusion*) *of the lips.* (action 2)

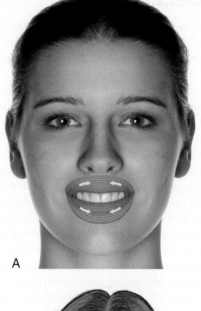

A

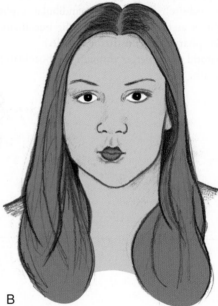

B

Figure 13-24 The orbicularis oris. **A,** Anterior view. **B,** Anterior view of the expression created by the contraction of orbicularis oris.

INNERVATION
☐ The Facial Nerve (CN VII)
  ☐ buccal and mandibular branches

ARTERIAL SUPPLY
☐ The Facial Artery (A Branch of the External Carotid Artery)

 PALPATION

1. With the client supine, wearing a finger cot or glove, place palpating fingers on the tissue of the lips.
2. Have the client pucker up the lips and feel for the contraction of the orbicularis oris.

Orbicularis Oris—*cont'd*

RELATIONSHIP TO OTHER STRUCTURES

☐ The orbicularis oris surrounds the mouth. The following muscles radiate outward from the orbicularis oris like spokes from a wheel: the depressor septi nasi, levator labii superioris alaeque nasi, levator labii superioris, zygomaticus minor, levator anguli oris, zygomaticus major, risorius, buccinator, depressor anguli oris, depressor labii inferioris, mentalis, and platysma.

☐ The orbicularis oris is involved with the deep front line myofascial meridian.

MISCELLANEOUS

1. In even more detail, the orbicularis oris has two layers, the *pars peripheralis* and the *pars marginalis,* in each of the four quadrants. Therefore the orbicularis oris actually has eight parts.

2. The orbicularis oris in humans is particularly well developed. This is necessary for the intricacies of speech.

3. Contraction of the orbicularis oris can also draw the angles (corners) of the mouth medially. This occurs because as the fibers of both sides of the orbicularis oris contract, they create a force that pulls the modiolus attachments toward each other.

4. The fibers of the orbicularis oris are reinforced by fibers of other muscles that blend into it. The levator labii superioris alaeque nasi, levator labii superioris, levator anguli oris, zygomaticus major, buccinator, depressor anguli oris, and depressor labii inferioris all blend into the orbicularis oris.

5. The contraction of the orbicularis oris causes the lips to close and protrude as in puckering the lips or whistling.

6. Six muscles attach into the modiolus: the zygomaticus major, levator anguli oris, risorius, depressor anguli oris, buccinator, and orbicularis oris.

7. The modiolus is a fibromuscular condensation approximately ¼ inch (0.5 cm) lateral to the angle of the mouth (see page 429).

13

Platysma

The name, platysma, *tells us that this muscle is broad and flat in shape.*

Derivation	☐ platysma: Gr. *broad, plate.*
Pronunciation	☐ pla-TIZ-ma

■ ATTACHMENTS

☐ **Subcutaneous Fascia of the Superior Chest**

   ☐ the pectoral and deltoid fascia

to the

☐ **Mandible and the Subcutaneous Fascia of the Lower Face**

■ FUNCTIONS

Concentric Mover Actions

1. **Draws Up the Skin of the Superior Chest and Neck, Creating Ridges of Skin of the Neck**
2. Depresses and Draws Laterally the Lower Lip
3. Depresses the Mandible at the Temporomandibular Joints

Mover Action Notes

- When both attachments of the platysma are fixed (i.e., the mandible is not allowed to move and the fascia of the chest is pulled taut and can only move just so far) and the platysma is contracted forcefully, the fibers of the platysma (attempting to move the attachments toward each other) tense, creating *ridges* of soft tissue in the skin of the neck. These ridges are usually easily visible. (The lower lip will also be seen to move). Note: Some sources describe this as *wrinkling the skin of the neck.* (action 1)
- The platysma attaches to the fascia of the lower lip. From there, its fibers run primarily inferiorly, and a bit laterally, toward the fascia of the superior chest. When the superior attachment to the fascia of the inferior face moves, the lower lip and angle (corner) of the mouth are drawn inferiorly and the angle of the mouth is drawn laterally. This creates the facial expression of horror, surprise, or disgust. (action 2)
- Given the attachment directly onto the mandible (and the attachment into the fascia overlying the mandible), and the fact that these fibers that attach into the mandible run vertically down to the chest, the platysma can pull the mandible down toward the chest, thus depressing the mandible at the temporomandibular joints (TMJs). (action 3)

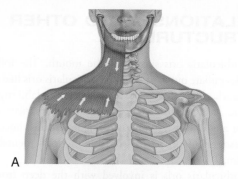

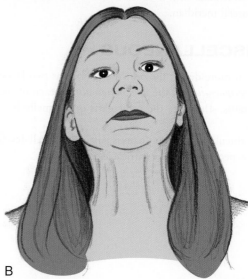

Figure 13-25 The platysma. **A,** Anterior view of the right platysma. **B,** Anterior view of the expression created by the bilateral contraction of the platysma.

INNERVATION
☐ Facial Nerve (CN VII)
   ☐ cervical branch

ARTERIAL SUPPLY
☐ The Facial Artery (a branch of the External Carotid Artery)
   ☐ and the transverse cervical artery (a branch of the thyrocervical trunk)

✋ PALPATION

1. With the client seated or supine, place palpating hand on the anterolateral neck.
2. Ask the client to forcefully contract the platysma by depressing and drawing the lower lip laterally, while keeping the mandible fixed in a position of slight depression. Observe and feel for the ridges of skin of the neck caused by the contraction of the platysma.

■ RELATIONSHIP TO OTHER STRUCTURES

☐ The platysma is superficial in the chest and neck. In the face, it is superficial to the depressor anguli oris, the depressor labii inferioris, and the risorius.

☐ The clavicle and parts of the deltoid, pectoralis major, sternocleidomastoid, infrahyoids, and suprahyoids are all deep to the platysma.

☐ The platysma is involved with the superficial front line and superficial front arm line myofascial meridians.

■ MISCELLANEOUS

1. The skeletal action of depression of the mandible at the temporomandibular joints (TMJs) by the platysma is extremely weak.

2. The platysma on one side blends with the contralateral platysma.

3. The platysma often blends with the other facial muscles in the lower face.

4. The platysma in humans is considered to be a remnant of a broader fascial muscle called the *panniculus carnosus* found in four-legged mammals. The panniculus carnosus is what enables a horse to shake off flies from its skin, and it is the same muscle that enables a cat to raise the hair on its back.

5. When the platysma contracts and the ridges or wrinkling of the skin of the neck occurs, it is reminiscent of the title character from the film *The Creature from the Black Lagoon*.

13

CHAPTER

14

Muscles of the Hip Joint

CHAPTER **OUTLINE**

CHAPTER **OVERVIEW**

The muscles addressed in this chapter are the muscles whose principal function is usually considered to be movement of the hip joint. Other muscles in the body can also move the hip joint, but they are placed in different chapters because their primary function is usually considered to be at another joint. These muscles are the hamstring group and rectus femoris of the quadriceps femoris group; they are covered in Chapter 15.

Overview of Structure

☐ Structurally, muscles of the hip joint are generally classified as being anterior, posterior, medial, or lateral. Actually, most hip joint muscles lie somewhere between, for example, anterolateral or anteromedial.

☐ The psoas major, iliacus, tensor fasciae latae, and sartorius are hip flexors and are located anteriorly (the rectus femoris of the quadriceps femoris group, also located anteriorly, is covered in Chapter 15).

☐ The adductor muscles of the hip joint are located medially.

☐ The gluteal group is located primarily laterally. The deep lateral rotator group is a group of six muscles that are deeply situated in the posterior buttock and are oriented horizontally. (The hamstring group, covered in Chapter 15, crosses the hip joint posteriorly with a vertical orientation.)

Overview of Function

The following general rules regarding actions can be stated for the functional groups of muscles of the hip joint:

☐ If a muscle crosses the hip joint anteriorly with a vertical direction to its fibers, it can flex the thigh at the hip joint by moving the anterior surface of the thigh toward the anterior surface of the pelvis. Or it can anteriorly tilt the pelvis at the hip joint by moving the anterior surface of the pelvis toward the anterior surface of the thigh.

☐ If a muscle crosses the hip joint posteriorly with a vertical direction to its fibers, it can extend the thigh at the hip joint by moving the posterior surface of the thigh toward the posterior surface of the pelvis. Or it can posteriorly tilt the pelvis at the hip joint by moving the posterior surface of the pelvis toward the posterior surface of the thigh.

☐ If a muscle crosses the hip joint laterally with a vertical direction to its fibers, it can abduct the thigh at the hip joint by moving the lateral surface of the thigh toward the lateral surface of the pelvis. Or it can depress (laterally tilt) the same-side (ipsilateral) pelvis at the hip joint by moving the lateral surface of the pelvis toward the lateral surface of the thigh.

☐ If a muscle crosses the hip joint medially, it can adduct the thigh at the hip joint by moving the medial surface of the thigh toward the medial surface of the pelvis. Or it can elevate the same-side (ipsilateral) pelvis at the hip joint by moving the medial surface of the pelvis toward the medial surface of the thigh.

☐ Medial rotators of the thigh wrap around the femur from medial to lateral, anterior to the hip joint. They can also ipsilaterally rotate the pelvis at the hip joint.

☐ Lateral rotators of the thigh wrap around the femur from medial to lateral, posterior to the hip joint. They can also contralaterally rotate the pelvis at the hip joint.

☐ Reverse actions are common at the hip joint and tend to occur when the foot is planted on the ground causing the distal attachment to be fixed and therefore the proximal attachment to be mobile and move toward the distal attachment. The reverse actions wherein the pelvis moves at the hip joint are often as important as, if not more important than, the typically thought of standard mover actions of the thigh at the hip joint.

14

Anterior Views of the Muscles of the Hip Joint—Superficial and Intermediate Views

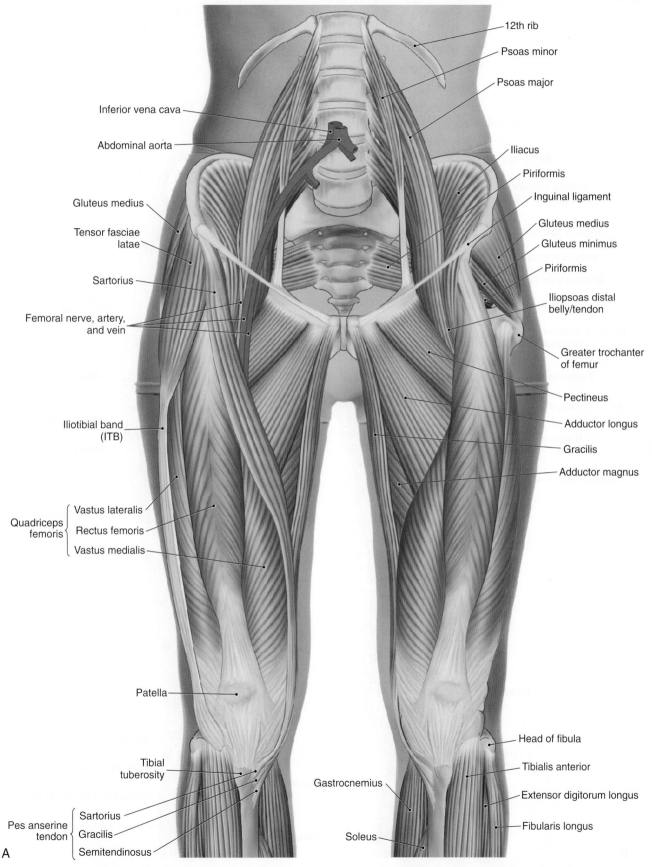

12th rib

Psoas minor

Psoas major

Inferior vena cava

Abdominal aorta

Iliacus

Piriformis

Inguinal ligament

Gluteus medius

Gluteus medius

Tensor fasciae latae

Gluteus minimus

Piriformis

Sartorius

Iliopsoas distal belly/tendon

Femoral nerve, artery, and vein

Greater trochanter of femur

Pectineus

Adductor longus

Iliotibial band (ITB)

Gracilis

Adductor magnus

Quadriceps femoris { Vastus lateralis Rectus femoris Vastus medialis

Patella

Tibial tuberosity

Head of fibula

Tibialis anterior

Gastrocnemius

Extensor digitorum longus

Pes anserine tendon { Sartorius Gracilis Semitendinosus

Soleus

Fibularis longus

A

14

Figure 14-1 Anterior views of the muscles of the hip joint. **A,** Superficial view on the right and an intermediate view on the left.

Anterior Views of the Muscles of the Hip Joint—Deep Views

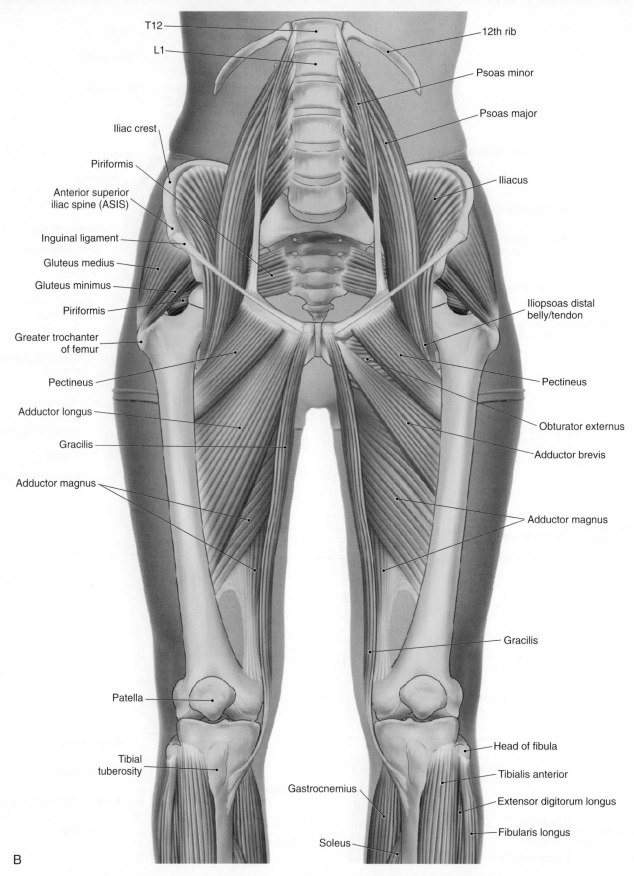

T12

L1

12th rib

Psoas minor

Psoas major

Iliac crest

Piriformis

Anterior superior
iliac spine (ASIS)

Iliacus

Inguinal ligament

Gluteus medius

Gluteus minimus

Piriformis

Iliopsoas distal
belly/tendon

Greater trochanter
of femur

Pectineus

Pectineus

Adductor longus

Gracilis

Obturator externus

Adductor brevis

Adductor magnus

Adductor magnus

Gracilis

Patella

Tibial
tuberosity

Head of fibula

Tibialis anterior

Gastrocnemius

Extensor digitorum longus

Fibularis longus

Soleus

14

B

Figure 14-1, cont'd B, Deep view on the right and deeper view on the left.

Posterior Views of the Muscles of the Hip Joint—Superficial and Intermediate Views

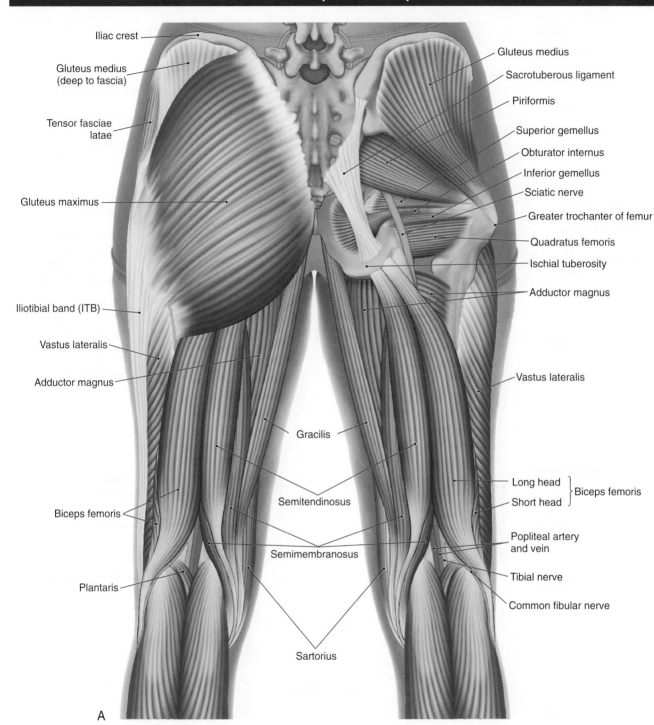

Figure 14-2 Posterior views of the muscles of the hip joint. **A,** Superficial view on the left and intermediate view on the right.

Posterior Views of the Muscles of the Hip Joint—Deep Views

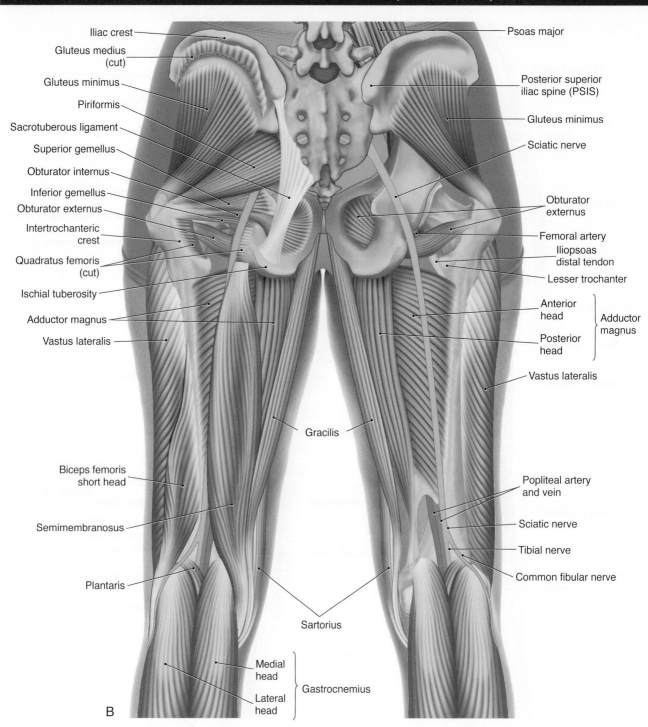

Iliac crest

Gluteus medius (cut)

Gluteus minimus

Piriformis

Sacrotuberous ligament

Superior gemellus

Obturator internus

Inferior gemellus

Obturator externus

Intertrochanteric crest

Quadratus femoris (cut)

Ischial tuberosity

Adductor magnus

Vastus lateralis

Gracilis

Biceps femoris short head

Semimembranosus

Plantaris

Sartorius

Medial head

Lateral head

Gastrocnemius

Psoas major

Posterior superior iliac spine (PSIS)

Gluteus minimus

Sciatic nerve

Obturator externus

Femoral artery

Iliopsoas distal tendon

Lesser trochanter

Anterior head

Posterior head

Adductor magnus

Vastus lateralis

Popliteal artery and vein

Sciatic nerve

Tibial nerve

Common fibular nerve

B

Figure 14-2, cont'd B, Deep view on the left and deeper view on the right.

14

Medial Views of the Muscles of the Right Hip Joint—Superficial and Deep Views

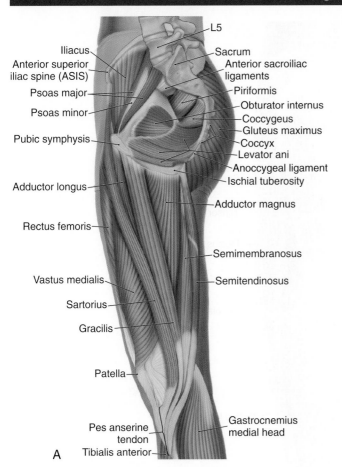

A

- L5
- Iliacus
- Anterior superior iliac spine (ASIS)
- Psoas major
- Psoas minor
- Pubic symphysis
- Sacrum
- Anterior sacroiliac ligaments
- Piriformis
- Obturator internus
- Coccygeus
- Gluteus maximus
- Coccyx
- Levator ani
- Anoccygeal ligament
- Ischial tuberosity
- Adductor longus
- Adductor magnus
- Rectus femoris
- Semimembranosus
- Vastus medialis
- Semitendinosus
- Sartorius
- Gracilis
- Patella
- Gastrocnemius medial head
- Pes anserine tendon
- Tibialis anterior

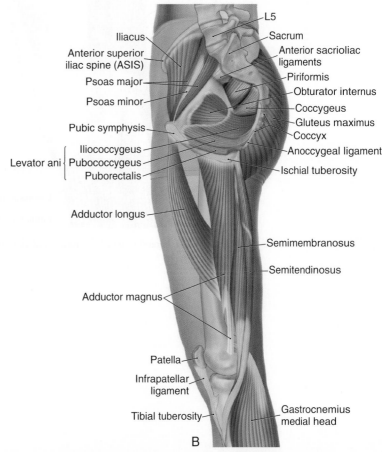

B

- L5
- Iliacus
- Anterior superior iliac spine (ASIS)
- Psoas major
- Psoas minor
- Pubic symphysis
- Levator ani { Iliococcygeus / Pubococcygeus / Puborectalis
- Sacrum
- Anterior scrioliac ligaments
- Piriformis
- Obturator internus
- Coccygeus
- Gluteus maximus
- Coccyx
- Anoccygeal ligament
- Ischial tuberosity
- Adductor longus
- Semimembranosus
- Semitendinosus
- Adductor magnus
- Patella
- Infrapatellar ligament
- Tibial tuberosity
- Gastrocnemius medial head

Figure 14-3 Medial views of the muscles of the right hip joint. **A,** Superficial. **B,** Deep.

14

Lateral View of the Muscles of the Right Hip Joint—Superficial View

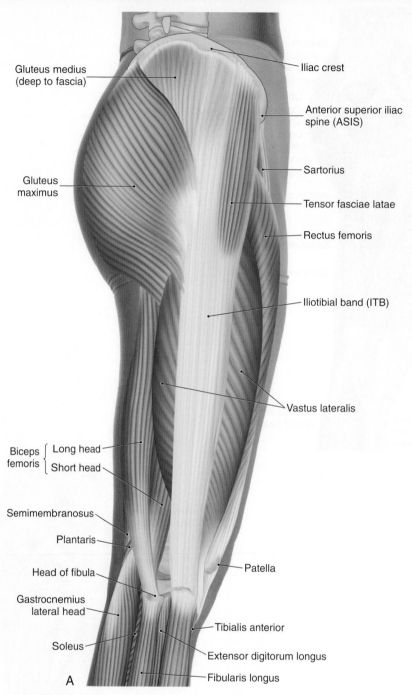

Gluteus medius
(deep to fascia)

Iliac crest

Gluteus
maximus

Anterior superior iliac
spine (ASIS)

Sartorius

Tensor fasciae latae

Rectus femoris

Iliotibial band (ITB)

Vastus lateralis

Biceps { Long head
femoris { Short head

Semimembranosus

Plantaris

Head of fibula

Gastrocnemius
lateral head

Soleus

Patella

Tibialis anterior

Extensor digitorum longus

Fibularis longus

A

Figure 14-4 Lateral views of the muscles of the right hip joint. **A,** Superficial.

14

Lateral View of the Muscles of the Right Hip Joint—Deep View

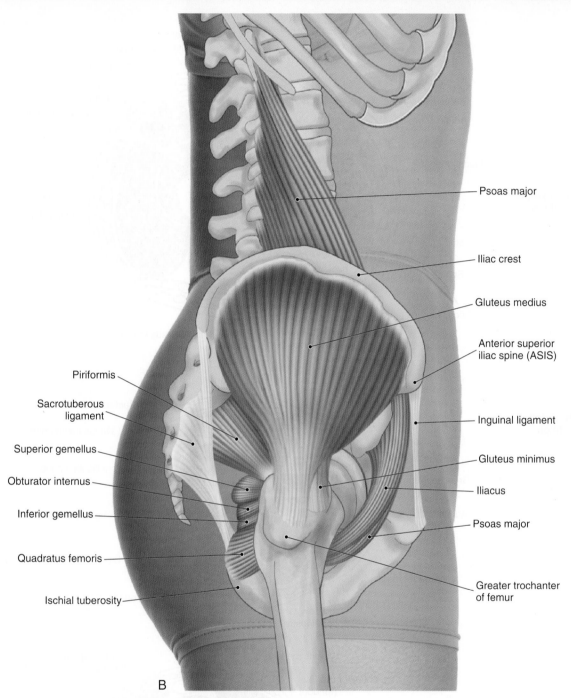

Piriformis

Sacrotuberous ligament

Superior gemellus

Obturator internus

Inferior gemellus

Quadratus femoris

Ischial tuberosity

Psoas major

Iliac crest

Gluteus medius

Anterior superior iliac spine (ASIS)

Inguinal ligament

Gluteus minimus

Iliacus

Psoas major

Greater trochanter of femur

B

Figure 14-4, cont'd B, Deep.

14

Transverse Plane Cross Sections of the Right Thigh

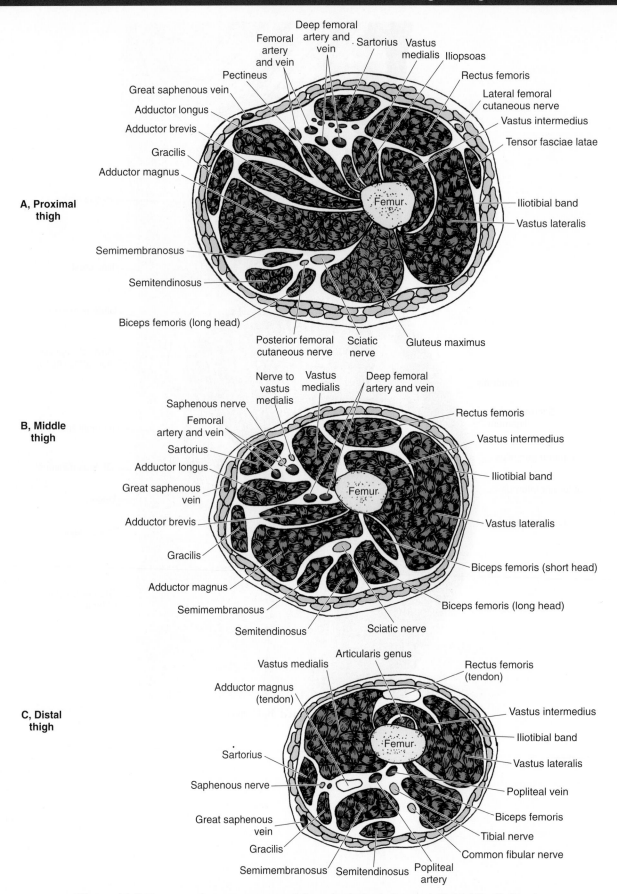

Figure 14-5 Transverse plane cross sections of the right thigh. **A,** Proximal. **B,** Middle. **C,** Distal. Perspective: Top is anterior; bottom is posterior; right is lateral; left is medial.

Psoas Major (of Iliopsoas)

The name, psoas major, *tells us that this muscle is located in the loin (low back) area and is large (larger than the psoas minor).*

Derivation	☐ psoas: Gr. *loin (low back).*
	major: L. *larger.*
Pronunciation	☐ SO-as, MAY-jor

■ ATTACHMENTS

☐ **Anterolateral Lumbar Spine**
  ☐ anterolaterally on the bodies of T12-L5 and the intervertebral discs between, and anteriorly on the TPs of L1-L5

to the

☐ **Lesser Trochanter of the Femur**

■ FUNCTIONS

CONCENTRIC (SHORTENING) MOVER ACTIONS	
Standard Mover Actions	**Reverse Mover Actions**
☐ **1. Flexes the thigh at the hip joint**	☐ **1. Flexes the trunk at the spinal joints**
☐ **2. Posteriorly tilts the pelvis at the LS joint**	☐ **2. Anteriorly tilts the pelvis at the hip joint**
☐ **3. Laterally rotates the thigh at the hip joint**	☐ 3. Contralaterally rotates the trunk and pelvis
☐ 4. Elevates the same-side pelvis at the LS joint	☐ 4. Laterally flexes the trunk at the spinal joints

LS joint = lumbosacral joint

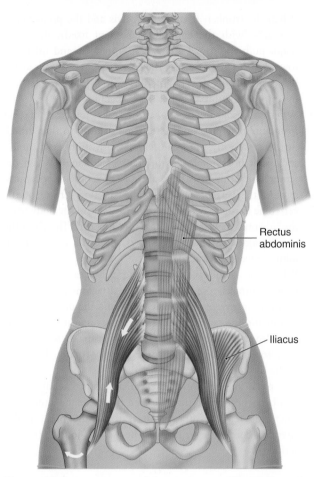

Figure 14-6 Anterior view of the psoas major. The left iliacus has been drawn in and the rectus abdominis has been ghosted in.

Labels: Rectus abdominis; Iliacus

Standard Mover Action Notes

• The psoas major crosses the hip joint anteriorly (with its fibers running vertically in the sagittal plane); therefore it flexes the thigh at the hip joint. (action 1)
• The iliopsoas is the prime mover (most powerful muscle) of flexion of the thigh (and anterior tilt of the pelvis) at the hip joint. (action 1)
• If the trunk is fixed and the psoas major pulls the thigh toward the trunk anteriorly, but the pelvis is fixed to the thigh, the psoas major pulls the thigh/pelvis as a unit toward the anterior trunk and can posteriorly tilt the pelvis at the LS joint. (action 2)
• The psoas major crosses the hip joint anteriorly in such a way that it wraps around from the vertebral column to attach onto the lesser trochanter of the femur (with its fibers running somewhat horizontally in the transverse plane). When the psoas major contracts, it pulls the lesser trochanter anterolaterally and laterally rotates the thigh at the hip joint. (action 3)
• Lateral rotation of the thigh at the hip joint is a very weak action of the psoas major. (action 3)

• The psoas major crosses the spinal joints laterally (with its fibers running vertically in the frontal plane); therefore when the spinal attachment is fixed, it pulls upward on the femoral attachment. If the femur is fixed to the pelvis, the pelvis will be elevated at the LS joint. (action 4)

Reverse Mover Action Notes

• The psoas major crosses the spinal joints anteriorly (with its fibers running vertically in the sagittal plane); therefore when the femoral attachment is fixed, the psoas major flexes the trunk at the spinal joints. (reverse action 1)
• There is controversy whether the psoas major flexes or extends the trunk at the spinal joints. Its line of pull passes anteriorly to the lower lumbar spinal joints so it certainly flexes the lower lumbar spine. However, as it ascends it may pass posteriorly to the upper spinal joints that it crosses; therefore it would extend the vertebrae at these joints. Keep in mind that the degree of lumbar lordosis would affect the line of pull of this muscle relative to the joints it crosses. (reverse action 1)

14

Psoas Major (of Iliopsoas)—*cont'd*

- When the trunk is fixed to the pelvis and the psoas major contracts (with the femoral attachment fixed), the psoas major pulls the spinal attachment anteriorly and inferiorly toward the femurs, causing the pelvis to anteriorly tilt at the hip joint. An excessively anteriorly tilted pelvis results in a hyperlordotic lumbar spine. (reverse action 2)
- When the psoas major crosses the spinal joints, it attaches from anterolaterally on the vertebral column to then attach further anteriorly onto the femur (with its fibers running somewhat horizontally in the transverse plane). When the femoral attachment is fixed and the psoas major contracts, it pulls the vertebrae, causing the anterior surface of the vertebrae to rotate toward the opposite side of the body from the side on which the psoas major is attached. Therefore the psoas major contralaterally rotates the trunk at the spinal joints. (reverse action 3)
- When the trunk is fixed to the pelvis, and the psoas major contracts, it pulls on the spinal attachment and rotates it in the transverse plane. The trunk and the pelvis move as a unit, and the pelvis rotates toward the opposite side of the body from the side on which the psoas major is attached. Therefore the psoas major contralaterally rotates the pelvis at the hip joint. (reverse action 3)
- The psoas major crosses the spinal joints laterally (with its fibers running vertically in the frontal plane); therefore when the femoral attachment is fixed, the psoas major laterally flexes the trunk at the spinal joints. (reverse action 4)

Eccentric Antagonist Functions

1. Restrains/slows thigh extension and pelvic posterior tilt at the hip joint
2. Restrains/slows thigh medial rotation and pelvic ipsilateral rotation at the hip joint
3. Restrains/slows lumbar spinal extension
4. Restrains/slows lumbar spinal lateral flexion to the opposite side
5. Restrains/slows ipsilateral rotation of the lumbar spine
6. Restrains/slows anterior tilt and depression of the same-side pelvis at the LS joint

Eccentric Antagonist Function Note

- A force of lateral rotation of the thigh at the hip joint prevents medial rotation of the entire lower extremity (thigh, leg, and talus) if the weight-bearing foot overly pronates (if the arch of the foot drops).

Isometric Stabilization Functions

1. Stabilizes the lumbar spine at the spinal joints
2. Stabilizes the pelvis at the LS and hip joints
3. Stabilizes the thigh at the hip joint

Isometric Stabilization Function Note

- Because the psoas major lies so close to the lumbar spine, its major stabilization function is at the spine.

INNERVATION
- Lumbar Plexus
  - **L1, L2,** L3

ARTERIAL SUPPLY
- The Lumbar Arteries (branches of the Aorta)
  - and the Iliolumbar Artery (a branch of the Internal Iliac Artery)

🖐 PALPATION

1. With the client supine with a pillow under the knees, place palpating hand on the abdomen between the iliac crest and the twelfth rib (lateral to the rectus abdominis, approximately halfway between the ASIS and the umbilicus).
2. Palpate slowly but deeply with even pressure directed postero-medially toward the spine.
3. Ask the client to flex the thigh at the hip joint a few degrees and feel for the contraction of the psoas major.
4. The distal belly of the psoas major is also palpable in the proximal anterior thigh between the pectineus and the sartorius. Note: Be careful with palpation in this region because the femoral nerve, artery, and vein lie over the iliopsoas and pectineus here.

■ RELATIONSHIP TO OTHER STRUCTURES

- The psoas major is deep in the abdomen and lies anteromedially to the quadratus lumborum.
- Distally, the psoas major tendon is joined by the iliacus tendon to attach onto the lesser trochanter of the femur.
- The psoas major lies deep to the inguinal ligament and directly anterior to the hip joint.
- The psoas minor lies directly anterior to the belly of the psoas major.
- The psoas major is located within the deep front line myofascial meridian.

■ MISCELLANEOUS

1. The psoas major and the iliacus muscle are sometimes considered to be the *iliopsoas* muscle because of their common distal attachment onto the lesser trochanter of the femur.
2. The proximal attachment of the psoas major on the spine arises by five separate slips of tissue.

14

Psoas Major (of Iliopsoas)—*cont'd*

3. There is a great deal of controversy regarding whether the psoas major flexes or extends the lumbar spine in the sagittal plane. To determine this, we must look at where the line of pull of the psoas major is relative to the axis of movement for each of the spinal joints that it crosses. Generally, the line of pull of the psoas major crosses anteriorly to the axis of motion of the lumbar spinal joints; therefore it pulls the vertebrae anteriorly. For this reason, the psoas major is considered to be a flexor of the lumbar spine. This is certainly true for the L5-S1 spinal joint. However, as we look further up the lumbar spine, the line of pull of the psoas major moves increasingly posterior. By the T12-L1 spinal joint, the psoas major's line of pull may actually cross posteriorly to the joint, thereby causing extension of the spine at that level (i.e., extension of T12 on L1). Another factor to consider is that if the posture of the lumbar spine changes, the line of pull of the psoas major relative to the axis of motion of the spinal joints changes. Specifically, if the lordotic curve of the lumbar spine increases, the line of pull of the psoas major will move farther posterior relative to the axis of motion for the spinal joints and the ability of the psoas major to extend the trunk at the lumbar spinal joints will increase. In this case the psoas major becomes an extensor of the lumbar spine. The danger of extension in the lumbar spine is that it increases the lordotic curve of the spine and may cause what is commonly called *swayback*.

4. There is another consideration when trying to determine the effect of the psoas major on the lumbar spine in the sagittal plane: whether or not the vertebrae superior to the vertebra that is being moved are fixed to it or not. If we accept that the psoas major crosses anteriorly to the axis of movement of whatever spinal joint it is crossing, a concentric contraction of the psoas major causes that vertebra to be pulled anteriorly; this will result in flexion of that vertebra on the vertebra that is inferior to it. Let's use the L3 vertebra as an example. When the psoas major contracts and pulls on L3, it will flex L3 on L4 at the L3-L4 spinal joint. If the vertebra directly superior to it, L2, is fixed to L3 (perhaps by deep extensor muscular contraction), L2 will move along with L3 and the lumbar spine will flex at the L3-L4 spinal joint. However, if L2 is not fixed to L3, the psoas major will pull L3 anteriorly and L2 will now be relatively posterior, thus causing L2 to be extended on L3 at the L2-L3 spinal joint. In this scenario, the psoas major is still flexing L3 at the L3-L4 spinal joint, but L2 is now extending at the L2-L3 spinal joint. Consequently the pull of the psoas major flexes the vertebra to which it is attached; however, the force of gravity on the weight of the vertebra directly superior causes it to extend. The danger of extension in the lumbar spine is that it increases the lordotic curve and may result in what is commonly called *swayback*.

5. With regard to posture, a chronically tight psoas major anteriorly tilts the pelvis at the hip joints, causing the lumbar curve to increase (*hyperlordosis,* also known as *swayback*). Straight-legged sit-ups tend to disproportionately strengthen the psoas major in comparison to the anterior abdominal wall muscles. To avoid this, it is recommended to do curl-ups, wherein the hip and knee joints are flexed and the trunk "curls" up (i.e., spinal flexion, not the pelvis anteriorly tilting at the hip joints) approximately 30 degrees. With the hip joint flexed to 90 degrees, the psoas major is slackened and will not be as readily engaged if the curl-up is restricted to approximately 30 degrees.

6. The roots of the lumbar plexus of nerves enter the psoas major muscle directly; the lumbar plexus itself is located within the belly of the psoas major, and the branches of the lumbar plexus then emerge from the psoas major muscle. Therefore a tight psoas major may entrap these nerves.

7. Tenderloin (also known as *filet mignon*) is the psoas major of a cow.

14

Iliacus (of Iliopsoas)

The name, iliacus, tells us that this muscle attaches onto the ilium.

Derivation	☐ iliacus: L. *refers to the ilium.*
Pronunciation	☐ i-lee-AK-us

■ ATTACHMENTS

☐ **Internal Ilium**
  ☐ the upper ⅔ of the iliac fossa, and the anterior inferior iliac spine (AIIS) and the sacral ala

  to the

☐ **Lesser Trochanter of the Femur**

■ FUNCTIONS

CONCENTRIC (SHORTENING) MOVER ACTIONS	
Standard Mover Actions	**Reverse Mover Actions**
☐ 1. Flexes the thigh at the hip joint	☐ 1. Anteriorly tilts the pelvis at the hip joint
☐ 2. Laterally rotates the thigh at the hip joint	☐ 2. Contralaterally rotates the pelvis at the hip joint

Standard Mover Action Notes

- The iliacus crosses the hip joint anteriorly (with its fibers running vertically in the sagittal plane); therefore it flexes the thigh at the hip joint. (action 1)
- The iliopsoas is the prime mover (most powerful muscle) of flexion of the thigh (and anterior tilt of the pelvis) at the hip joint. (action 1)
- The iliacus crosses the hip joint anteriorly in such a way that it wraps around from the internal ilium to attach onto the lesser trochanter of the femur (with its fibers running somewhat horizontally in the transverse plane). When the iliacus contracts, it pulls the lesser trochanter anterolaterally and laterally rotates the thigh at the hip joint. (action 2)
- Lateral rotation of the thigh at the hip joint is a very weak action of the iliacus. (action 2)

Reverse Mover Action Notes

- When the thigh is fixed and the iliacus contracts, it pulls the anterior surface of the pelvis toward the anterior thigh. Therefore it anteriorly tilts the pelvis at the hip joint. (reverse action 1)
- The iliacus crosses the hip joint anteriorly (with its fibers running somewhat horizontally in the transverse plane) in such a way that it wraps around from the femur to attach laterally onto the pelvis. When the femur is fixed and the iliacus contracts, it rotates the pelvis (in the transverse plane) away from the side of the body on which the iliacus is

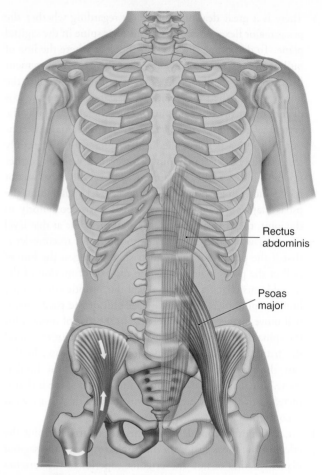

Figure 14-7 Anterior view of the iliacus. The left psoas major has been drawn in and the rectus abdominis has been ghosted in.

attached. Therefore the iliacus contralaterally rotates the pelvis at the hip joint. (reverse action 2)

Eccentric Antagonist Functions

1. Restrains/slows thigh extension and pelvic posterior tilt at the hip joint
2. Restrains/slows thigh medial rotation and pelvic ipsilateral rotation at the hip joint

Isometric Stabilization Functions

1. Stabilizes the thigh and pelvis at the hip joint

Isometric Stabilization Function Note

- A force of lateral rotation of the thigh at the hip joint prevents medial rotation of the entire lower extremity (thigh, leg, and talus) if the weight-bearing foot overly pronates (if the arch of the foot drops).

14

Iliacus (of Iliopsoas)—*cont'd*

Additional Note on Functions

1. Some sources state that the iliacus can abduct the thigh at the hip joint. If this is true, it would have to be the outermost (most lateral) fibers that have this ability because their line of pull may fall just lateral to the mechanical axis of the hip joint.

INNERVATION
- ☐ The Femoral Nerve
  - ☐ **L2,** L3

ARTERIAL SUPPLY
- ☐ The Iliolumbar Artery (a branch of the Internal Iliac Artery)
  - ☐ and the Obturator Artery (a branch of the Internal Iliac Artery)

 ### PALPATION

1. With the client supine with the thighs slightly passively flexed and laterally rotated at the hip joints (this can be accomplished by placing a small pillow under the client's knees), place palpating fingers on the anterior iliac crest and palpate into the iliac fossa by curling your fingertips around the iliac crest.
2. Have the client flex the thigh at the hip joint and feel for the contraction of the iliacus.
3. The distal belly of the iliacus is also somewhat palpable in the proximal anterior thigh between the pectineus and the sartorius. Note: Be careful with palpation in the anterior thigh region, because the femoral nerve, artery, and vein lie over the iliopsoas and pectineus here.

■ RELATIONSHIP TO OTHER STRUCTURES

- ☐ Distally the iliacus tendon joins the psoas major tendon to attach onto the lesser trochanter of the femur.
- ☐ The iliacus lies deep to the inguinal ligament and directly anterior to the hip joint.
- ☐ Distal to the inguinal ligament, the fibers of the distal belly of the iliacus lie lateral to the fibers of the distal psoas major.
- ☐ The iliacus is located within the deep front line myofascial meridian.

■ MISCELLANEOUS

1. The iliacus and the psoas major muscle are sometimes considered to be the *iliopsoas* muscle because of their common distal attachment onto the lesser trochanter of the femur.
2. The majority of the fibers of the distal iliacus actually attach into the psoas major's tendon (deep on the posterior side) to then attach onto the lesser trochanter.
3. With regard to posture, a chronically tight iliacus anteriorly tilts the pelvis, causing the lumbar curve to increase (*hyperlordosis*, also known as *swayback*). Straight-legged sit-ups tend to disproportionately strengthen the iliacus in comparison to the anterior abdominal wall muscles. To avoid this, it is recommended to do curl-ups, wherein the hip and knee joints are flexed and the trunk "curls" up (i.e., spinal flexion, not the pelvis anteriorly tilting at the hip joints) approximately 30 degrees. With the hip joint flexed to 90 degrees, the iliacus is slackened and will not be as readily engaged if the curl-up is restricted to approximately 30 degrees.

14

Tensor Fasciae Latae (TFL)

The name, tensor fasciae latae, *tells us that this muscle tenses the fascia lata. The fascia lata is the broad covering of fascia that envelops the musculature of the thigh.*

Derivation	☐ tensor: L. *stretcher.*
	fasciae: L. *band/bandage.*
	latae: L. *broad, refers to the side.*
Pronunciation	☐ TEN-sor, FASH-ee-a, LA-tee

■ ATTACHMENTS

☐ **Anterior Superior Iliac Spine (ASIS)**
  ☐ and the anterior iliac crest

to the

☐ **Iliotibial Band (ITB)**
  ☐ ⅓ of the way down the thigh

■ FUNCTIONS

CONCENTRIC (SHORTENING) MOVER ACTIONS	
Standard Mover Actions	**Reverse Mover Actions**
☐ 1. Flexes the thigh at the hip joint	☐ 1. Anteriorly tilts the pelvis at the hip joint
☐ 2. Abducts the thigh at the hip joint	☐ 2. Depresses the same-side pelvis at the hip joint
☐ 3. Medially rotates the thigh at the hip joint	☐ 3. Ipsilaterally rotates the pelvis at the hip joint
☐ 4. Extends the leg at the knee joint	☐ 4. Extends the thigh at the knee joint

Standard Mover Action Notes

- The TFL crosses the hip joint anteriorly (with its fibers running vertically in the sagittal plane); therefore it flexes the thigh at the hip joint. (action 1)
- The TFL crosses the hip joint laterally (with its fibers running vertically in the frontal plane); therefore it abducts the thigh at the hip joint. (action 2)
- The TFL crosses the hip joint laterally in such a way that it wraps from anteriorly on the pelvis to posteriorly into the ITB (with its fibers running somewhat horizontally in the transverse plane). When the TFL pulls on the iliotibial band, it pulls this lateral attachment antero-medially, causing the anterior thigh to face medially. There-fore the TFL medially rotates the thigh at the hip joint. (action 3)
- Because of its pull via the ITB (which attaches to the pro-ximal anterolateral tibia), the TFL crosses the knee joint anteriorly (with a vertical orientation to its pull in the sagit-tal plane); therefore it extends the leg at the knee joint. (action 4)

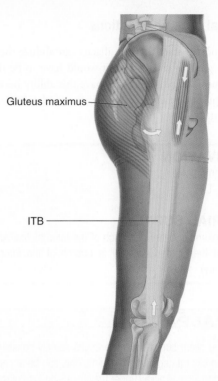

Figure 14-8 Lateral view of the right tensor fasciae latae (TFL). The glutueus maximus has been ghosted in. *ITB,* Iliotibial band.

Reverse Mover Action Notes

- If the TFL contracts and the femur is fixed, it pulls the anterior pelvis toward the anterior thigh. Therefore the TFL anteriorly tilts the pelvis at the hip joint. (reverse action 1)
- If the TFL contracts and the femur is fixed, it pulls the lateral pelvis toward the lateral thigh. Therefore the TFL depresses (laterally tilts) the same-side pelvis at the hip joint. Note: Depressing one side of the pelvis causes the other side to elevate. (reverse action 2)
- The TFL crosses the hip joint in such a way that it wraps from medially on the pelvis to laterally into the ITB (with its fibers running somewhat horizontally in the transverse plane). When the iliotibial band attachment is fixed and the TFL contracts, it pulls on the pelvis, causing the anterior pelvis to face toward the same side of the body on which the TFL is attached. Therefore the TFL ipsilaterally rotates the pelvis at the hip joint. (reverse action 3)
- If the leg is fixed, the TFL can extend the thigh at the knee joint via its ITB attachment which crosses the knee joint anteriorly (with a vertical orientation to its fibers in the sagittal plane). (reverse action 4)

Eccentric Antagonist Functions

1. Restrains/slows thigh extension and pelvic posterior tilt at the hip joint

14

Tensor Fasciae Latae (TFL)—*cont'd*

2. Restrains/slows thigh adduction and same-side pelvic elevation at the hip joint
3. Restrains/slows thigh lateral rotation and pelvic contralateral rotation at the hip joint
4. Restrains/slows knee joint flexion

Isometric Stabilization Functions

1. Stabilizes the thigh and pelvis at the hip joint
2. Stabilizes the knee joint

Isometric Stabilization Function Notes

- Same-side pelvic depression force on the support limb side prevents depression of pelvis to the opposite side (swing limb side) when walking. This is the most important function of the TFL.
- Given that both the TFL and the gluteus maximus attach into the ITB and the ITB crosses the knee joint anteriorly, both of these muscles in effect cross the knee joint anteriorly and therefore, theoretically, can extend the leg at the knee joint. However, there is controversy over their ability to actually do this. Certainly, extension of the leg at the knee joint is not one of their major actions. It is likely that the role of these two muscles and the ITB crossing the knee is primarily to help stabilize the knee joint.

Additional Notes on Functions

- The anteromedial fibers of the TFL are more active with flexion and abduction of the thigh at the hip joint and anterior tilt and depression of the pelvis at the hip joint.
- The posterolateral fibers of the TFL are more active with medial rotation of the thigh at the hip joint and ipsilateral rotation of the pelvis at the hip joint.

INNERVATION
- ☐ The Superior Gluteal Nerve
  - ☐ **L4, L5,** S1

ARTERIAL SUPPLY
- ☐ The Superior Gluteal Artery (a branch of the Internal Iliac Artery)
  - ☐ and the Deep Femoral Artery (a major branch of the Femoral Artery)

✋ PALPATION

1. With the client supine, place palpating fingers just distal and slightly lateral to the anterior superior iliac spine (ASIS).
2. Have the client actively hold the thigh in a position of flexion and medial rotation at the hip joint and palpate for the engagement of the TFL. Resistance can be added.
3. Continue palpating the TFL distally and slightly posteriorly toward the ITB attachment.

■ RELATIONSHIP TO OTHER STRUCTURES

- ☐ The TFL is posterior to the sartorius.
- ☐ The TFL is superficial to the anterior fibers of the gluteus medius and anterior to the middle fibers of the gluteus medius.
- ☐ The TFL is superficial to the vastus lateralis. At its proximal attachment, the TFL is superficial to the proximal attachment of the rectus femoris.
- ☐ The TFL is located within the lateral line and spiral line myofascial meridians.

■ MISCELLANEOUS

1. There are two muscles that attach into the ITB: the TFL and the gluteus maximus. Given that the TFL attaches into the ITB from one direction and the gluteus maximus attaches into the ITB from the opposite direction, they have opposite actions of rotation.
2. A chronically tight TFL can create the postural conditions of a *functional* short lower extremity (usually called a *short leg*) and a compensatory scoliosis. When the TFL is tight, it pulls on and depresses (laterally tilts) the pelvis toward the thigh on that side. This results in a *functional short leg* (as opposed to a *structural short leg*, wherein the femur and/or the tibia on one side is actually shorter than on the other side). Further, depressing the pelvis on one side creates an unlevel sacrum for the spine to sit on, and a compensatory scoliosis must occur to return the head to a level position. (Note: The head must be level for proper proprioceptive balance in the inner ear and for the eyes to be level for visual proprioception.)
3. The ITB is a thickening of the fascia lata in the lateral thigh.
4. If the TFL is tight, it can increase tension in the ITB, thereby increasing the likelihood of *ITB friction syndrome* at the greater trochanter or lateral condyle of the femur.

14

Sartorius

The name, sartorius, *tells us that this muscle performs the four actions necessary to create a cross-legged position that a "sartor" (Latin for tailor) sits in to do his or her work. These actions are flexion, abduction, and lateral rotation of the thigh at the hip joint and flexion of the leg at the knee joint.*

Derivation	☐ sartorius: L. *tailor.*
Pronunciation	☐ sar-TOR-ee-us

■ ATTACHMENTS

☐ **Anterior Superior Iliac Spine (ASIS)**

to the

☐ **Pes Anserine Tendon (at the Proximal Anteromedial Tibia)**

■ FUNCTIONS

CONCENTRIC (SHORTENING) MOVER ACTIONS	
Standard Mover Actions	**Reverse Mover Actions**
☐ **1. Flexes the thigh at the hip joint**	☐ **1. Anteriorly tilts the pelvis at the hip joint**
☐ **2. Abducts the thigh at the hip joint**	☐ 2. Depresses the same-side pelvis at the hip joint
☐ **3. Laterally rotates the thigh at the hip joint**	☐ 3. Contralaterally rotates the pelvis at the hip joint
☐ **4. Flexes the leg at the knee joint**	☐ 4. Flexes the thigh at the knee joint
☐ 5. Medially rotates the leg at the knee joint	☐ 5. Laterally rotates the thigh at the knee joint

Standard Mover Action Notes

- The sartorius crosses the hip joint anteriorly (with its fibers running vertically in the sagittal plane); therefore it flexes the thigh at the hip joint. (action 1)
- The sartorius crosses the hip joint laterally (with its fibers running vertically in the frontal plane); therefore it abducts the thigh at the hip joint. (action 2)
- The sartorius crosses the hip joint medially in such a way that it wraps from anteriorly on the pelvis to posteriorly on the leg (with its fibers running somewhat horizontally in the transverse plane). When the leg is fixed to the thigh and the sartorius pulls the leg, it rotates the thigh anterolaterally, causing the anterior thigh to face laterally. Therefore the sartorius laterally rotates the thigh at the hip joint. (action 3)
- The sartorius crosses the knee joint posteriorly (with its fibers running vertically in the sagittal plane); therefore it flexes the leg at the knee joint. (action 4)
- The sartorius crosses the knee joint medially from posterior to anterior (with its fibers running somewhat horizontally

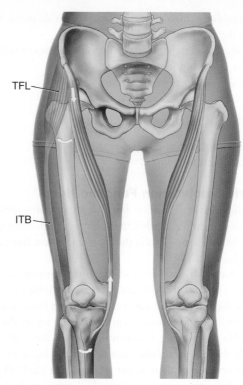

Figure 14-9 Anterior view of the sartorius. The tensor fasciae latae (TFL) and iliotibial band (ITB) have been ghosted in.

in the transverse plane) to attach into the pes anserine tendon at the medial tibia. When the sartorius pulls at the tibial attachment, the tibial attachment rotates posteromedially, causing the anterior tibia to face somewhat medially. Therefore the sartorius medially rotates the leg at the knee joint. (action 5)

Reverse Mover Action Notes

- With the distal attachment fixed, the sartorius, by pulling inferiorly on the anterior pelvis, anteriorly tilts the pelvis at the hip joint. (reverse action 1)
- With the distal attachment fixed, the sartorius, by pulling inferiorly on the lateral pelvis, depresses (laterally tilts) the pelvis on that side at the hip joint. Note: Depression of one side of the pelvis causes the other side to elevate. (reverse action 2)
- The sartorius crosses the hip joint in such a way that it wraps from laterally on the pelvis to medially onto the tibia (with its fibers running somewhat horizontally in the transverse plane). When the tibial attachment is fixed and the sartorius contracts, it pulls on the pelvis, causing the anterior pelvis to face the opposite side of the body from the side on which the sartorius is attached. Therefore the sartorius contralaterally rotates the pelvis at the hip joint. (reverse action 3)

Sartorius—*cont'd*

- The sartorius crosses the knee joint posteriorly (with its fibers running vertically in the sagittal plane). If the distal attachment is fixed, it flexes the thigh at the knee joint. (reverse action 4)
- Any muscle that medially rotates the leg at the knee joint can laterally rotate the thigh at the knee joint if the distal (leg) attachment is fixed. (reverse action 5)

Eccentric Antagonist Functions

1. Restrains/slows extension, adduction, and medial roation of the thigh at the hip joint
2. Restrains/slows posterior tilt, same-side elevation, and ipsilateral rotation of the pelvis at the hip joint
4. Restrains/slows knee joint extension
5. Restrains/slows lateral rotation of the leg and medial rotation of the thigh at the knee joint

Isometric Stabilization Functions

1. Stabilizes the thigh and pelvis at the hip joint
2. Stabilizes the knee joint

Isometric Stabilization Function Notes

- Same-side pelvic depression force on the support limb side prevents depression of the pelvis to the opposite side (swing limb side) when walking
- The distal tendon of the sartorius (along with the gracilis and semitendinosus muscles—the three pes anserine muscles) helps stabilize the medial knee joint against lateral to medial (valgus) forces that would buckle the knee joint medially.

Additional Note on Functions

1. All three pes anserine muscles (sartorius, gracilis, and semitendinosus) flex and medially rotate the leg at the knee joint.

INNERVATION
- ☐ The Femoral Nerve
  - ☐ L2, L3

ARTERIAL SUPPLY
- ☐ The Femoral Artery (the continuation of the External Iliac Artery)

🖐 PALPATION

1. With the client supine, place palpating fingers just distal and slightly medial to the anterior superior iliac spine (ASIS).
2. Have the client actively hold the thigh in a position of flexion and lateral rotation at the hip joint and palpate for the engagement of the sartorius. Resistance can be added.
3. Continue palpating the sartorius distally toward the pes anserine attachment.

■ RELATIONSHIP TO OTHER STRUCTURES

- ☐ The sartorius is superficial for its entire length.
- ☐ Proximally, the sartorius is located between the tensor fasciae latae (which is lateral to it) and the iliopsoas (which is medial to it).
- ☐ Deep to the sartorius are the rectus femoris, the vastus medialis, and the adductor longus.
- ☐ Of the three muscles that attach into the pes anserine tendon (sartorius, gracilis, semitendinosus), the sartorius' attachment is the most anterior and proximal.
- ☐ The sartorius is located within the superficial front line and ipsilateral functional line myofascial meridians.

■ MISCELLANEOUS

1. The sartorius is one of three muscles that attach into the pes anserine tendon. The other two muscles that attach here are the gracilis and the semitendinosus. *Pes anserine* means goose foot.
2. Think **SGS:** Of the muscles that attach into the pes anserine, the *sartorius* attaches the most anterior and proximal of the three, the *gracilis* is in the middle, and the *semitendinosus* attaches the most posterior and distal.
3. The sartorius is the longest muscle in the human body.
4. The medial border of the sartorius is the lateral border of the *femoral triangle* of the thigh. The femoral triangle is located between the medial borders of the sartorius and adductor longus and contains the femoral nerve, artery, and vein.
5. The lateral femoral cutaneous nerve sometimes pierces the sartorius. This can lead to entrapment of this nerve, causing *meralgia paresthetica*.

14

These muscles are grouped together, because they all adduct the thigh at the hip joint. There are five adductor muscles of the thigh: the pectineus, gracilis, adductor brevis, adductor longus, and adductor magnus.

ATTACHMENTS

Anatomically, the adductor muscle group of the thigh makes up the majority of the musculature of the medial thigh. Their relative anatomic relationships are as follows:

- Superficially, from the anterior perspective, from lateral to medial, one will see the pectineus, then the adductor longus, then the gracilis. The adductor brevis is deep to the adductor longus. The adductor magnus is the deepest (most posterior) of the entire group.
  - All three *adductor* muscles attach onto the linea aspera of the femur.
- The muscles of the adductor group are located within and/or involved with the deep front line, front functional line, and spiral line myofascial meridians.

FUNCTIONS

- The adductors all cross the hip joint medially, with their fibers running from proximal and medial on the pelvic bone to distal and lateral on the lower extremity. Therefore they all adduct the thigh at the hip joint.
- Their reverse action is to elevate the same-side (ipsilateral) pelvis at the hip joint. This will also depress the opposite-side (contralateral) pelvis at the hip joint.
- Four of the five adductors can also flex the thigh at the hip joint because they are anterior to the hip joint. The adductor magnus extends the thigh at the hip joint because it is posterior to the hip joint.
- Beyond 60 degrees of flexion of the thigh at the hip joint, the adductors' line of pull relative to the hip joint is posterior and they can all do extension of the thigh at the hip joint.
- There is some controversy about the role of all three *adductors* (adductor longus, adductor brevis, and adductor magnus) regarding rotation of the thigh at the hip joint. Some sources state that these three adductor muscles medi-

ally rotate the thigh at the hip joint; other sources state that they laterally rotate the thigh at the hip joint. Much of the confusion arises because of the difference between the shaft of the femur and the mechanical axis of the femur. Usually the mechanical axis of a long bone runs through its shaft. However, because of the change in angulation between the neck and the shaft of the femur and the natural curved shape of the femoral shaft (convex anteriorly), the mechanical axis of the femur lies posterior to its shaft. (The mechanical axis can be determined by drawing a line from the center of the femoral head to the midpoint between the femoral condyles.) When one first looks at the attachment of these three adductors onto the linea aspera of the femur, it seems that their attachment site is posterior to the axis of the femur and therefore they should laterally rotate the femur. However, considering that the mechanical axis is posterior to the shaft of the femur, the attachment of the adductors onto the linea aspera is actually anterior to the mechanical axis of the femur. For this reason the weight of the evidence favors the adductors' role as medial rotators of the thigh at the hip joint.

MISCELLANEOUS

- When the adductor muscles are strained and pain is felt at their proximal attachment, it is usually called a *groin pull* in lay terms.
- The gracilis muscle is also known as the *adductor gracilis*.

INNERVATION

☐ The adductors are innervated by the obturator nerve, except the pectineus, which is innervated by the femoral nerve. (The adductor magnus is innervated by the obturator nerve and the sciatic nerve.)

ARTERIAL SUPPLY

☐ The adductors receive the majority of their blood supply from the deep femoral artery.

Anterior Views of the Adductors of the Thigh—Superficial and Deep Views

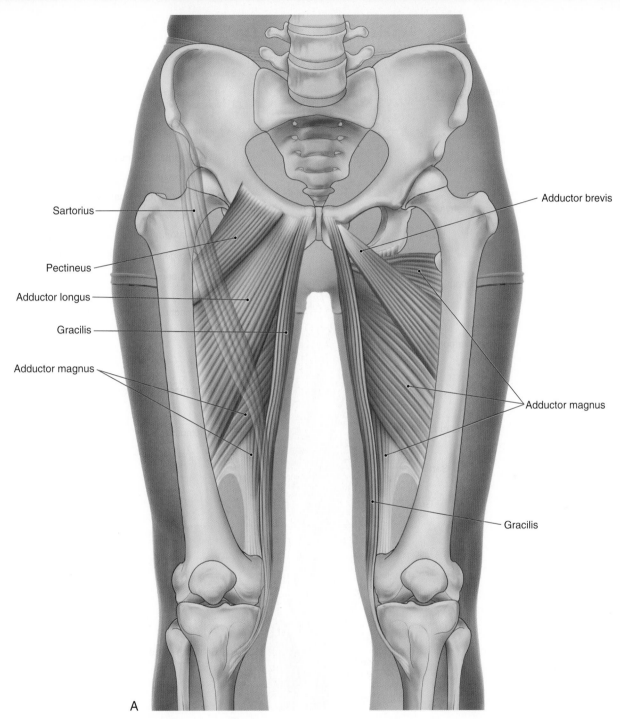

Sartorius

Pectineus

Adductor longus

Gracilis

Adductor magnus

Adductor brevis

Adductor magnus

Gracilis

A

Figure 14-10 Views of the adductor group. **A,** Anterior views. Superficial view on the right (the sartorius has been ghosted in) and deep view on the left.

14

Medial View of the Adductors of the Thigh

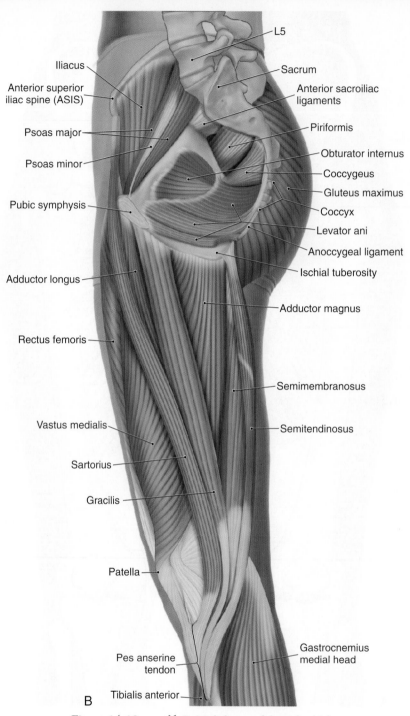

Figure 14-10, cont'd B, Medial view of the right thigh.

Posterior View of the Adductors of the Thigh

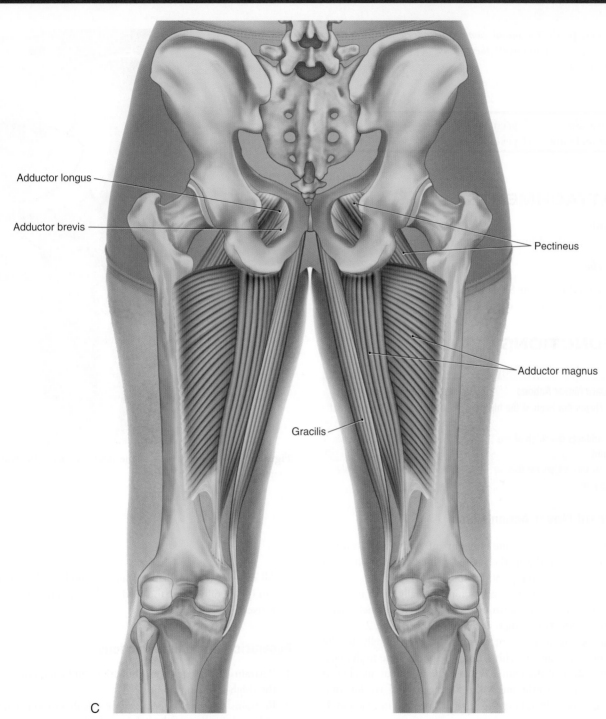

Adductor longus

Adductor brevis

Pectineus

Adductor magnus

Gracilis

C

Figure 14-10, cont'd C, Posterior view.

Pectineus (of Adductor Group)

The name, pectineus, *means comb. This muscle has a comblike appearance because its muscle fibers form a flat surface as they leave the pubic bone.*

Derivation	☐ pectineus: L. *comb.*
Pronunciation	☐ pek-TIN-ee-us

■ ATTACHMENTS

☐ **Pubis**
   ☐ the pectineal line on the superior pubic ramus

   to the

☐ **Proximal Posterior Shaft of the Femur**
   ☐ the pectineal line of the femur

■ FUNCTIONS

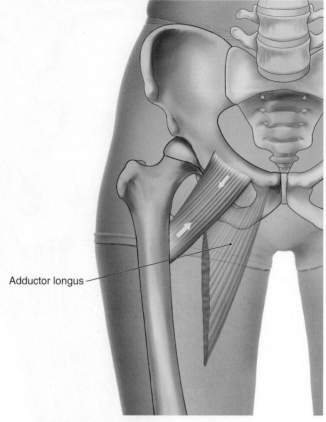

Figure 14-11 Anterior view of the right pectineus. The adductor longus has been cut and ghosted in.

Adductor longus

CONCENTRIC (SHORTENING) MOVER ACTIONS	
Standard Mover Actions	**Reverse Mover Actions**
☐ **1. Flexes the thigh at the hip joint**	☐ **1. Anteriorly tilts the pelvis at the hip joint**
☐ **2. Adducts the thigh at the hip joint**	☐ 2. Elevates the same-side pelvis at the hip joint
☐ 3. Medially rotates the thigh at the hip joint	☐ 3. Ipsilaterally rotates the pelvis at the hip joint

Standard Mover Action Notes

- The pectineus crosses the hip joint anteriorly (with its fibers running vertically in the sagittal plane); therefore it flexes the thigh at the hip joint. (action 1)
- The pectineus crosses the hip joint medially (with its fibers running somewhat horizontally in the frontal plane); therefore it adducts the thigh at the hip joint. (action 2)
- The pectineus is oriented somewhat horizontally in the transverse plane, attaching from the pubic bone to the posterior shaft of the femur. Because the pectineus attaches to the posterior femur anterior to the mechanical axis for rotation, it medially rotates the thigh at the hip joint. (action 3)

Reverse Mover Action Notes

- With the distal femoral attachment fixed, the pectineus, by pulling inferiorly on the anterior pelvis, anteriorly tilts the pelvis at the hip joint. (reverse action 1)
- With the distal femoral attachment fixed, the pectineus pulls the medial aspect of the pelvic bone inferiorly toward the medial thigh, resulting in elevation of the same-side pelvis at the hip joint. Note: Elevation of one side of the pelvis causes the other side to depress. (reverse action 2)

- All muscles that medially rotate the thigh at the hip joint can ipsilaterally rotate the pelvis at the hip joint (if the thigh is fixed). (reverse action 3)

Eccentric Antagonist Functions

1. Restrains/slows extension, abduction, and lateral rotation of the thigh at the hip joint
2. Restrains/slows posterior tilt, same-side depression, and contralateral rotation of the pelvis at the hip joint

Isometric Stabilization Functions

1. Stabilizes the thigh and pelvis at the hip joint

Additional Note on Functions

1. All five members of the adductors of the thigh group can, as their name implies, adduct the thigh (and elevate the same-side pelvis) at the hip joint.

14

Pectineus (of Adductor Group)—*cont'd*

INNERVATION

☐ The Femoral Nerve
   ☐ **L2**, L3

ARTERIAL SUPPLY

☐ The Femoral Artery (the continuation of the External Iliac Artery) and the Deep Femoral Artery (a major branch of the Femoral Artery)
   ☐ and the Obturator Artery (a branch of the Internal Iliac Artery)

✋ PALPATION

1. With the client supine, first locate the adductor longus tendon at the pubic bone (it is the most prominent tendon in the groin region).
2. Once located, drop laterally off the adductor longus and you are on the pectineus.
3. To bring out the pectineus, ask the client to adduct and/or flex the thigh at the hip joint against resistance. Keep in mind that these actions will cause all the thigh adductors to contract. (Note: Be careful with palpation in the proximal anterior thigh, because the femoral nerve, artery, and vein lie over the iliopsoas and pectineus here.)
4. The pectineus can be challenging to palpate because it sits a bit deeper than the adjacent adductor longus and iliopsoas.

■ RELATIONSHIP TO OTHER STRUCTURES

☐ In the proximal anteromedial thigh, part of the pectineus is superficial and lies medial to the iliopsoas and lateral to the adductor longus.
☐ The lateral part of the pectineus lies deep to the iliopsoas.
☐ From the anterior perspective, the obturator externus and the quadratus femoris are directly deep to the pectineus.
☐ The femoral nerve, artery, and vein lie over the lateral aspect of the pectineus.
☐ The pectineus is located within the deep front line myofascial meridian.

■ MISCELLANEOUS

1. Although some sources do not include it, the pectineus belongs in the adductor group of muscles (adductor longus, brevis, magnus, and gracilis). Note the similarity of the direction of fibers of the pectineus to the direction of fibers of the adductor longus.
2. The pectineus is a transitional muscle between the flexor muscles of the thigh and the adductor group of the thigh.
3. Do not confuse the pectineal line of the pubis (which is along the superior pubic ramus and is also known as the *pecten of the pubis*) with the pectineal line of the femur (which runs on the posterior femur between the lesser trochanter and the linea aspera of the femur).

14

Adductor Longus (of Adductor Group)

The name, adductor longus, *tells us that this muscle is an adductor and is long (longer than the adductor brevis).*

Derivation	☐ adductor: L. *a muscle that adducts a body part.*
	longus: L. *longer.*
Pronunciation	☐ ad-DUK-tor, LONG-us

■ ATTACHMENTS

☐ **Pubis**
  ☐ the anterior body

to the

☐ **Linea Aspera of the Femur**
  ☐ the middle ⅓ at the medial lip

■ FUNCTIONS

CONCENTRIC (SHORTENING) MOVER ACTIONS	
Standard Mover Actions	**Reverse Mover Actions**
☐ **1. Adducts the thigh at the hip joint**	☐ 1. Elevates the same-side pelvis at the hip joint
☐ **2. Flexes the thigh at the hip joint**	☐ **2. Anteriorly tilts the pelvis at the hip joint**
☐ 3. Medially rotates the thigh at the hip joint	☐ 3. Ipsilaterally rotates the pelvis at the hip joint

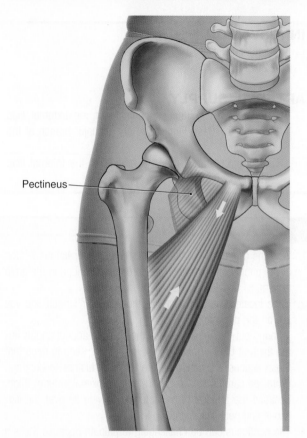

Pectineus

Figure 14-12 Anterior view of the right adductor longus. The pectineus has been cut and ghosted in.

Standard Mover Action Notes

- The adductor longus crosses the hip joint medially (with its fibers running somewhat horizontally in the frontal plane); therefore it adducts the thigh at the hip joint. (action 1)
- The adductor longus crosses the hip joint anteriorly (with its fibers running vertically in the sagittal plane); therefore it flexes the thigh at the hip joint. (action 2)
- Although the major sagittal plane action of the adductor longus is flexion of the thigh at the hip joint, if the thigh is flexed far enough in front of the body, the adductor longus' line of pull is now posterior to the sagittal plane axis of motion of the hip joint and it is now able to extend the thigh at the hip joint. This is important during the gait cycle to begin extension of the lower extremity that is flexed and in front of the body. (action 2)
- The adductor longus is oriented somewhat horizontally in the transverse plane, attaching from the pubic bone to the posterior shaft of the femur. Because the adductor longus attaches to the posterior femur anterior to the mechanical axis for rotation, it medially rotates the thigh at the hip joint. (action 3)

Reverse Mover Action Notes

- With the distal femoral attachment fixed, the adductor longus pulls the medial aspect of the pelvic bone inferiorly toward the medial thigh, resulting in elevation of the same-side pelvis at the hip joint. Note: Elevation of one side of the pelvis causes the other side to depress. (reverse action 1)
- With the distal femoral attachment fixed, the adductor longus, by pulling inferiorly on the anterior pelvis, anteriorly tilts the pelvis at the hip joint. (reverse action 2)
- All muscles that medially rotate the thigh at the hip joint can ipsilaterally rotate the pelvis at the hip joint (if the thigh is fixed). (reverse action 3)

Eccentric Antagonist Functions

1. Restrains/slows abduction, extension, and lateral rotation of the thigh at the hip joint
2. Restrains/slows same-side depression, posterior tilt, and contralateral rotation of the pelvis at the hip joint

14

Adductor Longus (of Adductor Group)—*cont'd*

Isometric Stabilization Functions

1. Stabilizes the thigh and pelvis at the hip joint

Additional Note on Functions

1. All five members of the adductors of the thigh group can, as their name implies, adduct the thigh (and elevate the same-side pelvis) at the hip joint.

INNERVATION
- The Obturator Nerve
  - **L2, L3,** L4

ARTERIAL SUPPLY
- The Femoral Artery (the continuation of the External Iliac Artery) and the Deep Femoral Artery (a major branch of the Femoral Artery)
  - and the Obturator Artery (a branch of the Internal Iliac Artery)

PALPATION

1. With the client supine, place palpating hand on the proximal anteromedial thigh, very close to the pubic bone.
2. Ask the client to actively adduct the thigh at the hip joint and feel for the proximal tendon of the adductor longus. It will be the most prominent tendon in the proximal anteromedial thigh.
3. Once located, try to follow the adductor longus distally as far as possible. At a certain point, the adductor longus will be posterior (deep) to the sartorius.

■ RELATIONSHIP TO OTHER STRUCTURES

- Much of the adductor longus is superficial in the proximal anteromedial thigh.
- The adductor longus is medial to the pectineus and lateral to the gracilis.
- From the anterior perspective, the adductor brevis is directly deep to the adductor longus. (The adductor magnus is directly deep to the adductor brevis.)
- All three *adductors* attach distally onto the linea aspera. The attachment of the adductor longus on the linea aspera is the most medial of the three adductor muscles.
- The vastus medialis attaches onto the medial lip of the linea aspera, medial to the adductor longus.
- The adductor longus is located within the deep front line and front functional line myofascial meridians.

■ MISCELLANEOUS

1. The adductor longus has the most prominent proximal tendon in the groin region, which can serve as a useful landmark for locating the pectineus, gracilis, and adductor magnus.
2. The attachment of the adductor longus at the linea aspera often blends with the attachment of the vastus medialis.
3. The medial border of the adductor longus is the medial border of the femoral triangle of the thigh. The femoral triangle is located between the medial borders of the sartorius and adductor longus and contains the femoral nerve, artery, and vein.

14

Gracilis (of Adductor Group)

The name, gracilis, *tells us that the shape of this muscle is slender and graceful.*

Derivation	☐ gracilis: L. *slender, graceful.*
Pronunciation	☐ gra-SIL-is

■ ATTACHMENTS

☐ **Pubis**

   ☐ the anterior body and the inferior ramus

to the

☐ **Pes Anserine Tendon (at the Proximal Anteromedial Tibia)**

■ FUNCTIONS

CONCENTRIC (SHORTENING) MOVER ACTIONS	
Standard Mover Actions	**Reverse Mover Actions**
☐ **1. Adducts the thigh at the hip joint**	☐ 1. Elevates the same-side pelvis at the hip joint
☐ **2. Flexes the thigh at the hip joint**	☐ **2. Anteriorly tilts the pelvis at the hip joint**
☐ **3. Flexes the leg at the knee joint**	☐ 3. Flexes the thigh at the knee joint
☐ 4. Medially rotates the leg at the knee joint	☐ 4. Laterally rotates the thigh at the knee joint
☐ 5. Medially rotates the thigh at the hip joint	☐ 5. Ipsilaterally rotates the pelvis at the hip joint

Standard Mover Action Notes

- The gracilis crosses the hip joint medially (with its fibers running somewhat horizontally in the frontal plane); therefore it adducts the thigh at the hip joint. This is the major action of the gracilis. (action 1)
- The gracilis crosses the hip joint anteriorly (with its fibers running vertically in the sagittal plane); therefore it flexes the thigh at the hip joint. (action 2)
- The gracilis crosses the knee joint posteriorly (with its fibers running vertically in the sagittal plane); therefore it flexes the leg at the knee joint. (action 3)
- The gracilis crosses the knee joint medially from posterior to anterior (with its fibers running somewhat horizontally in the transverse plane) to attach into the pes anserine tendon at the medial tibia. When the gracilis pulls at the tibial attachment, the tibial attachment rotates posteromedially, causing the anterior tibia to face somewhat medially. Therefore the gracilis medially rotates the leg at the knee joint. (action 4)
- If the knee joint is extended so that it does not allow rotation (and/or if the leg is fixed to the thigh), then when the gracilis pulls the leg into medial rotation, the thigh will follow and medially rotate at the hip joint. (action 5)

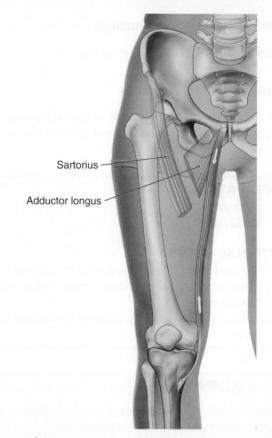

Figure 14-13 Anterior view of the right gracilis. The adductor longus and sartorius have been cut and ghosted in.

Reverse Mover Action Notes

- With the distal attachment fixed, the gracilis pulls the medial aspect of the pelvic bone inferiorly toward the medial thigh, resulting in elevation of the same-side pelvis at the hip joint. Note: Elevation of one side of the pelvis causes the other side to depress. (reverse action 1)
- With the distal attachment fixed, the gracilis, by pulling inferiorly on the anterior pelvis, anteriorly tilts the pelvis at the hip joint. (reverse action 2)
- The gracilis crosses the knee joint posteriorly (with its fibers running vertically in the sagittal plane). If the distal attachment is fixed and the pelvis is fixed to the thigh, the gracilis flexes the thigh at the knee joint. (reverse action 3)
- If the distal end of the gracilis on the tibia is fixed, the reverse action of medial rotation of the leg at the knee joint is lateral rotation of the thigh at the knee joint. (reverse action 4)
- All muscles that medially rotate the thigh at the hip joint can ipsilaterally rotate the pelvis at the hip joint (if the thigh is fixed). (reverse action 5)

Eccentric Antagonist Functions

1. Restrains/slows abduction, extension, and lateral rotation of the thigh at the hip joint

Gracilis (of Adductor Group)—*cont'd*

2. Restrains/slows same-side depression, posterior tilt, and contralateral rotation of the pelvis at the hip joint
3. Restrains/slows knee joint extension
4. Restrains/slows lateral rotation of the leg and medial rotation of the thigh at the knee joint

Isometric Stabilization Functions

1. Stabilizes the thigh and pelvis at the hip joint
2. Stabilizes the knee joint

Isometric Stabilization Function Note

- The distal tendon of the gracilis (along with the sartorius and semitendinosus muscles – the three pes anserine muscles) helps stabilize the medial knee joint against lateral to medial (valgus) forces that would buckle the knee joint medially.

Additional Notes on Functions

1. All five members of the adductors of the thigh group can, as their name implies, adduct the thigh (and elevate the same-side pelvis) at the hip joint.
2. All three pes anserine muscles (sartorius, gracilis, and semitendinosus) flex and medially rotate the leg at the knee joint.

INNERVATION
- ☐ The Obturator Nerve
  - ☐ L2, L3

ARTERIAL SUPPLY
- ☐ The Deep Femoral Artery (a major branch of the Femoral Artery)
  - ☐ and the Obturator Artery (a branch of the Internal Iliac Artery)

✋ PALPATION

1. With the client supine with the thighs on the table and the legs hanging off the table (the leg is flexed to 90 degrees at the knee joint), locate the adductor longus tendon at the pubic bone (it is the most prominent tendon in the groin region).
2. Then drop immediately off it posteriorly and you are on the gracilis.
3. Ask the client to actively flex the leg at the knee joint against the resistance of the table and the gracilis will engage.
4. Once located, continue palpating the gracilis distally toward the tibia.

■ RELATIONSHIP TO OTHER STRUCTURES

- ☐ The gracilis is located in the medial thigh and is superficial for its entire course.
- ☐ Proximally, the adductor longus is anterior and lateral to the gracilis. More distally, the sartorius is anterior to the gracilis.
- ☐ Proximally, the adductor magnus is posterior to the gracilis. More distally, the semimembranosus and the semitendinosus are posterior to the gracilis.
- ☐ The gracilis is one of three muscles that attach into the pes anserine tendon, and it attaches between the sartorius and the semitendinosus on the tibia.
- ☐ The gracilis is located within the deep front line myofascial meridian.

■ MISCELLANEOUS

1. The gracilis is also known as the *adductor gracilis.*
2. The gracilis is one of three muscles that attach into the pes anserine tendon. The other two muscles that attach here are the sartorius and the semitendinosus. *Pes anserine* means goose foot.
3. Think **SGS:** Of the muscles that attach into the pes anserine, the *sartorius* attaches the most anterior and proximal of the three, the *gracilis* is in the middle, and the *semitendinosus* attaches the most posterior and distal.
4. The gracilis is the only member of the adductor group that crosses the knee joint.
5. The gracilis is the second longest muscle in the human body. (The sartorius is the longest.)
6. The curve of the gracilis is an artifact of evolution. In bent-kneed quadrupeds, the gracilis runs in a straight line. As our knee joints extended (straightened out) with evolution, the gracilis stayed behind due to fascia that held it down.

14

Adductor Brevis (of Adductor Group)

The name, adductor brevis, *tells us that this muscle is an adductor and is short (shorter than the adductor longus).*

Derivation	☐ adductor: L. *a muscle that adducts a body part.*
	brevis: L. *shorter.*
Pronunciation	☐ ad-DUK-tor, BRE-vis

■ ATTACHMENTS

☐ **Pubis**
  ☐ the inferior ramus

to the

☐ **Linea Aspera of the Femur**
  ☐ the proximal ⅓

■ FUNCTIONS

CONCENTRIC (SHORTENING) MOVER ACTIONS	
Standard Mover Actions	**Reverse Mover Actions**
☐ **1. Adducts the thigh at the hip joint**	☐ 1. Elevates the same-side pelvis at the hip joint
☐ **2. Flexes the thigh at the hip joint**	☐ **2. Anteriorly tilts the pelvis at the hip joint**
☐ 3. Medially rotates the thigh at the hip joint	☐ 3. Ipsilaterally rotates the pelvis at the hip joint

Standard Mover Action Notes

- The adductor brevis crosses the hip joint medially (with its fibers running somewhat horizontally in the frontal plane); therefore it adducts the thigh at the hip joint. (action 1)
- The adductor brevis crosses the hip joint anteriorly (with its fibers running vertically in the sagittal plane); therefore it flexes the thigh at the hip joint. (action 2)
- Although the major sagittal plane action of the adductor brevis is flexion of the thigh at the hip joint, if the thigh is flexed far enough in front of the body, the adductor brevis' line of pull is now posterior to the axis of motion of the hip joint and it is now able to extend the thigh at the hip joint. This is important during the gait cycle to begin extension of the lower extremity that is flexed and in front of the body. (action 2)
- The adductor brevis is oriented somewhat horizontally in the transverse plane, attaching from the pubic bone to the posterior shaft of the femur. Because the adductor brevis attaches to the posterior femur anterior to the mechanical axis for rotation, it medially rotates the thigh at the hip joint. (action 3)

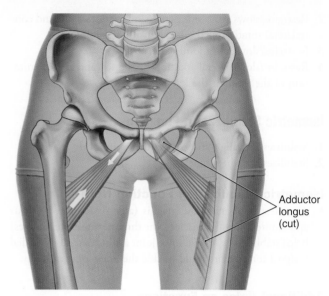

Figure 14-14 Anterior view of the right adductor brevis. The adductor longus has been cut and ghosted in on the left.

Reverse Mover Action Notes

- With the distal femoral attachment fixed, the adductor brevis pulls the medial aspect of the pelvic bone inferiorly toward the medial thigh, resulting in elevation of the same-side pelvis at the hip joint. Note: Elevation of one side of the pelvis causes the other side to depress. (reverse action 1)
- With the distal femoral attachment fixed, the adductor brevis, by pulling inferiorly on the anterior pelvis, anteriorly tilts the pelvis at the hip joint. (reverse action 2)
- All muscles that medially rotate the thigh at the hip joint can ipsilaterally rotate the pelvis at the hip joint (if the thigh is fixed). (reverse action 3)

Eccentric Antagonist Functions

1. Restrains/slows abduction, extension, and lateral rotation of the thigh at the hip joint
2. Restrains/slows same-side depression, posterior tilt, and contralateral rotation of the pelvis at the hip joint

Isometric Stabilization Functions

1. Stabilizes the thigh and pelvis at the hip joint

Additional Note on Functions

1. All five members of the adductors of the thigh group can, as their name implies, adduct the thigh (and elevate the same-side pelvis) at the hip joint.

14

Adductor Brevis (of Adductor Group)—*cont'd*

INNERVATION
- ☐ The Obturator Nerve
  - ☐ L2, L3

ARTERIAL SUPPLY
- ☐ The Femoral Artery (the continuation of the External Iliac Artery) and the Deep Femoral Artery (a major branch of the Femoral Artery)
  - ☐ and the Obturator Artery (a branch of the Internal Iliac Artery)

✋ PALPATION

1. With the client supine, place palpating hand on the proximal anteromedial thigh, very close to the pubic bone.
2. Ask the client to actively adduct the thigh at the hip joint and feel for the proximal tendon of the adductor longus. It will be the most prominent tendon in the proximal anteromedial thigh.
3. Once located, have the client relax and try to palpate deep to the adductor longus for the adductor brevis. (Note: It is very difficult to discern the adductor brevis from the adductor longus.)

■ RELATIONSHIP TO OTHER STRUCTURES

- ☐ From the anterior perspective, the adductor brevis is deep to the adductor longus and superficial to the adductor magnus.
- ☐ All three *adductors* attach distally onto the linea aspera. The adductor brevis attaches onto the linea aspera between the attachments of the adductor longus and adductor magnus.
- ☐ The adductor brevis is located within the deep front line and front functional line myofascial meridians.

■ MISCELLANEOUS

1. The adductor brevis is located between the adductor longus and the adductor magnus.

14

Adductor Magnus (of Adductor Group)

The name, adductor magnus, *tells us that this muscle is an adductor and is large (larger than the adductor longus and the adductor brevis).*

Derivation	□ adductor: L. *a muscle that adducts a body part.*
	magnus: L. *great, larger.*
Pronunciation	□ ad-DUK-tor, MAG-nus

■ ATTACHMENTS

□ **Pubis and Ischium**
  □ ANTERIOR HEAD: inferior pubic ramus and the ramus of the ischium
  □ POSTERIOR HEAD: ischial tuberosity

to the

□ **Linea Aspera of the Femur**
  □ ANTERIOR HEAD: gluteal tuberosity, linea aspera, and medial supracondylar line of the femur
  □ POSTERIOR HEAD: adductor tubercle of the femur

■ FUNCTIONS

CONCENTRIC (SHORTENING) MOVER ACTIONS	
Standard Mover Actions	**Reverse Mover Actions**
□ **1. Adducts the thigh at the hip joint**	□ 1. Elevates the same-side pelvis at the hip joint
□ **2. Extends the thigh at the hip joint**	□ **2. Posteriorly tilts the pelvis at the hip joint**
□ 3. Flexes the thigh at the hip joint	□ 3. Anteriorly tilts the pelvis at the hip joint
□ 4. Medially rotates the thigh at the hip joint	□ 4. Ipsilaterally rotates the pelvis at the hip joint

Standard Mover Action Notes

• The adductor magnus crosses the hip joint medially (with its fibers running somewhat horizontally in the frontal plane); therefore it adducts the thigh at the hip joint. (action 1)
• The adductor magnus crosses the hip joint posteriorly (with its fibers running vertically in the sagittal plane); therefore it extends the thigh at the hip joint. (action 2)
• Some sources state that the most anterior fibers (often termed the *adductor minimus*) of the adductor magnus can flex the thigh at the hip joint. This would be explained by their pubic attachment being slightly anterior to the femoral attachment. (action 3)
• The adductor magnus is oriented somewhat horizontally in the transverse plane, attaching from the pelvic bone to the posterior shaft of the femur. Because the adductor magnus attaches to the posterior femur anterior to the mechanical axis for rotation, it medially rotates the thigh at the hip joint. (action 4)

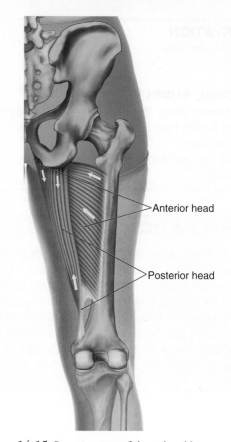

Figure 14-15 Posterior view of the right adductor magnus.

Reverse Mover Action Notes

• With the distal femoral attachment fixed, the adductor magnus pulls the medial aspect of the pelvic bone inferiorly toward the medial thigh, resulting in elevation of the same-side pelvis at the hip joint. Note: Elevation of one side of the pelvis causes the other side to depress. (reverse action 1)
• With the distal femoral attachment fixed, the adductor magnus, by pulling inferiorly on the posterior pelvis, posteriorly tilts the pelvis at the hip joint. (reverse action 2)
• All muscles that flex the thigh at the hip joint can anteriorly tilt the pelvis at the hip joint if the distal femoral attachment is fixed. (reverse action 3)
• All muscles that medially rotate the thigh at the hip joint can ipsilaterally rotate the pelvis at the hip joint (if the distal femoral attachment is fixed). (reverse action 4)

Eccentric Antagonist Functions

1. Restrains/slows abduction, flexion, extension, and lateral rotation of the thigh at the hip joint
2. Restrains/slows same-side depression, anterior tilt, posterior tilt, and contralateral rotation of the pelvis at the hip joint

14

Adductor Magnus (of Adductor Group)—*cont'd*

Isometric Stabilization Functions

1. Stabilizes the thigh and pelvis at the hip joint

Additional Notes on Functions

1. All five members of the adductors of the thigh group can, as their name implies, adduct the thigh (and elevate the same-side pelvis) at the hip joint.
2. The adductor magnus is the only member of the adductor group whose major sagittal plane actions are extension of the thigh and posterior tilt of the pelvis at the hip joint.

INNERVATION

☐ The Obturator Nerve and the Sciatic Nerve
  ☐ the obturator nerve innervates the anterior head
  ☐ the tibial branch of the sciatic nerve innervates the posterior head
  ☐ **L2, L3,** L4

ARTERIAL SUPPLY
Anterior Head
☐ The Femoral Artery (the continuation of the External Iliac Artery) and the Deep Femoral Artery (a major branch of the Femoral Artery)
  ☐ and the Obturator Artery (a branch of the Internal Iliac Artery)
Posterior Head
☐ The Deep Femoral Artery (a major branch of the Femoral Artery) and the Inferior Gluteal Artery (a branch of the Internal Iliac Artery)
  ☐ and the Obturator Artery (a branch of the Internal Iliac Artery) and branches of the Popliteal Artery (the continuation of the Femoral Artery)

✋ PALPATION

1. With the client supine with thighs on the table and legs hanging off the table, place your palpating fingers on the proximal medial thigh and ask the client to flex the leg at the knee joint against the resistance of the table.
2. This will engage the gracilis and medial hamstrings but not the adductor magnus, which is located between them.
3. To engage the adductor magnus, ask the client to either adduct the thigh at the hip joint against your resistance or to extend the thigh at the hip joint against the resistance of the table.

■ RELATIONSHIP TO OTHER STRUCTURES

☐ From the anterior perspective, the adductor magnus is deep to the pectineus, the adductor longus, and the adductor brevis. (There is a small portion of the adductor magnus that is superficial from the anterior perspective between the sartorius, adductor longus, and the gracilis.)
☐ From the posterior perspective, the adductor magnus is deep to all three hamstring muscles.
☐ Although the adductor magnus is primarily deep from the anterior and posterior perspectives, there is a large portion of it that is superficial medially.
☐ All three *adductors* attach distally onto the linea aspera. The adductor longus and adductor brevis attach directly medial to the adductor magnus on the linea aspera of the femur.
☐ The gluteus maximus and the short head of the biceps femoris attach directly lateral to the adductor magnus onto the femur. (They attach onto the gluteal tuberosity and the linea aspera of the femur, respectively.)
☐ The obturator externus and the quadratus femoris lie directly proximal to the adductor magnus.
☐ The adductor magnus is located within the deep front line and involved with the spiral line myofascial meridians.

■ MISCELLANEOUS

1. The adductor magnus has an *anterior head* and a *posterior head.*
2. The anterior head of the adductor magnus consists of two sections. The first section is often called the *adductor minimus* (it is also called the *horizontal fibers*); the second section is called the *oblique fibers.*
3. The posterior head of the adductor magnus is also called the *ischiocondylar section,* because it attaches from the ischial tuberosity to the adductor tubercle, which is on the medial condyle of the femur.
4. The anterior head of the adductor magnus arises from the inferior ramus of the pubis and the ramus of the ischium.
5. The anterior and posterior heads of the adductor magnus (the oblique fibers of the anterior head and the ischiocondylar section) are separated distally by a hiatus called the *adductor hiatus.*
6. The femoral artery and vein from the anterior thigh pass through the adductor hiatus, becoming the popliteal artery and vein in the distal posterior thigh.
7. The position of the adductor magnus in the medial thigh is such that from the anterior perspective it forms a floor that the other adductors sit on and from the posterior perspective it forms a floor that the hamstrings sit on.
8. The adductor magnus is a transitional muscle between the adductor group and the hamstring group.
9. Like the hamstring muscles, the adductor magnus attaches to the ischial tuberosity and can extend the thigh at the hip joint. For this reason, the adductor magnus (or more specifically the posterior head of the adductor magnus) is sometimes referred to as the *fourth hamstring.*

14

Gluteal Group

There are three muscles in the gluteal group: the gluteus maximus, medius, and minimus.

- All three gluteal muscles cross the hip joint, so they can move the thigh at the hip joint and/or move the pelvis at the hip joint.

- The gluteus medius and minimus are primarily important for stabilizing the pelvis when walking.

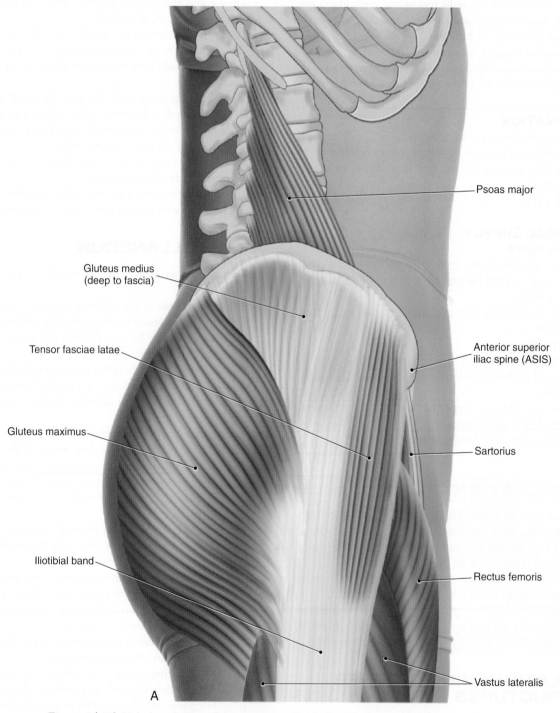

Psoas major

Gluteus medius (deep to fascia)

Tensor fasciae latae

Anterior superior iliac spine (ASIS)

Gluteus maximus

Sartorius

Iliotibial band

Rectus femoris

Vastus lateralis

A

Figure 14-16 Right lateral views of the gluteal muscles. **A,** Superficial view. The gluteus minimus is not seen.

14

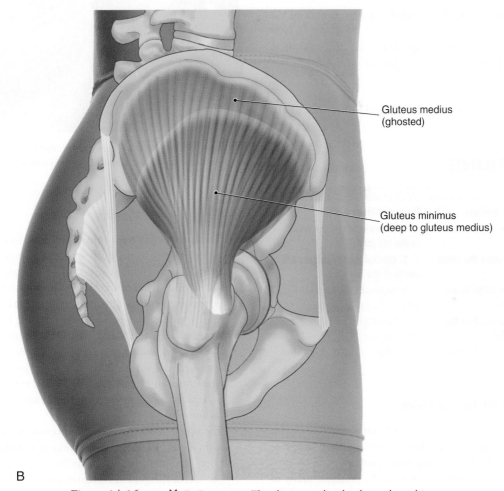

Gluteus medius
(ghosted)

Gluteus minimus
(deep to gluteus medius)

B

Figure 14-16, cont'd B, Deep view. The gluteus medius has been ghosted in.

14

Gluteus Maximus (of Gluteal Group)

The name, gluteus maximus, *tells us that this muscle is located in the gluteal (i.e., buttock) region and is large (larger than the gluteus medius and the gluteus minimus).*

Derivation	☐ gluteus: Gr. *buttocks.*
	maximus: L. *greatest.*
Pronunciation	☐ GLOO-tee-us, MAX-i-mus

■ ATTACHMENTS

☐ **Posterior Iliac Crest, the Posterolateral Sacrum, and the Coccyx**

   ☐ and the sacrotuberous ligament, the thoracolumbar fascia, and the fascia over the gluteus medius

  to the

☐ **Iliotibial Band (ITB) and the Gluteal Tuberosity of the Femur**

■ FUNCTIONS

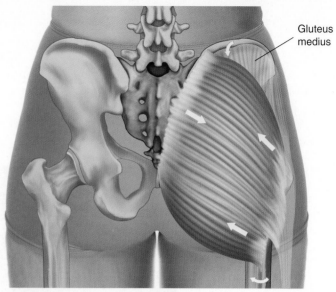

Figure 14-17 Posterior view of the right gluteus maximus. The tensor fasciae latae, fascia over the gluteus medius, and iliotibial band have been ghosted in.

CONCENTRIC (SHORTENING) MOVER ACTIONS	
Standard Mover Actions	**Reverse Mover Actions**
☐ **1. Extends the thigh at the hip joint**	☐ **1. Posteriorly tilts the pelvis at the hip joint**
☐ **2. Laterally rotates the thigh at the hip joint**	☐ **2. Contralaterally rotates the pelvis at the hip joint**
☐ **3. Abducts the thigh at the hip joint (upper ⅓)**	☐ 3. Depresses the same-side pelvis at the hip joint (upper ⅓)
☐ **4. Adducts the thigh at the hip joint (lower ⅔)**	☐ 4. Elevates the same-side pelvis at the hip joint (lower ⅔)
☐ 5. Extends the leg at the knee joint	☐ 5. Extends the thigh at the knee joint

Standard Mover Action Notes

• The gluteus maximus crosses the hip joint posteriorly (with its fibers running vertically in the sagittal plane); therefore it extends the thigh at the hip joint. (action 1)

• The gluteus maximus wraps around the posterior pelvis to attach laterally onto the iliotibial band and femur (with its fibers running somewhat horizontally in the transverse plane). When the gluteus maximus contracts, it pulls this lateral attachment posteromedially, causing the anterior surface of the thigh to face laterally. Therefore the gluteus maximus laterally rotates the thigh at the hip joint. (action 2)

• If a person is standing and pinches the buttocks together (i.e., contracts the gluteus maximus muscles), an interesting postural effect occurs. The contraction of the gluteus maximus muscles should cause lateral rotation of the thighs at the hip joints. However, because of the friction between the bottom of the feet and the floor, the thighs cannot freely laterally rotate. Therefore the rotatory force on the thighs is

translated all the way to the talus of the foot which laterally rotates relative to the calcaneus at the subtalar joint. Lateral rotation is a component action of foot supination, which lifts up the arches of the feet. A conclusion from this might be that if a person's gluteus maximus muscles are well developed and therefore have a stronger resting baseline tone, the arches of their feet may gain extra support. (action 2)

• The gluteus maximus, albeit the largest extensor and/or lateral rotator of the thigh at the hip joint, only contracts when forceful extension and/or lateral rotation of the thigh is required, such as running, jumping, or climbing stairs. (actions 1, 2)

• The upper ⅓ of the gluteus maximus crosses the hip joint from medial to lateral above the center of the joint (with its fibers running vertically in the frontal plane). Therefore this portion of the gluteus maximus abducts the thigh at the hip joint. (Note the similarity of the direction of these fibers of the gluteus maximus to the direction of fibers of the nearby gluteus medius.) (action 3)

• The lower ⅔ of the gluteus maximus crosses the hip joint from medial to lateral below the center of the joint (with its fibers running somewhat horizontally in the frontal plane). Therefore this portion of the gluteus maximus adducts the thigh at the hip joint. (action 4)

• Because of its pull via the iliotibial band (which attaches to the proximal anterolateral tibia), the gluteus maximus crosses the knee joint anteriorly (with a vertical orientation to its pull in the sagittal plane). Therefore the gluteus maximus extends the leg at the knee joint. (action 5)

14

Gluteus Maximus (of Gluteal Group)—*cont'd*

Reverse Mover Action Notes

- When the thigh is fixed, the gluteus maximus, by pulling down on the posterior pelvis, posteriorly tilts the pelvis at the hip joint. This action is important during walking, running, and returning to an upright position from a stooped position. (reverse action 1)
- The gluteus maximus crosses the hip joint posteriorly (with its fibers running somewhat horizontally in the transverse plane). When the femoral attachment is fixed and the gluteus maximus contracts, it pulls on the pelvis, causing the anterior pelvis to face the opposite side of the body from the side on which the gluteus maximus is attached. Therefore the gluteus maximus contralaterally rotates the pelvis at the hip joint. (reverse action 2)
- Contralateral rotation of the pelvis at the hip joint is important whenever a foot is planted on the ground and the pelvis is rotated to the opposite side, such as when planting and cutting in sports. (reverse action 2)
- The upper ⅓ of the gluteus maximus' fibers cross the hip joint laterally. If the distal attachment is fixed, the lateral surface of the pelvis will be pulled down toward the lateral surface of the thigh. Therefore, the upper ⅓ of the gluteus maximus depresses the same-side (ipsilateral) pelvis at the hip joint. This action is important because it prevents depression of pelvis to the opposite side when walking. (reverse action 3)
- The lower ⅔ of the gluteus maximus' fibers cross the hip joint on the medial side (below the center of the joint). If the distal attachment is fixed, the medial pelvis is pulled down toward the medial thigh, causing elevation of the same-side pelvis at the hip joint. (reverse action 4)
- Via its iliotibial band attachment, the gluteus maximus crosses the knee joint anteriorly (with its fibers running vertically in the sagittal plane). If the distal attachment is fixed, it extends the thigh at the knee joint. (reverse action 5)

Eccentric Antagonist Functions

1. Restrains/slows flexion, medial rotation, adduction, and abduction of the thigh at the hip joint
2. Restrains/slows anterior tilt, ipsilateral rotation, same-side elevation and same-side depression of the pelvis at the hip joint
3. Restrains/slows knee joint flexion

Isometric Stabilization Functions

1. Stabilizes the thigh and pelvis at the hip joint
2. Stabilizes the knee joint
3. Stabilizes the subtalar joint

Isometric Stabilization Function Notes

- Given that both the gluteus maximus and the tensor fasciae latae attach into the iliotibial band and the iliotibial band crosses the knee joint anterolaterally, both of these muscles in effect cross the knee joint anteriorly and therefore, theoretically, can extend the leg at the knee joint. However, there is controversy over their ability to actually do this. Certainly, extension of the leg at the knee joint is not one of their major actions. It is likely that the role of these two muscles and the iliotibial band crossing the knee joint is primarily to help stabilize the knee joint.
- Lateral rotation of the thigh at the hip joint acts to prevent medial rotation of the thigh and entire lower extremity, including the talus at the subtalar joint. This can stabilize the subtalar joint and prevent excessive pronation (dropping of the arch) of the foot.

INNERVATION
☐ The Inferior Gluteal Nerve
  ☐ **L5, S1,** S2

ARTERIAL SUPPLY
☐ The Superior Gluteal Artery and the Inferior Gluteal Artery (branches of the Internal Iliac Artery)

14

✋ PALPATION

1. With the client prone, place your palpating hand on the posterior gluteal region, just lateral to the sacrum.
2. Have the client laterally rotate and extend the thigh at the hip joint and feel for the contraction of the gluteus maximus. Resistance can be added to the distal thigh.
3. Palpate the gluteus maximus distally and laterally to its distal attachment on the iliotibial band and femur.

■ RELATIONSHIP TO OTHER STRUCTURES

☐ The gluteus maximus is superficial in the posterior pelvis and covers the posteroinferior portion of the gluteus medius. The gluteus maximus also covers the entire piriformis, superior gemellus, obturator internus, inferior gemellus, obturator externus, quadratus femoris, and ischial tuberosity.
☐ The attachment of the gluteus maximus onto the gluteal tuberosity of the femur is between the vastus lateralis and adductor magnus attachments.
☐ The gluteus maximus is located within the lateral line and back functional line myofascial meridians.

■ MISCELLANEOUS

1. Two muscles attach into the iliotibial band (ITB): the gluteus maximus and the tensor fasciae latae (TFL). Given that the gluteus maximus attaches into the ITB from one direction and the TFL attaches into the ITB from the opposite direction, they have opposite actions of rotation.

2. It can be helpful to think of the gluteus maximus as the *speed skater's muscle.* The gluteus maximus is powerful in extending, abducting, and laterally rotating the thigh at the hip joint, which are all actions that are necessary when speed skating.

3. The gluteus maximus is the largest muscle in the human body.

14

Gluteus Medius (of Gluteal Group)

The name, gluteus medius, *tells us that this muscle is located in the gluteal (i.e., buttock) region and is medium sized (smaller than the gluteus maximus and larger than the gluteus minimus).*

Derivation	☐ gluteus: Gr. *buttocks.*
	medius: L. *middle.*
Pronunciation	☐ GLOO-tee-us, MEED-ee-us

■ ATTACHMENTS

☐ **External Ilium**
    ☐ inferior to the iliac crest and between the anterior and posterior gluteal lines

to the

☐ **Greater Trochanter of the Femur**
    ☐ the lateral surface

■ FUNCTIONS

CONCENTRIC (SHORTENING) MOVER ACTIONS	
Standard Mover Actions	**Reverse Mover Actions**
☐ **1. Abducts the thigh at the hip joint (entire muscle)**	☐ **1. Depresses the same-side pelvis at the hip joint**
☐ **2. Extends the thigh at the hip joint (posterior fibers)**	☐ **2. Posteriorly tilts the pelvis at the hip joint**
☐ **3. Flexes the thigh at the hip joint (anterior fibers)**	☐ **3. Anteriorly tilts the pelvis at the hip joint**
☐ **4. Laterally rotates the thigh at the hip joint (posterior fibers)**	☐ **4. Contralaterally rotates the pelvis at the hip joint**
☐ **5. Medially rotates the thigh at the hip joint (anterior fibers)**	☐ 5. Ipsilaterally rotates the pelvis at the hip joint

Standard Mover Action Notes

- The gluteus medius crosses the hip joint laterally above the center of the joint (with its fibers running vertically in the frontal plane). Therefore the gluteus medius abducts the thigh at the hip joint. (action 1)
- The posterior fibers of the gluteus medius cross the hip joint posteriorly (running vertically in the sagittal plane); therefore they extend the thigh at the hip joint. (action 2)
- The anterior fibers of the gluteus medius cross the hip joint anteriorly (running vertically in the sagittal plane); therefore they flex the thigh at the hip joint. (action 3)
- The posterior fibers of the gluteus medius wrap around the posterior pelvis to attach laterally onto the greater trochanter (running somewhat horizontally in the transverse plane). When the posterior fibers contract, they pull the greater trochanter posteromedially, causing the anterior surface of the thigh to face laterally. Therefore the gluteus medius laterally rotates the thigh at the hip joint. Note the similarity of the direction of posterior fibers of the gluteus medius to the direction of fibers of the neighboring piriformis. (action 4)

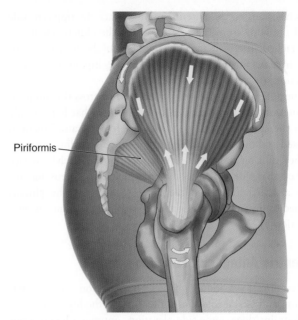

Piriformis

Figure 14-18 Lateral view of the right gluteus medius. The piriformis has been ghosted in.

- The anterior fibers of the gluteus medius wrap around the anterior pelvis to attach laterally onto the greater trochanter (running somewhat horizontally in the transverse plane). When the anterior fibers contract, they pull the greater trochanter anteromedially, causing the anterior surface of the thigh to face medially. Therefore the gluteus medius medially rotates the thigh at the hip joint. Note the similarity of the direction of anterior fibers of the gluteus medius to the direction of fibers of the neighboring tensor fasciae latae. (action 5)

Reverse Mover Action Notes

- When the femoral attachment is fixed, the gluteus medius, by pulling inferiorly on the pelvis laterally, depresses (i.e., laterally tilts) the same-side (ipsilateral) pelvis at the hip joint. Note: Depression of one side of the pelvis causes the other side of the pelvis to elevate. (reverse action 1)
- Ipsilateral pelvic depression force on the support-limb side when walking prevents depression of the pelvis to the opposite unsupported swing-limb side. (reverse action 1)
- When the femoral attachment is fixed and the posterior fibers of the gluteus medius contract, they pull inferiorly on the posterior pelvis, posteriorly tilting the pelvis at the hip joint. (reverse action 2)
- When the femoral attachment is fixed and the anterior fibers of the gluteus medius contract, they pull inferiorly on the anterior pelvis, anteriorly tilting the pelvis at the hip joint. (reverse action 3)
- The posterior fibers of the gluteus medius cross the hip joint posteriorly (running somewhat horizontally in the transverse plane). When the femoral attachment is fixed and the posterior fibers of the gluteus medius contract, they pull on the

14

pelvis, causing the anterior pelvis to face the opposite side of the body from the side on which the gluteus medius is attached. Therefore the posterior fibers of the gluteus medius contralaterally rotate the pelvis at the hip joint. (reverse action 4)

- The anterior fibers of the gluteus medius cross the hip joint anteriorly (with their fibers running somewhat horizontally in the transverse plane). When the femoral attachment is fixed and the anterior fibers of the gluteus medius contract, they pull on the pelvis, causing the anterior pelvis to face the same side of the body on which the gluteus medius is attached. Therefore the anterior fibers of the gluteus medius ipsilaterally rotate the pelvis at the hip joint. (reverse action 5)

Eccentric Antagonist Functions

1. Restrains/slows adduction, flexion, extension, medial rotation, and lateral rotation of the thigh at the hip joint
2. Restrains/slows same-side elevation, anterior tilt, posterior tilt, ipsilateral rotation, and contralateral rotation of the pelvis at the hip joint

Isometric Stabilization Functions

1. Stabilizes the thigh and pelvis at the hip joint
2. Stabilizes the subtalar joint

Isometric Stabilization Function Notes

- Same-side (ipsilateral) pelvic depression (lateral tilt) force by the gluteus medius is actually its most important function. When one foot is lifted off the floor, the pelvis should fall to that side because it is now unsupported. However, this is prevented by the gluteus medius on the support-limb side, which contracts and creates a force of ipsilateral depression of the pelvis. Depressing the pelvis on the support-limb side prevents the pelvis from falling (depressing) to the other unsupported swing-limb side. Therefore the pelvis remains level. With every step that a person takes when walking, contraction of the gluteus medius on the support side occurs. Therefore, the gluteus medius is important and necessary for proper gait by isometrically contracting to stabilize the pelvis.
- The gluteus medius contracts to create a force of same-side pelvic depression (lateral tilt) not only when a foot is lifted off the floor to walk (see note above) but also when weight is simply shifted to one foot. Therefore the habitual practice of standing with all or most of the body weight on one side tends to cause the gluteus medius on that side to become overused and tight.
- Thigh lateral rotation action prevents medial rotation of the thigh and entire lower extremity, including the talus at the subtalar joint, if the foot overly pronates (if the arch of the foot collapses).

Additional Notes on Functions

1. Note how the gluteus medius fans around the hip joint. It crosses the hip joint posteriorly, laterally, and anteriorly. Therefore some sources consider the gluteus medius to have three sections: posterior, middle, and anterior. This orientation is similar to the orientation of the deltoid to the glenohumeral joint. Therefore both of these muscles can do the same actions at their respective joints. The gluteus medius can abduct, extend, flex, laterally rotate, and medially rotate the thigh at the hip joint. The deltoid can abduct, extend, flex, laterally rotate, and medially rotate the arm at the glenohumeral joint

2. Because the posterior portion of the gluteus medius is the thickest part, its actions are the strongest. Therefore the strongest actions of the gluteus medius are abduction, extension, and lateral rotation of the thigh at the hip joint.

INNERVATION
- ☐ The Superior Gluteal Nerve
  - ☐ **L4, L5,** S1

ARTERIAL SUPPLY
- ☐ The Superior Gluteal Artery (a branch of the Internal Iliac Artery)

✋ PALPATION

1. With the client side lying, place your palpating fingers immediately distal to the middle of the iliac crest.
2. Have the client abduct the thigh into the air and feel for the contraction of the gluteus medius. Resistance can be added.
3. The posterior and anterior fibers of the gluteus medius are deep to the gluteus maximus and tensor fasciae latae, respectively, and can be difficult to discern from these overlying muscles.

■ RELATIONSHIP TO OTHER STRUCTURES

- ☐ The posterior ⅓ of the gluteus medius is deep to the gluteus maximus. A portion of the anterior gluteus medius is deep to the tensor fasciae latae.
- ☐ The middle portion of the gluteus medius is superficial.
- ☐ The anterior fibers of the gluteus medius lie next to and deep to the tensor fasciae latae (with essentially an identical fiber direction), and the posterior fibers of the gluteus medius lie next to the piriformis (with essentially an identical fiber direction).
- ☐ Deep to the gluteus medius is the gluteus minimus.

Gluteus Medius (of Gluteal Group)—*cont'd*

☐ The gluteus medius is located within the lateral line myofascial meridian.

■ MISCELLANEOUS

1. There is usually a thick layer of fascia overlying the gluteus medius muscle called the *gluteal fascia* or the *gluteal aponeurosis.*

2. A chronically tight gluteus medius can create the postural conditions of a *functional* short lower extremity (usually called a *short leg*) and a compensatory scoliosis. When the gluteus medius is tight, it pulls on and depresses (laterally tilts) the pelvis toward the thigh on that side. This results in a *functional short leg* (as opposed to a *structural short leg* wherein the femur and/or the tibia on one side is actually shorter than on the other side). Further, depressing the pelvis on one side creates an unlevel sacrum for the spine to sit on and a compensatory scoliosis must occur to return the head to a level position. (Note: The head must be level for proper proprioceptive balance in the inner ear and for the eyes to be level for visual proprioception.)

3. Understanding the role of the gluteus medius as a same-side pelvis depressor whenever a person lifts a foot off the floor or simply shifts his or her weight to one side gives us another easy way to palpate the gluteus medius. Stand and rock your weight back and forth from one foot to the other while palpating both gluteus medius muscles. The gluteus medius muscle on the support-limb side (the side that you are bearing weight on) will clearly be felt as it contracts.

14

Gluteus Minimus (of Gluteal Group)

The name, gluteus minimus, *tells us that this muscle is located in the gluteal (i.e., buttock) region and is small (smaller than the gluteus maximus and the gluteus medius).*

Derivation	□ gluteus: Gr. *buttocks.*
	minimus: L. *least.*
Pronunciation	□ GLOO-tee-us, MIN-i-mus

■ ATTACHMENTS

□ **External Ilium**
  □ between the anterior and inferior gluteal lines

to the

□ **Greater Trochanter of the Femur**
  □ the anterior surface

■ FUNCTIONS

CONCENTRIC (SHORTENING) MOVER ACTIONS	
Standard Mover Actions	**Reverse Mover Actions**
□ 1. Abducts the thigh at the hip joint (entire muscle)	□ 1. Depresses the same-side pelvis at the hip joint
□ 2. Flexes the thigh at the hip joint (anterior fibers)	□ 2. Anteriorly tilts the pelvis at the hip joint
□ 3. Extends the thigh at the hip joint (posterior fibers)	□ 3. Posteriorly tilts the pelvis at the hip joint
□ 4. Medially rotates the thigh at the hip joint (anterior fibers)	□ 4. Ipsilaterally rotates the pelvis at the hip joint
□ 5. Laterally rotates the thigh at the hip joint (posterior fibers)	□ 5. Contralaterally rotates the pelvis at the hip joint

Standard Mover Action Notes

- The gluteus minimus has the same standard (and reverse) mover actions as the gluteus medius. One difference is that the thickest and most powerful aspect of the gluteus minimus is its anterior aspect. Therefore its actions of abduction, flexion, and medial rotation are its most powerful actions. The other difference is that the gluteus medius fans out more anteriorly and posteriorly around the hip joint; therefore it is much more powerful than the gluteus minimus because of its greater size and greater coverage around the joint. (actions 1, 2, 3, 4, 5)
- The gluteus minimus crosses the hip joint laterally above the center of the joint (with its fibers running vertically in the frontal plane). Therefore the gluteus minimus abducts the thigh at the hip joint. (action 1)
- The anterior fibers of the gluteus minimus cross the hip joint anteriorly (running vertically in the sagittal plane); therefore they flex the thigh at the hip joint. (action 2)
- The posterior fibers of the gluteus minimus cross the hip joint posteriorly (running vertically in the sagittal plane); therefore they extend the thigh at the hip joint. (action 3)

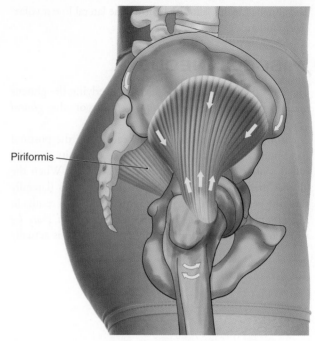

Piriformis

Figure 14-19 Lateral view of the right gluteus minimus. The piriformis has been ghosted in.

- The anterior fibers of the gluteus minimus wrap around the anterior pelvis to attach laterally onto the greater trochanter (running somewhat horizontally in the transverse plane). When the anterior fibers contract, they pull the greater trochanter anteromedially, causing the anterior surface of the thigh to face medially. Therefore the gluteus minimus medially rotates the thigh at the hip joint. Note the similarity of the direction of anterior fibers of the gluteus minimus to the direction of fibers of the neighboring tensor fasciae latae. (action 4)
- The posterior fibers of the gluteus minimus wrap around the posterior pelvis to attach laterally onto the greater trochanter (running somewhat horizontally in the transverse plane). When the posterior fibers contract, they pull the greater trochanter posteromedially, causing the anterior surface of the thigh to face laterally. Therefore the gluteus minimus laterally rotates the thigh at the hip joint. Note the similarity of the direction of posterior fibers of the gluteus minimus to the direction of fibers of the neighboring piriformis. (action 1)

Reverse Mover Action Notes

- The gluteus minimus has the same standard and reverse mover actions as the gluteus medius. The only difference is that the thickest and most powerful aspect of the gluteus minimus is its anterior aspect. Therefore its reverse actions of same-side depression, anterior tilt, and ipsilateral rotation of the pelvis are its most powerful reverse actions. (reverse actions 1, 2, 3, 4, 5)
- When the femoral attachment is fixed, the gluteus minimus, by pulling inferiorly on the pelvis laterally, depresses (i.e.,

14

Gluteus Minimus (of Gluteal Group)—*cont'd*

laterally tilts) the same-side (ipsilateral) pelvis at the hip joint. Note: Depression of one side of the pelvis causes the other side of the pelvis to elevate. (reverse action 1)

- Ipsilateral pelvic depression force on the support-limb side when walking prevents depression of the pelvis to the opposite unsupported swing-limb side. (reverse action 1)
- When the femoral attachment is fixed and the anterior fibers of the gluteus minimus contract, they pull inferiorly on the anterior pelvis, anteriorly tilting the pelvis at the hip joint. (reverse action 2)
- When the femoral attachment is fixed and the posterior fibers of the gluteus minimus contract, they pull inferiorly on the posterior pelvis, posteriorly tilting the pelvis at the hip joint. (reverse action 3)
- The anterior fibers of the gluteus minimus cross the hip joint anteriorly (with their fibers running somewhat horizontally in the transverse plane). When the femoral attachment is fixed and the anterior fibers of the gluteus minimus contract, they pull on the pelvis, causing the anterior pelvis to face the same on which the gluteus minimus is attached. Therefore the anterior fibers of the gluteus minimus ipsilaterally rotate the pelvis at the hip joint. (reverse action 4)
- The posterior fibers of the gluteus mimimus cross the hip joint posteriorly (running somewhat horizontally in the transverse plane). When the femoral attachment is fixed and the posterior fibers of the gluteus minimus contract, they pull on the pelvis, causing the anterior pelvis to face the opposite side of the body from the side on which the gluteus minimus is attached. Therefore the posterior fibers of the gluteus minimus contralaterally rotate the pelvis at the hip joint. (reverse action 5)

Eccentric Antagonist Functions

1. Restrains/slows adduction, extension, flexion, lateral rotation, and medial rotation of the thigh at the hip joint
2. Restrains/slows same-side elevation, posterior tilt, anterior tilt, contralateral rotation, and ipsilateral rotation of the pelvis at the hip joint

Isometric Stabilization Functions

1. Stabilizes the thigh and pelvis at the hip joint
2. Stabilizes the subtalar joint

Isometric Stabilization Function Notes

- As with the gluteus medius, same-side (ipsilateral) pelvic depression (lateral tilt) force by the gluteus minimus is actually its most important function because it stabilizes the pelvis by preventing it from depressing (falling) to the unsupported side when walking.
- The gluteus minimus also contracts to stabilize the pelvis when a person has the habitual practice of standing with all or most of their body weight on one side. Overuse for this function can cause the gluteus minimus to become tight.

- Thigh lateral rotation action prevents medial rotation of the thigh and entire lower extremity, including the talus at the subtalar joint, if the foot overly pronates (if the arch of the foot collapses).

Additional Note on Functions

1. Like the gluteus medius, the gluteus minimus fans around the hip joint and has three sections: anterior, middle, and posterior. This orientation is similar to the orientation of the deltoid to the glenohumeral joint. Therefore both of these muscles can do the same actions at their respective joints. The gluteus minimus can abduct, flex, extend, medially rotate, and laterally rotate the thigh at the hip joint. The deltoid can abduct, flex, extend, medially rotate, and laterally rotate the arm at the glenohumeral joint.

INNERVATION

- ☐ The Superior Gluteal Nerve
  - ☐ **L4, L5,** S1

ARTERIAL SUPPLY

- ☐ The Superior Gluteal Artery (a branch of the Internal Iliac Artery)

✋ PALPATION

1. It is extremely difficult to differentiate the gluteus minimus from the gluteus medius because the gluteus medius entirely overlies the gluteus minimus and they have identical actions. The thickest part of the gluteus minimus is the anterior portion.
2. To palpate, follow the same procedure as for the gluteus medius and try to palpate deeper for the gluteus minimus.
3. If the superficial gluteus medius is relaxed and the gluteus minimus is very tight, it may be possible to feel and distinguish the gluteus minimus.

■ RELATIONSHIP TO OTHER STRUCTURES

- ☐ The gluteus minimus is deep to the gluteus medius.
- ☐ Deep to the gluteus minimus are the joint capsule of the hip joint and the ilium.
- ☐ The gluteus minimus is directly superior to the piriformis.
- ☐ The gluteus minimus is involved with the lateral line myofascial meridian.

■ MISCELLANEOUS

1. A chronically tight gluteus minimus can contribute to the related biomechanical postural conditions of a functional *short lower extremity* (usually called a *short leg*) with a compensatory scoliosis (see Miscellaneous section of gluteus medius).

Deep Lateral Rotator Group

Deep to the gluteus maximus, there is a second layer of muscles that laterally rotates the thigh at the hip joint. These muscles are usually grouped together and called the *deep lateral rotators* or the *deep six*.

The deep lateral rotator muscles are the following (from superior to inferior): the piriformis, superior gemellus, obturator internus, inferior gemellus, obturator externus, and quadratus femoris.

■ ATTACHMENTS

- On observation, it is clear that all the deep lateral rotators have a nearly identical direction of fibers. They lie approximately horizontal in the transverse plane, and they attach laterally onto or near the greater trochanter of the femur.
- From a posterior perspective, all these muscles are at the same depth (except for the obturator externus, which lies deep to the quadratus femoris and is either entirely covered or nearly entirely covered by it).
- The piriformis and obturator internus both arise from the internal surface of the pelvis. All the other muscles of the deep lateral rotator group arise from the external surface of the pelvis.

■ FUNCTIONS

- When the deep lateral rotators of the thigh pull the femur toward their more medial attachment in the posterior buttock region, they cause lateral rotation of the thigh at the hip joint.
- A force of lateral rotation of the thigh prevents medial rotation of the thigh and entire lower extremity, including the talus at the subtalar joint, if the foot overly pronates (if the arch of the foot collapses).
- When the femoral attachment of the deep lateral rotators of the thigh is fixed, the pelvis rotates instead of the femur. This rotation causes the pelvis to rotate away from the side of the body on which these muscles are attached. Therefore these muscles contralaterally rotate the pelvis at the hip joint. (Note: All muscles that laterally rotate the thigh at the hip joint can also contralaterally rotate the pelvis at the hip joint.)

- This reverse action of contralateral rotation of the pelvis at the hip joint is important when a person is walking or running and plants the foot to change the direction of movement. In sports, this is called *planting and cutting*.
- An important function of the deep lateral rotator group is to stabilize the hip joint. Their line of pull is largely horizontal, pulling the femoral head into the acetabulum. In this regard they are analogous to the rotator cuff group of the glenohumeral joint.

■ MISCELLANEOUS

- The two largest muscles of the deep lateral rotator group are the piriformis and quadratus femoris.
- The gluteus maximus can also laterally rotate the thigh at the hip joint, but it is superficial to this group.
- Although it is at the same depth, the gluteus medius is usually not included in this group. The posterior fibers of the gluteus medius have the same direction as the piriformis, which lies directly inferior to it, and these fibers laterally rotate the thigh at the hip joint.
- The posterior fibers of the gluteus minimus can also laterally rotate the thigh at the hip joint, but the gluteus minimus is considered to be at a third deeper layer of musculature in the posterior pelvis.
- As a rule, because of their horizontal orientation, the deep lateral rotators do not fit well into the longitudinally oriented myofascial meridians. They may be considered to be involved with the deep front line myofascial meridian.

INNERVATION
☐ The deep lateral rotators are innervated by branches of the lumbosacral plexus, except for the obturator externus, which is innervated by the obturator nerve.

ARTERIAL SUPPLY
☐ The deep lateral rotators receive their arterial supply from the superior and inferior gluteal arteries and the obturator artery.

14

Posterior Views of the Deep Lateral Rotator Group

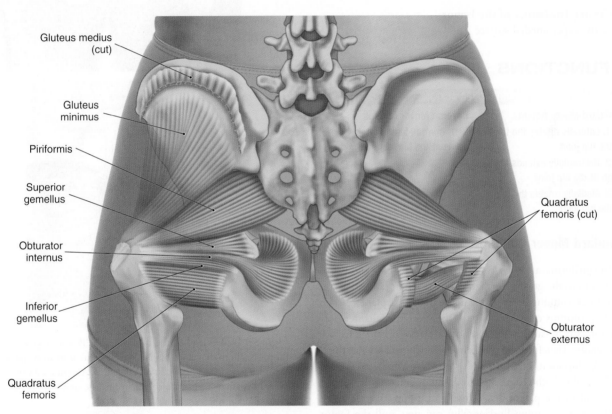

Gluteus medius
(cut)

Gluteus
minimus

Piriformis

Superior
gemellus

Obturator
internus

Inferior
gemellus

Quadratus
femoris

Quadratus
femoris (cut)

Obturator
externus

Figure 14-20 Views of the deep lateral rotator group. The deep lateral rotator group is shown on the left; the gluteus minimus has been ghosted in. The quadratus femoris has been cut on the right to show the obturator externus.

14

Piriformis (of Deep Lateral Rotator Group)

The name, piriformis, *tells us that this muscle is shaped like a pear.*

Derivation	☐ piriformis: L. *pear shaped.*
Pronunciation	☐ pi-ri-FOR-mis

■ ATTACHMENTS

☐ **Anterior Sacrum**
    ☐ and the anterior surface of the sacrotuberous ligament

to the

☐ **Greater Trochanter of the Femur**
    ☐ the superomedial surface

■ FUNCTIONS

CONCENTRIC (SHORTENING) MOVER ACTIONS	
Standard Mover Actions	**Reverse Mover Actions**
☐ 1. **Laterally rotates the thigh at the hip joint**	☐ 1. **Contralaterally rotates the pelvis at the hip joint**
☐ 2. **Horizontally extends the thigh at the hip joint**	
☐ 3. **Medially rotates the thigh at the hip joint**	☐ 2. Ipsilaterally rotates the pelvis at the hip joint

Standard Mover Action Notes

- The piriformis attaches from the sacrum medially and wraps around to the greater trochanter of the femur laterally (with its fibers running horizontally in the transverse plane). When the piriformis contracts, it pulls the greater trochanter posteromedially, causing the anterior surface of the thigh to face laterally. Therefore the piriformis laterally rotates the thigh at the hip joint. (action 1)
- When the thigh is already flexed, the orientation of the line of pull of the piriformis relative to the hip joint changes. The fibers (running horizontally) can now pull the femur away from the midline in the frontal plane. Therefore the piriformis horizontally extends the thigh at the hip joint. Note: Horizontal extension is also known as horizontal abduction, hence the piriformis is often said to abduct the hip joint. (action 2)
- When the thigh is already flexed, the orientation of the line of pull of the piriformis relative to the hip joint changes. When the thigh is not in flexion, the fibers of the piriformis wrap around the posterior side of the femur to attach onto the greater trochanter. However, if the thigh is sufficiently flexed (sources state a minimum of 60 degrees is needed), the fibers of the piriformis now wrap around the anterior side of the femur to attach onto the greater trochanter. Given this direction of fibers relative to the hip joint, the piriformis now pulls the greater trochanter anteromedially instead of posteromedially. Therefore the piriformis medially rotates

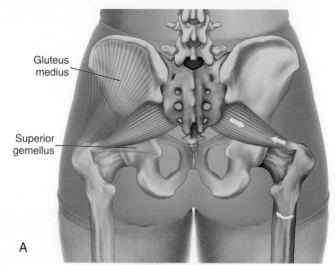

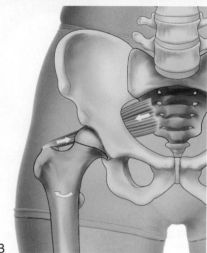

Figure 14-21 Views of the piriformis. **A,** Posterior view. The piriformis has been drawn on both sides. The gluteus medius and superior gemellus have been ghosted in on the left. **B,** Anterior view of the right piriformis, showing its attachment onto the anterior surface of the sacrum.

the thigh at the hip joint instead of laterally rotating the thigh at the hip joint. The best way to visualize this is to place a string where the piriformis attaches, flex the thigh to approximately 90 degrees, and look from above at where the string is located relative to the hip joint before and after the thigh is flexed. (action 3)

Reverse Mover Action Notes

- The piriformis crosses the hip joint posteriorly (with its fibers running somewhat horizontally in the transverse plane). When the femoral attachment is fixed and the piriformis contracts, it pulls on the pelvis, causing the anterior pelvis to face the opposite side of the body from the side of the body on which the piriformis is attached. Therefore the

Piriformis (of Deep Lateral Rotator Group)—*cont'd*

piriformis contralaterally rotates the pelvis at the hip joint. (reverse action 1)

- Contralateral rotation of the pelvis at the hip joint is important whenever a foot is planted on the ground and the pelvis is rotated to the opposite side, such as when planting and cutting in sports. (reverse action 1)
- If the piriformis changes its line of pull at the hip joint to become a medial rotator of the thigh, then its reverse action changes to be ipsilateral rotation of the pelvis. (reverse action 2)

Eccentric Antagonist Functions

1. Restrains/slows medial rotation, horizontal flexion, and lateral rotation of the thigh at the hip joint
2. Restrains/slows ipsilateral rotation and contralateral rotation of the pelvis at the hip joint

Isometric Stabilization Functions

1. Stabilizes the thigh and pelvis at the hip joint
2. Stabilizes the sacrum at the sacroiliac and lumbosacral joints
3. Stabilizes the subtalar joint

Isometric Stabilization Function Note

- A force of lateral rotation of the thigh prevents medial rotation of the thigh and entire lower extremity, including the talus at the subtalar joint, if the foot overly pronates (if the arch of the foot collapses).

Additional Notes on Functions

1. All six members of the deep lateral rotator group can, as their name implies, laterally rotate the thigh (and contralaterally rotate the pelvis) at the hip joint.
2. The piriformis, superior gemellus, obturator internus, and inferior gemellus can all horizontally extend (horizontally abduct) the thigh at the hip joint if the thigh is flexed.

INNERVATION
- ☐ Nerve to Piriformis (of the Lumbosacral Plexus)
  - ☐ L5, **S1**, S2

ARTERIAL SUPPLY
- ☐ The Superior and Inferior Gluteal Arteries (branches of the Internal Iliac Artery)

✋ PALPATION

1. With the client prone, place palpating hand just lateral to the sacrum, at a point halfway between the posterior superior iliac spine (PSIS) and the apex of the sacrum.
2. Flex the client's leg at the knee joint to 90 degrees. Then have the client laterally rotate the thigh at the hip joint against gentle resistance and feel for the contraction of the piriformis. (Note: Lateral rotation of the thigh at the hip joint involves the client's foot moving medially, toward the opposite side of the body.)
3. Continue palpating the piriformis laterally toward the greater trochanter of the femur.

■ RELATIONSHIP TO OTHER STRUCTURES

- ☐ The piriformis is deep to the gluteus maximus.
- ☐ The piriformis is located between the gluteus medius (which is superior to it) and the superior gemellus (which is inferior to it).
- ☐ The piriformis is involved with the deep front line myofascial meridian.

■ MISCELLANEOUS

1. Probably the most common method to stretch the piriformis is to have the client supine with the foot flat on the table (i.e., the thigh flexed at the hip joint and the leg flexed at the knee joint); then horizontally flex (horizontally adduct) the client's thigh toward the opposite side of the body.
2. The piriformis can change from being a lateral rotator of the thigh at the hip joint to a medial rotator of the thigh at the hip joint (if the thigh is first flexed at the hip joint); therefore the method of stretching the piriformis varies with the position of the client's thigh. If the client's thigh is flexed, lateral rotation must be used to stretch the piriformis. If the client's thigh is not flexed, medial rotation would be used. The thigh must be flexed to at least 60 degrees for the piriformis to become a medial rotator of the thigh.
3. The piriformis sometimes blends with the gluteus medius.
4. The piriformis often protectively tightens when the client's sacroiliac joint is sprained.
5. The relationship of the sciatic nerve to the piriformis varies. The sciatic nerve normally exits from the pelvis between the piriformis and the superior gemellus. However, in approximately 10% to 20% of individuals, the common fibular portion of the sciatic nerve (occasionally even the entire sciatic nerve) may pierce the piriformis muscle, exiting through the middle of it. Some sources believe this makes the sciatic nerve more susceptible to being compressed if the piriformis is tight; others do not. When the piriformis does compress the sciatic nerve, regardless of the relationship between the piriformis and the sciatic nerve, this condition is called *piriformis syndrome* and can result in symptoms of *sciatica*.

14

Superior Gemellus (of Deep Lateral Rotator Group)

The name, superior gemellus, *tells us that this muscle is the more superior muscle of a pair of similar muscles.*

Derivation	☐ superior: L. *upper.*
	gemellus: L. *twin.*
Pronunciation	☐ su-PEE-ree-or, jee-MEL-us

■ ATTACHMENTS

☐ **Ischial Spine**

to the

☐ **Greater Trochanter of the Femur**
   ☐ the medial surface

■ FUNCTIONS

CONCENTRIC (SHORTENING) MOVER ACTIONS	
Standard Mover Actions	**Reverse Mover Actions**
☐ **1. Laterally rotates the thigh at the hip joint**	☐ **1. Contralaterally rotates the pelvis at the hip joint**
☐ 2. Horizontally extends the thigh at the hip joint	

Standard Mover Action Notes

- The superior gemellus wraps around the posterior pelvis to attach laterally onto the greater trochanter of the femur (with its fibers running horizontally in the transverse plane). When the superior gemellus contracts, it pulls the greater trochanter posteromedially, causing the anterior surface of the thigh to face laterally. Therefore the superior gemellus laterally rotates the thigh at the hip joint. (Note the similarity of the direction of fibers of the superior gemellus to the direction of fibers of the piriformis.) (action 1)
- As with the piriformis, if the thigh is already flexed, the orientation of the line of pull of the superior gemellus to the femur changes. The fibers (running horizontally) can now pull the femur away from the midline in the frontal plane. Therefore the superior gemellus horizontally extends (i.e., horizontally abducts) the thigh at the hip joint. (action 2)

Reverse Mover Action Note

- The superior gemellus crosses the hip joint posteriorly (with its fibers running somewhat horizontally in the transverse plane). When the femoral attachment is fixed and the superior gemellus contracts, it pulls on the pelvis, causing the anterior pelvis to face the opposite side of the body from the side of the body on which the superior gemellus is attached. Therefore the superior gemellus contralaterally rotates the pelvis at the hip joint. Contralateral rotation of the pelvis is functionally important when a person is walking or running and changes direction. (reverse action 1)

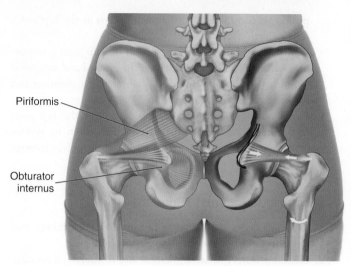

Figure 14-22 Posterior view. The superior gemellus is shown on both sides. The piriformis and obturator internus have been ghosted in on the left.

Eccentric Antagonist Functions

1. Restrains/slows medial rotation and horizontal flexion of the thigh at the hip joint
2. Restrains/slows ipsilateral rotation of the pelvis at the hip joint

Isometric Stabilization Functions

1. Stabilizes the thigh and pelvis at the hip joint
2. Stabilizes the subtalar joint

Isometric Stabilization Function Note

- A force of lateral rotation of the thigh at the hip joint prevents medial rotation of the thigh and entire lower extremity, including the talus at the subtalar joint, if the foot overly pronates (if the arch of the foot collapses).

Additional Notes on Functions

1. All six members of the deep lateral rotator group can, as their name implies, laterally rotate the thigh (and contralaterally rotate the pelvis) at the hip joint.
2. The piriformis, superior gemellus, obturator internus, and inferior gemellus can all horizontally extend (horizontally abduct) the thigh at the hip joint if the thigh is flexed.

INNERVATION
☐ Nerve to Obturator Internus (of the Lumbosacral Plexus)
   ☐ L5, S1

ARTERIAL SUPPLY
☐ The Inferior Gluteal Artery (a branch of the Internal Iliac Artery)

Superior Gemellus (of Deep Lateral Rotator Group)—*cont'd*

PALPATION

1. With the client prone, place palpating fingers just inferior to the piriformis.
2. Flex the client's leg at the knee joint to 90 degrees.
3. Then have the client laterally rotate the thigh at the hip joint against gentle resistance and feel for the contraction of the superior gemellus. It is difficult to discern the superior gemellus from the other nearby deep lateral rotators. (Note: Lateral rotation of the thigh at the hip joint involves the client's foot moving medially, toward the opposite side of the body.)

■ RELATIONSHIP TO OTHER STRUCTURES

☐ The superior gemellus lies between the piriformis (which is superior to it) and the obturator internus (which is inferior to it).
☐ The sciatic nerve normally exits the pelvis between the piriformis and the superior gemellus.
☐ The superior gemellus is involved with the deep front line myofascial meridian.

■ MISCELLANEOUS

1. The lateral tendons of the superior gemellus, obturator internus, and inferior gemellus usually blend together.

14

Obturator Internus (of Deep Lateral Rotator Group)

The name, obturator internus, *tells us that this muscle attaches to the internal surface of the obturator foramen.*

Derivation	☐ obturator: L. *to stop up, obstruct (refers to the obturator foramen).*
	internus: L. *inner.*
Pronunciation	☐ ob-too-RAY-tor, in-TER-nus

■ ATTACHMENTS

☐ **Internal Surface of the Pelvic Bone Surrounding the Obturator Foramen**
  ☐ the internal surfaces of the margin of the obturator foramen, the obturator membrane, the ischium, the pubis, and the ilium

to the

☐ **Greater Trochanter of the Femur**
  ☐ the medial surface

■ FUNCTIONS

CONCENTRIC (SHORTENING) MOVER ACTIONS	
Standard Mover Actions	**Reverse Mover Actions**
☐ 1. Laterally rotates the thigh at the hip joint	☐ 1. Contralaterally rotates the pelvis at the hip joint
☐ 2. Horizontally extends the thigh at the hip joint	

Standard Mover Action Notes

- The obturator internus wraps around the posterior pelvis to attach laterally onto the greater trochanter of the femur (with its fibers running horizontally in the transverse plane). When the obturator internus contracts, it pulls the greater trochanter posteromedially, causing the anterior surface of the thigh to face laterally. Therefore the obturator internus laterally rotates the thigh at the hip joint. (Note the similarity of the direction of fibers of the obturator internus to the direction of fibers of the other deep lateral rotators.) (action 1)
- As with the piriformis and the superior gemellus, if the thigh is already flexed, the orientation of the line of pull of the obturator internus to the femur changes. The fibers (running horizontally) can now pull the femur away from the midline in the frontal plane. Therefore the obturator internus horizontally extends (i.e., horizontally abducts) the thigh at the hip joint. (action 2)

Reverse Mover Action Note

- The obturator internus crosses the hip joint posteriorly (with its fibers running somewhat horizontally in the transverse plane). When the femoral attachment is fixed and the obtu-

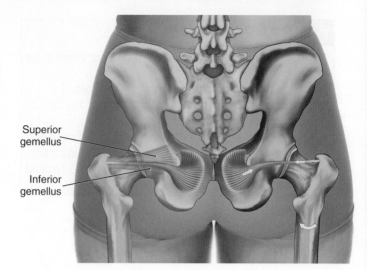

Superior gemellus

Inferior gemellus

Figure 14-23 Posterior view. The obturator internus is shown on both sides. The superior gemellus and inferior gemellus have been ghosted in on the left.

rator internus contracts, it pulls on the pelvis, causing the anterior pelvis to face the opposite side of the body from the side of the body to which the obturator internus is attached. Therefore the obturator internus contralaterally rotates the pelvis at the hip joint. Contralateral rotation of the pelvis is functionally important when a person is walking or running and changes direction. (reverse action 1)

Eccentric Antagonist Functions

1. Restrains/slows medial rotation and horizontal flexion of the thigh at the hip joint
2. Restrains/slows ipsilateral rotation of the pelvis at the hip joint

Isometric Stabilization Functions

1. Stabilizes the thigh and pelvis at the hip joint
2. Stabilizes the subtalar joint

Isometric Stabilization Function Note

- A force of lateral rotation of the thigh at the hip joint prevents medial rotation of the thigh and entire lower extremity, including the talus at the subtalar joint, if the foot overly pronates (if the arch of the foot collapses).

Additional Notes on Functions

1. All six members of the deep lateral rotator group can, as their name implies, laterally rotate the thigh (and contralaterally rotate the pelvis) at the hip joint.
2. The piriformis, superior gemellus, obturator internus, and inferior gemellus can all horizontally extend (horizontally abduct) the thigh at the hip joint if the thigh is flexed.

14

Obturator Internus (of Deep Lateral Rotator Group)—*cont'd*

INNERVATION
- ☐ Nerve to Obturator Internus (of the Lumbosacral Plexus)
  - ☐ L5, **S1**

ARTERIAL SUPPLY
- ☐ The Superior and Inferior Gluteal Arteries (branches of the Internal Iliac Artery)
  - ☐ and the Obturator Artery (a branch of the Internal Iliac Artery)

✋ PALPATION

1. With the client prone, place palpating fingers inferior to the piriformis and the superior gemellus.
2. Flex the client's leg at the knee joint to 90 degrees. Then have the client laterally rotate the thigh at the hip joint against gentle resistance and feel for the contraction of the obturator internus. It is difficult to discern the obturator internus from the other nearby deep lateral rotators. (Note: Lateral rotation of the thigh at the hip joint involves the client's foot moving medially, toward the opposite side of the body.)

■ RELATIONSHIP TO OTHER STRUCTURES

- ☐ The obturator internus begins inside the pelvis and exits the pelvis through the lesser sciatic foramen. It wraps around the ischium between the ischial spine and the ischial tuberosity to join the other lateral rotators of the thigh.
- ☐ The obturator internus lies between the two gemelli muscles. It is directly inferior to the superior gemellus and directly superior to the inferior gemellus.
- ☐ The obturator internus is involved with the deep front line myofascial meridian.

■ MISCELLANEOUS

1. *Obturator* means to stop up or obstruct. The obturator foramen is obstructed by the obturator membrane, as well as by the obturator internus and obturator externus.
2. The lateral tendons of the superior gemellus, obturator internus, and inferior gemellus usually blend together.
3. The obturator internus has a much larger pelvic attachment than the obturator externus.
4. The obturator internus has a tendon that makes an abrupt turn of 90 degrees or more. (Other muscles that do this are the fibularis longus, tibialis posterior, flexor digitorum longus, flexor hallucis longus, tensor palati, and superior oblique.)
5. If the opportunity to attend a cadaver lab workshop occurs, it can be an invaluable experience to actually see and feel the muscles and other tissues of the body that are abstractly studied in books. In cadaver dissection, the obturator internus can usually be readily identified and discerned from the other muscles of the deep lateral rotators of the thigh group by the shiny appearance of its lateral tendon.
6. The obturator internus is multipennate.

14

Inferior Gemellus (of Deep Lateral Rotator Group)

The name, inferior gemellus, *tells us that this muscle is the more inferior muscle of a pair of similar muscles.*

Derivation	☐ inferior: L. *lower.*
	gemellus: L. *twin.*
Pronunciation	☐ in-FEE-ree-or, jee-MEL-us

■ ATTACHMENTS

☐ **Ischial Tuberosity**
   ☐ the superior aspect

to the

☐ **Greater Trochanter of the Femur**
   ☐ the medial surface

■ FUNCTIONS

CONCENTRIC (SHORTENING) MOVER ACTIONS	
Standard Mover Actions	**Reverse Mover Actions**
☐ 1. Laterally rotates the thigh at the hip joint	☐ 1. Contralaterally rotates the pelvis at the hip joint
☐ 2. Horizontally extends the thigh at the hip joint	

Standard Mover Action Notes

- The inferior gemellus wraps around the posterior pelvis to attach laterally onto the greater trochanter (with its fibers running horizontally in the transverse plane). When the inferior gemellus contracts, it pulls the greater trochanter posteromedially, causing the anterior surface of the thigh to face laterally. Therefore the inferior gemellus laterally rotates the thigh at the hip joint. (Note the similarity of the direction of fibers of the inferior gemellus to the direction of fibers of the other deep lateral rotators.) (action 1)
- As with the piriformis, superior gemellus, and obturator internus, if the thigh is already flexed, the orientation of the line of pull of the inferior gemellus to the femur changes. The fibers (running horizontally) can now pull the femur away from the midline in the frontal plane. Therefore the inferior gemellus horizontally extends (i.e., horizontally abducts) the thigh at the hip joint. (action 2)

Reverse Mover Action Note

- The inferior gemellus crosses the hip joint posteriorly (with its fibers running somewhat horizontally in the transverse plane). When the femoral attachment is fixed, and the inferior gemellus contracts, it pulls on the pelvis, causing the anterior pelvis to face the opposite side of the body from the side to which the inferior gemellus is attached. Therefore the inferior gemellus contralaterally rotates the pelvis at the hip

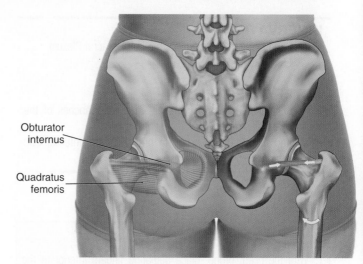

Figure 14-24 Posterior view. The inferior gemellus is shown on both sides. The obturator internus and quadratus femoris have been ghosted in on the left.

Obturator internus

Quadratus femoris

joint. Contralateral rotation of the pelvis is functionally important when a person is walking or running and changes direction. (reverse action 1)

Eccentric Antagonist Functions

1. Restrains/slows medial rotation and horizontal flexion of the thigh the hip joint
2. Restrains/slows ipsilateral rotation of the pelvis at the hip joint

Isometric Stabilization Functions

1. Stabilizes the thigh and pelvis at the hip joint
2. Stabilizes the subtalar joint

Isometric Stabilization Function Note

- A force of lateral rotation of the thigh at the hip joint prevents medial rotation of the thigh and entire lower extremity, including the talus at the subtalar joint, if the foot overly pronates (if the arch of the foot collapses).

Additional Notes on Functions

1. All six members of the deep lateral rotator group can, as their name implies, laterally rotate the thigh (and contralaterally rotate the pelvis) at the hip joint.
2. The piriformis, superior gemellus, obturator internus, and inferior gemellus can all horizontally extend (horizontally abduct) the thigh at the hip joint if the thigh is flexed.

Inferior Gemellus (of Deep Lateral Rotator Group)—*cont'd*

INNERVATION
☐ Nerve to Quadratus Femoris (of the Lumbosacral Plexus)
  ☐ L5, S1

ARTERIAL SUPPLY
☐ The Inferior Gluteal Artery (a branch of the Internal Iliac Artery)
  ☐ and the Obturator Artery (a branch of the Internal Iliac Artery)

🖑 PALPATION

1. With the client prone, place palpating fingers just lateral and slightly superior to the superior margin of the ischial tuberosity.
2. Flex the client's leg at the knee joint to 90 degrees. Then have the client laterally rotate the thigh at the hip joint against gentle resistance and feel for the contraction of the inferior gemellus. It is difficult to discern the inferior gemellus from the other nearby deep lateral rotators. (Note: Lateral rotation of the thigh at the hip joint involves the client's foot moving medially, toward the opposite side of the body.)

■ RELATIONSHIP TO OTHER STRUCTURES

☐ The inferior gemellus is inferior to the obturator internus.
☐ The inferior gemellus is superior to the obturator externus and the quadratus femoris.
☐ The inferior gemellus is involved with the deep front line myofascial meridian.

■ MISCELLANEOUS

1. The lateral tendons of the superior gemellus, obturator internus, and inferior gemellus usually blend together.

14

Obturator Externus (of Deep Lateral Rotator Group)

The name, obturator externus, *tells us that this muscle attaches to the external surface of the obturator foramen.*

Derivation	☐ obturator: L. *to stop up, obstruct (refers to the obturator foramen).*
	externus: L. *outer.*
Pronunciation	☐ ob-too-RAY-tor, ex-TER-nus

■ ATTACHMENTS

☐ **External Surface of the Pelvic Bone Surrounding the Obturator Foramen**
  ☐ the external surfaces of the margin of the obturator foramen on the ischium and the pubis, and the obturator membrane

to the

☐ **Trochanteric Fossa of the Femur**

■ FUNCTIONS

CONCENTRIC (SHORTENING) MOVER ACTIONS	
Standard Mover Actions	**Reverse Mover Actions**
☐ 1. Laterally rotates the thigh at the hip joint	☐ 1. Contralaterally rotates the pelvis at the hip joint
☐ 2. Adducts the thigh at the hip joint	☐ 2. Elevates the same-side pelvis at the hip joint

Standard Mover Action Notes

• The obturator externus wraps around the posterior pelvis to attach laterally onto the femur (with its fibers running horizontally in the transverse plane). When the obturator externus contracts, it pulls the greater trochanter posteromedially, causing the anterior surface of the thigh to face laterally. Therefore the obturator externus laterally rotates the thigh at the hip joint. (Note the similarity of the direction of fibers of the obturator externus to the direction of fibers of the other deep lateral rotators.) (action 1)

• The obturator externus attaches far enough distally to be below the center of the hip joint. Therefore it can adduct the thigh at the hip joint. (action 2)

Reverse Mover Action Notes

• The obturator externus crosses the hip joint posteriorly (with its fibers running somewhat horizontally in the transverse plane). When the femoral attachment is fixed and the obturator externus contracts, it pulls on the pelvis, causing the anterior pelvis to face the opposite side of the body from the side to which the obturator externus is attached. Therefore the obturator externus contralaterally rotates the pelvis at the

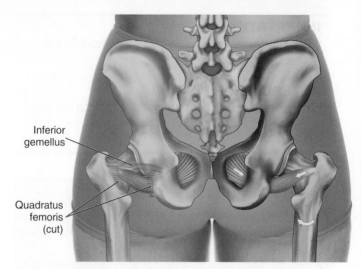

Figure 14-25 Posterior view. The obturator externus is shown on both sides. The inferior gemellus and quadratus femoris (cut) have been ghosted in on the left.

hip joint. Contralateral rotation of the pelvis is functionally important when a person is walking or running and changes direction. (reverse action 1)

• With the distal femoral attachment fixed, the obturator externus pulls the medial aspect of the pelvic bone inferiorly toward the medial thigh, resulting in elevation of the same-side pelvis at the hip joint. Note: Elevation of one side of the pelvis causes the other side to depress. (reverse action 2)

Eccentric Antagonist Functions

1. Restrains/slows medial rotation and abduction of the thigh at the hip joint
2. Restrains/slows ipsilateral rotation and depression of the same-side pelvis at the hip joint

Isometric Stabilization Functions

1. Stabilizes the thigh and pelvis at the hip joint
2. Stabilizes the subtalar joint

Isometric Stabilization Function Note

• A force of lateral rotation of the thigh at the hip joint prevents medial rotation of the thigh and entire lower extremity, including the talus at the subtalar joint, if the foot overly pronates (if the arch of the foot collapses).

Additional Note on Functions

1. All six members of the deep lateral rotator group can, as their name implies, laterally rotate the thigh (and contralaterally rotate the pelvis) at the hip joint.

Obturator Externus (of Deep Lateral Rotator Group)—*cont'd*

INNERVATION
☐ The Obturator Nerve
   ☐ L3, **L4**

ARTERIAL SUPPLY
☐ The Obturator Artery (a branch of the Internal Iliac Artery)

✋ PALPATION

1. With the client prone, place palpating fingers slightly lateral to the superior margin of the ischial tuberosity.
2. Flex the client's leg at the knee joint to 90 degrees. Then have the client laterally rotate the thigh at the hip joint against gentle resistance and feel for the contraction of the obturator externus. It is difficult to discern the obturator externus from the other nearby deep lateral rotators. (Note: Lateral rotation of the thigh at the hip joint will involve the client's foot moving medially, toward the opposite side of the body.)

■ RELATIONSHIP TO OTHER STRUCTURES

☐ The obturator externus is directly inferior to the inferior gemellus.
☐ From the posterior perspective, the obturator externus is deep to the quadratus femoris and is either entirely covered or nearly entirely covered by it.
☐ From the anterior perspective, the obturator externus is directly deep to the pectineus.
☐ The obturator externus is involved with the deep front line myofascial meridian.

■ MISCELLANEOUS

1. *Obturator* means to stop up or obstruct. The obturator foramen is obstructed by the obturator membrane, as well as by the obturator internus and obturator externus.
2. The obturator externus is the only muscle of the deep lateral rotator group that is not visible in the second layer of the posterior pelvic muscles. It is either entirely covered or nearly entirely covered by the quadratus femoris. When the obturator externus is visible in this layer, it is located between the inferior gemellus and the quadratus femoris.
3. The obturator externus is the only deep lateral rotator that is not innervated by the lumbosacral plexus. It is innervated by the obturator nerve.

14

Quadratus Femoris (of Deep Lateral Rotator Group)

The name, quadratus femoris, *tells us that this muscle is square in shape and attaches to the femur.*

Derivation	□ quadratus: L. *squared.*
	femoris: L. *refers to the femur.*
Pronunciation	□ kwod-RATE-us, FEM-o-ris

■ ATTACHMENTS

□ **Ischial Tuberosity**
  □ the lateral border

to the

□ **Intertrochanteric Crest of the Femur**

■ FUNCTIONS

CONCENTRIC (SHORTENING) MOVER ACTIONS	
Standard Mover Actions	**Reverse Mover Actions**
□ **1. Laterally rotates the thigh at the hip joint**	□ **1. Contralaterally rotates the pelvis at the hip joint**
□ 2. Adducts the thigh at the hip joint	□ 2. Elevates the same-side pelvis at the hip joint

Standard Mover Action Notes

• The quadratus femoris wraps around the posterior pelvis to attach laterally onto the femur (with its fibers running horizontally in the transverse plane). When the quadratus femoris contracts, it pulls the greater trochanter posteromedially, causing the anterior surface of the thigh to face laterally. Therefore the quadratus femoris laterally rotates the thigh at the hip joint. (Note the similarity of the direction of fibers of the quadratus femoris to the direction of fibers of the other deep lateral rotators.) (action 1)

• The quadratus femoris attaches sufficiently inferior on the pelvis and distal on the femur to cross the hip joint medially below the center of the joint (with its fibers running horizontally in the frontal plane). When the quadratus femoris contracts, it pulls the lateral attachment (i.e., the thigh) medially in the frontal plane. Therefore the quadratus femoris adducts the thigh at the hip joint. (action 2)

Reverse Mover Action Notes

• The quadratus femoris crosses the hip joint posteriorly (with its fibers running somewhat horizontally in the transverse plane). When the femoral attachment is fixed and the quadratus femoris contracts, it pulls on the pelvis, causing the anterior pelvis to face the opposite side of the body from the side to which the quadratus femoris is attached. Therefore the quadratus femoris contralaterally rotates the pelvis at the hip joint. (reverse action 1)

• Contralateral rotation of the pelvis at the hip joint is important whenever a foot is planted on the ground and the pelvis

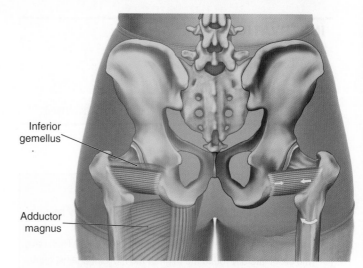

Figure 14-26 Posterior view. The quadratus femoris is shown on both sides. The inferior gemellus and adductor magnus have been ghosted in on the left.

is rotated to the opposite side, such as when planting and cutting in sports. (reverse action 1)

• With the distal femoral attachment fixed, the quadratus femoris pulls the medial aspect of the pelvic bone inferiorly toward the medial thigh, resulting in elevation of the same-side pelvis at the hip joint. Note: Elevation of one side of the pelvis causes the other side to depress. (reverse action 2)

Eccentric Antagonist Functions

1. Restrains/slows medial rotation and abduction of the thigh at the hip joint
2. Restrains/slows ipsilateral rotation and depression of the same-side pelvis at the hip joint

Isometric Stabilization Functions

1. Stabilizes the thigh and pelvis at the hip joint
2. Stabilizes the subtalar joint

Isometric Stabilization Function Note

• A force of lateral rotation of the thigh at the hip joint prevents medial rotation of the thigh and entire lower extremity, including the talus at the subtalar joint, if the foot overly pronates (if the arch of the foot collapses).

Additional Notes on Functions

1. All six members of the deep lateral rotator group can, as their name implies, laterally rotate the thigh (and contralaterally rotate the pelvis) at the hip joint.
2. If the thigh is in a position of flexion at the hip joint, the quadratus femoris can extend the thigh back to anatomical position.

14

Quadratus Femoris (of Deep Lateral Rotator Group)—*cont'd*

INNERVATION
- ☐ Nerve to Quadratus Femoris (of the Lumbosacral Plexus)
  - ☐ L5, S1

ARTERIAL SUPPLY
- ☐ The Inferior Gluteal Artery (a branch of the Internal Iliac Artery)
  - ☐ and the Obturator Artery (a branch of the Internal Iliac Artery)

✋ PALPATION

1. With the client prone, place palpating fingers on the lateral side of the ischial tuberosity.
2. Flex the client's leg at the knee joint to 90 degrees. Then have the client laterally rotate the thigh at the hip joint against gentle resistance and feel for the contraction of the quadratus femoris. (Note: Lateral rotation of the thigh at the hip joint will involve the client's foot moving medially, toward the opposite side of the body.)
3. Be aware that the sciatic nerve usually courses over the quadratus femoris.

■ RELATIONSHIP TO OTHER STRUCTURES

- ☐ The quadratus femoris is directly inferior to the inferior gemellus and directly superior to the adductor magnus.
- ☐ From the posterior perspective, the quadratus femoris is superficial to and either entirely covers or nearly entirely covers the obturator externus.
- ☐ The sciatic nerve runs vertically, superficial to the quadratus femoris.
- ☐ The quadratus femoris is involved with the deep front line myofascial meridian.

■ MISCELLANEOUS

1. The quadratus femoris is a fairly massive muscle; it is usually larger than the superior gemellus, obturator internus, and inferior gemellus combined. It is often larger than the piriformis.

14

Muscles of the Knee Joint

CHAPTER OUTLINE

CHAPTER OVERVIEW

The muscles addressed in this chapter are the muscles whose principal function is usually considered to be movement of the knee joint. Other muscles in the body can also move the knee joint, but they are placed in different chapters because their primary function is usually considered to be at another joint. These muscles are the sartorius and gracilis (covered in Chapter 14) and the gastrocnemius and plantaris (covered in Chapter 16). Note: The hamstring group and the rectus femoris of the quadriceps femoris group (covered in this chapter) also cross the hip joint and therefore move the thigh and pelvis at the hip joint.

Overview of Structure
- Structurally, muscles of the knee joint are generally classified as being either anterior or posterior. The quadriceps femoris group and the articularis genus are located anteriorly. The hamstring group and the popliteus are located posteriorly.

Overview of Function
The following general rules regarding actions can be stated for the functional groups of muscles of the knee joint:
- If a muscle crosses the knee joint anteriorly with a vertical direction to its fibers, it can extend the leg at the knee joint by moving the anterior surface of the leg toward the anterior surface of the thigh.
- If a muscle crosses the knee joint posteriorly with a vertical direction to its fibers, it can flex the leg at the knee joint by moving the posterior surface of the leg toward the posterior surface of the thigh.
- If a muscle wraps around the knee joint, it can rotate the knee joint (the knee joint can only rotate if it is first flexed). Medial rotators attach to the medial side of the leg.
- The biceps femoris is the only lateral rotator and attaches to the lateral side of the leg.
- Reverse actions are common at the knee joint and tend to occur when the foot is planted on the ground, causing the distal attachment to be fixed and therefore the proximal attachment (the thigh) to be mobile and move toward the distal attachment (the leg).
- The reverse action of extension of the leg at the knee joint is extension of the thigh at the knee joint in which the anterior surface of the thigh moves toward the anterior surface of the leg. This occurs every time we stand up from a seated position.
- The reverse action of flexion of the leg at the knee joint is flexion of the thigh at the knee joint in which the posterior surface of the thigh moves toward the posterior surface of the leg.
- The reverse action of medial rotation of the leg at the knee joint is lateral rotation of the thigh at the knee joint; the reverse action of lateral rotation of the leg at the knee joint is medial rotation of the thigh at the knee joint.

Review the muscles and bones from this chapter on the enclosed CD!

Anterior Views of the Muscles of the Knee Joint

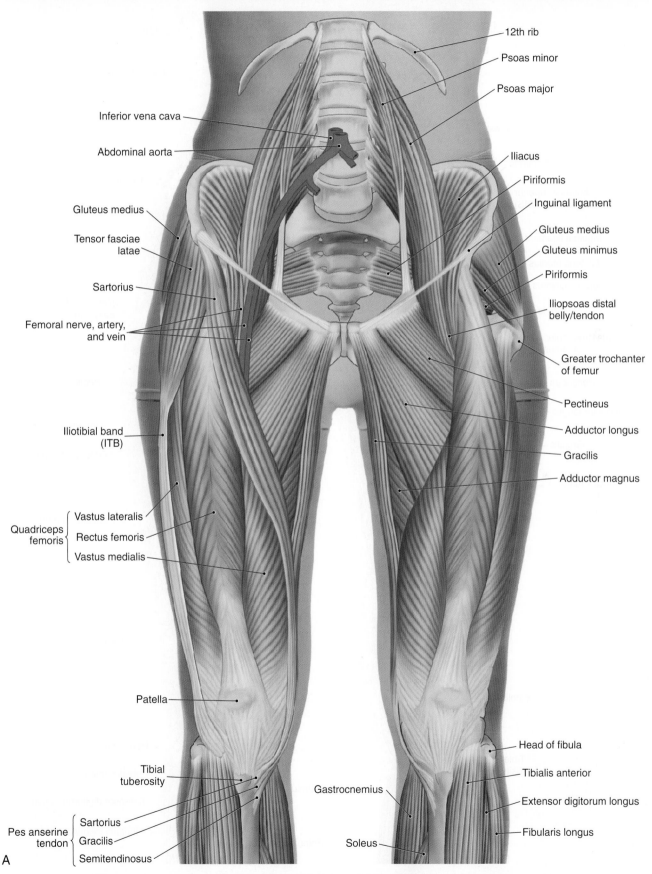

Figure 15-1 Anterior views of the muscles of the knee joint. **A,** Superficial and intermediate views.

Anterior Views of the Muscles of the Knee Joint—*cont'd*

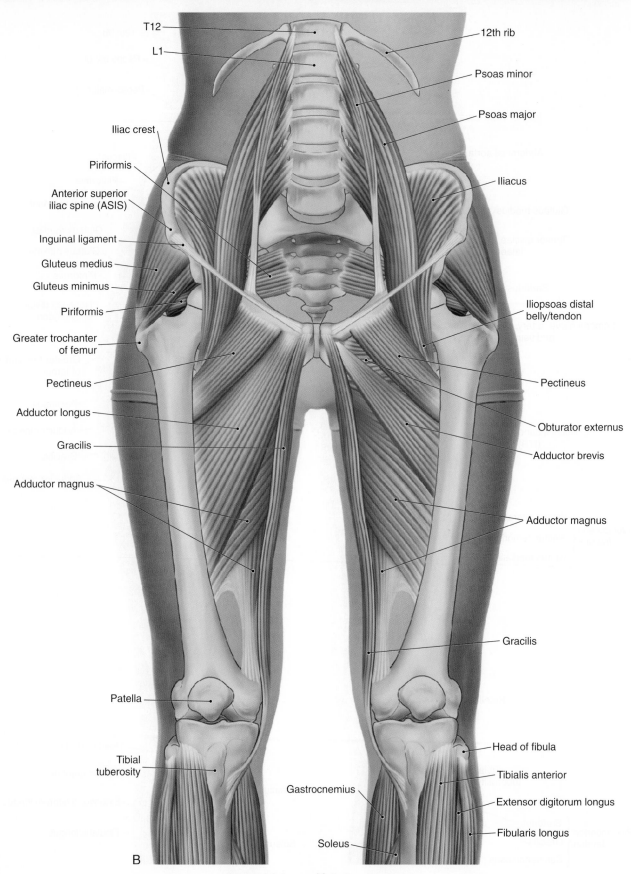

15

T12

L1

Iliac crest

Piriformis

Anterior superior
iliac spine (ASIS)

Inguinal ligament

Gluteus medius

Gluteus minimus

Piriformis

Greater trochanter
of femur

Pectineus

Adductor longus

Gracilis

Adductor magnus

Patella

Tibial
tuberosity

Gastrocnemius

Soleus

12th rib

Psoas minor

Psoas major

Iliacus

Iliopsoas distal
belly/tendon

Pectineus

Obturator externus

Adductor brevis

Adductor magnus

Gracilis

Head of fibula

Tibialis anterior

Extensor digitorum longus

Fibularis longus

B

Figure 15-1, cont'd B, Deeper views.

Posterior Views of the Muscles of the Knee Joint

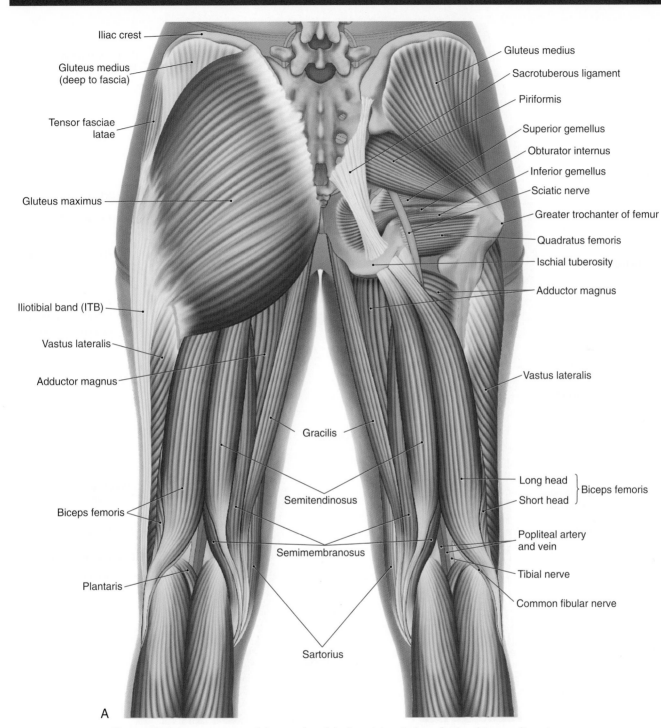

Iliac crest

Gluteus medius
(deep to fascia)

Tensor fasciae
latae

Gluteus maximus

Iliotibial band (ITB)

Vastus lateralis

Adductor magnus

Biceps femoris

Plantaris

Gluteus medius

Sacrotuberous ligament

Piriformis

Superior gemellus

Obturator internus

Inferior gemellus

Sciatic nerve

Greater trochanter of femur

Quadratus femoris

Ischial tuberosity

Adductor magnus

Vastus lateralis

Gracilis

Semitendinosus

Semimembranosus

Sartorius

Long head ⎫
            ⎬ Biceps femoris
Short head ⎭

Popliteal artery
and vein

Tibial nerve

Common fibular nerve

A

Figure 15-2 Posterior views of the muscles of the knee joint. **A,** Superficial and intermediate views.

Posterior Views of the Muscles of the Knee Joint—*cont'd*

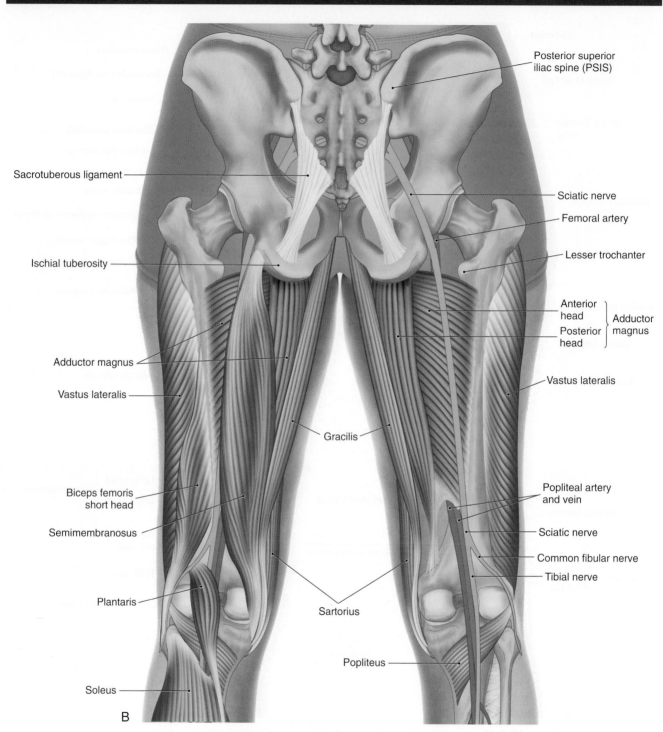

Figure 15-2, cont'd B, Deeper views.

Lateral Views of the Muscles of the Right Knee Joint

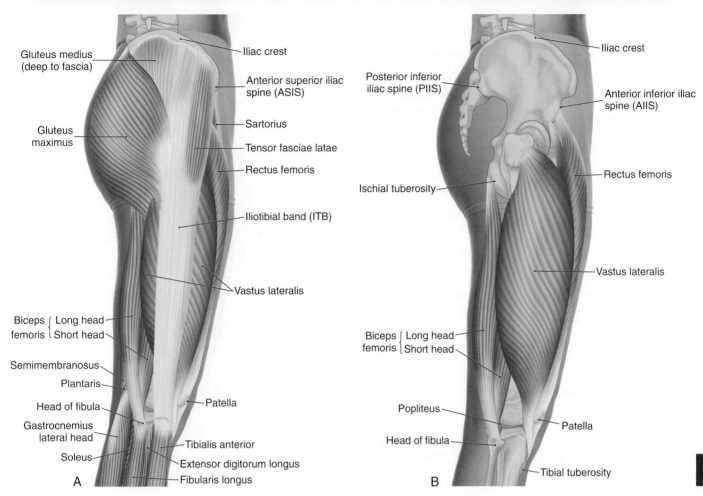

Figure 15-3 Lateral views of the muscles of the right knee joint. **A,** Superficial. **B,** Deep.

15

Medial Views of the Muscles of the Right Knee Joint

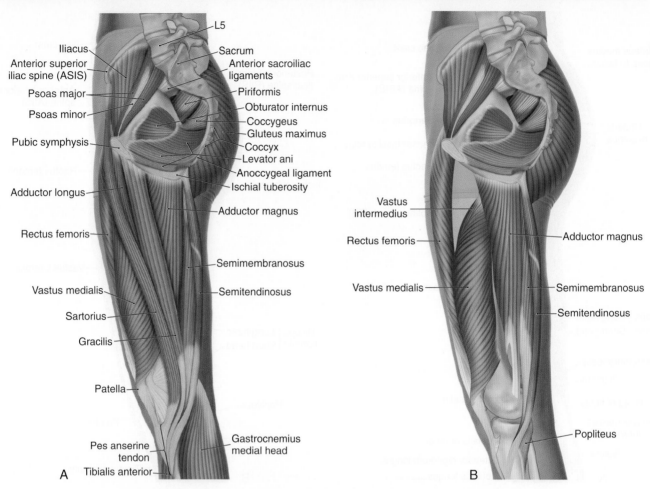

Figure 15-4 Medial views of the muscles of the right knee joint. **A,** Superficial. **B,** Deep.

Transverse Plane Cross Sections of the Muscles of the Right Thigh

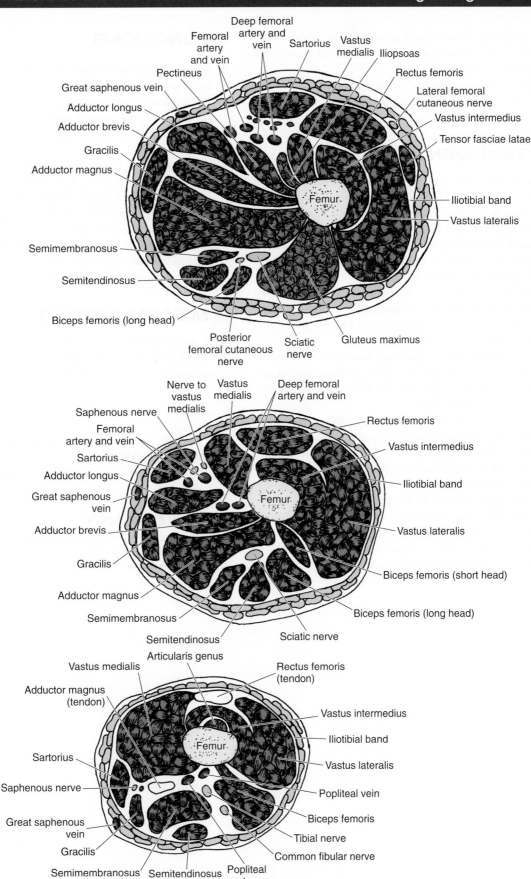

Figure 15-5 Transverse plane cross sections of the muscles of the right thigh. **A,** Proximal. **B,** Middle. **C,** Distal.

Quadriceps Femoris Group (Quads)

- The quadriceps femoris are a group of muscles that wrap around nearly the entire shaft of the femur and are superficial in the anterior thigh.
- There are four quadriceps femoris muscles: the rectus femoris, vastus lateralis, vastus medialis, and vastus intermedius.

■ ATTACHMENTS

- These muscles are grouped together as the quadriceps femoris, because they all attach distally onto the patella and then onto the tibial tuberosity via the patellar ligament. The patella is a sesamoid bone that formed within the distal tendon of the quadriceps femoris group. Therefore the patellar ligament is actually a continuation of the distal tendon of the quadriceps femoris.
- The quadriceps femoris have additional distal fibers (primarily from the vastus lateralis, vastus medialis, and vastus intermedius) called *retinacular fibers* that attach onto the lateral and medial condyles of the tibia.
- Keep in mind that *vastus* quadriceps femoris muscles attach onto the linea aspera. Therefore although these muscles are superficial anteriorly, they are also located in the lateral, medial, and posterior thigh.
- The names of the quadriceps femoris muscles generally refer to where they are located relative to each other. The vastus lateralis is more lateral, the vastus medialis is more medial, and the vastus intermedius is between the other two. The rectus femoris is straight (*rectus* means straight) up and down (proximal to distal) over the femur.
- From the anterior perspective, the rectus femoris is the most superficial of the quadriceps femoris muscles.
- All four quadriceps femoris muscles are located within the superficial front line myofascial meridian.

■ FUNCTIONS

- As a group, all four quadriceps femoris muscles extend the leg at the knee joint.
- Because it is the only quadriceps femoris muscle that crosses the hip joint, the rectus femoris is the only one that can move the thigh at the hip joint and/or move the pelvis at the hip joint.
- The reason that the quadriceps femoris are so large and strong is not just to move the leg into extension at the knee joint but rather to do the reverse action, in other words, move the thigh into extension at the knee joint. This happens every time a person stands up from a seated position. To move the thigh at the knee joint requires moving the entire body along with the thigh; hence the quadriceps femoris group needs to be very large and strong.

■ MISCELLANEOUS

- If the quadriceps femoris group is considered to be one muscle, it is the largest muscle in the human body (being appreciably larger than the gluteus maximus).

INNERVATION
- The quadriceps femoris group is innervated by the femoral nerve.

ARTERIAL SUPPLY
- The quadriceps femoris group receives its blood supply from the femoral artery and the deep femoral artery.

Views of the Quadriceps Femoris Group

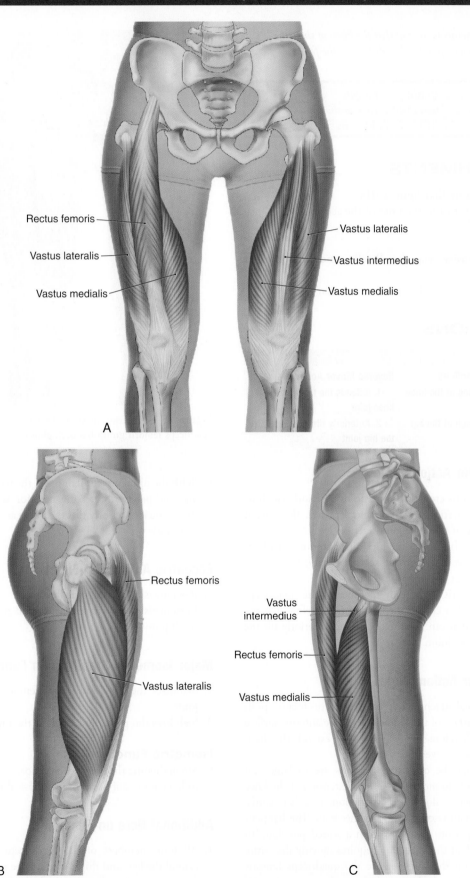

Figure 15-6 Views of the quadriceps femoris group. **A,** Anterior views; superficial on the right and deep on the left. **B,** Lateral view of the right thigh. **C,** Medial view of the right thigh.

15

Rectus Femoris (of Quadriceps Femoris Group)

The name, rectus femoris, *tells us that the fibers of this muscle run straight up and down (proximal to distal) on the femur.*

Derivation	☐ rectus: L. *straight.* femoris: L. *refers to the femur.*
Pronunciation	☐ REK-tus, FEM-o-ris

■ ATTACHMENTS

☐ **Anterior Inferior Iliac Spine (AIIS)**
 ☐ and just superior to the brim of the acetabulum

 to the

☐ **Tibial Tuberosity via the Patella and the Patellar Ligament**
 ☐ and the tibial condyles via the retinacular fibers

■ FUNCTIONS

CONCENTRIC (SHORTENING) MOVER ACTIONS	
Standard Mover Actions	**Reverse Mover Actions**
☐ 1. Extends the leg at the knee joint	☐ 1. Extends the thigh at the knee joint
☐ 2. Flexes the thigh at the hip joint	☐ 2. Anteriorly tilts the pelvis at the hip joint

Standard Mover Actions Notes

- The rectus femoris crosses the knee joint anteriorly (with its fibers running vertically in the sagittal plane); therefore it extends the leg at the knee joint. (action 1)
- The rectus femoris crosses the hip joint anteriorly (with its fibers running vertically in the sagittal plane); therefore it flexes the thigh at the hip joint. (action 2)
- The rectus femoris is the only member of the quadriceps femoris group that crosses the hip joint. Therefore it is the only member that can flex the thigh (and anteriorly tilt the pelvis) at the hip joint. (action 2)

Reverse Mover Actions Notes

- If the distal tibial attachment is fixed, the rectus femoris pulls the anterior surface of the femur toward the anterior surface of the tibia. Therefore, the rectus femoris extends the thigh at the knee joint. (reverse action 1)
- The reason that the quadriceps femoris are so large and strong is not just to move the leg into extension at the knee joint but rather to do the reverse action, in other words, move the thigh into extension at the knee joint. This happens every time a person stands up from a seated position. To move the thigh at the knee joint requires moving the entire body along with the thigh; hence the quadriceps femoris group needs to be very large and strong. (reverse action 1)

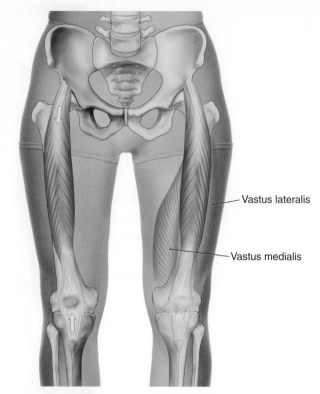

Vastus lateralis

Vastus medialis

Figure 15-7 Anterior views of the rectus femoris. The rest of the quadriceps femoris group has been ghosted in on the left.

- With the distal attachment fixed, the rectus femoris pulls the anterior pelvis toward the anterior surface of the femur. Therefore it anteriorly tilts the pelvis at the hip joint. (reverse action 2)

Eccentric Antagonist Functions

1. Restrains/slows knee joint flexion
2. Restrains/slows thigh extension and pelvic posterior tilt at the hip joint

Major Isometric Stabilization Functions

1. Stabilizes the knee joint (tibiofemoral and patellofemoral joints)
2. Stabilizes the pelvis and thigh at the hip joint

Isometric Function Note

- Strengthening the quadriceps femoris group is a major factor in knee joint stabilization for physical rehabilitation work.

Additional Note on Functions

1. All four members of the quadriceps femoris group can extend the leg (and thigh) at the knee joint. Only the rectus femoris crosses and moves the hip joint.

15

Rectus Femoris (of Quadriceps Femoris Group)—*cont'd*

INNERVATION
☐ The Femoral Nerve
  ☐ L2, **L3, L4**

ARTERIAL SUPPLY
☐ The Femoral Artery (the continuation of the External Iliac Artery) and the Deep Femoral Artery (a major branch of the Femoral Artery)

PALPATION

1. With the client supine with a pillow under the knees, place palpating hand just proximal to the patella.
2. Resist the client from extending the leg at the knee joint and feel for the contraction of the rectus femoris.
3. Continue palpating the rectus femoris toward the anterior inferior iliac spine (AIIS).

■ RELATIONSHIP TO OTHER STRUCTURES

☐ The rectus femoris is superficial for its entire course except proximally, where it is deep to the sartorius and the tensor fasciae latae.
☐ Deep to the rectus femoris is the vastus intermedius.
☐ The rectus femoris is primarily located between the vastus lateralis (laterally) and the vastus medialis (medially), but it slightly overlies the two.
☐ The rectus femoris is located within the superficial front line myofascial meridian.

■ MISCELLANEOUS

1. The proximal attachment of the rectus femoris onto the anterior inferior iliac spine (AIIS) is known as the *straight tendon.*
2. The proximal attachment of the rectus femoris, which attaches just superior to the brim of the acetabulum, is known as the *reflected tendon.*
3. Because of the difference in leverage, the rectus femoris is more powerful at the knee joint than at the hip joint.
4. The rectus femoris is bipennate.

15

Vastus Lateralis (of Quadriceps Femoris Group)

The name, vastus lateralis, *tells us that this muscle is vast in size and located laterally.*

Derivation	☐ vastus: L. *vast.*
	laterilis: L. *lateral.*
Pronunciation	☐ VAS-tus, lat-er-A-lis

■ ATTACHMENTS

☐ **Linea Aspera of the Femur**
　☐ the lateral lip of the linea aspera of the femur, and the intertrochanteric line and gluteal tuberosity of the femur

to the

☐ **Tibial Tuberosity via the Patella and the Patellar Ligament**
　☐ and the tibial condyles via the retinacular fibers

■ FUNCTIONS

CONCENTRIC (SHORTENING) MOVER ACTIONS	
Standard Mover Actions	**Reverse Mover Actions**
☐ 1. Extends the leg at the knee joint	☐ 1. Extends the thigh at the knee joint

Standard Mover Actions Note

- The vastus lateralis crosses the knee joint anteriorly (with its fibers running vertically in the sagittal plane); therefore it extends the leg at the knee joint. (action 1)

Reverse Mover Actions Notes

- If the distal tibial attachment is fixed, the vastus lateralis pulls the anterior surface of the femur toward the anterior surface of the tibia. Therefore, the rectus femoris extends the thigh at the knee joint. (reverse action 1)
- The reason that the quadriceps femoris are so large and strong is not just to move the leg into extension at the knee joint but rather to do the reverse action, in other words, move the thigh into extension at the knee joint. This happens every time a person stands up from a seated position. To move the thigh at the knee joint requires moving the entire body along with the thigh; hence the quadriceps femoris group needs to be very large and strong. (reverse action 1)

Eccentric Antagonist Function

1. Restrains/slows knee joint flexion

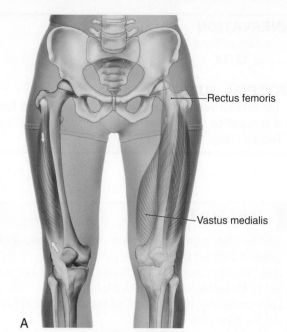

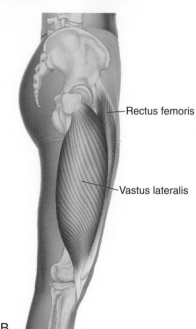

Figure 15-8 Views of the vastus lateralis. **A,** Anterior views. The rest of the quadriceps femoris group has been ghosted in on the left. **B,** Right lateral view. The rectus femoris has been drawn in.

Isometric Stabilization Function

1. Stabilizes the knee joint (tibiofemoral and patellofemoral joints)

Isometric Function Note

- Strengthening the quadriceps femoris group is a major factor in knee joint stabilization for physical rehabilitation work.

Vastus Lateralis (of Quadriceps Femoris Group)—*cont'd*

Additional Notes on Functions

1. The fibers of the vastus lateralis are oriented somewhat horizontally, which creates a line of pull on the patella that can pull it slightly laterally at the patellofemoral joint, in addition to proximally, when it contracts to extend the leg at the knee joint. Similarly, the vastus medialis can pull the patella slightly medially as the leg extends at the knee joint. The counterbalancing forces of the vastus lateralis and the vastus medialis help ensure that the patella tracks correctly on the femur at the patellofemoral joint as the knee (tibiofemoral) joint extends and flexes.

2. All four members of the quadriceps femoris group can extend the leg (and thigh) at the knee joint.

INNERVATION
- The Femoral Nerve
  - L2, **L3, L4**

ARTERIAL SUPPLY
- The Femoral Artery (the continuation of the External Iliac Artery) and the Deep Femoral Artery (a major branch of the Femoral Artery)
  - and branches of the Popliteal Artery (the continuation of the Femoral Artery)

✋ PALPATION

1. With the client supine, place palpating hand just distal to the greater trochanter.
2. Have the client extend the leg at the knee joint against your resistance and feel for the contraction of the vastus lateralis.
3. Continue palpating the vastus lateralis toward the patella in the lateral, posterolateral, and anterolateral thigh.

■ RELATIONSHIP TO OTHER STRUCTURES

- Anteriorly, the vastus lateralis is lateral and partially deep to the rectus femoris.
- In the lateral thigh, the vastus lateralis is deep to the tensor fasciae latae and the iliotibial band (ITB).
- Posteriorly, the vastus lateralis is superficial between the iliotibial band and the biceps femoris of the hamstring group.
- From the lateral perspective, the vastus intermedius and the femur are deep to the vastus lateralis.
- The vastus lateralis is located within the back functional line and involved with the superficial front line myofascial meridians.

■ MISCELLANEOUS

1. The vastus lateralis is the largest of the four quadriceps femoris muscles.
2. Pain attributed to the ITB is often caused by tightness of the vastus lateralis, which is deep to the ITB.
3. The vastus lateralis is pennate.

15

Vastus Medialis (of Quadriceps Femoris Group)

The name, vastus medialis, *tells us that this muscle is vast in size and located medially.*

Derivation	☐ vastus: L. *vast.*
	medialis: L. *medial.*
Pronunciation	☐ VAS-tus, mee-dee-A-lis

■ ATTACHMENTS

☐ **Linea Aspera of the Femur**
  ☐ the medial lip of the linea aspera, and the intertrochanteric line and the medial supracondylar line of the femur

  to the

☐ **Tibial Tuberosity via the Patella and the Patellar Ligament**
  ☐ and the tibial condyles via the retinacular fibers

■ FUNCTIONS

CONCENTRIC (SHORTENING) MOVER ACTIONS	
Standard Mover Actions	**Reverse Mover Actions**
☐ 1. Extends the leg at the knee joint	☐ 1. Extends the thigh at the knee joint

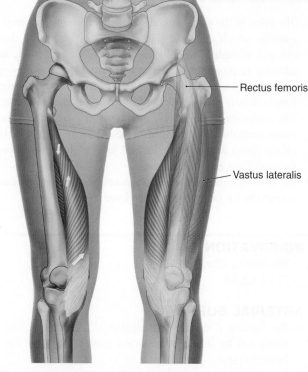

Figure 15-9 Anterior views of the vastus medialis. The rest of the quadriceps femoris group has been ghosted in on the left.

— Rectus femoris

— Vastus lateralis

Standard Mover Actions Note

• The vastus medialis crosses the knee joint anteriorly (with its fibers running vertically in the sagittal plane); therefore it extends the leg at the knee joint. (action 1)

Reverse Mover Actions Notes

• If the distal tibial attachment is fixed, the vastus medialis pulls the anterior surface of the femur toward the anterior surface of the tibia. Therefore, the rectus femoris extends the thigh at the knee joint. (reverse action 1)

• The reason that the quadriceps femoris are so large and strong is not just to move the leg into extension at the knee joint but rather to do the reverse action, in other words, move the thigh into extension at the knee joint. This happens every time a person stands up from a seated position. To move the thigh at the knee joint requires moving the entire body along with the thigh; hence the quadriceps femoris group needs to be very large and strong. (reverse action 1)

Eccentric Antagonist Function

1. Restrains/slows knee joint flexion

Isometric Stabilization Function

1. Stabilizes the knee joint (tibiofemoral and patellofemoral joints)

Isometric Function Note

• Strengthening the quadriceps femoris group is a major factor in knee joint stabilization for physical rehabilitation work.

Additional Notes on Functions

1. The fibers of the vastus medialis are oriented somewhat horizontally, which creates a line of pull on the patella that can pull it slightly medially at the patellofemoral joint, in addition to proximally, when it contracts to extend the leg at the knee joint. Similarly, the vastus lateralis can pull the patella slightly laterally as the leg extends at the knee joint. The counterbalancing forces of the vastus medialis and the vastus lateralis help ensure that the patella tracks correctly on the femur at the patellofemoral joint as the knee (tibiofemoral) joint extends and flexes.

2. All four members of the quadriceps femoris group can extend the leg (and thigh) at the knee joint.

15

Vastus Medialis (of Quadriceps Femoris Group)—*cont'd*

INNERVATION
☐ The Femoral Nerve
   ☐ L2, **L3, L4**

ARTERIAL SUPPLY
☐ The Femoral Artery (the continuation of the External Iliac Artery)

✋ PALPATION

1. With the client supine, place palpating hand just proximal and medial to the patella.
2. Have the client extend the leg at the knee joint against your resistance and feel for the contraction of the vastus medialis.
3. Continue palpating the vastus medialis proximally as far as possible.

■ RELATIONSHIP TO OTHER STRUCTURES

☐ Anteriorly, the vastus medialis is medial and slightly deep to the rectus femoris. It is also deep to the sartorius.
☐ The vastus medialis is anterior to the adductor group.
☐ From the medial perspective, the femur is deep to the vastus medialis.
☐ The vastus medialis is involved with the superficial front line myofascial meridian.

■ MISCELLANEOUS

1. The most distal aspect of the vastus medialis is the bulkiest and may form a bulge in well-toned individuals.
2. Some sources refer to the upper fibers of the vastus medialis as the *vastus medialis longus (VML)* and the lower fibers as the *vastus medialis oblique (VMO)* because of the drastic difference in the direction of the upper fibers compared with the lower fibers.
3. The vastus medialis is pennate.

15

Vastus Intermedius (of Quadriceps Femoris Group)

The name, vastus intermedius, tells us that this muscle is vast in size and located between the two other vastus muscles.

Derivation	☐ vastus: L. *vast.*
	inter: L. *between.*
	medius: L. *middle.*
Pronunciation	☐ VAS-tus, in-ter-MEE-dee-us

■ ATTACHMENTS

☐ **Anterior Shaft and Linea Aspera of the Femur**
  ☐ the anterior and lateral surfaces of the femur and the lateral lip of the linea aspera

to the

☐ **Tibial Tuberosity via the Patella and the Patellar Ligament**
  ☐ and the tibial condyles via the retinacular fibers

■ FUNCTIONS

CONCENTRIC (SHORTENING) MOVER ACTIONS	
Standard Mover Actions	**Reverse Mover Actions**
☐ 1. Extends the leg at the knee joint	☐ 1. Extends the thigh at the knee joint

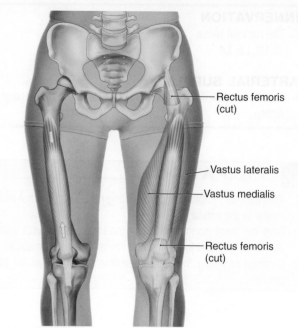

Figure 15-10 Anterior views of the vastus intermedius. The rest of the quadriceps femoris group has been ghosted in on the left.

Rectus femoris (cut)

Vastus lateralis

Vastus medialis

Rectus femoris (cut)

Standard Mover Actions Notes

• The vastus intermedius crosses the knee joint anteriorly (with its fibers running vertically in the sagittal plane); therefore it extends the leg at the knee joint. (action 1)

Reverse Mover Actions Notes

• If the distal tibial attachment is fixed, the vastus intermedius pulls the anterior surface of the femur toward the anterior surface of the tibia. Therefore, the rectus femoris extends the thigh at the knee joint. (reverse action 1)
• The reason that the quadriceps femoris are so large and strong is not just to move the leg into extension at the knee joint but rather to do the reverse action, in other words, move the thigh into extension at the knee joint. This happens every time a person stands up from a seated position. To move the thigh at the knee joint requires moving the entire body along with the thigh; hence the quadriceps femoris group needs to be very large and strong. (reverse action 1)

Eccentric Antagonist Function

1. Restrains/slows knee joint flexion

Isometric Stabilization Function

1. Stabilizes the knee joint (tibiofemoral and patellofemoral joints)

Isometric Function Note

• Strengthening the quadriceps femoris group is a major factor in knee joint stabilization for physical rehabilitation work.

Additional Note on Functions

1. All four members of the quadriceps femoris group can extend the leg (and thigh) at the knee joint.

INNERVATION
☐ The Femoral Nerve
  ☐ L2, **L3, L4**

ARTERIAL SUPPLY
☐ The Deep Femoral Artery (a major branch of the Femoral Artery)

15

Vastus Intermedius (of Quadriceps Femoris Group)—*cont'd*

 PALPATION

1. With the client supine, place palpating hand just proximal to the patella.
2. If the rectus femoris can be lifted and/or moved aside, the distal vastus intermedius may be palpated deep to the rectus femoris when approached from either the medial or the lateral side.
3. To feel the vastus intermedius deep to the rectus femoris, make sure that the direction of your pressure is oriented toward the middle of the femur.

■ RELATIONSHIP TO OTHER STRUCTURES

☐ The vastus intermedius is deep to the rectus femoris and the vastus lateralis.
☐ From the anterior perspective, a small muscle called the *articularis genus* and the femur are deep to the vastus intermedius.
☐ From the lateral perspective, the femur is deep to the vastus intermedius.

■ MISCELLANEOUS

1. The vastus intermedius somewhat blends into the vastus lateralis and the vastus medialis.
2. The vastus intermedius sometimes blends with the articularis genus.
3. The vastus intermedius is pennate.

15

Articularis Genus

The name, articularis genus, *tells us that this muscle is involved with the knee joint.*

Derivation	articularis: L. *refers to a joint.*
	genu: L. *referes to the knee.*
Pronunciation	ar-TIK-you-LA-ris, JE-new

■ ATTACHMENTS

☐ **Anterior Distal Femoral Shaft**

to the

☐ **Knee Joint Capsule**

■ FUNCTIONS

CONCENTRIC (SHORTENING) MOVER ACTIONS	
Standard Mover Actions	**Reverse Mover Actions**
☐ **1. Tenses and pulls the knee joint capsule proximally**	☐ 1. The reverse action of moving the femur is unlikely to occur

Standard Mover Action Notes

- The articularis genus (with its fibers oriented vertically) pulls its distal attachment, the joint capsule of the knee joint, toward its proximal attachment, the anterior distal shaft of the femur. (action 1)
- The action of the articularis genus tensing and pulling the knee joint capsule proximally couples with the contraction of the quadriceps femoris group contracting and pulling the patella proximally when the knee joint extends. Pulling the knee joint capsule proximally when the patella moves proximally prevents the capsule from being pinched between the patella and femur. (action 1)

Eccentric Antagonist Function

1. Restrains/slows distal movement of the knee joint capsule

Isometric Stabilization Function

1. Stabilizes the position of the knee joint capsule

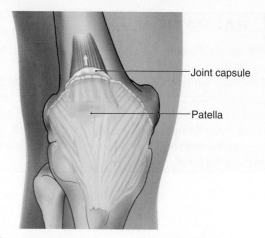

Figure 15-11 Anterior view of the right articularus genus.

INNERVATION
☐ The Femoral Nerve
  ☐ L2, **L3, L4**

ARTERIAL SUPPLY
☐ The Deep Femoral Artery (a major branch of the Femoral Artery)

✋ PALPATION

☐ The articularis genus is a small muscle deep to the rectus femoris and vastus intermedius and is extremely difficult, if not impossible, to palpate and distinguish from the adjacent musculature.

■ RELATIONSHIP TO OTHER STRUCTURES

☐ The articularis genus is deep to the vastus intermedius.
☐ Deep to the articularis genus is the femur.
☐ The articularis genus is involved with the superficial front line myofascial meridian.

■ MISCELLANEOUS

1. The articularis genus is sometimes a distinct muscle and sometimes it blends with the vastus intermedius.

15

Hamstring Group

The hamstrings are a group of muscles in the posterior thigh. There are three hamstring muscles: the biceps femoris, semitendinosus, and semimembranosus.

■ ATTACHMENTS

- These muscles are grouped together as the hamstrings, because they all attach proximally onto the ischial tuberosity.
- The semitendinosus and the semimembranosus are located medially in the posterior thigh and are sometimes referred to as the *medial hamstrings.*
- The biceps femoris is located laterally in the posterior thigh and is sometimes referred to as the *lateral hamstrings.* (*Hamstrings* is plural because the biceps femoris has two heads.)
- The semitendinosus and long head of the biceps femoris are superficial; the semimembranosus and short head of the biceps femoris are deeper.
- All three hamstring muscles are located within the superficial back line myofascial meridian.

■ FUNCTIONS

- As a group, all three hamstrings flex the leg (or thigh) at the knee joint.
- Because of the difference in leverage, the hamstrings are more powerful at the hip joint than they are at the knee joint.

- As a group, all three hamstrings (except the short head of the biceps femoris) extend the thigh at the hip joint and/or posteriorly tilt the pelvis at the hip joint.

■ MISCELLANEOUS

- The *hamstrings,* as a group, were given this name because butchers used to hang the carcass of a pig by the hamstring tendons.

INNERVATION

- ☐ The three hamstrings are innervated by the sciatic nerve. They are all innervated by the tibial branch of the sciatic nerve except for the short head of the biceps femoris, which is innervated by the common fibular branch of the sciatic nerve.

ARTERIAL SUPPLY

- ☐ The upper ⅓ of the hamstrings receives its arterial supply from the inferior gluteal artery and the obturator artery.
- ☐ The middle ⅓ of the hamstrings receives its arterial supply from perforating branches of the deep femoral artery.
- ☐ The distal ⅓ of the hamstrings receives its arterial supply from the popliteal artery.

15

Posterior Views of the Hamstring Group

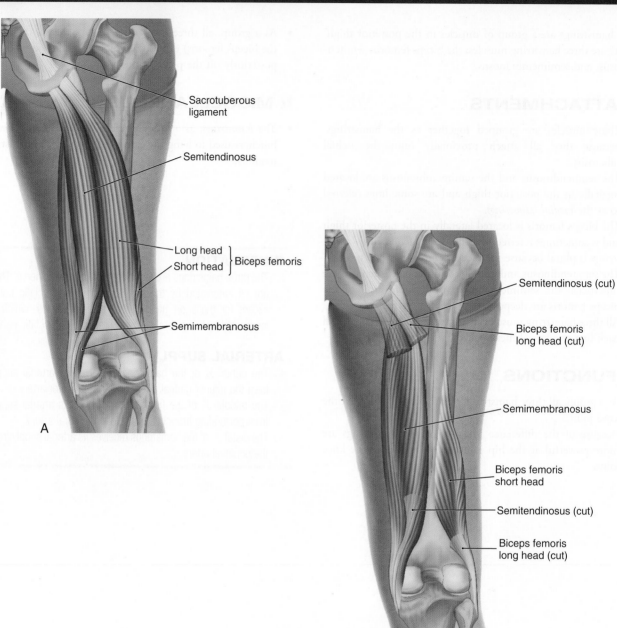

Sacrotuberous ligament

Semitendinosus

Long head
Short head } Biceps femoris

Semimembranosus

A

Semitendinosus (cut)

Biceps femoris
long head (cut)

Semimembranosus

Biceps femoris
short head

Semitendinosus (cut)

Biceps femoris
long head (cut)

B

Figure 15-12 Posterior views of the right hamstring group. **A,** Superificial. **B,** Deep.

15

Biceps Femoris (of Hamstring Group)

The name, biceps femoris, *tells us that this muscle has two heads and lies over the femur.*

Derivation	☐ biceps: L. *two heads.*
	femoris: L. *refers to the femur.*
Pronunciation	☐ BY-seps, FEM-o-ris

■ ATTACHMENTS

☐ **LONG HEAD: Ischial Tuberosity**
  ☐ and the sacrotuberous ligament
☐ **SHORT HEAD: Linea Aspera**
  ☐ and the lateral supracondylar line of the femur

  to the

☐ **Head of the Fibula**
  ☐ and the lateral tibial condyle

■ FUNCTIONS

CONCENTRIC (SHORTENING) MOVER ACTIONS	
Standard Mover Actions	**Reverse Mover Actions**
☐ **1. Flexes the leg at the knee joint**	☐ 1. Flexes the thigh at the knee joint
☐ **2. Extends the thigh at the hip joint**	☐ **2. Posteriorly tilts the pelvis at the hip joint**
☐ 3. Laterally rotates the leg at the knee joint	☐ 3. Medially rotates the thigh at the knee joint
☐ 4. Laterally rotates the thigh at the hip joint	☐ 4. Contralaterally rotates the pelvis at the hip joint
☐ 5. Adducts the thigh at the hip joint	☐ 5. Elevates the same-side pelvis at the hip joint

Standard Mover Action Notes

- The biceps femoris crosses the knee joint posteriorly (with its fibers running vertically in the sagittal plane); therefore it flexes the leg at the knee joint. (action 1)
- The long head of the biceps femoris crosses the hip joint posteriorly (with its fibers running vertically in the sagittal plane); therefore it extends the thigh at the hip joint. The short head cannot extend the thigh at the hip joint because it does not cross the hip joint. (action 2)
- The biceps femoris crosses the knee joint laterally from posterior to anterior (with its fibers running somewhat horizontally in the transverse plane) and attaches to the lateral leg. When the biceps femoris pulls at the leg attachment, the attachment is pulled posteriorly, causing the anterior leg to face somewhat laterally. Therefore the biceps femoris laterally rotates the leg at the knee joint. (Note: The knee joint can only rotate if it is first flexed.) (action 3)
- The biceps femoris is the only muscle that can laterally rotate the leg (and medially rotate the thigh) at the knee joint. (action 3)

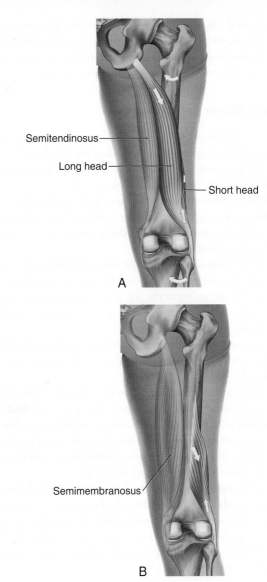

Figure 15-13 Posterior views of the right biceps femoris. **A,** The long and short heads of the biceps femoris are drawn in. The semitendinosus has been ghosted in. **B,** The short head of the biceps femoris. The semimembranosus has been ghosted in.

- The long head of the biceps femoris crosses the hip joint laterally, wrapping around the thigh from posteriorly on the pelvis to more anteriorly onto the leg (with its fibers running somewhat horizontally in the transverse plane). If the leg is fixed to the thigh and the long head of the biceps femoris pulls on the leg, the leg and thigh are pulled posterolaterally, causing the anterior thigh to face laterally. Therefore the biceps femoris laterally rotates the thigh at the hip joint. (action 4)
- The long head of the biceps femoris crosses the hip joint posteriorly (with its fibers running somewhat horizontally in

15

Biceps Femoris (of Hamstring Group)—cont'd

the frontal plane) below the center of the hip joint from medial on the pelvis to laterally on the leg. Therefore when the biceps femoris pulls its lateral attachment (the leg) medially, it adducts the thigh at the hip joint. (action 5)

Reverse Mover Action Notes

• Reverse actions of the biceps femoris usually occur when the foot is planted on the ground, making the distal attachment relatively more fixed so that the proximal attachment moves instead. (reverse actions 1, 2, 3, 4, 5)

• The biceps femoris crosses the knee joint posteriorly (with its fibers running vertically in the sagittal plane). If the distal attachment is fixed, the thigh flexes toward the leg at the knee joint. (reverse action 1)

• With the distal attachment fixed, the long head of the biceps femoris, by pulling inferiorly on the posterior pelvis, posteriorly tilts the pelvis at the hip joint. The short head does not cross the hip joint; therefore it cannot move the pelvis at the hip joint. (reverse action 2)

• The reverse action of lateral rotation of the leg at the knee joint is medial rotation of the thigh at the knee joint. (reverse action 3)

• The long head of the biceps femoris runs slightly horizontally (in the transverse plane) across the hip joint. If the distal attachment is fixed, the pelvis will be pulled such that its anterior surface comes to face the opposite side of the body. Therefore, the biceps femoris contralaterally rotates the pelvis at the hip joint. (reverse action 4)

• With the distal attachment fixed, the long head of the biceps femoris pulls inferiorly on the ischial tuberosity, causing the iliac crest on that side to elevate. Therefore the long head of the biceps femoris elevates the same-side pelvis at the hip joint. Note: If one side of the pelvis elevates, the other side depresses. (reverse action 5)

Eccentric Antagonist Functions

1. Restrains/slows knee joint extension and medial rotation of the leg and lateral rotation of the thigh at the knee joint
2. Restrains/slows flexion, medial rotation, and abduction of the thigh at the hip joint
3. Restrains/slows anterior tilt, , ipsilateral rotation, and same-side depression of the pelvis at the hip joint

Isometric Stabilization Functions

1. Stabilizes the thigh and pelvis at the hip joint
2. Stabilizes the knee joint

Additional Note on Functions

1. All three hamstring muscles (biceps femoris, semitendinosus, and semimembranosus) flex the knee joint.

INNERVATION

☐ The Sciatic Nerve
  ☐ the tibial nerve and the common fibular nerve; L5, **S1**, S2

ARTERIAL SUPPLY

Long Head

☐ The Inferior Gluteal Artery (a branch of the Internal Iliac Artery) and perforating branches of the Deep Femoral Artery (a major branch of the Femoral Artery)
  ☐ and the Obturator Artery (a branch of the Internal Iliac Artery) and branches of the Popliteal Artery (the continuation of the Femoral Artery)

Short Head

☐ Perforating branches of the Deep Femoral Artery (a major branch of the Femoral Artery)
  ☐ and branches of the Popliteal Artery (the continuation of the Femoral Artery)

✋ PALPATION

1. With the client prone with the leg partially flexed at the knee joint, place palpating hand just distal and slightly lateral to the ischial tuberosity.
2. Resist the client from performing further flexion of the leg at the knee joint and palpate the biceps femoris toward the head of the fibula.

■ RELATIONSHIP TO OTHER STRUCTURES

☐ The biceps femoris is a lateral hamstring muscle.
☐ The biceps femoris is superficial in the posterolateral thigh, except proximally where it is deep to the gluteus maximus.
☐ The proximal attachment of the short head begins immediately distal to the femoral attachment of the gluteus maximus.
☐ All fibers of the short head of the biceps femoris are deep to the long head except distally near the knee, where some of the fibers of the short head are superficial, lateral to the long head of the biceps femoris.
☐ The biceps femoris is just lateral to the semitendinosus and just medial (and also superficial) to the vastus lateralis.
☐ The biceps femoris is located within the superficial back line and spiral line myofascial meridians.

■ MISCELLANEOUS

1. The proximal attachment of the biceps femoris' long head blends with the proximal attachment of the semitendinosus.
2. Some sources state that short head of the biceps femoris is not a true hamstring muscle because it does not attach to the ischial tuberosity, does not cross the hip joint, and is not innervated by the tibial nerve branch of the sciatic nerve.

Semitendinosus (of Hamstring Group)

The name, semitendinosus, *tells us that this muscle has a long, slender (distal) tendon.*

Derivation	☐ semitendinosus: L. *refers to its long tendon.*
Pronunciation	☐ SEM-i-TEN-di-NO-sus

■ ATTACHMENTS

☐ **Ischial Tuberosity**

to the

☐ **Pes Anserine Tendon (at the Proximal Anteromedial Tibia)**

■ FUNCTIONS

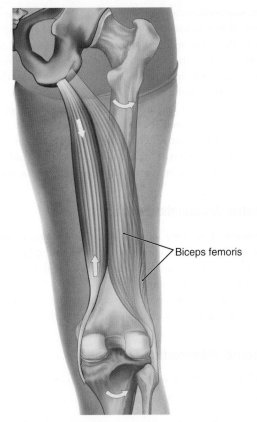

Biceps femoris

Figure 15-14 Posterior view of the right semitendinosus. The biceps femoris has been ghosted in.

CONCENTRIC (SHORTENING) MOVER ACTIONS	
Standard Mover Actions	**Reverse Mover Actions**
☐ **1. Flexes the leg at the knee joint**	☐ 1. Flexes the thigh at the knee joint
☐ **2. Extends the thigh at the hip joint**	☐ **2. Posteriorly tilts the pelvis at the hip joint**
☐ 3. Medially rotates the leg at the knee joint	☐ 3. Laterally rotates the thigh at the knee joint
☐ 4. Medially rotates the thigh at the hip joint	☐ 4. Ipsilaterally rotates the pelvis at the hip joint
☐ 5. Adducts the thigh at the hip joint	☐ 5. Elevates the same-side pelvis at the hip joint

Standard Mover Actions Notes

• The semitendinosus crosses the knee joint posteriorly (with its fibers running vertically in the sagittal plane); therefore it flexes the leg at the knee joint. (action 1)

• The semitendinosus crosses the hip joint posteriorly (with its fibers running vertically in the sagittal plane); therefore it extends the thigh at the hip joint. (action 2)

• The semitendinosus crosses the knee joint medially from posterior to anterior (with its fibers running somewhat horizontally in the transverse plane) to attach into the pes anserine tendon at the medial tibia. When the semitendinosus pulls at the leg attachment, the attachment is pulled posteriorly, causing the anterior tibia to face somewhat medially. Therefore the semitendinosus medially rotates the leg at the knee joint. (Note: The knee joint can only rotate if it is first flexed.) (action 3)

• The semitendinosus crosses the hip joint medially, wrapping around the thigh from posteriorly on the pelvis to more anteriorly onto the leg (with its fibers running somewhat horizontally in the transverse plane). If the leg is fixed to the thigh, and the semitendinosus pulls on the leg, the thigh rotates posteromedially, causing the anterior thigh to face

medially. Therefore the semitendinosus medially rotates the thigh at the hip joint. (action 4)

• The semitendinosus crosses the hip joint posteriorly (with its fibers running somewhat horizontally in the frontal plane) from medial on the pelvis to slightly laterally on the leg. Therefore when the semitendinosus pulls its lateral attachment (the leg) medially, it adducts the thigh at the hip joint. (action 5)

Reverse Mover Actions Notes

• Reverse actions of the semitendinosus usually occur when the foot is planted on the ground, making the distal attachment relatively more fixed so that the proximal attachment moves instead. (reverse actions 1, 2, 3, 4, 5)

• The semitendinosus crosses the knee joint posteriorly (with its fibers running vertically in the sagittal plane). If the distal attachment is fixed, the thigh flexes toward the leg at the knee joint. (reverse action 1)

• With the distal attachment fixed, the semitendinosus, by pulling inferiorly on the posterior pelvis, posteriorly tilts the pelvis at the hip joint. (reverse action 2)

• The reverse action of medial rotation of the leg at the knee joint is lateral rotation of the thigh at the knee joint. (reverse action 3)

15

Semitendinosus (of Hamstring Group)—*cont'd*

- The semitendinosus runs slightly horizontally (in the transverse plane) across the hip joint. If the distal attachment is fixed, the pelvis will be pulled such that its anterior surface comes to face the same side of the body. Therefore, the semitendinosus ipsilaterally rotates the pelvis at the hip joint. (reverse action 4)
- With the distal attachment fixed, the semitendinosus pulls inferiorly on the ischial tuberosity, causing the iliac crest on that side to elevate. Therefore the semitendinosus elevates the same-side pelvis at the hip joint. Note: If one side of the pelvis elevates, the other side depresses. (reverse action 5)

Eccentric Antagonist Functions

1. Restrains/slows knee joint extension and lateral rotation of the leg and medial rotation of the thigh at the knee joint
2. Restrains/slows flexion, lateral rotation, and abduction of the thigh at the hip joint
3. Restrains/slows anterior tilt, contralateral rotation, and same-side depression of the pelvis at the hip joint

Isometric Stabilization Functions

1. Stabilizes the thigh and pelvis at the hip joint
2. Stabilizes the knee joint

Isometric Function Note

- The distal tendon of the semitendinosus (along with the sartorius and gracilis muscles) helps stabilize the medial knee joint against lateral to medial (valgus) forces that would buckle the knee joint medially.

Additional Notes on Actions

1. All three hamstring muscles (biceps femoris, semitendinosus, and semimembranosus) flex the knee joint.
2. All three pes anserine muscles (sartorius, gracilis, and semitendinosus) flex and medially rotate the leg at the knee joint (or flex and laterally rotate the thigh at the knee joint).

INNERVATION
- ☐ The Sciatic Nerve
  - ☐ the tibial nerve; L5, **S1,** S2

ARTERIAL SUPPLY
- ☐ The Inferior Gluteal Artery (a branch of the Internal Iliac Artery) and perforating branches of the Deep Femoral Artery (a major branch of the Femoral Artery)
  - ☐ and the Obturator Artery (a branch of the Internal Iliac Artery) and branches of the Popliteal Artery (the continuation of the Femoral Artery)

✋ PALPATION

1. With the client prone with the leg partially flexed at the knee joint, place palpating hand just distal and slightly medial to the ischial tuberosity.
2. Resist the client from performing further flexion of the leg at the knee joint and palpate the semitendinosus toward the pes anserine tendon.

■ RELATIONSHIP TO OTHER STRUCTURES

- ☐ The semitendinosus is the more superficial medial hamstring muscle.
- ☐ The proximal attachment of the semitendinosus is deep to the gluteus maximus.
- ☐ The biceps femoris is lateral to the semitendinosus. More distally, a portion of the semimembranosus is lateral to the semitendinosus.
- ☐ Medial to the semitendinosus is the adductor magnus and a portion of the semimembranosus.
- ☐ The majority of the semimembranosus is deep to the semitendinosus.
- ☐ Of the three muscles that attach into the pes anserine tendon, the semitendinosus' attachment is the most posterior and distal.
- ☐ The semitendinosus is located within the superficial back line myofascial meridian.

■ MISCELLANEOUS

1. The semitendinosus is named for its long distal tendon.
2. The semitendinosus is one of three muscles that attach into the pes anserine tendon. The other two muscles that attach here are the sartorius and the gracilis.
3. Think **SGS:** Of the muscles that attach into the pes anserine, the *sartorius* attaches the most anteriorly and proximally of the three, the *gracilis* is in the middle, and the *semitendinosus* attaches the most posteriorly and distally.
4. *Pes anserine* means goose foot.
5. The proximal tendon of the semitendinosus blends with the proximal tendon of the biceps femoris.
6. The semitendinosus often has a fibrous septum that divides it into distinct proximal and distal portions.

Semimembranosus (of Hamstring Group)

The name, semimembranosus, *tells us that this muscle has a flattened, membranous (proximal) attachment.*

Derivation	☐ semimembranosus: L. *refers to its flattened, membranous tendon.*
Pronunciation	☐ SEM-i-MEM-bra-NO-sus

■ ATTACHMENTS

☐ **Ischial Tuberosity**

to the

☐ **Posterior Surface of the Medial Condyle of the Tibia**

■ FUNCTIONS

CONCENTRIC (SHORTENING) MOVER ACTIONS	
Standard Mover Actions	**Reverse Mover Actions**
☐ **1. Flexes the leg at the knee joint**	☐ 1. Flexes the thigh at the knee joint
☐ **2. Extends the thigh at the hip joint**	☐ **2. Posteriorly tilts the pelvis at the hip joint**
☐ 3. Medially rotates the leg at the knee joint	☐ 3. Laterally rotates the thigh at the knee joint
☐ 4. Medially rotates the thigh at the hip joint	☐ 4. Ipsilaterally rotates the pelvis at the hip joint
☐ 5. Adducts the thigh at the hip joint	☐ 5. Elevates the same-side pelvis at the hip joint

Standard Mover Actions Notes

- The semimembranosus crosses the knee joint posteriorly (with its fibers running vertically in the sagittal plane); therefore it flexes the leg at the knee joint. (action 1)
- The semimembranosus crosses the hip joint posteriorly (with its fibers running vertically in the sagittal plane); therefore it extends the thigh at the hip joint. (action 2)
- The semimembranosus crosses the knee joint medially from posterior to anterior (with its fibers running somewhat horizontally in the transverse plane) to attach into the posterior surface of the medial tibial condyle. When the semimembranosus pulls at the leg attachment, the attachment is pulled posteriorly, causing the anterior tibia to face somewhat medially. Therefore the semimembranosus medially rotates the leg at the knee joint. (Note: The knee joint can only rotate if it is first flexed.) (action 3)
- The semimembranosus crosses the hip joint medially, wrapping around the thigh from posteriorly on the pelvis to more anteriorly onto the leg (with its fibers running somewhat horizontally in the transverse plane). If the leg is fixed to the thigh, and the semimembranosus pulls on the leg, the thigh

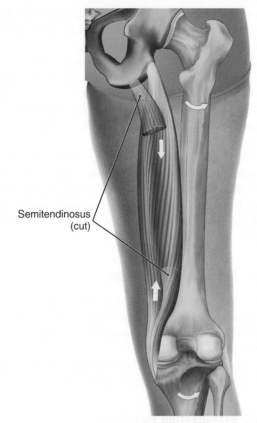

Figure 15-15 Posterior view of the right semimembranosus. The proximal and distal tendons of the semitendinosus have been cut and ghosted in.

rotates posteromedially, causing the anterior thigh to face medially. Therefore the semimembranosus medially rotates the thigh at the hip joint. (action 4)
- The semimembranosus crosses the hip joint posteriorly (with its fibers running somewhat horizontally in the frontal plane) from medial on the pelvis to slightly laterally on the leg. Therefore when the semimembranosus pulls its lateral attachment (the leg) medially, it adducts the thigh at the hip joint. (action 5)

Reverse Mover Actions Notes

- Reverse actions of the semimembranosus usually occur when the foot is planted on the ground, making the distal attachment relatively more fixed so that the proximal attachment moves instead. (reverse actions 1, 2, 3, 4, 5)
- The semimembranosus crosses the knee joint posteriorly (with its fibers running vertically in the sagittal plane). If the distal attachment is fixed, the thigh flexes toward the leg at the knee joint. (reverse action 1)
- With the distal attachment fixed, the semimembranosus, by pulling inferiorly on the posterior pelvis, posteriorly tilts the pelvis at the hip joint. (reverse action 2)

Semitendinosus (cut)

- The reverse action of medial rotation of the leg at the knee joint is lateral rotation of the thigh at the knee joint. (reverse action 3)
- The semimembranosus runs slightly horizontally (in the transverse plane) across the hip joint. If the distal attachment is fixed, the pelvis will be pulled such that its anterior surface comes to face the same side of the body. Therefore, the semimembranosus ipsilaterally rotates the pelvis at the hip joint. (reverse action 4)
- With the distal attachment fixed, the semimembranosus pulls inferiorly on the ischial tuberosity, causing the iliac crest on that side to elevate. Therefore the semimembranosus elevates the same-side pelvis at the hip joint. Note: If one side of the pelvis elevates, the other side depresses. (reverse action 5)

Eccentric Antagonist Functions

1. Restrains/slows knee joint extension and lateral rotation of the leg and medial rotation of the thigh at the knee joint
2. Restrains/slows flexion, lateral rotation, and abduction of the thigh at the hip joint
3. Restrains/slows anterior tilt, contralateral rotation, and same-side depression of the pelvis at the hip joint

Isometric Stabilization Functions

1. Stabilizes the thigh and pelvis at the hip joint
2. Stabilizes the knee joint

Additional Note on Functions

1. All three hamstring muscles (biceps femoris, semitendinosus, and semimembranosus) flex the knee joint.

INNERVATION
- The Sciatic Nerve
  - the tibial nerve; L5, **S1**, S2

ARTERIAL SUPPLY
- The Inferior Gluteal Artery (a branch of the Internal Iliac Artery) and perforating branches of the Deep Femoral Artery (a major branch of the Femoral Artery)
  - and the Obturator Artery (a branch of the Internal Iliac Artery) and branches of the Popliteal Artery (the continuation of the Femoral Artery)

PALPATION

1. With the client prone with the leg partially flexed at the knee joint, place palpating hand on the posteromedial thigh.
2. Resist the client from performing further flexion of the leg at the knee joint and feel for the contraction of the semimembranosus. It is medial to the semitendinosus and on either side of the distal tendon of the semitendinosus. (Keep in mind that this will also make the semitendinosus and the biceps femoris contract.)

■ RELATIONSHIP TO OTHER STRUCTURES

- The semimembranosus is the deeper medial hamstring muscle.
- The semimembranosus is generally deep to the semitendinosus. However, part of it is superficial, and found medial to the semitendinosus. More distally, the muscle belly of the semimembranosus is superficial and located on both sides of the distal tendon of the semitendinosus.
- The proximal attachment of the semimembranosus is deep to the gluteus maximus.
- Even though the semimembranosus is a medial hamstring muscle, its proximal attachment on the ischial tuberosity is located more laterally than the proximal attachments of the semitendinosus and biceps femoris.
- Superior to the proximal attachment of the semimembranosus on the ischial tuberosity are the medial attachments of the quadratus femoris and the inferior gemellus.
- Deep to the semimembranosus from the posterior perspective is the adductor magnus.
- The semimembranosus is located within the superficial back line myofascial meridian.

■ MISCELLANEOUS

1. The semimembranosus is named for its flattened, membranous proximal tendon.
2. The semimembranosus is the largest of the three hamstring muscles.
3. The semimembranosus also attaches into the medial meniscus of the knee joint.
4. The medial meniscus attachment of the semimembranosus facilitates the posterior movement of the medial meniscus during knee flexion. This helps to prevent impingement of the medial meniscus between the femur and tibia during flexion of the knee joint. (Note: The popliteus has the same action with regard to the lateral meniscus.)

15

Popliteus

The name, popliteus, *tells us that this muscle is located in the posterior knee.*

Derivation	☐ popliteus: L. *ham of the knee (refers to the posterior knee).*
Pronunciation	☐ pop-LIT-ee-us

■ ATTACHMENTS

☐ **Distal Posterolateral Femur**
  ☐ the lateral surface of the lateral condyle of the femur

to the

☐ **Proximal Posteromedial Tibia**

■ FUNCTIONS

CONCENTRIC (SHORTENING) MOVER ACTIONS	
Standard Mover Actions	**Reverse Mover Actions**
☐ 1. Medially rotates the leg at the knee joint	☐ 1. Laterally rotates the thigh at the knee joint
☐ 2. Flexes the leg at the knee joint	☐ 2. Flexes the thigh at the knee joint

Standard Mover Actions Notes

- At the posterior knee, the popliteus wraps around the knee joint from the lateral femur to the medial tibia (with its fibers running horizontally in the transverse plane). When the popliteus contracts, it pulls the tibial attachment posterolaterally toward the femoral attachment. This causes the anterior leg to face somewhat medially. Therefore the popliteus medially rotates the leg at the knee joint. (action 1)
- The popliteus crosses the knee joint posteriorly (with its fibers running somewhat vertically in the sagittal plane); therefore it flexes the leg at the knee joint. (action 2)

Reverse Mover Actions Notes

- Reverse actions of the popliteus usually occur when the foot is planted on the ground, making the distal attachment relatively more fixed so that the proximal attachment, the thigh moves instead. (reverse actions 1, 2)
- Because the popliteus crosses the knee joint horizontally in the transverse plane, it can rotate the knee joint. When its distal attachment on the leg is fixed (e.g., when the foot is planted on the ground), instead of rotating the leg medially, the popliteus pulls on the thigh, causing its anterior surface to face laterally. Therefore the popliteus laterally rotates the thigh at the knee joint. (reverse action 1)
- The popliteus crosses the knee joint posteriorly (with its fibers running vertically in the sagittal plane). If the distal

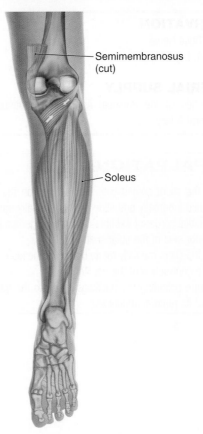

Figure 15-16 Posterior view of the right popliteus. The soleus and cut distal tendon of the semimembranosus have been ghosted in.

attachment is fixed, the thigh will flex toward the leg at the knee joint. (reverse action 2)

Eccentric Antagonist Functions

1. Restrains/slows lateral rotation of the leg and medial rotation of the thigh at the knee joint
2. Restrains/slows knee joint extension

Isometric Stabilization Function

1. Stabilizes the knee joint

Additional Note on Functions

1. To flex a fully extended knee joint, medial rotation of the leg at the knee joint and/or lateral rotation of the thigh at the knee joint is required. Of all muscles that can do these actions, the popliteus is considered to be the most important at creating this initial knee joint rotation and is said to *unlock* the extended knee joint.

15

Popliteus—*cont'd*

INNERVATION
- ☐ The Tibial Nerve
  - ☐ L4, L5, S1

ARTERIAL SUPPLY
- ☐ Branches of the Popliteal Artery (the continuation of the Femoral Artery)

✋ PALPATION

1. With the client seated with the feet flat on the floor, locate the tibial tuberosity and slide around medially until you are on the medial border of the tibia; curl your fingertips around to the posterior side of the tibial shaft.
2. Have the client medially rotate the leg at the knee joint and feel for the contraction of the popliteus.
3. Continue palpating the popliteus (deep to the gastrocnemius) toward its femoral attachment.

■ RELATIONSHIP TO OTHER STRUCTURES

- ☐ The popliteus is deep to the plantaris and the lateral head of the gastrocnemius.
- ☐ The popliteus is proximal to the soleus.
- ☐ Deep to the popliteus are the femur and the tibia.
- ☐ The proximal tendon of the popliteus arises from the femur within the joint capsule of the knee (i.e., it is intra-articular).
- ☐ The popliteus is located within the deep front line and involved with the superficial back line myofascial meridians.

■ MISCELLANEOUS

1. The popliteus is located in the deep posterior compartment of the leg.
2. The proximal tendon of the popliteus is located within the knee joint (i.e., it is intra-articular). The only other muscle that has an intra-articular tendon is the (long head of the) biceps brachii at the glenohumeral joint.
3. The popliteus also attaches into the lateral meniscus of the knee joint. This attachment facilitates the posterior movement of the lateral meniscus during knee flexion. This helps to prevent impingement of the lateral meniscus between the femur and tibia during flexion of the knee joint. (Note: The semimembranosus has the same action with regard to the medial meniscus.)

15

NOTES

15

16

Muscles of the Ankle and Subtalar Joints

CHAPTER OUTLINE

CHAPTER OVERVIEW

The muscles addressed in this chapter are the muscles whose principal function is usually considered to be movement of the ankle and subtalar joints. Other muscles in the body can also move the ankle and subtalar joints, but they are placed in different chapters because their primary function is usually considered to be at other joints. These muscles are the extrinsic muscles of the toes covered in Chapter 17; they are the extensor digitorum longus, extensor hallucis longus, flexor digitorum longus, and flexor hallucis longus.

Overview of Structure
□ Structurally, muscles of the ankle and subtalar joints have their bellies in the leg and are located in one of four distinct compartments. These four compartments of the leg are the anterior, lateral, superficial posterior, and deep posterior compartments and are shown in Figure 16-5.
□ The anterior compartment contains the tibialis anterior, extensor digitorum longus, extensor hallucis longus, and fibularis tertius.
□ The lateral compartment contains the fibularis longus and fibularis brevis.

□ The superficial posterior compartment contains the gastrocnemius, soleus, and plantaris.
□ The deep posterior compartment contains the tibialis posterior, flexor digitorum longus, flexor hallucis longus, and popliteus. Some of these muscles are addressed in other chapters.
□ The location by compartment helps determine the actions of these muscles. For example, all muscles of the anterior compartment do dorsiflexion; all muscles of the lateral and posterior compartments do plantarflexion. All muscles of the lateral compartment do eversion. The final determination of exactly what the actions of a muscle of the ankle and subtalar joints will be is where the distal tendon of that muscle crosses these joints (for example, the tibialis anterior is located in the anterolateral leg, but its tendon crosses the subtalar joint medially so it inverts the foot).

Overview of Function
The following general rules regarding actions can be stated for the functional groups of muscles of the ankle and subtalar joints:

Review the muscles and bones from this chapter on the enclosed CD!

☐ If a muscle crosses the ankle joint anteriorly with a vertical direction to its fibers, it can dorsiflex the foot at the ankle joint by moving the dorsum of the foot toward the anterior (dorsal) surface of the leg.

☐ If a muscle crosses the ankle joint posteriorly with a vertical direction to its fibers, it can plantarflex the foot at the ankle joint by moving the plantar surface of the foot toward the posterior surface of the leg.

☐ If a muscle crosses the subtalar joint laterally, it can evert the foot at the subtalar joint by moving the lateral surface of the foot toward the lateral surface of the leg. Note: Eversion is the principle component of pronation.

☐ If a muscle crosses the subtalar joint medially, it can invert the foot at the subtalar joint by moving the medial surface of the foot toward the medial surface of the leg. Note: Inversion is the principle component of supination.

☐ Reverse actions occur when the foot is planted on the ground and the leg must move relative to the foot. The same terms can be used to describe these reverse actions. For example, when the anterior (dorsal) surface of the leg moves toward the dorsum of the foot, it is called dorsiflexion of the leg at the ankle joint.

16

Anterior View of the Muscles of the Right Ankle and Subtalar Joints

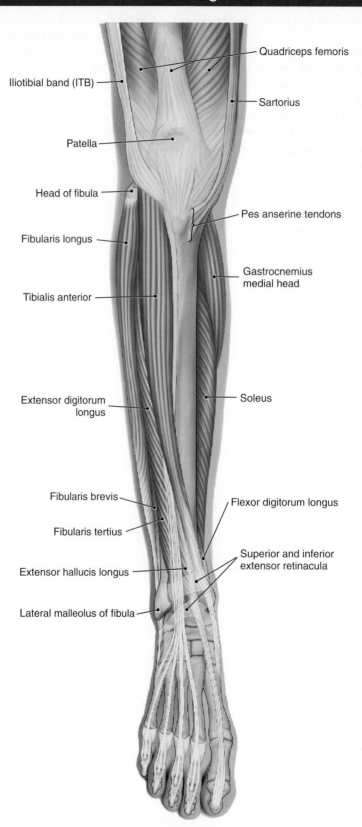

Figure 16-1 Anterior view of the muscles of the right ankle and subtalar joints.

16

Posterior View of the Muscles of the Right Ankle and Subtalar Joints—Superficial View

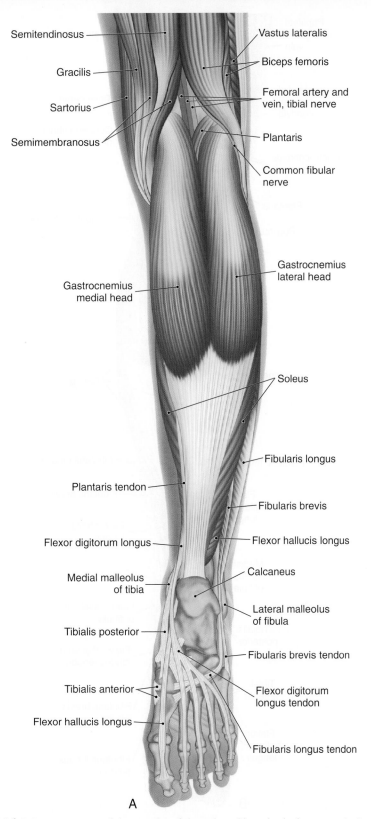

A

Figure 16-2 Posterior views of the muscles of the right ankle and subtalar joints. **A,** Superficial.

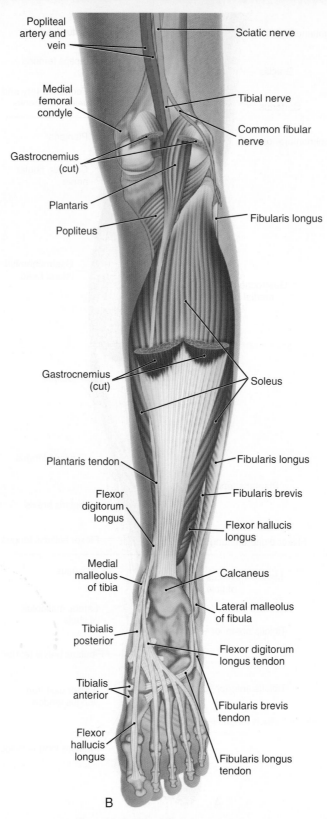

Popliteal artery and vein

Sciatic nerve

Medial femoral condyle

Tibial nerve

Common fibular nerve

Gastrocnemius (cut)

Plantaris

Popliteus

Fibularis longus

Gastrocnemius (cut)

Soleus

Plantaris tendon

Fibularis longus

Flexor digitorum longus

Fibularis brevis

Flexor hallucis longus

Medial malleolus of tibia

Calcaneus

Lateral malleolus of fibula

Tibialis posterior

Flexor digitorum longus tendon

Tibialis anterior

Fibularis brevis tendon

Flexor hallucis longus

Fibularis longus tendon

B

Figure 16-2, cont'd B, Intermediate.

16

Posterior View of the Muscles of the Right Ankle and Subtalar Joints—Deep View

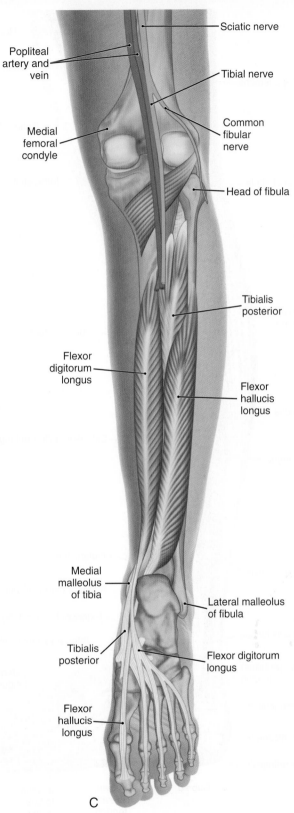

C

Figure 16-2, cont'd C, Deep.

Lateral View of the Muscles of the Right Ankle and Subtalar Joints

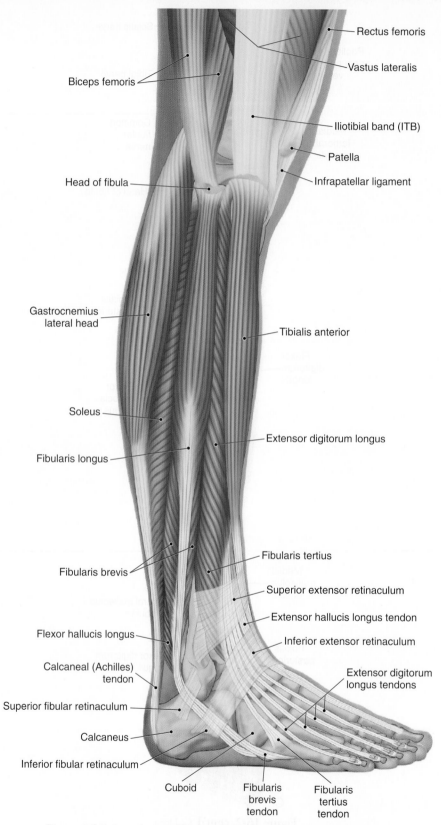

Rectus femoris

Vastus lateralis

Biceps femoris

Iliotibial band (ITB)

Patella

Head of fibula

Infrapatellar ligament

Gastrocnemius
lateral head

Tibialis anterior

Soleus

Extensor digitorum longus

Fibularis longus

Fibularis tertius

Fibularis brevis

Superior extensor retinaculum

Extensor hallucis longus tendon

Flexor hallucis longus

Inferior extensor retinaculum

Calcaneal (Achilles)
tendon

Extensor digitorum
longus tendons

Superior fibular retinaculum

Calcaneus

Inferior fibular retinaculum

Cuboid

Fibularis
brevis
tendon

Fibularis
tertius
tendon

16

Figure 16-3 Lateral view of the muscles of the right ankle and subtalar joints.

Medial Views of the Muscles of the Right Ankle and Subtalar Joints

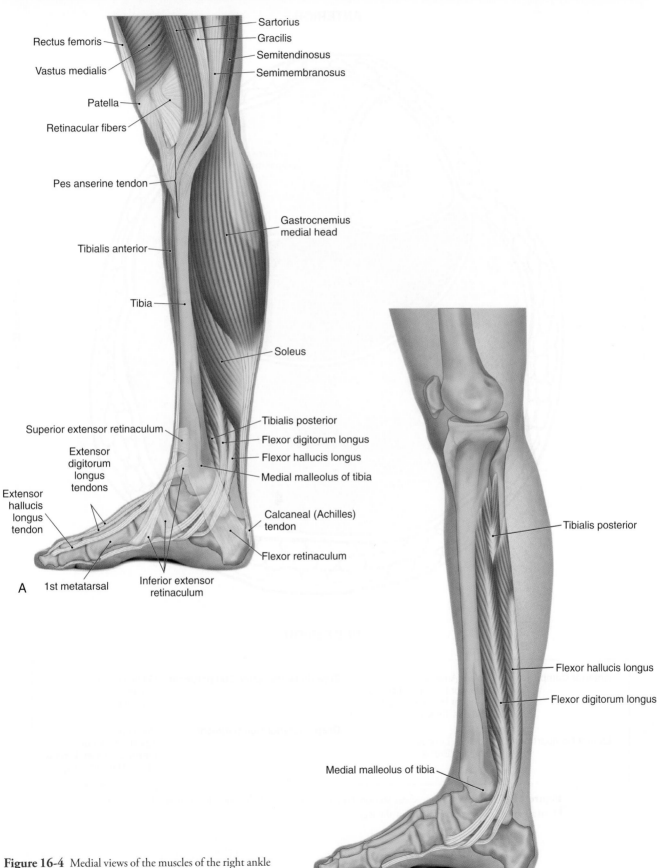

Figure 16-4 Medial views of the muscles of the right ankle and subtalar joints. **A,** Superficial. **B,** Deep.

Transverse Plane Cross Section of the Right Leg—Compartments

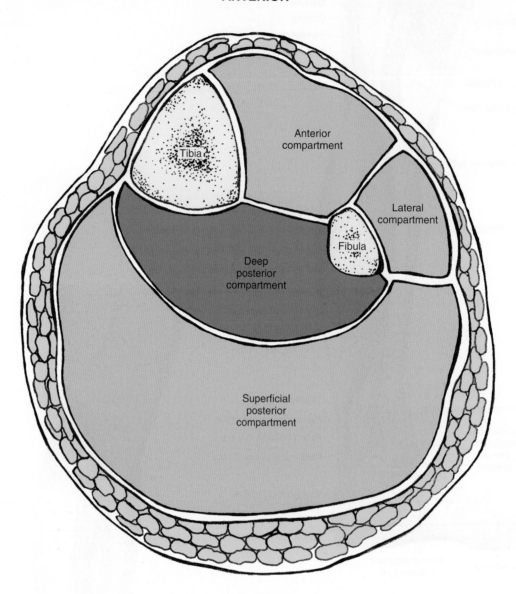

Figure 16-5 Transverse plane cross section (approximately ⅓ of the way distal to the knee joint), illustrating the four compartments of the leg.

Anterior Compartment:	Tibialis Anterior	Superficial Posterior Compartment:	Gastrocnemius
	Extensor Digitorum Longus		Soleus
	Extensor Hallucis Longus		Plantaris
	Fibularis Tertius		
		Deep Posterior Compartment:	Popliteus
Lateral Compartment:	Fibularis Longus		Tibialis Posterior
	Fibularis Brevis		Flexor Digitorum Longus
			Flexor Hallucis Longus

Transverse Plane Cross Section of the Right Leg—Muscles

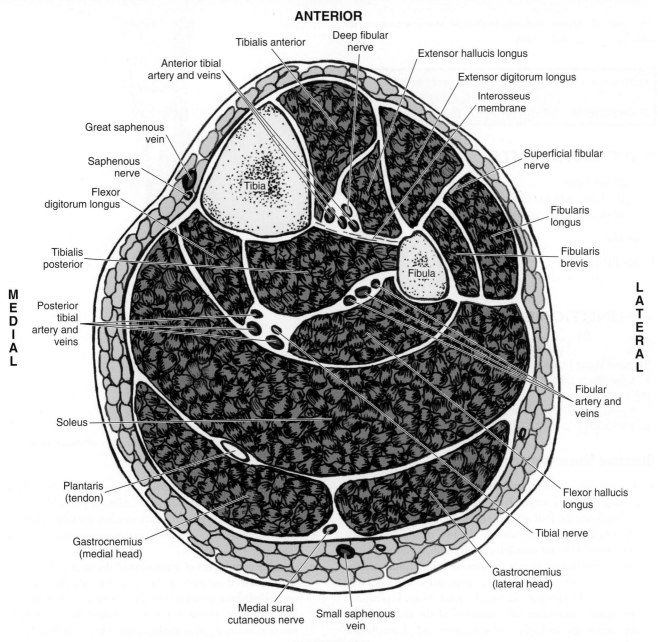

ANTERIOR

Tibialis anterior

Deep fibular nerve

Anterior tibial artery and veins

Extensor hallucis longus

Extensor digitorum longus

Interosseus membrane

Great saphenous vein

Saphenous nerve

Flexor digitorum longus

Tibialis posterior

Tibia

Fibula

Superficial fibular nerve

Fibularis longus

Fibularis brevis

MEDIAL

LATERAL

Posterior tibial artery and veins

Soleus

Plantaris (tendon)

Gastrocnemius (medial head)

Gastrocnemius (lateral head)

Fibular artery and veins

Flexor hallucis longus

Tibial nerve

Medial sural cutaneous nerve

Small saphenous vein

16

POSTERIOR

Figure 16-6 Transverse plane cross section (approximately ⅓ of the way distal to the knee joint), illustrating the muscles within the compartments of the leg.

Tibialis Anterior

The name, tibialis anterior, *tells us that this muscle attaches to the tibia and is located anteriorly.*

Derivation	☐ tibialis: L. *refers to the tibia.*
	anterior: L. *before, in front of.*
Pronunciation	☐ tib-ee-A-lis, an-TEE-ri-or

■ ATTACHMENTS

☐ **Anterior Tibia**
  ☐ the lateral tibial condyle, the proximal ⅔ of the anterior tibia, and the proximal ⅔ of the interosseus membrane

  to the

☐ **Medial Foot**
  ☐ the first cuneiform and first metatarsal

■ FUNCTIONS

CONCENTRIC (SHORTENING) MOVER ACTIONS	
Standard Mover Actions	**Reverse Mover Actions**
☐ **1. Dorsiflexes the foot at the ankle joint**	☐ 1. Dorsiflexes the leg at the ankle joint
☐ 2. Inverts (supinates) the foot at the subtalar joint	☐ 2. Inverts (supinates) the talus at the subtalar joint

Standard Mover Actions Notes

• The tibialis anterior crosses the ankle joint anteriorly (with its fibers running vertically in the sagittal plane); therefore it dorsiflexes the foot at the ankle joint. (action 1)
• The tibialis anterior crosses into the foot medial to the axis of motion of the subtalar joint (with its fibers running vertically in the frontal plane); therefore it inverts/supinates the foot (more specifically, it inverts/supinates the calcaneus relative to the talus) at the subtalar joint. Note: Inversion is the major component of supination of the foot; subtalar supination also includes medial rotation and plantarflexion of the foot. (action 2)

Reverse Mover Action Notes

• Reverse actions at the ankle and subtalar joints usually occur when the foot is planted on the ground so that the proximal attachment moves toward the distal one. (reverse actions 1, 2)
• The tibialis anterior crosses the ankle joint anteriorly (with its fibers running vertically in the sagittal plane). If the distal attachment is fixed, the tibialis anterior pulls the anterior (dorsal) surface of the leg toward the dorsum of the foot, therefore it dorsiflexes the leg at the ankle joint. This action occurs during the gait cycle when our foot is planted on the ground. (reverse action 1)

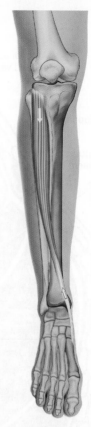

Figure 16-7 Anterior view of the right tibialis anterior.

• The reverse action of inversion of the foot at the subtalar joint is inversion of the leg at the subtalar joint. Moving the leg at the subtalar joint involves moving the talus relative to the calcaneus. Inversion is the major component of supination. (reverse action 2)
• Another component of supination of the talus at the subtalar joint is lateral rotation of the talus. Because the ankle and (extended) knee joints do not allow rotation, when the talus laterally rotates, the entire lower extremity follows with lateral rotation of the thigh at the hip joint. (reverse action 2)

Eccentric Antagonist Functions

1. Restrains/slows ankle joint plantarflexion
2. Restrains/slows eversion (pronation) at the subtalar joint

Eccentric Antagonist Function Note

• The eccentric action of restraining/slowing eversion (pronation) of the foot at the subtalar joint is extremely important during the gait cycle (from heel-strike to foot-flat) so that the arch does not entirely collapse.

Isometric Stabilization Functions

1. Stabilizes the ankle and subtalar joints

16

Tibialis Anterior—*cont'd*

Isometric Function Note

- As one of the two stirrup muscles, the tibialis anterior plays an important role in supporting and stabilizing the arches (including the subtalar joint) of the foot.

Additional Notes on Functions

- All four muscles in the anterior compartment of the leg can dorsiflex the foot (and leg) at the ankle joint.
- The tibialis anterior and the tibialis posterior both invert the foot (at the subtalar joint). However, because the tibialis anterior is anterior, it can also dorsiflex the foot at the ankle joint, whereas the tibialis posterior, being posterior, can plantarflex the foot at the ankle joint.

INNERVATION

- ☐ The Deep Fibular Nerve
  - ☐ **L4**, L5

ARTERIAL SUPPLY

- ☐ The Anterior Tibial Artery (a terminal branch of the Popliteal Artery)

✋ PALPATION

1. With the client seated or supine, have the client dorsiflex and invert the foot (resistance can be added) and look for and then palpate the distal tendon of the tibialis anterior as it crosses the ankle joint anteromedially.
2. Continue palpating the tibialis anterior proximally on the lateral side of the tibia.
3. Note: So that the extensors digitorum and hallucis longus do not contract, make sure that the client is not extending the toes.

■ RELATIONSHIP TO OTHER STRUCTURES

- ☐ The tibialis anterior is superficial in the anterolateral leg.
- ☐ The tibialis anterior lies just lateral to the tibia.
- ☐ The extensor digitorum longus is lateral to the tibialis anterior, more distally, the extensor hallucis longus is lateral to the tibialis anterior.
- ☐ Deep to the belly of the tibialis anterior are the extensor digitorum longus and the extensor hallucis longus.
- ☐ The tibialis anterior is located within the superficial front line and spiral line myofascial meridians.

■ MISCELLANEOUS

1. The tibialis anterior is located in the anterior compartment of the leg.
2. The tibialis anterior has a very prominent distal tendon.
3. The tibialis anterior and the fibularis longus are known as the *stirrup muscles*. These two muscles both attach at the same location on the medial foot (first cuneiform and first metatarsal) and may be viewed as a stirrup to support the arch (medial longitudinal arch) of the foot. The tibialis anterior is also credited with supporting the transverse arch and the lateral longitudinal arch of the foot.
4. When the tibialis anterior is tight and painful, especially along its tibial attachment, this condition is usually called *shin splints* or *anterior shin splints*. (Note: *Shin splints* is a general term that is applied to most any painful condition that occurs in the leg [i.e., between the knee and the ankle]. Shin splints due to a painful tibialis anterior is probably the most common form of shin splints.)

16

Fibularis Tertius

The name, fibularis tertius, *tells us that this muscle attaches to the fibula and is the third fibularis muscle. The first two fibularis muscles are the fibularis longus and fibularis brevis.*

Derivation	☐ fibularis: L. *refers to the fibula.*
	tertius: L. *third.*
Pronunciation	☐ fib-you-LA-ris, TER-she-us

■ ATTACHMENTS

☐ **Distal Anterior Fibula**
  ☐ the distal ⅓ of the anterior fibula and the distal ⅓ of the interosseus membrane

  to the

☐ **Fifth Metatarsal**
  ☐ the dorsal surface of the base of the fifth metatarsal

■ FUNCTIONS

CONCENTRIC (SHORTENING) MOVER ACTIONS	
Standard Mover Actions	**Reverse Mover Actions**
☐ **1. Dorsiflexes the foot at the ankle joint**	☐ 1. Dorsiflexes the leg at the ankle joint
☐ 2. Everts (pronates) the foot at the subtalar joint	☐ 2. Everts (pronates) the talus at the subtalar joint

Standard Mover Actions Notes

- The fibularis tertius crosses the ankle joint anteriorly (with its fibers running vertically in the sagittal plane); therefore it dorsiflexes the foot at the ankle joint. (action 1)
- The fibularis tertius crosses into the foot lateral to the axis of motion of the subtalar joint (with its fibers running vertically in the frontal plane); therefore it everts/pronates the foot (more specifically, it everts/pronates the calcaneus relative to the talus) at the subtalar joint. Note: Eversion is the major component of pronation of the foot; subtalar pronation also includes lateral rotation and dorsiflexion of the foot. (action 2)

Reverse Mover Action Notes

- Reverse actions at the ankle and subtalar joints usually occur when the foot is planted on the ground so that the proximal attachment moves toward the distal one. (reverse actions 1, 2)
- The fibularis tertius crosses the ankle joint anteriorly (with its fibers running vertically in the sagittal plane). If the distal attachment is fixed, the fibularis tertius pulls the anterior (dorsal) surface of the leg toward the dorsum of the foot, therefore it dorsiflexes the leg at the ankle joint. This action occurs during the gait cycle when our foot is planted on the ground. (reverse action 1)

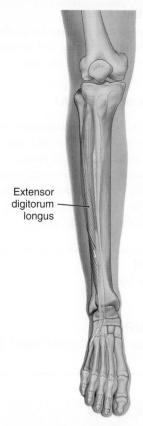

Extensor digitorum longus

Figure 16-8 Anterior view of the right fibularis tertius. The extensor digitorum longus has been ghosted in.

- The reverse action of eversion of the foot at the subtalar joint is eversion of the leg at the subtalar joint. Moving the leg at the subtalar joint involves moving the talus relative to the calcaneus. Eversion is the major component of pronation. (reverse action 2)
- Another component of pronation of the talus at the subtalar joint is medial rotation of the talus. Because the ankle and (extended) knee joints do not allow rotation, when the talus medially rotates, the entire lower extremity follows with medial rotation of the thigh at the hip joint. (reverse action 2)

Eccentric Antagonist Functions

1. Restrains/slows ankle joint plantarflexion
2. Restrains/slows inversion (supination) at the subtalar joint

Eccentric Antagonist Function Note

- The eccentric action of restraining/slowing plantarflexion of the foot is important during the gait cycle (from heel-strike to foot-flat).

Isometric Stabilization Functions

1. Stabilizes the ankle and subtalar joints

16

Fibularis Tertius—*cont'd*

Additional Notes on Functions

1. All four muscles in the anterior compartment of the leg can dorsiflex the foot (and leg) at the ankle joint.
2. The three fibularis muscles are grouped together, because they all evert the subtalar joint.

INNERVATION
- ☐ The Deep Fibular Nerve
  - ☐ L5, S1

ARTERIAL SUPPLY
- ☐ The Anterior Tibial Artery (a terminal branch of the Popliteal Artery)

🖐 PALPATION

1. With the client seated or supine, first locate the tendon of the extensor digitorum longus that goes to the little (fifth) toe. If not visible, it can usually be palpated by strumming perpendicular across it as the client extends the little toe.
2. Once located, look and palpate immediately lateral to it for the tendon of the fibularis tertius running approximately parallel and going to the base of the fifth metatarsal as the client everts and dorsiflexes the foot (resistance can be added).
3. Note: The fibularis tertius is sometimes missing.

■ RELATIONSHIP TO OTHER STRUCTURES

- ☐ The fibularis tertius is actually part of the extensor digitorum longus. It comprises the most distal part of the belly of the extensor digitorum longus, which becomes the most lateral tendon (and attaches to the fifth metatarsal).
- ☐ The distal tendon of the fibularis tertius is located just lateral to the tendon of the extensor digitorum longus that goes to the little toe.
- ☐ Deep to the fibularis tertius is the fibula.
- ☐ The fibularis tertius is located within the superficial front line myofascial meridian.

■ MISCELLANEOUS

1. The fibularis tertius is located in the anterior compartment of the leg.
2. The fibularis tertius was formerly named the *peroneus tertius*.
3. The fibularis tertius is actually the most distal and lateral part of the extensor digitorum longus. Its fibers do not attach onto a digit (a phalanx); for this reason the fibularis tertius is given a separate name and considered to be a separate muscle from the extensor digitorum longus.
4. The fibularis tertius is homologous to the extensor digiti minimi of the forearm/hand.
5. The fibularis tertius is sometimes missing.
6. The fibularis tertius is pennate.

16

Fibularis Longus

The name, fibularis longus, *tells us that this muscle attaches to the fibula and is long (longer than the fibularis brevis).*

Derivation	☐ fibularis: L. *refers to the fibula.*
	longus: L. *longer.*
Pronunciation	☐ fib-you-LA-ris, LONG-us

■ ATTACHMENTS

☐ **Proximal Lateral Fibula**
   ☐ the head of the fibula and the proximal ½ of the lateral fibula

to the

☐ **Medial Foot**
   ☐ the first cuneiform and first metatarsal

■ FUNCTIONS

CONCENTRIC (SHORTENING) MOVER ACTIONS	
Standard Mover Actions	**Reverse Mover Actions**
☐ **1. Everts (pronates) the foot at the subtalar joint**	☐ 1. Everts (pronates) the talus at the subtalar joint
☐ **2. Plantarflexes the foot at the ankle joint**	☐ 2. Plantarflexes the leg at the ankle joint

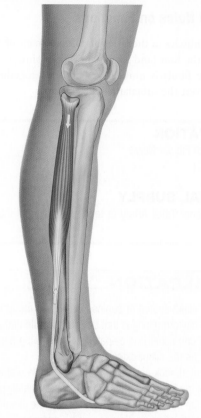

Figure 16-9 Lateral view of the right fibularis longus.

Standard Mover Actions Notes

• The fibularis longus crosses onto the foot laterally (with its fibers running vertically in the frontal plane); therefore it everts/pronates the foot (more specifically, it everts/pronates the calcaneus relative to the talus) at the subtalar joint. Note: Eversion is the major component of subtalar pronation; subtalar pronation also includes lateral rotation and dorsiflexion of the foot. (action 1)

• The fibularis longus crosses the ankle joint posteriorly (with its fibers running vertically in the sagittal plane); therefore it plantarflexes the foot at the ankle joint. (action 2)

Reverse Mover Action Notes

• Reverse actions at the ankle and subtalar joints usually occur when the foot is planted on the ground so that the proximal attachment moves toward the distal one. (reverse actions 1, 2)

• The reverse action of eversion of the foot at the subtalar joint is eversion of the leg at the subtalar joint. Moving the leg at the subtalar joint involves moving the talus relative to the calcaneus. Eversion is the major component of pronation. (reverse action 1)

• Another component of pronation of the talus at the subtalar joint is medial rotation of the talus. Because the ankle and (extended) knee joints do not allow rotation, when the talus

medially rotates, the entire lower extremity follows with medial rotation of the thigh at the hip joint. (reverse action 1)

• The fibularis longus crosses the ankle joint posteriorly (with its fibers running vertically in the sagittal plane). If the distal attachment is fixed, the fibularis longus pulls the posterior surface of the leg toward the plantar surface of the foot, therefore it plantarflexes the leg at the ankle joint. (reverse action 2)

Eccentric Antagonist Functions

1. Restrains/slows inversion (supination) at the subtalar joint
2. Restrains/slows ankle joint dorsiflexion

Isometric Stabilization Functions

1. Stabilizes the ankle and subtalar joints

Isometric Function Notes

• The action of eversion is important in preventing inversion sprains of the ankle; therefore to help stabilize the ankle joint, it is important to strengthen the fibularis longus in clients who have a history of inversion sprains.

16

Fibularis Longus—cont'd

- As one of the two stirrup muscles, the fibularis longus plays an important role in supporting and stabilizing the arches (and the subtalar joint) of the foot.

Additional Notes on Functions

1. Both muscles in the lateral compartment of the leg (fibularis longus and brevis) can evert (pronate) the foot (and leg) at the subtalar joint.
2. The three fibularis muscles are grouped together because they all evert the subtalar joint.

INNERVATION
- ☐ The Superficial Fibular Nerve
  - ☐ L5, S1

ARTERIAL SUPPLY
- ☐ The Fibular Artery (a branch of the Posterior Tibial Artery)

✋ PALPATION

1. With the client prone, supine, or side lying, place palpating hand on the proximal lateral leg just distal to the head of the fibula.
2. Ask the client to actively evert the foot and feel for the contraction of the belly of the fibularis longus from the head of the fibula to the point where it becomes tendon halfway down the leg.
3. Continue palpating the distal tendon to the posterior side of the lateral malleolus of the fibula.
4. Distal to the lateral malleolus, the tendon of the fibularis longus is challenging to palpate as it runs toward the cuboid. In the plantar foot, the distal tendon is usually not palpable.
5. Note: The distal tendon of the fibularis brevis is usually prominent distal to the lateral malleolus as it runs to the base of the fifth metatarsal. Do not mistake the fibularis brevis tendon for the fibularis longus tendon.

■ RELATIONSHIP TO OTHER STRUCTURES

- ☐ Proximally, the fibularis longus is posterior (lateral) to the tibialis anterior and the extensor digitorum longus.
- ☐ Proximally, the fibularis longus is superficial to the extensor digitorum longus. Distally, the fibularis longus is superficial to the fibularis brevis.
- ☐ The fibularis longus is anterior to the soleus.
- ☐ The distal tendon of the fibularis longus is very deep and found in the fourth layer of muscles of the plantar surface of the foot.
- ☐ The fibularis longus is located within the lateral line and spiral line myofascial meridians.

■ MISCELLANEOUS

1. The fibularis longus is located in the lateral compartment of the leg.
2. The fibularis longus becomes tendon halfway down the leg.
3. The distal tendon of the fibularis longus follows an unusual path; it crosses posterior to the lateral malleolus to enter the lateral side of the foot, where it crosses posterior to the cuboid and then dives deep into the plantar side of the foot. It finally attaches onto the medial side of the foot at the same location as the attachment of the tibialis anterior (first cuneiform and first metatarsal).
4. The three fibularis muscles are grouped together, because they all evert the foot at the subtalar joint.
5. The fibularis longus and the fibularis brevis both cross posterior to the lateral malleolus; therefore they both plantarflex the foot at the ankle joint. The fibularis tertius crosses anterior to the lateral malleolus; therefore it dorsiflexes the foot at the ankle joint.
6. The fibularis longus has a tendon that makes an abrupt turn of approximately 90 degrees.
7. The fibularis longus was formerly named the *peroneus longus.*
8. The fibularis longus and the tibialis anterior are known as the *stirrup muscles.* These two muscles both attach at the same location on the medial foot (first cuneiform and first metatarsal) and may be viewed to act as a stirrup to support the arch (medial longitudinal arch) of the foot. The fibularis longus is also credited with supporting the transverse arch and the lateral longitudinal arch of the foot.
9. The fibularis longus and the fibularis brevis should be strengthened in people who have had inversion sprains of the ankle joint.

16

Fibularis Brevis

The name, fibularis brevis, *tells us that this muscle attaches onto the fibula and is short (shorter than the fibularis longus).*

Derivation	☐ fibularis: L. *refers to the fibula.*
	brevis: L. *shorter.*
Pronunciation	☐ fib-you-LA-ris, BRE-vis

■ ATTACHMENTS

☐ **Distal Lateral Fibula**
   ☐ the distal ½ of the lateral fibula

to the

☐ **Fifth Metatarsal**
   ☐ the lateral side of the base of the fifth metatarsal

■ FUNCTIONS

CONCENTRIC (SHORTENING) MOVER ACTIONS	
Standard Mover Actions	**Reverse Mover Actions**
☐ **1. Everts (pronates) the foot at the subtalar joint**	☐ 1. Everts (pronates) the talus at the subtalar joint
☐ **2. Plantarflexes the foot at the ankle joint**	☐ 2. Plantarflexes the leg at the ankle joint

Standard Mover Actions Notes

- The fibularis brevis crosses onto the foot laterally (with its fibers running vertically in the frontal plane); therefore it everts/pronates the foot (more specifically, it everts/pronates the calcaneus relative to the talus) at the subtalar joint. Note: Eversion is the major component of subtalar pronation; subtalar pronation also includes lateral rotation and dorsiflexion of the foot. (action 1)
- The fibularis brevis crosses the ankle joint posteriorly (with its fibers running vertically in the sagittal plane); therefore it plantarflexes the foot at the ankle joint. (action 2)

Reverse Mover Action Notes

- Reverse actions at the ankle and subtalar joints usually occur when the foot is planted on the ground so that the proximal attachment moves toward the distal one. (reverse actions 1, 2)
- The reverse action of eversion of the foot at the subtalar joint is eversion of the leg at the subtalar joint. Moving the leg at the subtalar joint involves moving the talus relative to the calcaneus. Eversion is the major component of pronation. (reverse action 1)
- Another component of pronation of the talus at the subtalar joint is medial rotation of the talus. Because the ankle and (extended) knee joints do not allow rotation, when the talus medially rotates, the entire lower extremity follows with medial rotation of the thigh at the hip joint. (reverse action 1)

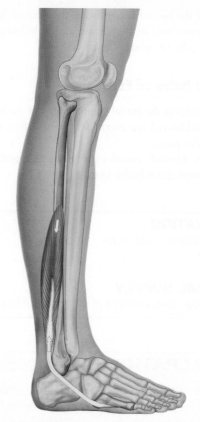

Figure 16-10 Lateral view of the right fibularis brevis.

- The fibularis brevis crosses the ankle joint posteriorly (with its fibers running vertically in the sagittal plane). If the distal attachment is fixed, the fibularis brevis pulls the posterior surface of the leg toward the plantar surface of the foot, therefore it plantarflexes the leg at the ankle joint. (reverse action 2)

Eccentric Antagonist Functions

1. Restrains/slows inversion (supination) at the subtalar joint
2. Restrains/slows ankle joint dorsiflexion

Isometric Stabilization Functions

1. Stabilizes the ankle and subtalar joints

Isometric Function Note

- The action of eversion is important in preventing inversion sprains of the ankle; therefore to help stabilize the ankle joint, it is important to strengthen the fibularis brevis in clients who have a history of inversion sprains.

16

Fibularis Brevis—*cont'd*

Additional Notes on Functions

1. Both muscles in the lateral compartment of the leg (fibularis longus and brevis) can evert (pronate) the foot (and leg) at the subtalar joint.
2. The three fibularis muscles are grouped together because they all evert the subtalar joint.

INNERVATION
☐ The Superficial Fibular Nerve
  ☐ L5, S1

ARTERIAL SUPPLY
☐ The Fibular Artery (a branch of the Posterior Tibial Artery)

✋ PALPATION

1. With the client prone, supine, or side lying, place palpating hand on the distal lateral leg.
2. Have the client evert the foot (resistance can be added) and feel for the belly of the fibularis brevis on either side (especially the posterior side) of the fibularis longus' distal tendon. Keep in mind that this will make both the fibularis longus and the fibularis brevis stand out.
3. Distal to the lateral malleolus, the distal tendon of the fibularis brevis is easily palpable and usually visible all the way to its attachment onto the base of the fifth metatarsal.

■ RELATIONSHIP TO OTHER STRUCTURES

☐ The fibularis brevis is deep to the fibularis longus, but it is not entirely covered by the fibularis longus.
☐ The fibularis brevis is posterior to the extensor digitorum longus.
☐ The fibularis brevis is anterior to the soleus.
☐ Deep to the fibularis brevis is the fibula.
☐ The fibularis brevis is located within the lateral line myofascial meridian.

■ MISCELLANEOUS

1. The fibularis brevis is located in the lateral compartment of the leg.
2. The distal tendon of the fibularis brevis travels with the distal tendon of the fibularis longus. Together they both cross posterior to the lateral malleolus. Therefore they both plantarflex the foot at the ankle joint.
3. The fibularis brevis was formerly named the *peroneus brevis.*

16

Gastrocnemius (*Gastrocs*) (of Triceps Surae Group)

The name, gastrocnemius, *tells us that this muscle gives the posterior leg its belly shape. (The contour of the posterior leg is the result of the two bellies of the gastrocnemius.)*

Derivation	☐ gastro: Gr. *stomach.*
	nemius: Gr. *leg.*
Pronunciation	☐ GAS-trok-NEE-me-us

◼ ATTACHMENTS

☐ **Medial and Lateral Femoral Condyles**
    ☐ and the distal posteromedial femur and the distal posterolateral femur

to the

☐ **Calcaneus via the Calcaneal (Achilles) Tendon**
    ☐ the posterior surface

◼ FUNCTIONS

CONCENTRIC (SHORTENING) MOVER ACTIONS	
Standard Mover Actions	**Reverse Mover Actions**
☐ **1. Plantarflexes the foot at the ankle joint**	☐ 1. Plantarflexes the leg at the ankle joint
☐ **2. Flexes the leg at the knee joint**	☐ 2. Flexes the thigh at the knee joint
☐ 3. Inverts (supinates) the foot at the subtalar joint	☐ 3. Inverts (supinates) the talus at the subtalar joint

Standard Mover Actions Notes

- The gastrocnemius crosses the ankle joint posteriorly (with its fibers running vertically in the sagittal plane); therefore it plantarflexes the foot at the ankle joint. Plantarflexion of the foot at the ankle joint is an important action during the gait cycle when pushing off the ground (toe-off phase). (action 1)
- The gastrocnemius crosses the knee joint posteriorly (with its fibers running vertically in the sagittal plane); therefore it flexes the leg at the knee joint. (action 2)
- The gastrocnemius crosses into the foot to attach onto the calcaneus medial to the axis of the subtalar joint. Therefore the gastrocnemius inverts/supinates the foot (more specifically, it inverts/supinates the calcaneus relative to the talus) at the subtalar joint. Note: Inversion is the major component of subtalar supination; subtalar supination also includes medial rotation and plantarflexion of the foot. (action 3)

Reverse Mover Action Notes

- Reverse actions at the ankle and subtalar joints usually occur when the foot is planted on the ground so that the proximal attachment moves toward the distal one. (reverse actions 1, 2, 3)

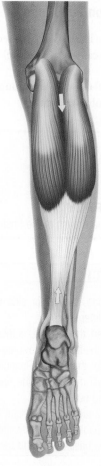

Figure 16-11 Posterior view of the right gastrocnemius.

- The gastrocnemius crosses the ankle joint posteriorly (with its fibers running vertically in the sagittal plane). If the distal attachment is fixed, the gastrocnemius pulls the posterior surface of the leg toward the plantar surface of the foot, therefore it plantarflexes the foot at the ankle joint. (reverse action 1)
- The gastrocnemius crosses the knee joint posteriorly (with its fibers running vertically in the sagittal plane). If the distal attachment is fixed, the gastrocnemius pulls the posterior surface of the thigh toward the posterior surface of the leg, therefore it flexes the thigh at the knee joint. (reverse action 2)
- The reverse action of inversion of the foot at the subtalar joint is inversion of the leg at the subtalar joint. Moving the leg at the subtalar joint involves moving the talus relative to the calcaneus. Inversion is the major component of supination. (reverse action 3)
- Another component of supination of the talus at the subtalar joint is lateral rotation of the talus. Because the ankle and (extended) knee joints do not allow rotation, when the talus laterally rotates, the entire lower extremity follows with lateral rotation of the thigh at the hip joint. (reverse action 3)

16

Gastrocnemius (*Gastrocs*) (of Triceps Surae Group)—*cont'd*

Eccentric Antagonist Functions

1. Restrains/slows ankle joint dorsiflexion
2. Restrains/slows knee joint extension
3. Restrains/slows eversion (pronation) at the subtalar joint

Eccentric Antagonist Function Note

- Restraining/slowing dorsiflexion of the leg at the ankle joint is important when standing and bending forward (at the ankle, knee, and hip joints).

Isometric Stabilization Functions

1. Stabilizes the ankle, subtalar, and knee joints

Additional Notes on Functions

1. Even though plantarflexion of the foot at the ankle joint is a very important action during walking, there is very little gastrocnemius activity in walking. The gastrocnemius is not appreciably recruited unless one walks uphill or up stairs, on an unstable surface (such as sand), runs, jumps, or tiptoes.
2. All three muscles in the superficial posterior compartment of the leg (gastrocnemius, soleus, and plantaris) can plantarflex the foot (and leg) at the ankle joint.

INNERVATION
- ☐ The Tibial Nerve
  - ☐ S1, S2

ARTERIAL SUPPLY
- ☐ Sural branches of the Popliteal Artery (the continuation of the Femoral Artery)

✋ PALPATION

1. With the client prone with the leg extended at the knee joint, place palpating hand on the proximal posterior leg.
2. Have the client plantarflex the foot at the ankle joint (resistance can be given) and feel for the contraction of the gastrocnemius. It can be palpated from its proximal attachments to its distal attachment on the calcaneus via the calcaneal (Achilles) tendon.

■ RELATIONSHIP TO OTHER STRUCTURES

- ☐ The gastrocnemius is superficial in the posterior leg.
- ☐ The soleus is deep to the gastrocnemius and is largely, but not entirely, covered by it.
- ☐ The distal belly and tendon of the biceps femoris is superficial to the proximal attachment of the lateral gastrocnemius.
- ☐ The gastrocnemius is located within the superficial back line myofascial meridian.

■ MISCELLANEOUS

1. The gastrocnemius is located in the superficial posterior compartment of the leg.
2. The gastrocnemius and the soleus together are sometimes called the *triceps surae*. *Triceps* refers to having three heads (medial gastrocnemius, lateral gastrocnemius, and soleus) and *surae* (SUR-eye) refers to the calf of the leg. They are grouped together as the triceps surae because they all attach to the calcaneus via the calcaneal (Achilles) tendon.
3. Given that the distal tendon of the plantaris is directly next to (and often melds with) the calcaneal (Achilles) tendon, the plantaris is often grouped with the gastrocnemius and the soleus. This group is sometimes called the *quadriceps surae*.
4. The Achilles tendon derives its name from the Greek myth in which Achilles went into battle to rescue Helen of Troy. When he was young, to make him invulnerable to poison arrows, his mother dipped him into the River Styx. However, she held him by his posterior ankle (i.e., heel). Therefore he was vulnerable in that one spot; hence, the expression *Achilles' heel* denoting a person's weakness. Unfortunately, Paris hit him with a poison arrow in his heel and he died. The relevance to anatomy is that the muscles of the triceps surae are the prime movers of foot plantarflexion, which is needed to push the foot off the ground when walking or running. If the Achilles tendon ruptures, one loses the ability to walk and/or run, which makes one vulnerable and weak.
5. The gastrocnemius becomes tendon approximately halfway down the leg.
6. Excessive use of high-heeled shoes can result in chronic shortened triceps surae muscles.
7. The fact that the gastrocnemius crosses the knee joint and the soleus does not cross the knee joint gives us the ability to preferentially stretch one of these muscles without stretching the other. For either muscle, stretching is accomplished by doing dorsiflexion at the ankle joint, because these muscles are plantarflexors. The key to stretching the gastrocnemius alone is to keep the knee joint straight (i.e., in extension) so that it is stretched across both the knee and ankle joints. Note: This stretch is usually called the *runner's stretch* and is done leaning up against a wall. For the gastrocnemius, the heel must be kept down on the ground and the knee joint must be in extension.

16

Soleus (of Triceps Surae Group)

The name, soleus, *tells us that this muscle attaches onto the sole (calcaneus) of the foot.*

Derivation	☐ soleus: L. *sole of the foot.*
Pronunciation	☐ SO-lee-us

■ ATTACHMENTS

☐ **Posterior Tibia and Fibula**
   ☐ the soleal line of the tibia and the head and proximal ⅓ of the fibula

to the

☐ **Calcaneus via the Calcaneal (Achilles) Tendon**
   ☐ the posterior surface

■ FUNCTIONS

CONCENTRIC (SHORTENING) MOVER ACTIONS	
Standard Mover Actions	**Reverse Mover Actions**
☐ **1. Plantarflexes the foot at the ankle joint**	☐ 1. Plantarflexes the leg at the ankle joint
☐ 2. Inverts (supinates) the foot at the subtalar joint	☐ 2. Inverts (supinates) the talus at the subtalar joint

Standard Mover Actions Notes

- The soleus crosses the ankle joint posteriorly (with its fibers running vertically in the sagittal plane); therefore it plantarflexes the foot at the ankle joint. Plantarflexion of the foot at the ankle joint is an important action during the gait cycle when pushing off the ground (toe-off phase). (action 1)
- The soleus crosses into the foot to attach onto the calcaneus medial to the axis of the subtalar joint. Therefore the soleus inverts/supinates the foot (more specifically, it inverts/supinates the calcaneus relative to the talus) at the subtalar joint. Note: Inversion is the major component of subtalar supination; subtalar supination also includes medial rotation and plantarflexion of the foot. (action 2)

Reverse Mover Action Notes

- Reverse actions at the ankle and subtalar joints usually occur when the foot is planted on the ground so that the proximal attachment moves toward the distal one. (reverse actions 1, 2)
- The soleus crosses the ankle joint posteriorly (with its fibers running vertically in the sagittal plane). If the distal attachment is fixed, the soleus pulls the posterior surface of the leg toward the plantar surface of the foot, therefore it plantarflexes the leg at the ankle joint. (reverse action 1)
- The reverse action of inversion of the foot at the subtalar joint is inversion of the leg at the subtalar joint. Moving the

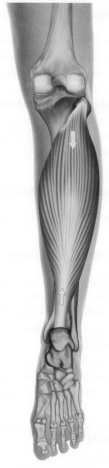

Figure 16-12 Posterior view of the right soleus.

leg at the subtalar joint involves moving the talus relative to the calcaneus. Inversion is the major component of supination. (reverse action 2)
- Another component of supination of the talus at the subtalar joint is lateral rotation of the talus. Because the ankle and (extended) knee joints do not allow rotation, when the talus laterally rotates, the entire lower extremity follows with lateral rotation of the thigh at the hip joint. (reverse action 2)

Eccentric Antagonist Functions

1. Restrains/slows ankle joint dorsiflexion
2. Restrains/slows eversion (pronation) at the subtalar joint

Eccentric Antagonist Function Note

- Restraining/slowing dorsiflexion of the leg at the ankle joint is important when standing and bending forward (bending at the ankle, knee, and hip joints).

16

Soleus (of Triceps Surae Group)—cont'd

Isometric Stabilization Functions

1. Stabilizes the ankle and subtalar joints

Additional Note on Function

1. All three muscles in the superficial posterior compartment of the leg (gastrocnemius, soleus, and plantaris) can plantarflex the foot (and leg) at the ankle joint.

INNERVATION
- ☐ The Tibial Nerve
  - ☐ S1, S2

ARTERIAL SUPPLY
- ☐ Sural branches of the Popliteal Artery (the continuation of the Femoral Artery)

✋ PALPATION

1. With the client prone with the leg flexed to 90 degrees at the knee joint, place palpating hand on the proximal posterior leg.
2. Have the client plantarflex the foot at the ankle joint against mild resistance and feel for the contraction of the soleus through the gastrocnemius.
3. The soleus is superficial and can be palpated on either side of the belly of the gastrocnemius, especially on the lateral side of the leg.

■ RELATIONSHIP TO OTHER STRUCTURES

- ☐ Posteriorly, the soleus is deep to the gastrocnemius and the plantaris, but medially and laterally the soleus is superficial.
- ☐ Medially, the soleus is located between the gastrocnemius and the tibia.
- ☐ Laterally, the soleus is located between the gastrocnemius and the fibularis longus.
- ☐ The soleus is superficial to the three deep muscles of the posterior leg: the tibialis posterior, the flexor digitorum longus, and the flexor hallucis longus (the *Tom, Dick, and Harry* muscles).

☐ The soleus is located within the superficial back line myofascial meridian.

■ MISCELLANEOUS

1. The soleus is located in the superficial posterior compartment of the leg.
2. The soleus and the gastrocnemius together are sometimes called the *triceps surae. Triceps* refers to having three heads (the medial gastrocnemius, the lateral gastrocnemius, and the soleus) and *surae* (SUR-eye) refers to the calf of the leg. They are grouped together as the triceps surae, because they all attach to the calcaneus via the calcaneal (Achilles) tendon.
3. Given that the distal tendon of the plantaris is directly next to (and often melds with) the calcaneal (Achilles) tendon, the plantaris is often grouped with the gastrocnemius and the soleus. This group is sometimes called the *quadriceps surae.*
4. The Achilles tendon derives its name from the Greek myth in which Achilles went into battle to rescue Helen of Troy. When he was young, to make him invulnerable to poison arrows, his mother dipped him into the River Styx. However, she held him by his posterior ankle (i.e., heel). Therefore he was vulnerable in that one spot, hence, the expression *Achilles' heel* denoting a person's weakness. Unfortunately, Paris hit him with a poison arrow in his heel and he died. The relevance to anatomy is that the triceps surae are the prime movers of foot plantarflexion, which is needed to push the foot off the ground when walking or running. If the Achilles tendon ruptures, one loses the ability to walk and/or run, which makes one vulnerable and weak.
6. The soleus becomes tendon much farther distally in the leg than the gastrocnemius.
7. The soleus is a thick muscle, largely accounting for the contours of the gastrocnemius being so visible. ("Behind every great gastrocnemius is a great soleus." ☺)
8. Excessive use of high-heeled shoes can result in chronic shortened triceps surae muscles.
9. The fact that the soleus does not cross the knee joint and that the gastrocnemius does cross the knee joint gives us the ability to preferentially stretch one of these muscles without stretching the other. For either muscle, stretching is accomplished by doing dorsiflexion at the ankle joint, because these muscles are plantarflexors. The key to stretching the soleus alone is to have the knee joint partially flexed so that the gastrocnemius is slackened across the knee joint. Note: This stretch is usually called the *runner's stretch* and is done leaning up against a wall. For the soleus, the heel must be kept down on the ground and the knee joint must be partially flexed.

16

Plantaris

The name, plantaris, *tells us that this muscle attaches onto the calcaneus, a bone of the plantar surface of the foot.*

Derivation	☐ plantaris: L. *refers to the plantar side of the foot.*
Pronunciation	☐ plan-TA-ris

■ ATTACHMENTS

☐ **Distal Posterolateral Femur**
    ☐ the lateral condyle and the distal lateral supracondylar line of the femur

to the

☐ **Calcaneus**
    ☐ the posterior surface

■ FUNCTIONS

CONCENTRIC (SHORTENING) MOVER ACTIONS	
Standard Mover Actions	**Reverse Mover Actions**
☐ **1. Plantarflexes the foot at the ankle joint**	☐ 1. Plantarflexes the leg at the ankle joint
☐ **2. Flexes the leg at the knee joint**	☐ 2. Flexes the thigh at the knee joint
☐ 3. Inverts (supinates) the foot at the subtalar joint	☐ 3. Inverts (supinates) the talus at the subtalar joint

Standard Mover Actions Notes

- The plantaris crosses the ankle joint posteriorly (with its fibers running vertically in the sagittal plane); therefore it plantarflexes the foot at the ankle joint. Plantarflexion of the foot at the ankle joint is an important action during the gait cycle when pushing off the ground (toe-off phase). (action 1)
- The plantaris crosses the knee joint posteriorly (with its fibers running vertically in the sagittal plane); therefore it flexes the leg at the knee joint. (action 2)
- The plantaris crosses into the foot to attach onto the calcaneus medial to the axis of the subtalar joint. Therefore the plantaris inverts/supinates the foot (more specifically, it inverts/supinates the calcaneus relative to the talus) at the subtalar joint. Note: Inversion is the major component of subtalar supination; subtalar supination also includes medial rotation and plantarflexion of the foot. (action 3)

Reverse Mover Action Notes

- Reverse actions at the ankle and subtalar joints usually occur when the foot is planted on the ground so that the proximal attachment moves toward the distal one. (reverse actions 1, 2, 3)

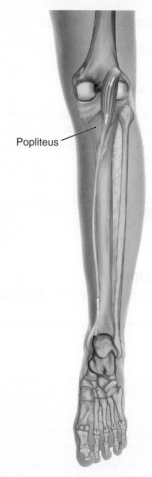

Popliteus

Figure 16-13 Posterior view of the right plantaris. The popliteus has been ghosted in.

- The plantaris crosses the ankle joint posteriorly (with its fibers running vertically in the sagittal plane). If the distal attachment is fixed, the plantaris pulls the posterior surface of the leg toward the plantar surface of the foot, therefore it plantarflexes the foot at the ankle joint. (reverse action 1)
- The plantaris crosses the knee joint posteriorly (with its fibers running vertically in the sagittal plane). If the distal attachment is fixed, the plantaris pulls the posterior surface of the thigh toward the posterior surface of the leg, therefore it flexes the thigh at the knee joint. (reverse action 2)
- The reverse action of inversion of the foot at the subtalar joint is inversion of the leg at the subtalar joint. Moving the leg at the subtalar joint involves moving the talus relative to the calcaneus. Inversion is the major component of supination. (reverse action 3)
- Another component of supination of the talus at the subtalar joint is lateral rotation of the talus. Because the ankle and (extended) knee joints do not allow rotation, when the talus laterally rotates, the entire lower extremity follows with lateral rotation of the thigh at the hip joint. (reverse action 3)

16

Plantaris—cont'd

Eccentric Antagonist Functions

1. Restrains/slows ankle joint dorsiflexion
2. Restrains/slows knee joint extension
3. Restrains/slows eversion (pronation) at the subtalar joint

Isometric Stabilization Functions

1. Stabilizes the ankle, subtalar, and knee joints

Additional Notes on Functions

1. All three muscles in the superficial posterior compartment of the leg (gastrocnemius, soleus, and plantaris) can plantarflex the foot (and leg) at the ankle joint.
2. The plantaris muscle is so weak that many sources consider its function to be negligible.

INNERVATION
□ The Tibial Nerve
  □ S1, S2

ARTERIAL SUPPLY
□ Sural branches of the Popliteal Artery (the continuation of the Femoral Artery)

PALPATION

1. With the client prone with the leg extended at the knee joint, place palpating fingers on the proximal posterior leg, at the lateral border of the popliteal fossa (just medial to the proximal attachment of the lateral head of the gastrocnemius).
2. Ask the client to actively flex the leg at the knee joint and plantarflex the foot at the ankle joint and feel for the contraction of the belly of the plantaris. (Distinguishing the plantaris from the lateral head of the gastrocnemius will be difficult given that the gastrocnemius will also contract with these two actions.)
3. The long distal tendon of the plantaris is extremely difficult to palpate and discern.

■ RELATIONSHIP TO OTHER STRUCTURES

□ The plantaris attaches proximally just medial to the lateral head of the gastrocnemius and the distal tendon of the biceps femoris.
□ Much of the belly of the plantaris is superficial in the posterior knee just medial to the lateral head of the gastrocnemius. Here the plantaris is superficial to the popliteus.
□ The rest of the belly and the proximal ½ of the long distal tendon of the plantaris are sandwiched between the gastrocnemius and the soleus. (The tendon is deep to the gastrocnemius and superficial to the soleus.)
□ The distal ½ of the long distal tendon is superficial just medial to the medial margin of the distal tendon of the gastrocnemius.
□ The plantaris is located within the superficial back line myofascial meridian.

■ MISCELLANEOUS

1. The plantaris is located in the superficial posterior compartment of the leg.
2. After crossing the knee joint, the plantaris becomes a very long, thin tendon that runs the entire length of the leg and attaches to the calcaneus.
3. The distal tendon of the plantaris often joins with the calcaneal (Achilles) tendon of the gastrocnemius and soleus.
4. Given that the distal tendon of the plantaris is directly next to (and often melds with) the calcaneal (Achilles) tendon, the plantaris is often grouped with the gastrocnemius and the soleus. This group is sometimes called the *quadriceps surae.*
5. The plantaris of the leg is considered to be analogous to the palmaris longus of the forearm.
6. The name *plantaris* is misleading, because this muscle does not attach onto the plantar surface of the foot in humans (although it does attach onto the posterior calcaneus, which is near the plantar surface). In other primates, the plantaris curves around the calcaneus to attach into the plantar fascia, thereby actually attaching onto the plantar surface of the foot.

16

Tibialis Posterior (*Tom* of *Tom, Dick, and Harry* Group)

The name, tibialis posterior, *tells us that this muscle attaches to the tibia and is located in the posterior leg.*

Derivation	☐ tibialis: L. *refers to the tibia.*
	posterior: L. *behind, toward the back.*
Pronunciation	☐ tib-ee-A-lis, pos-TEE-ri-or

■ ATTACHMENTS

☐ **Posterior Tibia and Fibula**
  ☐ the proximal ⅔ of the posterior tibia, fibula, and interosseus membrane

to the

☐ **Navicular Tuberosity**
  ☐ and metatarsals two through four and all the tarsal bones except the talus

■ FUNCTIONS

CONCENTRIC (SHORTENING) MOVER ACTIONS	
Standard Mover Actions	**Reverse Mover Actions**
☐ **1. Plantarflexes the foot at the ankle joint**	☐ 1. Plantarflexes the leg at the ankle joint
☐ **2. Inverts (supinates) the foot at the subtalar joint**	☐ 2. Inverts (supinates) the talus at the subtalar joint

Standard Mover Actions Notes

- The tibialis posterior crosses the ankle joint posteriorly (with its fibers running vertically in the sagittal plane); therefore it plantarflexes the foot at the ankle joint. Plantarflexion of the foot at the ankle joint is an important action during the gait cycle when pushing off the ground (toe-off phase). (action 1)
- The tibialis posterior crosses onto the foot on the medial side (with its fibers running vertically in the frontal plane), therefore it inverts/supinates the foot (more specifically, it inverts/supinates the calcaneus relative to the talus) at the subtalar joint. Note: Inversion is the major component of subtalar supination; subtalar supination also includes medial rotation and plantarflexion of the foot. (action 2)

Reverse Mover Action Notes

- Reverse actions at the ankle and subtalar joints usually occur when the foot is planted on the ground so that the proximal attachment moves toward the distal one. (reverse actions 1, 2)
- The tibialis posterior crosses the ankle joint posteriorly (with its fibers running vertically in the sagittal plane). If the distal attachment is fixed, the tibialis posterior pulls the posterior

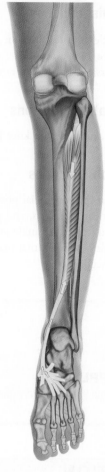

Figure 16-14 Posterior view of the right tibialis posterior.

surface of the leg toward the plantar surface of the foot, therefore it plantarflexes the leg at the ankle joint. (reverse action 1)
- The reverse action of inversion of the foot at the subtalar joint is inversion of the leg at the subtalar joint. Moving the leg at the subtalar joint involves moving the talus relative to the calcaneus. Inversion is the major component of supination. (reverse action 2)
- Another component of supination of the talus at the subtalar joint is lateral rotation of the talus. Because the ankle and (extended) knee joints do not allow rotation, when the talus laterally rotates, the entire lower extremity follows with lateral rotation of the thigh at the hip joint. (reverse action 2)

Eccentric Antagonist Functions

1. Restrains/slows ankle joint dorsiflexion
2. Restrains/slows eversion (pronation) at the subtalar joint

16

Tibialis Posterior (*Tom* of *Tom, Dick, and Harry* Group)—*cont'd*

Eccentric Antagonist Function Note

- Restraining/slowing dorsiflexion of the leg at the ankle joint is important when standing and bending forward (bending at the ankle, knee, and hip joints).

Isometric Stabilization Functions

1. Stabilizes the ankle and subtalar joints

Isometric Function Note

- The tibialis posterior plays an important role in supporting and stabilizing the arches (and the subtalar joint) of the foot.

Additional Note on Functions

1. Because the tendons of the Tom, Dick, and Harry group cross into the foot posterior to the medial malleolus, their line of pull is posteromedial. Therefore all three Tom, Dick, and Harry muscles plantarflex and invert the foot (at the ankle and subtalar joints respectively).

INNERVATION
- ☐ The Tibial Nerve
  - ☐ L4, L5

ARTERIAL SUPPLY
- ☐ The Posterior Tibial Artery (a terminal branch of the Popliteal Artery)

 PALPATION

1. With the client seated or supine, have the client plantarflex and invert the foot (resistance can be given) and look and palpate for the distal tendon of tibialis posterior immediately posterior to the medial malleolus of the tibia.
2. Once located, continue palpating the tibialis posterior distally to the navicular tuberosity and proximally into the posterior leg.
3. Note: Asking the client to extend all five toes will help eliminate contraction of the flexor digitorum longus and the flexor hallucis longus.

■ RELATIONSHIP TO OTHER STRUCTURES

- ☐ The tibialis posterior, flexor digitorum longus, and flexor hallucis longus are the deepest muscles in the posterior leg.

Where these muscles overlap, the tibialis posterior is the deepest of the three.
- ☐ The tibialis posterior is deep to the soleus.
- ☐ Deep to the tibialis posterior are the tibia, the fibula, and the interosseus membrane.
- ☐ Lateral to the belly of the tibialis posterior is the flexor hallucis longus, and medial to the belly of the tibialis posterior is the flexor digitorum longus.
- ☐ The distal tendon of the tibialis posterior crosses posterior to the medial malleolus along with the distal tendons of the flexor digitorum longus and the flexor hallucis longus. Of the three, the tendon of the tibialis posterior is the closest to the medial malleolus.
- ☐ Beyond the navicular tuberosity, the distal tendon of the tibialis posterior is very deep and found in the fourth layer of muscles of the plantar surface of the foot.
- ☐ The tibialis posterior is located within the deep front line myofascial meridian.

■ MISCELLANEOUS

1. The tibialis posterior is located in the deep posterior compartment of the leg.
2. The **T**ibialis posterior is *Tom* of the *Tom, Dick, and Harry* muscles. The Tom, Dick, and Harry muscles are the tibialis posterior, flexor digitorum longus, and flexor hallucis longus. Tom, Dick, and Harry are grouped together, because they are all deep in the posterior leg and their distal tendons cross posterior to the medial malleolus of the tibia (in order from anterior to posterior, Tom, Dick, and Harry).
3. It is worth noting that the location of the muscle bellies of the Tom, Dick, and Harry muscles in the posterior leg is, from medial to lateral, Dick, Tom, and Harry (i.e., flexor digitorum longus, tibialis posterior, and flexor hallucis longus).
4. The tibialis posterior has a tendon that makes an abrupt turn of approximately 90 degrees.
5. In the ankle region, the distal tendon of the tibialis posterior travels through the tarsal tunnel along with the distal tendon of the flexor digitorum longus.
6. Because the tibialis posterior helps support the arch (medial longitudinal arch) of the foot, some sources consider it to be the medial *stirrup muscle,* instead of the tibialis anterior.
7. When the tibialis posterior is tight and painful, this condition is often called *shin splints* or *posterior shin splints.*
8. The tibialis posterior is pennate.

16

CHAPTER

17

Extrinsic Muscles of the Toe Joints

CHAPTER **OUTLINE**

CHAPTER **OVERVIEW**

The muscles addressed in this chapter are the extrinsic muscles of the foot that move the toes. These muscles attach proximally to the leg and then travel distally to enter and attach to the foot. These extrinsic toe muscles also cross the ankle and subtalar joints; therefore they also move these joints. See Chapter 16 for the muscles of the ankle and subtalar joints. Note: Intrinsic muscles of the foot that also move the toes are addressed in Chapter 18.

Overview of Structure

☐ Structurally, extrinsic muscles of the foot that move the toes can be divided into two groups: flexors and extensors. The extensors are the extensor digitorum longus and extensor hallucis longus (*digitorum* refers to toes two through five; *hallucis* means big toe), located in the anterior compartment of the leg. The flexors are the flexor digitorum longus and flexor hallucis longus, located in the deep posterior compartment of the leg.

Overview of Function

The following general rules regarding actions can be stated for the functional groups of extrinsic toe muscles:

☐ Toes two through five can move at three joints: the metatarsophalangeal (MTP), proximal interphalangeal (PIP), and distal interphalangeal (DIP) joints.

☐ If a muscle crosses only the MTP joint, it can move the toe only at the MTP joint.

☐ If the muscle crosses the MTP and PIP joints, it can move the toe at both of these joints.

☐ If the muscle crosses the MTP, PIP, and DIP joints, it can move the toe at all three joints.

☐ The big toe (toe one) can move at two joints: the metatarsophalangeal (MTP) and interphalangeal (IP) joints. Similarly, a muscle can move the big toe at one or both joints that it crosses.

☐ If a muscle crosses the MTP, PIP, DIP, or IP joints of the toes on the plantar side, it can flex the toe at the joint(s) crossed; if a muscle crosses the MTP, PIP, DIP, or IP joints of the toes on the dorsal side, it can extend the toe at the joint(s) crossed.

☐ Reverse actions involve the proximal attachment moving toward the distal one. This occurs when the distal end of the foot is fixed, usually when the foot is planted on the ground (for example, when we toe-off during the gait cycle, the metatarsals of the toes extend, and therefore the foot extends toward the toes at the MTP joints).

☐ Because extrinsic toe muscles attach proximally to the leg, they also cross the ankle and subtalar joints so they can move the foot (or leg) at these joints.

Review the muscles and bones from this chapter on the enclosed CD!

☐ If a muscle crosses the ankle joint anteriorly to enter the foot, it can dorsiflex the foot (or leg) at the ankle joint; if it crosses the ankle joint posteriorly to enter the foot, it can plantarflex the foot (or leg) at the ankle joint.

☐ If a muscle crosses the subtalar joint on the lateral (fibular) side to enter the foot, it can evert the foot (or leg) at the subtalar joint; if it crosses the subtalar joint on the medial (tibial) side to enter the foot, it can invert the foot (or leg) at the subtalar joint.

17

Anterior View of the Extrinsic Muscles of the Toes of the Right Foot—Superficial View

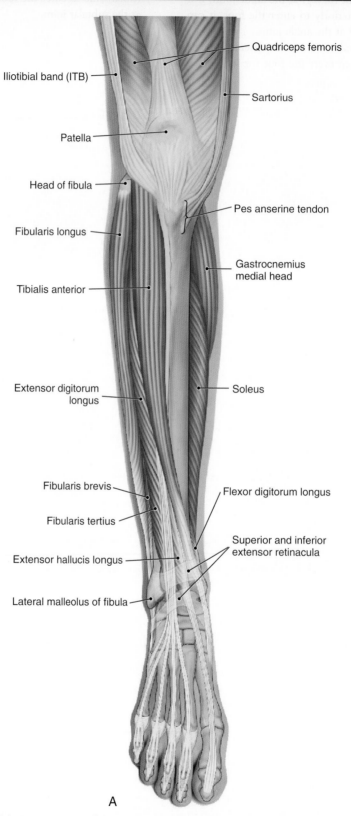

Quadriceps femoris

Iliotibial band (ITB)

Sartorius

Patella

Head of fibula

Pes anserine tendon

Fibularis longus

Gastrocnemius
medial head

Tibialis anterior

Extensor digitorum
longus

Soleus

Fibularis brevis

Flexor digitorum longus

Fibularis tertius

Superior and inferior
extensor retinacula

Extensor hallucis longus

Lateral malleolus of fibula

A

Figure 17-1 Anterior views of the extrinsic muscles of the toes at the right foot. **A,** Superficial.

17

Anterior View of the Extrinsic Muscles of the Toes of the Right Foot—Deep View

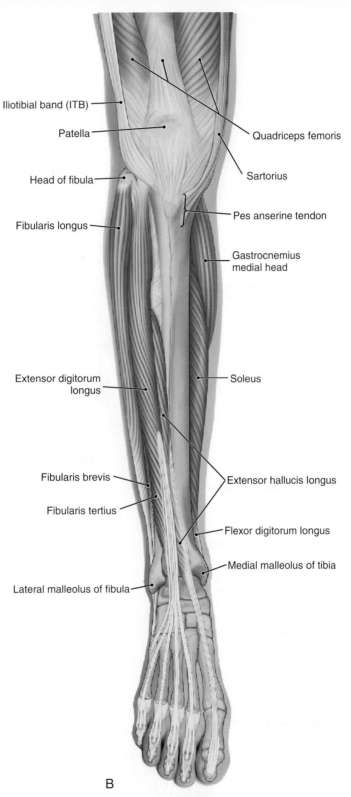

Iliotibial band (ITB)

Patella

Head of fibula

Fibularis longus

Extensor digitorum longus

Fibularis brevis

Fibularis tertius

Lateral malleolus of fibula

Quadriceps femoris

Sartorius

Pes anserine tendon

Gastrocnemius medial head

Soleus

Extensor hallucis longus

Flexor digitorum longus

Medial malleolus of tibia

B

Figure 17-1, cont'd B, Deep.

17

Posterior View of the Extrinsic Muscles of the Toes of the Right Foot—Superficial View

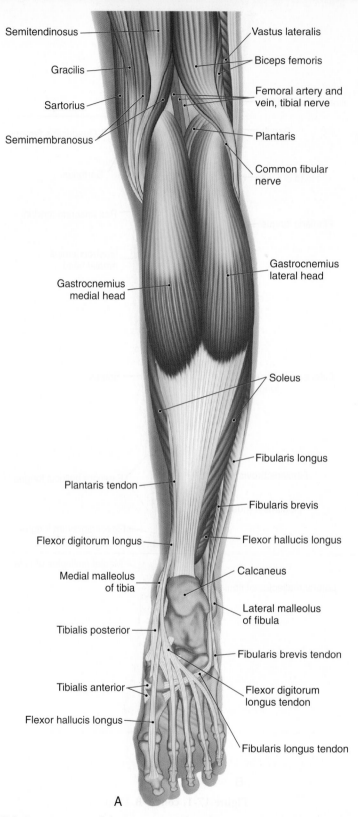

Semitendinosus

Gracilis

Sartorius

Semimembranosus

Vastus lateralis

Biceps femoris

Femoral artery and vein, tibial nerve

Plantaris

Common fibular nerve

Gastrocnemius medial head

Gastrocnemius lateral head

Soleus

Fibularis longus

Plantaris tendon

Fibularis brevis

Flexor digitorum longus

Flexor hallucis longus

Medial malleolus of tibia

Calcaneus

Lateral malleolus of fibula

Tibialis posterior

Fibularis brevis tendon

Tibialis anterior

Flexor digitorum longus tendon

Flexor hallucis longus

Fibularis longus tendon

A

17

Figure 17-2 Posterior views of the extrinsic muscles of the toes of the right foot. **A,** Superficial.

Posterior Views of the Extrinsic Muscles of the Toes of the Right Foot—Intermediate and Deep Views

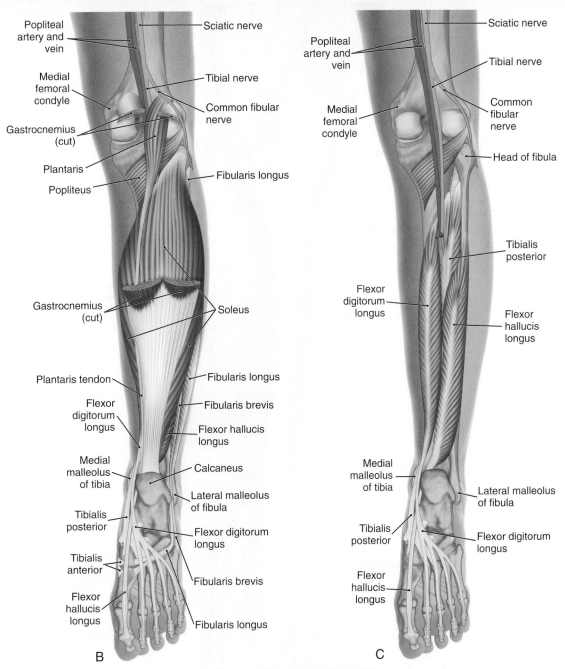

Figure 17-2, cont'd B, Intermediate. **C,** Deep.

Medial View of the Extrinsic Muscles of the Toes of the Right Foot—Superficial View

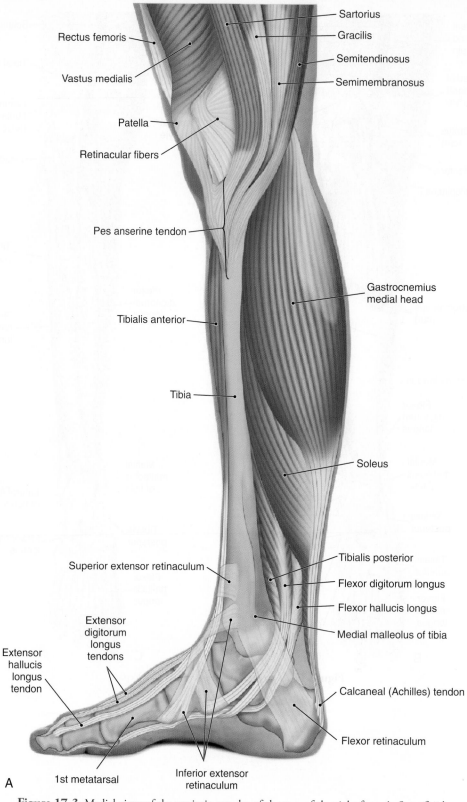

Sartorius

Gracilis

Semitendinosus

Semimembranosus

Rectus femoris

Vastus medialis

Patella

Retinacular fibers

Pes anserine tendon

Gastrocnemius
medial head

Tibialis anterior

Tibia

Soleus

Superior extensor retinaculum

Tibialis posterior

Flexor digitorum longus

Flexor hallucis longus

Medial malleolus of tibia

Extensor
digitorum
longus
tendons

Extensor
hallucis
longus
tendon

Calcaneal (Achilles) tendon

Flexor retinaculum

A

1st metatarsal

Inferior extensor
retinaculum

Figure 17-3 Medial views of the extrinsic muscles of the toes of the right foot. **A,** Superficial.

17

Medial View of the Extrinsic Muscles of the Toes of the Right Foot—Deep View

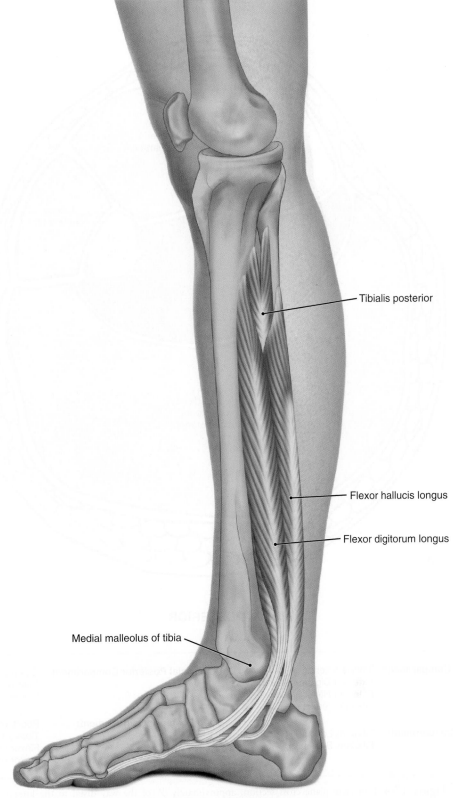

Tibialis posterior

Flexor hallucis longus

Flexor digitorum longus

Medial malleolus of tibia

B

Figure 17-3, cont'd B, Deep.

17

Transverse Plane Cross Section of the Right Leg Compartments

ANTERIOR

MEDIAL

LATERAL

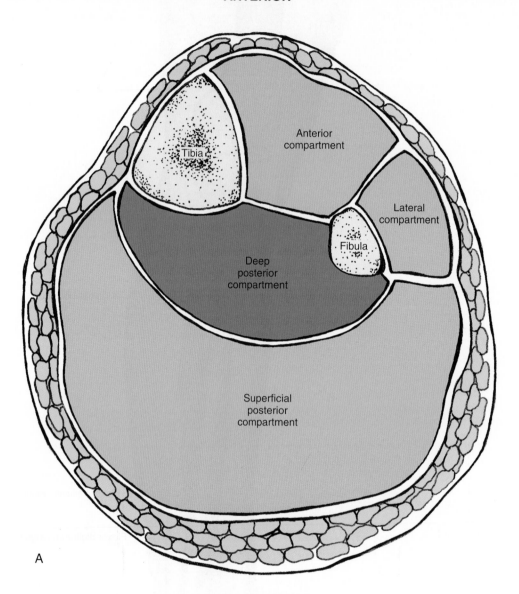

Anterior compartment

Lateral compartment

Tibia

Fibula

Deep posterior compartment

Superficial posterior compartment

A

POSTERIOR

Anterior Compartment:	Tibialis Anterior	**Superficial Posterior Compartment:**	Gastrocnemius
	Extensor Digitorum Longus		Soleus
	Extensor Hallucis Longus		Plantaris
	Fibularis Tertius		
		Deep Posterior Compartment:	Popliteus
Lateral Compartment:	Fibularis Longus		Tibialis Posterior
	Fibularis Brevis		Flexor Digitorum Longus
			Flexor Hallucis Longus

Figure 17-4 Transverse plane cross section, approximately ⅓ of the way distal to the knee joint. **A,** The four compartments of the leg.

17

Transverse Plane Cross Section of the Right Leg Muscles

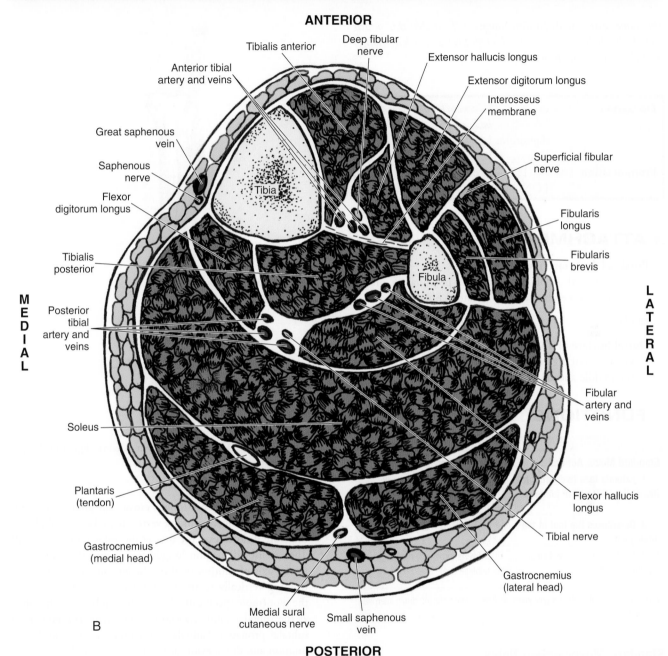

ANTERIOR

Tibialis anterior

Deep fibular nerve

Anterior tibial artery and veins

Extensor hallucis longus

Extensor digitorum longus

Interosseus membrane

Great saphenous vein

Saphenous nerve

Flexor digitorum longus

Superficial fibular nerve

Tibia

Fibularis longus

Tibialis posterior

Fibularis brevis

Fibula

M E D I A L

L A T E R A L

Posterior tibial artery and veins

Fibular artery and veins

Soleus

Plantaris (tendon)

Flexor hallucis longus

Tibial nerve

Gastrocnemius (medial head)

Gastrocnemius (lateral head)

B

Medial sural cutaneous nerve

Small saphenous vein

POSTERIOR

Figure 17-4, cont'd B, The muscles within the compartments of the leg.

17

Extensor Digitorum Longus

The name, extensor digitorum longus, *tells us that this muscle extends the digits (i.e., toes two through five) and is long (longer than the extensor digitorum brevis).*

Derivation	□ extensor: L. *a muscle that extends a body part.*
	digitorum: L. *refers to a digit* (toe).
	longus: L. *longer.*
Pronunciation	□ eks-TEN-sor, dij-i-TOE-rum, LONG-us

■ ATTACHMENTS

□ **Proximal Anterior Fibula**
  □ the proximal ⅔ of the fibula, the proximal ⅓ of the interosseus membrane, and the lateral tibial condyle

to the

□ **Dorsal Surface of Toes Two through Five**
  □ via its dorsal digital expansion onto the dorsal surface of the middle and distal phalanges

■ FUNCTIONS

CONCENTRIC (SHORTENING) MOVER ACTIONS	
Standard Mover Actions	**Reverse Mover Actions**
□ **1. Extends toes two through five at the MTP and IP joints**	□ 1. Extends metatarsals at the MTP joints and extends the more proximal phalanges at the IP joints
□ **2. Dorsiflexes the foot at the ankle joint**	□ 2. Dorsiflexes the leg at the ankle joint
□ 3. Everts (pronates) the foot at the subtalar joint	□ 3. Everts (pronates) the talus at the subtalar joint

MTP joints = metatarsophalangeal joints; IP joints = (proximal and distal) interphalangeal joints

Standard Mover Action Notes

• The extensor digitorum longus crosses toe joints two through five dorsally (with its fibers running horizontally in the sagittal plane); therefore it extends toes two through five. Given that it attaches all the way onto the distal phalanges, it crosses the MTP joint and the proximal and distal IP joints of toes two through five. Therefore the extensor digitorum longus extends toes two through five at all of these joints. (action 1)

• More specifically, extending toes at the MTP and IP joints refers to extending the proximal phalanges of the toes at the MTP joints, extending the middle phalanges at the proximal interphalangeal (PIP) joints, and extending the distal phalanges at the distal interphalangeal (DIP) joints. (action 1)

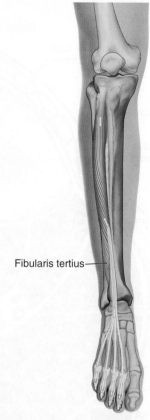

Fibularis tertius—

Figure 17-5 Anterior view of the right extensor digitorum longus. The fibularis tertius has been ghosted in.

• The extensor digitorum longus crosses the ankle joint anteriorly (with its fibers running vertically in the sagittal plane); therefore it dorsiflexes the foot at the ankle joint. (action 2)

• The extensor digitorum longus crosses into the foot lateral to the axis of motion of the subtalar joint (with its fibers running vertically in the frontal plane), therefore it everts the foot (more specifically the calcaneus relative to the talus) at the subtalar joint. Eversion is the major component of subtalar pronation (subtalar pronation also includes lateral rotation and dorsiflexion of the foot). (action 3)

Reverse Mover Action Notes

• Reverse actions within the lower extremity occur when the distal end is fixed (usually due to the foot being planted on the ground) so that the proximal attachment moves instead. (reverse actions 1, 2, 3)

• If the more distal attachment is fixed, the extensor digitorum longus extends the metatarsal relative to the proximal phalanx (at the MTP joint). The reverse action of metatarsal extension at the MTP joint happens during the gait cycle at toe-off. (reverse action 1)

• Extending the more proximal phalanges at the IP joints refers to extending the proximal phalanges at the proximal

17

Extensor Digitorum Longus—*cont'd*

interphalangeal (PIP) joints and extending the middle phalanges at the distal interphalangeal (DIP) joints. (reverse action 1)

- The extensor digitorum longus crosses the ankle joint anteriorly with a vertical direction to its fibers (in the sagittal plane). If the foot is fixed by being planted on the ground, the leg is dorsiflexed at the ankle joint by bringing the anterior (dorsal) surface of the leg toward the dorsal surface of the foot. This action occurs during the gait cycle (from foot-flat to toe-off). (reverse action 2)
- The reverse action of eversion of the foot at the subtalar joint is eversion of the leg at the subtalar joint. Moving the leg at the subtalar joint involves moving the talus relative to the calcaneus. Eversion is the principle component of pronation. (reverse action 3)
- Another component of pronation of the talus at the subtalar joint is medial rotation of the talus. Because the ankle and (extended) knee joints do not allow rotation, when the talus medially rotates, the entire lower extremity follows with medial rotation of the thigh at the hip joint. (reverse action 3)

Eccentric Antagonist Functions

1. Restrains/slows flexion of toes two through five at the MTP and IP joints, and metatarsals two through five at the MTP joints
2. Restrains/slows ankle joint plantarflexion
3. Restrains/slows inversion (supination) at the subtalar joint

Eccentric Antagonist Function Note

- The eccentric action of restraining/slowing plantarflexion of the foot is important during the gait cycle (from heel-strike to foot-flat).

Isometric Stabilization Functions

1. Stabilizes the ankle, subtalar, and MTP and IP joints of toes two through five

Additional Note on Functions

1. All four muscles in the anterior compartment of the leg can dorsiflex the foot (and leg) at the ankle joint.

INNERVATION
- The Deep Fibular Nerve
  - L5, S1

ARTERIAL SUPPLY
- The Anterior Tibial Artery (a terminal branch of the Popliteal Artery)

PALPATION

1. With the client seated or supine, place palpating fingers on the dorsum of the foot.
2. Have the client extend toes two through five (resistance can be added) and look and feel for the tensing of the tendons of the extensor digitorum longus.
3. Follow the extensor digitorum longus proximally as far as possible. The belly of the extensor digitorum longus can be palpated between the tibialis anterior and the fibularis longus.

■ RELATIONSHIP TO OTHER STRUCTURES

- The tibialis anterior and the extensor hallucis longus are medial to the extensor digitorum longus. The fibularis longus and the fibularis brevis are lateral to the extensor digitorum longus.
- The extensor digitorum longus is superficial, except proximally, where it is deep to the tibialis anterior and the fibularis longus.
- Deep to the extensor digitorum longus is the fibula.
- The fibers of the most distal and lateral part of the extensor digitorum longus (that arise from the distal ⅓ of the fibula) do not attach onto digits (i.e., toes) but rather onto the fifth metatarsal. This portion of the muscle is given a separate name, the *fibularis tertius*.
- The extensor digitorum longus is located within the superficial front line myofascial meridian.

■ MISCELLANEOUS

1. The extensor digitorum longus is located in the anterior compartment of the leg.
2. The distal attachment of the extensor digitorum longus spreads out to become a fibrous aponeurotic expansion that covers the dorsal, medial, and lateral sides of the proximal phalanx of toes two through five. It then continues distally to attach onto the dorsal sides of the middle and distal phalanges of these toes. This structure is called the *dorsal digital expansion*. The dorsal digital expansion also serves as an attachment site for the extensor digitorum brevis, lumbricals pedis, dorsal interossei pedis, and plantar interossei muscles.
3. The most distal and lateral part of the extensor digitorum longus (that arises from the distal ⅓ of the fibula) does not attach onto the digits (toes); therefore it is given a separate name, the *fibularis tertius*.
4. The extensor digitorum longus is pennate.

Extensor Hallucis Longus

The name, extensor hallucis longus, *tells us that this muscle extends the big toe and is long (longer than the extensor hallucis brevis).*

Derivation	☐ extensor: L. *a muscle that extends a body part.*
	hallucis: L. *refers to the big toe.*
	longus: L. *longer.*
Pronunciation	☐ eks-TEN-sor, hal-OO-sis, LONG-us

■ ATTACHMENTS

☐ **Middle Anterior Fibula**
  ☐ the middle ⅓ of the anterior fibula and the middle ⅓ of the interosseus membrane

to the

☐ **Dorsal Surface of the Big Toe (Toe One)**
  ☐ the distal phalanx

■ FUNCTIONS

CONCENTRIC (SHORTENING) MOVER ACTIONS	
Standard Mover Actions	**Reverse Mover Actions**
☐ **1. Extends the big toe (toe one) at the MTP and IP joints**	☐ 1. Extends the metatarsal at the MTP joint and extends the proximal phalanx at the IP joint
☐ **2. Dorsiflexes the foot at the ankle joint**	☐ 2. Dorsiflexes the leg at the ankle joint
☐ 3. Inverts (supinates) the foot at the subtalar joint	☐ 3. Inverts (supinates) the talus at the subtalar joint

MTP joint = metatarsophalangeal joint; IP joint = interphalangeal joint

Standard Mover Action Notes

- The extensor hallucis longus crosses the big toe dorsally (with its fibers running horizontally in the sagittal plane); therefore it extends the big toe. Because it attaches onto the distal phalanx, it crosses both the MTP and the IP joints of the big toe. Therefore the extensor hallucis longus extends the big toe at both of these joints. (action 1)
- More specifically, extending the big toe at the MTP and IP joints refers to extending the proximal phalanx at the MTP joint and extending the distal phalanx at the IP joint. (action 1)
- The extensor hallucis longus crosses the ankle joint anteriorly (with its fibers running vertically in the sagittal plane); therefore it dorsiflexes the foot at the ankle joint. (action 2)
- The extensor hallucis longus crosses into the foot medial to the axis of motion of the subtalar joint (with its fibers running vertically in the frontal plane), therefore it inverts

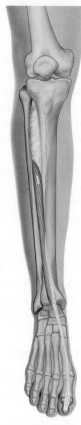

Figure 17-6 Anterior view of the right extensor hallucis longus.

the foot (more specifically the calcaneus relative to the talus) at the subtalar joint. Inversion is the major component of subtalar supination (subtalar supination also includes medial rotation and plantarflexion of the foot). (action 3)

Reverse Mover Action Notes

- Reverse actions within the lower extremity occur when the distal end is fixed (usually due to the foot being planted on the ground) so that the proximal attachment moves instead. (reverse actions 1, 2, 3)
- If the more distal attachment is fixed, the extensor hallucis longus extends the metatarsal of the big toe toward the proximal phalanx (at the MTP joint); and extends the proximal phalanx of the big toe toward the distal phalanx (at the IP joint). (reverse action 1)
- The reverse action of metatarsal extension at the MTP joint happens during the gait cycle at toe-off. (reverse action 1)
- The extensor hallucis longus crosses the ankle joint anteriorly with a vertical direction to its fibers (in the sagittal plane). If the foot is fixed by being planted on the ground, the leg is dorsiflexed at the ankle joint by bringing the anterior (dorsal) surface of the leg toward the dorsal surface of the foot. This action occurs during the gait cycle (from foot-flat to toe-off). (reverse action 2)

17

Extensor Hallucis Longus—*cont'd*

- The reverse action of inversion of the foot at the subtalar joint is inversion of the leg at the subtalar joint. Moving the leg at the subtalar joint involves moving the talus relative to the calcaneus. Inversion is the principle component of supination. (reverse action 3)
- Another component of supination of the talus at the subtalar joint is lateral rotation of the talus. Because the ankle and (extended) knee joints do not allow rotation, when the talus laterally rotates, the entire lower extremity follows with lateral rotation of the thigh at the hip joint. (reverse action 3)

Eccentric Antagonist Functions

1. Restrains/slows flexion of the big toe at the MTP and IP joints, and the metatarsal at the MTP joint
2. Restrains/slows ankle joint plantarflexion
3. Restrains/slows eversion at the subtalar joint

Eccentric Antagonist Function Note

- The eccentric action of restraining/slowing plantarflexion of the foot is important during the gait cycle (from heel-strike to foot-flat).

Isometric Stabilization Functions

1. Stabilizes the ankle and subtalar joints, and the MTP and IP joints of the big toe

Additional Note on Functions

1. All four muscles in the anterior compartment of the leg can dorsiflex the foot (and leg) at the ankle joint.

INNERVATION
- ☐ The Deep Fibular Nerve
  - ☐ **L5,** S1

ARTERIAL SUPPLY
- ☐ The Anterior Tibial Artery (a terminal branch of the Popliteal Artery)

✋ PALPATION

1. With the client either sitting or supine, place palpating fingers on the dorsum of the foot.
2. Have the client extend the big toe (resistance can be added) and look and feel for the tensing of the tendon of the extensor hallucis longus.
3. Follow the extensor hallucis longus proximally. It may be palpated superficially in the distal leg between the tibialis anterior tendon and the extensor digitorum longus.
4. With careful palpation, the belly of the extensor hallucis longus can be palpated deep to overlying musculature when the client extends the big toe.

■ RELATIONSHIP TO OTHER STRUCTURES

- ☐ The extensor hallucis longus arises between the tibialis anterior and the extensor digitorum longus and is deep to these muscles proximally.
- ☐ A small portion of the belly of the extensor hallucis longus is superficial in the distal half of the leg between the tendons of the tibialis anterior and the extensor digitorum longus.
- ☐ The distal tendon of the extensor hallucis longus becomes superficial and lies just lateral to the distal tendon of the tibialis anterior in the foot.
- ☐ Deep to the extensor hallucis longus is the fibula.
- ☐ The extensor hallucis longus is located within the superficial front line myofascial meridian.

■ MISCELLANEOUS

1. The extensor hallucis longus is located in the anterior compartment of the leg.
2. The extensor hallucis longus is pennate.

17

Flexor Digitorum Longus (*Dick* of *Tom, Dick, and Harry* Group)

The name, flexor digitorum longus, *tells us that this muscle flexes the digits (i.e., toes) and is long (longer than the flexor digitorum brevis).*

Derivation	☐ flexor:	L. *a muscle that flexes a body part.*
	digitorum:	L. *refers to a digit* (toe).
	longus:	L. *longer.*
Pronunciation	☐ FLEKS-or, dij-i-TOE-rum, LONG-us	

■ ATTACHMENTS

☐ **Middle Posterior Tibia**
  ☐ the middle ⅓ of the posterior tibia

to the

☐ **Plantar Surface of Toes Two through Five**
  ☐ the distal phalanges

■ FUNCTIONS

CONCENTRIC (SHORTENING) MOVER ACTIONS	
Standard Mover Actions	**Reverse Mover Actions**
☐ **1. Flexes toes two through five at the MTP and IP joints**	☐ 1. Flexes metatarsals at the MTP joints and flexes the more proximal phalanges at the IP joints
☐ **2. Plantarflexes the foot at the ankle joint**	☐ 2. Plantarflexes the leg at the ankle joint
☐ **3. Inverts (supinates) the foot at the subtalar joint**	☐ 3. Inverts (supinates) the talus at the subtalar joint

MTP joints = metatarsophalangeal joints; IP joints = (proximal and distal) interphalangeal joints

Standard Mover Action Notes

- The flexor digitorum longus crosses the toe joints on the plantar side (with its fibers running horizontally in the sagittal plane); therefore it flexes toes two through five. Given that the flexor digitorum longus attaches onto the distal phalanges, it crosses the MTP joint and the proximal and distal IP joints of toes two through five. Therefore the flexor digitorum longus flexes the toes at all of these joints. (action 1)
- More specifically, flexing toes at the MTP and IP joints refers to flexing the proximal phalanges at the MTP joints, flexing the middle phalanges at the proximal interphalangeal (PIP) joints, and flexing the distal phalanges at the distal interphalangeal (DIP) joints. (action 1)
- The flexor digitorum longus crosses the ankle joint posteriorly (with its fibers running vertically in the sagittal plane); therefore it plantarflexes the foot at the ankle joint. (action 2)
- The flexor digitorum longus enters the foot and crosses the subtalar joint on the medial side (with its fibers running

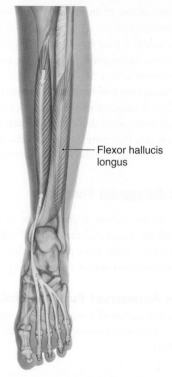

Figure 17-7 Posterior view of the right flexor digitorum longus. The flexor hallucis longus has been ghosted in.

Flexor hallucis longus

vertically in the frontal plane), therefore it inverts the foot (more specifically, the calcaneus relative to the talus) at the subtalar joint. Inversion is the major component of subtalar supination (subtalar supination also includes medial rotation and plantarflexion of the foot). (action 3)

Reverse Mover Action Notes

- Reverse actions within the lower extremity occur when the distal end is fixed (usually due to the foot being planted on the ground) so that the proximal attachment moves instead. (reverse actions 1, 2, 3)
- Reverse actions of the toes involve the metatarsal moving at the MTP joint, the proximal phalanx moving at the proximal interphalangeal (PIP) joint, and middle phalanx moving at the distal interphalangeal (DIP) joint. (reverse action 1)
- The flexor digitorum longus crosses the ankle joint posteriorly with a vertical direction to its fibers (in the sagittal plane). If the foot is fixed by being planted on the ground, the leg is plantarflexed at the ankle joint by bringing the posterior surface of the leg toward the plantar surface of the foot. (reverse action 2)
- The reverse action of inversion of the foot at the subtalar joint is inversion of the leg at the subtalar joint. Moving the leg at the subtalar joint involves moving the talus relative to the calcaneus. Inversion is the principle component of supination. (reverse action 3)

17

Flexor Digitorum Longus (*Dick* of *Tom, Dick, and Harry* Group)—*cont'd*

- Another component of supination of the talus at the subtalar joint is lateral rotation of the talus. Because the ankle and (extended) knee joints do not allow rotation, when the talus laterally rotates, the entire lower extremity follows with lateral rotation of the thigh at the hip joint. (reverse action 3)

Eccentric Antagonist Functions

1. Restrains/slows extension of toes two through five at the MTP and IP joints, and metatarsals two through five at the MTP joints.
2. Restrains/slows ankle joint dorsiflexion
3. Restrains/slows eversion of the subtalar joint

Eccentric Antagonist Function Note

- Restraining/slowing dorsiflexion of the leg at the ankle joint is important when standing and bending forward (bending at the ankle, knee, and hip joints).

Isometric Stabilization Functions

1. Stabilizes the ankle, subtalar, and MTP and IP joints of toes two through five

Isometric Stabilization Function Note

- The flexor digitorum longus helps support and stabilize the arches (and the subtalar joint) of the foot

Additional Note on Functions

1. Because the tendons of the Tom, Dick, and Harry group cross into the foot posterior to the medial malleolus, their line of pull is posteromedial. Therefore all three Tom, Dick, and Harry muscles plantarflex and invert the foot (at the ankle and subtalar joints, respectively).

INNERVATION
- ☐ The Tibial Nerve
  - ☐ L5, **S1, S2**

ARTERIAL SUPPLY
- ☐ The Posterior Tibial Artery (a terminal branch of the Popliteal Artery)

✋ PALPATION

1. With the client seated or supine, place palpating fingers posterior to the medial malleolus.
2. Have the client flex toes two through five (resistance can be added) and feel for the tensing of the distal tendon of the flexor digitorum longus.
3. Continue palpating the flexor digitorum longus proximally into the posteromedial leg between the soleus and tibia.

■ RELATIONSHIP TO OTHER STRUCTURES

- ☐ The flexor digitorum longus, tibialis posterior, and flexor hallucis longus are the deepest muscles in the posterior leg. Where these muscles overlap, the tibialis posterior is the deepest of the three.
- ☐ The flexor digitorum longus is deep to the soleus.
- ☐ Deep to the flexor digitorum longus is the tibia.
- ☐ The belly of the flexor digitorum longus is medial to the tibialis posterior and the flexor hallucis longus.
- ☐ The distal tendon of the flexor digitorum longus crosses posterior to the medial malleolus, along with the distal tendons of the tibialis posterior and the flexor hallucis longus.
- ☐ The flexor digitorum longus is located within the deep front line myofascial meridian.

■ MISCELLANEOUS

1. The flexor digitorum longus is located in the deep posterior compartment of the leg.
2. The flexor **D**igitorum longus is *Dick* of the *Tom, Dick, and Harry* group. The Tom, Dick, and Harry muscles are the tibialis posterior, flexor digitorum longus, and flexor hallucis longus. Tom, Dick, and Harry are grouped together, because they are all deep in the posterior leg and all of their distal tendons cross posterior to the medial malleolus of the tibia (in order from anterior to posterior, Tom, Dick, and Harry).
3. It is worth noting that the location of the muscle bellies of the Tom, Dick, and Harry muscles in the posterior leg is, from medial to lateral, Dick, Tom, and Harry (i.e., flexor digitorum longus, tibialis posterior, and flexor hallucis longus).
4. The flexor digitorum longus has a tendon that makes an abrupt turn of approximately 90 degrees.
5. In the ankle region, the distal tendon of the flexor digitorum longus travels through the tarsal tunnel along with the distal tendon of the tibialis posterior.
6. The distal tendons of the flexor digitorum longus reach their attachment site on the distal phalanges in an unusual manner. The tendons of the flexor digitorum brevis (an instrinsic muscle of the foot) lie superficial to the tendons of the flexor digitorum longus. The tendons of the flexor digitorum brevis split, and the tendons of the flexor digitorum longus then pass through these splits to continue on to the distal phalanges. (This is essentially identical to the arrangement of the flexor digitorum superficialis and flexor digitorum profundus of the upper extremity.)
7. Because the four individual distal tendons of the flexor digitorum longus split from one common distal tendon, the flexor digitorum longus does not allow for individual control of toes two through five.
8. The flexor digitorum longus is pennate.

17

Flexor Hallucis Longus (*Harry* of *Tom, Dick, and Harry* Group)

The name, flexor hallucis longus, tells us that this muscle flexes the big toe and is long (longer than the flexor hallucis brevis).

Derivation	☐ flexor:	L. *a muscle that flexes a body part.*
	hallucis:	L. *the big toe.*
	longus:	L. *longer.*
Pronunciation	☐ FLEKS-or, hal-OO-sis, LONG-us	

■ ATTACHMENTS

☐ **Distal Posterior Fibula**
  ☐ the distal ⅔ of the posterior fibula and the distal ⅔ of the interosseus membrane

to the

☐ **Plantar Surface of the Big Toe (Toe One)**
  ☐ the distal phalanx

■ FUNCTIONS

CONCENTRIC (SHORTENING) MOVER ACTIONS

Standard Mover Actions	**Reverse Mover Actions**
☐ **1. Flexes the big toe at the MTP and IP joints**	☐ 1. Flexes the metatarsal at the MTP joint and flexes the proximal phalanx at the IP joint
☐ **2. Plantarflexes the foot at the ankle joint**	☐ 2. Plantarflexes the leg at the ankle joint
☐ **3. Inverts (supinates) the foot at the subtalar joint**	☐ 3. Inverts (supinates) the talus at the subtalar joint

MTP joint = metatarsophalangeal joint; IP joint = interphalangeal joint.

17

Standard Mover Action Notes

- The flexor hallucis longus crosses the big toe on the plantar side (with its fibers running horizontally in the sagittal plane); therefore it flexes the big toe. Given that the flexor hallucis longus attaches onto the distal phalanx, it crosses both the MTP joint and IP joint of the big toe. Therefore the flexor hallucis longus flexes the big toe at both of these joints. (action 1)
- More specifically, flexing the big toe at the MTP and IP joints refers to flexing the proximal phalanx at the MTP joint and flexing the distal phalanx at the IP joint. (action 1)
- Flexion of the big toe at the MTP and IP joints contributes to toe-off during the gait cycle. (action 1)
- The flexor hallucis longus crosses the ankle joint posteriorly (with its fibers running vertically in the sagittal plane); therefore it plantarflexes the foot at the ankle joint. (action 2)
- The flexor hallucis longus enters the foot and crosses the subtalar joint on the medial side (with its fibers running vertically in the frontal plane), therefore it inverts the foot

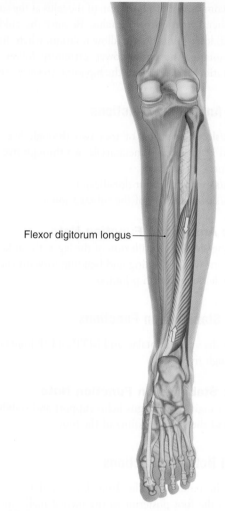

Flexor digitorum longus ——

Figure 17-8 Posterior view of the right flexor hallucis longus. The flexor digitorum longus has been ghosted in.

at the subtalar joint. Inversion is the major component of subtalar supination (subtalar supination also includes medial rotation and plantarflexion of the foot). (action 3)

Reverse Mover Action Notes

- Reverse actions within the lower extremity occur when the distal end is fixed (usually due to the foot being planted on the ground) so that the proximal attachment moves instead. (reverse actions 1, 2, 3)
- The reverse actions of flexion of the big toe involve the metatarsal moving at the MTP joint and the proximal phalanx moving at the IP joint. (reverse action 1)
- The flexor hallucis longus crosses the ankle joint posteriorly with a vertical direction to its fibers (in the sagittal plane). If the foot is fixed by being planted on the ground, the leg is plantarflexed at the ankle joint by bringing the posterior

Flexor Hallucis Longus (*Harry* of *Tom, Dick, and Harry* Group)—*cont'd*

surface of the leg toward the plantar surface of the foot. (reverse action 2)

- The reverse action of inversion of the foot at the subtalar joint is inversion of the leg at the subtalar joint. Moving the leg at the subtalar joint involves moving the talus relative to the calcaneus. Inversion is the principle component of supination. (reverse action 3)
- Another component of supination of the talus at the subtalar joint is lateral rotation of the talus. Because the ankle and (extended) knee joints do not allow rotation, when the talus laterally rotates, the entire lower extremity follows with lateral rotation of the thigh at the hip joint. (reverse action 3)

Eccentric Antagonist Functions

1. Restrains/slows extension of the big toe at the MTP and IP joints, and the metatarsal at the MTP joint
2. Restrains/slows ankle joint dorsiflexion
3. Restrains/slows eversion at the subtalar joint

Eccentric Antagonist Function Note

- Restraining/slowing dorsiflexion of the leg at the ankle joint is important when standing and bending forward (bending at the ankle, knee, and hip joints).

Isometric Stabilization Functions

1. Stabilizes the ankle, subtalar, and MTP and IP joints of the big toe

Additional Notes on Functions

1. The flexor hallucis longus is actually quite large and powerful; it is larger and stronger than the flexor digitorum longus. One reason for the size and strength of this muscle is to increase our propulsive force when we push off (*toe-off*) the ground by flexing the big toe when walking and running.
2. Because the tendons of the Tom, Dick, and Harry group cross into the foot posterior to the medial malleolus, their line of pull is posteromedial. Therefore all three Tom, Dick, and Harry muscles plantarflex and invert the foot (at the ankle and subtalar joints, respectively).

INNERVATION
☐ The Tibial Nerve
   ☐ L5, **S1, S2**

ARTERIAL SUPPLY
☐ The Posterior Tibial Artery (a terminal branch of the Popliteal Artery)

✋ PALPATION

1. With the client seated or supine, place palpating hand immediately posterior to the distal shaft of the tibia in the medial leg.
2. Have the client flex the big toe (resistance can be added) and feel for the tensing of the distal belly of the flexor hallucis longus.
3. Continue palpating the flexor hallucis longus distally into the foot and proximally into the posterior leg.

■ RELATIONSHIP TO OTHER STRUCTURES

☐ The flexor hallucis longus, flexor digitorum longus, and tibialis posterior are the deepest muscles in the posterior leg. Where these muscles overlap, the tibialis posterior is the deepest of the three.
☐ The flexor hallucis longus is deep to the soleus.
☐ Deep to the flexor hallucis longus are the fibula and the interosseus membrane.
☐ Even though the flexor hallucis longus ends up on the big toe in the medial foot, proximally, its belly is lateral in the posterior leg. The belly of the flexor hallucis longus is lateral to the bellies of the tibialis posterior and the flexor digitorum longus.
☐ Lateral to the flexor hallucis longus is the fibularis longus.
☐ The distal tendon of the flexor hallucis longus crosses posterior to the medial malleolus, along with the distal tendons of the tibialis posterior and the flexor digitorum longus. Of the three tendons, the flexor hallucis longus is the farthest from the medial malleolus (and most difficult to palpate).
☐ The flexor hallucis longus is located within the deep front line myofascial meridian.

■ MISCELLANEOUS

1. The flexor hallucis longus is located in the deep posterior compartment of the leg.
2. The flexor **H**allucis longus is *Harry* of the *Tom, Dick, and Harry* group. The Tom, Dick, and Harry muscles are the tibialis posterior, flexor digitorum longus, and flexor hallucis longus. Tom, Dick, and Harry are grouped together, because they are all deep in the posterior leg and all of their distal tendons cross posterior to the medial malleolus of the tibia (in order from anterior to posterior, Tom, Dick, and Harry).
3. It is worth noting that the location of the muscle bellies of the Tom, Dick, and Harry muscles in the posterior leg is, from medial to lateral, Dick, Tom, and Harry (i.e., flexor digitorum longus, tibialis posterior, and flexor hallucis longus).
4. The flexor hallucis longus has a tendon that makes an abrupt turn of approximately 90 degrees.

17

Intrinsic Muscles of the Toe Joints

CHAPTER OUTLINE

CHAPTER OVERVIEW

The muscles addressed in this chapter are the intrinsic muscles of the foot that move the toes. Intrinsic muscles of the foot are wholly located within the foot; in other words, they begin and end in the foot. Extrinsic muscles of the foot that also move the toes are covered in Chapter 17 (extrinsic muscles of the foot attach proximally to the thigh or leg and then travel distally to enter and attach to the foot).

Overview of Structure

☐ Structurally, intrinsic muscles of the foot that move the toes can be divided into two major groups: those on the dorsal side and those on the plantar side. The plantar intrinsic muscles are further subdivided into four groups/layers from superficial to deep, named with Roman numerals I, II, III, and IV, respectively.

☐ Layer I contains the abductor hallucis, abductor digiti minimi pedis, and flexor digitorum brevis. Layer II contains the quadratus plantae and lumbricals pedis. Layer III contains the flexor hallucis brevis, flexor digiti minimi pedis,

and adductor hallucis. Layer IV contains the plantar interossei and dorsal interossei pedis. *Hallucis* means big toe and *digiti minimi* refers to the little toe. Even though these layers are arranged from superficial to deep, each layer does not entirely cover the layer that is deep to it. So some muscles in the deeper layers may actually be superficial.

☐ It is useful to note the symmetry between Layers I and III. Layer I contains two abductors (of big toe and little toe) and a flexor, and Layer III contains two flexors (of big toe and little toe) and an adductor. Layer IV, being the deepest, contains the muscles that, as their names imply, are located between the metatarsal bones, the plantar interossei and dorsal interossei pedis.

Overview of Function

The following general rules regarding actions can be stated for the functional groups of intrinsic toe muscles:

☐ Toes two through five can move at three joints: the metatarsophalangeal (MTP), proximal interphalangeal (PIP), and

    Review the muscles and bones from this chapter on the enclosed CD!

distal interphalangeal (DIP) joints. If a muscle crosses only the MTP joint, it can move the toe only at the MTP joint. If the muscle crosses the MTP and PIP joints, it can move the toe at both of these joints. If the muscle crosses the MTP, PIP, and DIP joints, it can move the toe at all three joints.

☐ The big toe (toe number one) can move at two joints: the MTP and interphalangeal (IP) joints. Similarly, a muscle can only move the big toe at a joint or joints that it crosses.

☐ If a muscle crosses the MTP, PIP, DIP, or IP joints of a toe on the plantar side, it can flex the toe at the joint(s) crossed; if a muscle crosses the MTP, PIP, DIP, or IP joints of a toe on the dorsal side, it can extend the toe at the joint(s) crossed.

☐ If a muscle crosses the MTP joint of toes one, three, four, or five on the side that faces the second toe, it can adduct the toe at the MTP joint; if a muscle crosses the MTP joint of toes one, two, three, four, or five on the side that is away from the (center of the) second-toe side, it can abduct the toe at the MTP joint (the second toe abducts in both directions, tibial and fibular abduction). Note: The axis for abduction/adduction of the toes at the MTP joints is an imaginary line that runs through the center of the second toe when it is in anatomic position.

☐ There is a dorsal digital expansion in the foot formed by the distal tendons of the extensor digitorum longus. It is similar to the dorsal digital expansion of the hand; however, it is not as well developed. Similar to the hand, the lumbricals and interossei muscles attach into the dorsal digital expansion and can therefore do flexion of toes at the MTP joints and extension at the IP joints.

☐ Regarding motion of the toes, to be more specific, the proximal phalanx of the toe moves at the MTP joint, the middle phalanx moves at the PIP joint, and the distal phalanx moves at the DIP joint. For the big toe, the proximal phalanx moves at the MTP joint and the distal phalanx moves at the IP joint.

☐ Reverse actions involve the proximal attachment moving toward the distal one. This usually occurs when the toes are planted on the ground and fixed. Reverse actions of the toes involve the metatarsal moving at the MTP joint (relative to a fixed proximal phalanx), the proximal phalanx moving at the PIP joint (relative to a fixed middle phalanx), and the middle phalanx moving at the DIP joint (relative to a fixed distal phalanx).

18

Plantar View of the Right Foot—Superficial Fascial View

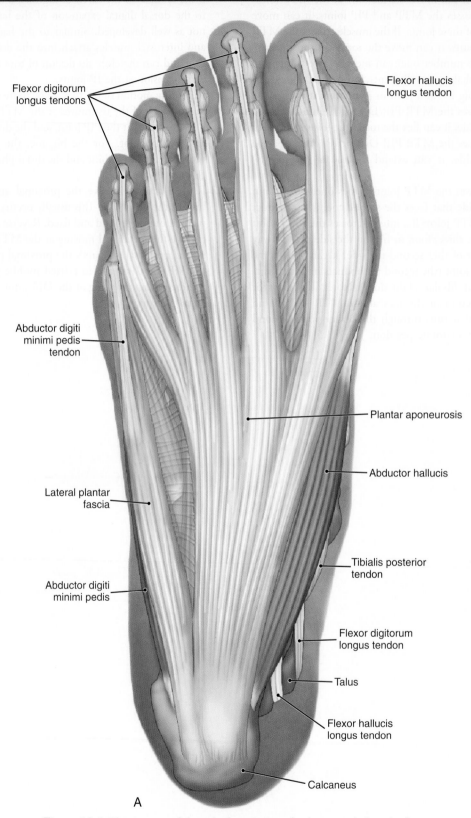

Flexor digitorum longus tendons

Flexor hallucis longus tendon

Abductor digiti minimi pedis tendon

Plantar aponeurosis

Abductor hallucis

Lateral plantar fascia

Tibialis posterior tendon

Abductor digiti minimi pedis

Flexor digitorum longus tendon

Talus

Flexor hallucis longus tendon

Calcaneus

A

Figure 18-1 Plantar views of the right foot. **A,** Superficial view, including the fascia.

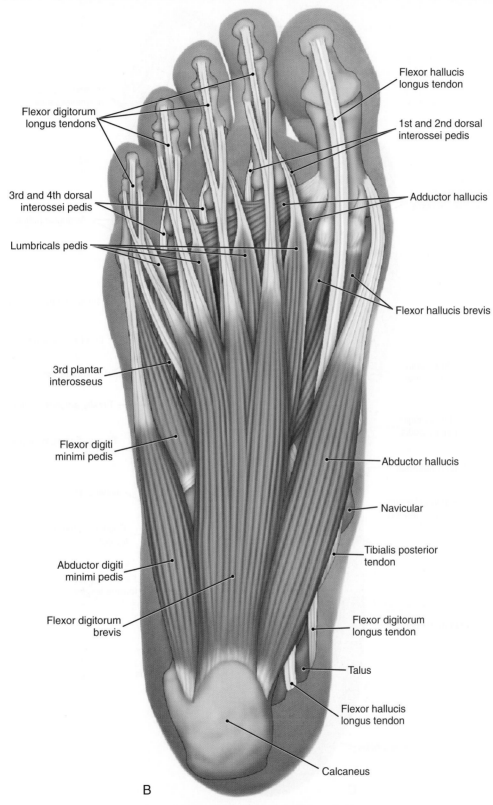

B

Figure 18-1, cont'd B, Superficial muscular view.

Plantar View of the Right Foot—Intermediate View

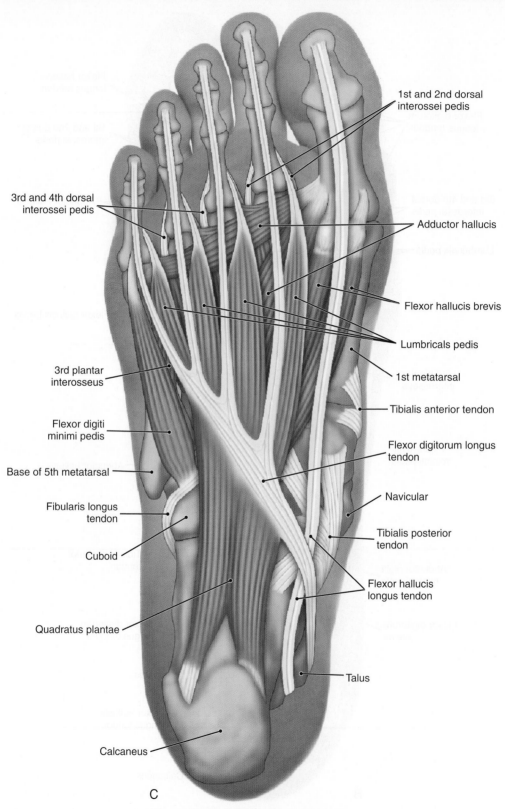

1st and 2nd dorsal interossei pedis

3rd and 4th dorsal interossei pedis

Adductor hallucis

Flexor hallucis brevis

Lumbricals pedis

1st metatarsal

3rd plantar interosseus

Tibialis anterior tendon

Flexor digiti minimi pedis

Flexor digitorum longus tendon

Base of 5th metatarsal

Navicular

Fibularis longus tendon

Tibialis posterior tendon

Cuboid

Flexor hallucis longus tendon

Quadratus plantae

Talus

Calcaneus

C

Figure 18-1, cont'd C, Intermediate view.

Plantar View of the Right Foot—Deep View

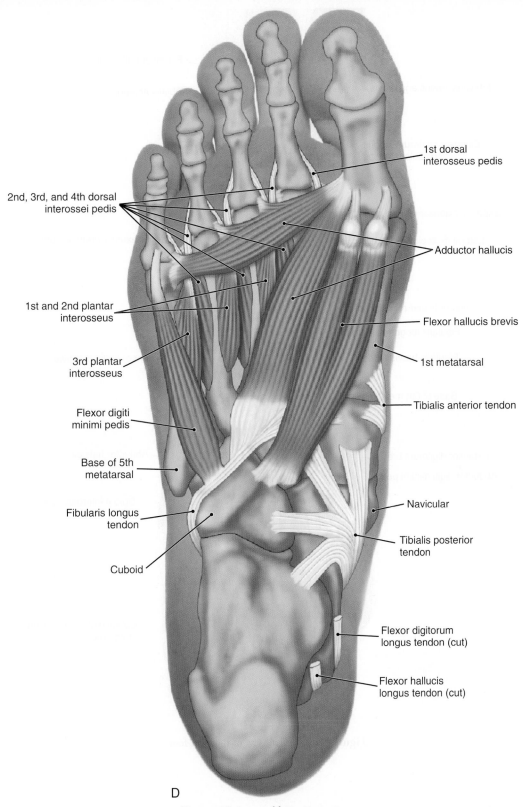

1st dorsal interosseus pedis

2nd, 3rd, and 4th dorsal interossei pedis

Adductor hallucis

1st and 2nd plantar interosseus

Flexor hallucis brevis

3rd plantar interosseus

1st metatarsal

Flexor digiti minimi pedis

Tibialis anterior tendon

Base of 5th metatarsal

Navicular

Fibularis longus tendon

Tibialis posterior tendon

Cuboid

Flexor digitorum longus tendon (cut)

Flexor hallucis longus tendon (cut)

D

Figure 18-1, cont'd D, Deep view.

18

Dorsal View of the Muscles of the Right Foot

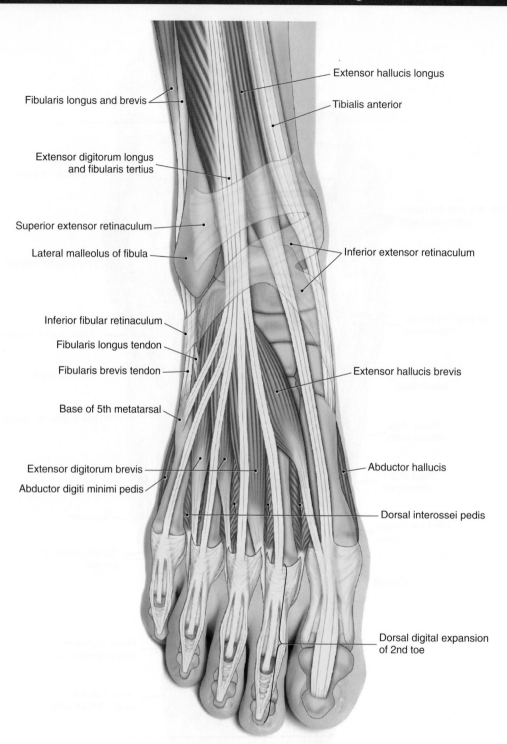

Fibularis longus and brevis

Extensor digitorum longus
and fibularis tertius

Superior extensor retinaculum

Lateral malleolus of fibula

Inferior fibular retinaculum

Fibularis longus tendon

Fibularis brevis tendon

Base of 5th metatarsal

Extensor digitorum brevis

Abductor digiti minimi pedis

Extensor hallucis longus

Tibialis anterior

Inferior extensor retinaculum

Extensor hallucis brevis

Abductor hallucis

Dorsal interossei pedis

Dorsal digital expansion
of 2nd toe

Figure 18-2 Dorsal view of the right foot.

Lateral View of the Muscles of the Right Foot

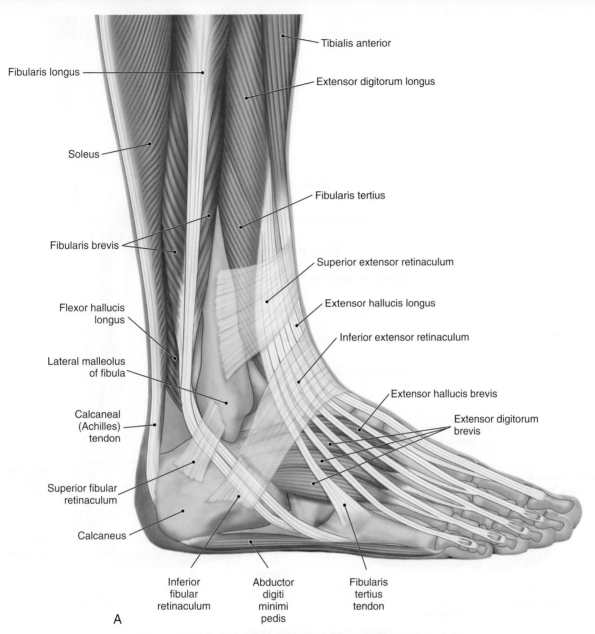

Tibialis anterior

Fibularis longus

Extensor digitorum longus

Soleus

Fibularis tertius

Fibularis brevis

Superior extensor retinaculum

Flexor hallucis longus

Extensor hallucis longus

Inferior extensor retinaculum

Lateral malleolus of fibula

Extensor hallucis brevis

Calcaneal (Achilles) tendon

Extensor digitorum brevis

Superior fibular retinaculum

Calcaneus

Inferior fibular retinaculum

Abductor digiti minimi pedis

Fibularis tertius tendon

A

18

Figure 18-3 Lateral and medial views of the right foot. **A,** Lateral view.

Medial View of the Muscles of the Right Foot

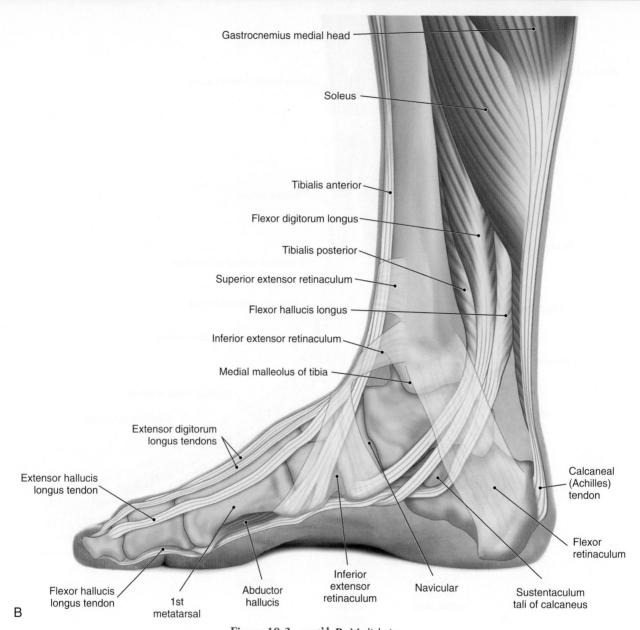

Gastrocnemius medial head

Soleus

Tibialis anterior

Flexor digitorum longus

Tibialis posterior

Superior extensor retinaculum

Flexor hallucis longus

Inferior extensor retinaculum

Medial malleolus of tibia

Extensor digitorum longus tendons

Extensor hallucis longus tendon

Calcaneal (Achilles) tendon

Flexor retinaculum

Flexor hallucis longus tendon

1st metatarsal

Abductor hallucis

Inferior extensor retinaculum

Navicular

Sustentaculum tali of calcaneus

B

Figure 18-3, cont'd B, Medial view.

18

Cross Section through the Right Foot

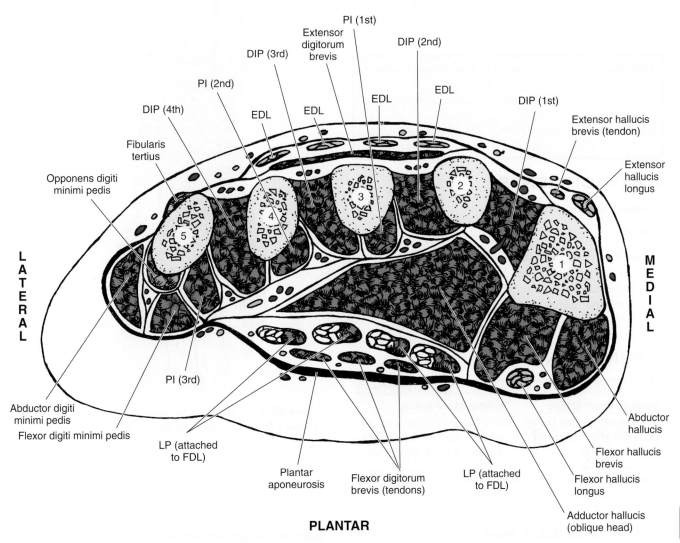

DORSAL

PI (1st)

Extensor
digitorum
brevis

DIP (2nd)

DIP (3rd)

PI (2nd)

EDL

DIP (1st)

DIP (4th)

EDL

EDL

EDL

Extensor hallucis
brevis (tendon)

Fibularis
tertius

Extensor
hallucis
longus

Opponens digiti
minimi pedis

5

4

3

2

1

L A T E R A L

M E D I A L

PI (3rd)

Abductor digiti
minimi pedis

Abductor
hallucis

Flexor digiti minimi pedis

LP (attached
to FDL)

Flexor hallucis
brevis

Plantar
aponeurosis

Flexor digitorum
brevis (tendons)

LP (attached
to FDL)

Flexor hallucis
longus

Adductor hallucis
(oblique head)

PLANTAR

Figure 18-4 Cross section through the right foot. This is a distal view (looking from distal to proximal). An opponens digiti minimi pedis, an anomalous muscle, is shown. DIP, dorsal interosseus pedis; EDL, extensor digitorum longus; FDL, flexor digitorum longus; LP, lumbricals pedis; PI, plantar interosseus.

18

DORSAL SURFACE
Extensor Digitorum Brevis

The name, extensor digitorum brevis, *tells us that this muscle extends the digits (i.e., toes) and is short (shorter than the extensor digitorum longus).*

Derivation	☐ extensor: L. *a muscle that extends a body part.*
	digitorum: L. *refers to a digit* (toe).
	brevis: L. *shorter.*
Pronunciation	☐ eks-TEN-sor, dij-i-TOE-rum, BRE-vis

■ ATTACHMENTS

☐ **Dorsal Surface of the Calcaneus**

to the

☐ **Toes Two through Four**
  ☐ the lateral side of the distal tendons of the extensor digitorum longus muscle of toes two through four (via the dorsal digital expansion into the middle and distal phalanges)

■ FUNCTIONS

CONCENTRIC (SHORTENING) MOVER ACTIONS	
Standard Mover Actions	**Reverse Mover Actions**
☐ 1. Extends toes two through four at the MTP, PIP, and DIP joints	☐ 1. Extends metatarsal at the MTP joint and extends the more proximal phalanges at the PIP and DIP joints

MTP joints = metatarsophalangeal joints; PIP joints = proximal interphalangeal joints; DIP joints = distal interphalangeal joints

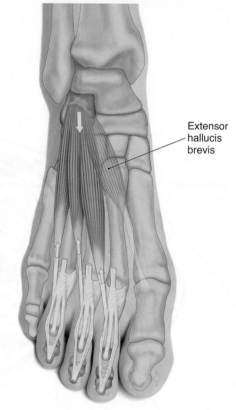

Extensor hallucis brevis

Figure 18-5 Dorsal view of the right extensor digitorum brevis. The extensor hallucis brevis has been ghosted in.

Standard Mover Action Notes

• The extensor digitorum brevis crosses toe joints two through four dorsally (with its fibers running horizontally in the sagittal plane); therefore it extends toes two through four. By attaching onto the distal tendon of the extensor digitorum longus of toes two through four (which attaches onto the distal phalanges of toes two through four), the extensor digitorum brevis pulls these tendons as if the belly of the extensor digitorum longus muscle itself had contracted. Therefore the extensor digitorum brevis has the same actions at toes two through four in the foot as the extensor digitorum longus muscle has, namely, extension of toes two through four at the MTP, PIP, and DIP joints of toes two through four. (action 1)

• More specifically, extending toes at the MTP, PIP, and DIP joints refers to extending the proximal phalanges of the toes at the MTP joints, extending the middle phalanges at the PIP joints, and extending the distal phalanges at the DIP joints. (action 1)

Reverse Mover Action Notes

• The reverse actions involve the distal attachment being fixed and the more proximal bone moving instead; in other words, extension of the metatarsal at the MTP joint, extension of the proximal phalanx at the PIP joint, and extension of the middle phalanx at the DIP joint. (reverse action 1)

• The reverse action of metatarsal extension happens during the gait cycle at toe-off. (reverse action 1)

Eccentric Antagonist Functions

1. Restrains/slows flexion of toes two through four at the MTP, PIP, and DIP joints, and flexion of metatarsals two through four at the MTP joints

Isometric Stabilization Functions

1. Stabilizes the MTP, PIP, and DIP joints of toes two through four

18

Extensor Digitorum Brevis—*cont'd*

INNERVATION

☐ The Deep Fibular Nerve
  ☐ L5, S1

ARTERIAL SUPPLY

☐ The Dorsalis Pedis Artery (the continuation of the Anterior Tibial Artery)

✋ PALPATION

1. With the client seated or supine, place palpating fingers approximately 1 inch (2 to 3 cm) distal to the lateral malleolus on the dorsum of the foot.
2. Have the client extend the toes (two through four) and feel for the contraction of the belly of the extensor digitorum brevis. Resistance can be added.

■ RELATIONSHIP TO OTHER STRUCTURES

☐ The extensor digitorum brevis is superficial except where the distal tendons of the extensor digitorum longus and the fibularis tertius cross superficially to it.

☐ Deep to the extensor digitorum brevis are the tarsal and metatarsal bones.
☐ The extensor digitorum brevis is lateral to the extensor hallucis brevis.
☐ The extensor digitorum brevis is located within the superficial front line myofascial meridian.

■ MISCELLANEOUS

1. The extensor digitorum brevis and the extensor hallucis brevis are the only intrinsic foot muscles located on the dorsal side.
2. The extensor digitorum brevis and extensor hallucis brevis are actually one muscle. However, the most medial part of extensor digitorum brevis does not attach onto a *digit*, therefore it is given a separate name, the *extensor hallucis brevis*. The term *digit* in the name of a muscle of the lower extremity is reserved for toes two through five, not toe number one, the big toe.
3. The common belly of the extensors digitorum and hallucis brevis is often visible on the proximal lateral surface of the dorsum of the foot.

18

Extensor Hallucis Brevis

The name, extensor hallucis brevis, *tells us that this muscle extends the big toe and is short (shorter than the extensor hallucis longus).*

Derivation	☐ extensor: L. *a muscle that extends a body part.*
	hallucis: L. *refers to the big toe.*
	brevis: L. *shorter.*
Pronunciation	☐ eks-TEN-sor, hal-OO-sis, BRE-vis

■ ATTACHMENTS

☐ **Dorsal Surface of the Calcaneus**

   to the

☐ **Dorsal Surface of the Big Toe (Toe One)**
   ☐ the base of the proximal phalanx of the big toe

■ FUNCTIONS

CONCENTRIC (SHORTENING) MOVER ACTIONS	
Standard Mover Actions	**Reverse Mover Actions**
☐ **1. Extends the big toe at the MTP joint**	☐ 1. Extends the metatarsal of the big toe at the MTP joint

MTP joint = metatarsophalangeal joint

Standard Mover Action Notes

• The extensor hallucis brevis crosses the MTP joint of the big toe (toe number one) dorsally (with its fibers running horizontally in the sagittal plane) to attach onto the proximal phalanx of the big toe. Therefore it extends the big toe at the MTP joint. (action 1)
• More specifically, extending the big toe at the MTP joint refers to extending the proximal phalanx of the big toe at the MTP joint. (action 1)

Reverse Mover Action Notes

• The reverse action of metatarsal extension at the MTP joint happens when the distal attachment (the proximal phalanx) is fixed and the proximal attachment (the metatarsal) moves. This occurs during the gait cycle at toe-off. (reverse action 1)

Eccentric Antagonist Function

1. Restrains/slows flexion of the MTP joint of the big toe

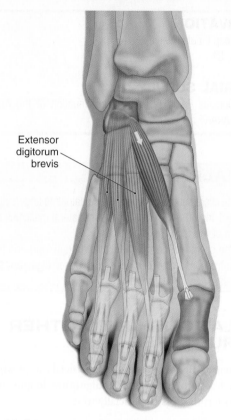

Extensor digitorum brevis

Figure 18-6 Dorsal view of the right extensor hallucis brevis. The extensor digitorum brevis has been ghosted in.

Isometric Stabilization Function

1. Stabilizes the MTP joint of the big toe

Additional Note on Functions

1. Given that the extensor hallucis brevis crosses the MTP joint of the big toe from lateral on the foot to medial on the big toe, this muscle should have the ability to adduct the big toe at the MTP joint.

INNERVATION
☐ The Deep Fibular Nerve
   ☐ L5, S1

ARTERIAL SUPPLY
☐ The Dorsalis Pedis Artery (the continuation of the Anterior Tibial Artery)

Extensor Hallucis Brevis—*cont'd*

 PALPATION

1. With the client seated or supine, place palpating fingers approximately 1 inch (2 to 3 cm) distal to the lateral malleolus on the dorsum of the foot.
2. Have the client extend the big toe and feel for the contraction of the belly of the extensor hallucis brevis. It will be medial to the extensor digitorum brevis. Resistance can be added.

■ RELATIONSHIP TO OTHER STRUCTURES

☐ The extensor hallucis brevis is superficial, except where the distal tendons of the extensor digitorum longus and the fibularis tertius cross superficially to it.
☐ Deep to the extensor hallucis brevis are the tarsal and metatarsal bones.
☐ The extensor hallucis brevis is medial to the extensor digitorum brevis.

☐ The extensor hallucis brevis is located within the superficial front line myofascial meridian.

■ MISCELLANEOUS

1. The extensor hallucis brevis and the extensor digitorum brevis are the only intrinsic foot muscles located on the dorsal side.
2. The extensor hallucis brevis is actually the most medial part of the extensor digitorum brevis. The extensor hallucis brevis is differentiated from the rest of the extensor digitorum brevis and given a separate name, because this part of the muscle does not attach onto a *digit*. Instead it attaches onto the big toe (the *hallux*). Therefore this portion of the extensor digitorum brevis is called the *extensor hallucis brevis*. The term *digit* in the name of a muscle of the lower extremity is reserved for toes two through five, not toe number one, the big toe.

PLANTAR SURFACE: LAYER I

Abductor Hallucis

The name, abductor hallucis, *tells us that this muscle abducts the big toe.*

Derivation	☐ abductor: L. *a muscle that abducts a body part.*
	hallucis: L. *refers to the big toe.*
Pronunciation	☐ ab-DUK-tor, hal-OO-sis

■ ATTACHMENTS

☐ **Tuberosity of the Calcaneus**
  ☐ and the flexor retinaculum and plantar fascia

to the

☐ **Big Toe (Toe One)**
  ☐ the medial plantar side of the base of the proximal phalanx

■ FUNCTIONS

CONCENTRIC (SHORTENING) MOVER ACTIONS	
Standard Mover Actions	**Reverse Mover Actions**
☐ **1. Abducts the big toe at the MTP joint**	☐ 1. Abducts the metatarsal of the big toe at the MTP joint
☐ 2. Flexes the big toe at the MTP joint	☐ 2. Flexes the metatarsal of the big toe at the MTP joint
MTP joint = metatarsophalangeal joint	

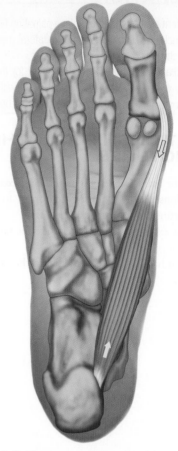

Figure 18-7 Plantar view of the right abductor hallucis.

Standard Mover Action Notes

• The abductor hallucis crosses the MTP joint to attach onto the proximal phalanx of the big toe (toe number one) on the medial side (with its fibers running horizontally). Therefore when the abductor hallucis contracts, it pulls the big toe medially away from the second toe (which is the axis of abduction/adduction of the toes). Therefore the abductor hallucis abducts the big toe at the MTP joint. (action 1)

• The abductor hallucis crosses the MTP joint to attach onto the proximal phalanx of the big toe on the plantar side (with its fibers running horizontally in the sagittal plane). Therefore when the abductor hallucis pulls on the big toe, it flexes the big toe at the MTP joint. (action 2)

• More specifically, abduction and flexion of the big toe at the MTP joint refers to abduction and flexion of the proximal phalanx of the big toe relative to the first metatarsal at the MTP joint. (actions 1, 2)

Reverse Mover Action Notes

• Reverse actions usually occur when the distal attachment is fixed and the proximal attachment moves instead. The reverse actions of the abductor hallucis involve abduction and flexion of the metatarsal of the big toe relative to a fixed

proximal phalanx at the MTP joint. These reverse actions are not likely to occur. (reverse actions 1, 2)

Eccentric Antagonist Functions

1. Restrains/slows adduction of the MTP joint of the big toe
2. Restrains/slows extension of the MTP joint of the big toe

Isometric Stabilization Function

1. Stabilizes the MTP joint of the big toe.

INNERVATION
☐ The Medial Plantar Nerve
  ☐ S1, S2

ARTERIAL SUPPLY
☐ The Medial Plantar Artery (a branch of the Posterior Tibial Artery)

Abductor Hallucis—*cont'd*

 PALPATION

1. With the client prone or supine, place palpating fingers along the proximal half of the plantar foot on the medial side.
2. Have the client abduct the big toe at the metatarsophalangeal joint and feel for the contraction of the abductor hallucis. Resistance can be added.
3. Continue palpating proximally and distally toward its attachments.

■ RELATIONSHIP TO OTHER STRUCTURES

☐ The abductor hallucis is located in the first plantar layer of intrinsic muscles of the foot along with the abductor digiti minimi pedis and the flexor digitorum brevis (and the plantar fascia).

☐ The abductor hallucis is medial to the plantar fascia and the flexor digitorum brevis (which is deep to the plantar fascia).
☐ The abductor hallucis is located within the superficial back line myofascial meridian.

■ MISCELLANEOUS

• All three muscles in the 1st plantar layer of intrinsic muscles of the foot attach proximally onto the tuberosity of the calcaneus and the plantar fascia, and attach distally onto the toes.

18

Abductor Digiti Minimi Pedis

The name, abductor digiti minimi pedis, *tells us that this muscle abducts the little toe.*

Derivation	☐ abductor: L. *a muscle that abducts a body part.*
	digiti: L. *refers to a digit* (toe).
	minimi: L. *least.*
	pedis: L. *refers to the foot.*
Pronunciation	☐ ab-DUK-tor, DIJ-i-tee, MIN-i-mee, PEED-us

■ ATTACHMENTS

☐ **Tuberosity of the Calcaneus**
  ☐ and the plantar fascia

to the

☐ **Little Toe (Toe Five)**
  ☐ the lateral plantar side of the base of the proximal phalanx

■ FUNCTIONS

CONCENTRIC (SHORTENING) MOVER ACTIONS	
Standard Mover Actions	**Reverse Mover Actions**
☐ **1. Abducts the little toe at the MTP joint**	☐ 1. Abducts the metatarsal of the little toe at the MTP joint
☐ 2. Flexes the little toe at the MTP joint	☐ 2. Flexes the metatarsal of the little toe at the MTP joint

MTP joint = metatarsophalangeal joint

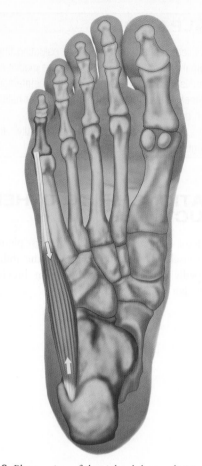

Figure 18-8 Plantar view of the right abductor digiti minimi pedis.

Standard Mover Action Notes

- The abductor digiti minimi pedis crosses the MTP joint to attach onto the proximal phalanx of the little toe (toe number five) on the lateral side (with its fibers running horizontally). When the abductor digiti minimi pedis contracts, it pulls the little toe laterally away from the second toe (which is the axis of abduction/adduction of the toes); therefore the abductor digiti minimi pedis abducts the little toe at the MTP joint. (action 1)
- The abductor digiti minimi pedis crosses the MTP joint to attach onto the proximal phalanx of the little toe on the plantar side (with its fibers running horizontally in the sagittal plane); therefore when it pulls on the little toe, the abductor digiti minimi pedis flexes the little toe at the MTP joint. (action 2)
- More specifically, abduction and flexion of the little toe at the MTP joint refer to abduction and flexion of the proximal phalanx of the little toe relative to a fixed fifth metatarsal at the MTP joint. (actions 1, 2)

Reverse Mover Action Notes

- Reverse actions usually occur when the distal attachment is fixed and the proximal attachment moves instead. Reverse actions of the abductor digiti minimi pedis involve abduction or flexion of the fifth metatarsal relative to the fixed proximal phalanx of the little toe at the MTP joint. These reverse actions are not very likely to occur. (reverse action 1)

Eccentric Antagonist Functions

1. Restrains/slows adduction of the MTP joint of the little toe
2. Restrains/slows extension of the MTP joint of the little toe

Isometric Stabilization Function

1. Stabilizes the MTP joint of the little toe

18

Abductor Digiti Minimi Pedis—*cont'd*

INNERVATION

☐ The Lateral Plantar Nerve
　☐ S2, S3

ARTERIAL SUPPLY

☐ The Lateral Plantar Artery (a branch of the Posterior Tibial Artery)

 PALPATION

1. With the client prone or supine, place palpating fingers on the lateral side of the plantar surface of the foot.
2. Have the client abduct the little toe and feel for the contraction of the abductor digiti minimi pedis. Resistance can be added.
3. Continue palpating proximally and distally toward its attachments.

■ RELATIONSHIP TO OTHER STRUCTURES

☐ The abductor digiti minimi pedis is located in the first plantar layer of intrinsic muscles of the foot along with the abductor hallucis and the flexor digitorum brevis (and the plantar fascia).
☐ The abductor digiti minimi pedis is lateral to the plantar fascia and the flexor digitorum brevis (which is deep to the plantar fascia).
☐ The abductor digiti minimi pedis is located within the superficial back line myofascial meridian.

■ MISCELLANEOUS

1. The abductor digiti minimi pedis is also known as the *abductor digiti minimi.* However, this allows for confusion with the abductor digiti minimi manus of the hand, which abducts the little finger of the hand.
2. All three muscles in the first plantar layer of intrinsic muscles of the foot attach proximally onto the tuberosity of the calcaneus and the plantar fascia, and attach distally onto the toes.

18

Flexor Digitorum Brevis

The name, flexor digitorum brevis, *tells us that this muscle flexes the digits (i.e., toes) and is short (shorter than the flexor digitorum longus).*

Derivation	☐ flexor:	L. *a muscle that flexes a body part.*
	digitorum:	L. *refers to a digit* (toe).
	brevis:	L. *shorter.*
Pronunciation	☐ FLEKS-or, dij-i-TOE-rum, BRE-vis

■ ATTACHMENTS

☐ **Tuberosity of the Calcaneus**
  ☐ and the plantar fascia

to the

☐ **Toes Two through Five**
  ☐ the medial and lateral sides of the middle phalanges

■ FUNCTIONS

CONCENTRIC (SHORTENING) MOVER ACTIONS	
Standard Mover Actions	**Reverse Mover Actions**
☐ 1. Flexes toes two through five at the MTP and PIP joints	☐ 1. Flexes the metatarsals at the MTP joints and flexes the proximal phalanges at the PIP joints

MTP joints = metatarsophalangeal joints; PIP joints = proximal interphalangeal joints

Standard Mover Action Notes

- The flexor digitorum brevis crosses both the MTP and PIP joints of toes two through five on the plantar side (with its fibers running horizontally in the sagittal plane) to then attach onto the medial and lateral sides of the middle phalanges of toes two through five. Because the flexor digitorum brevis crosses these joints on the plantar side, it flexes the MTP and the PIP joints of toes two through five. (action 1)
- More specifically, flexing toes at the MTP and PIP joints refers to flexing the proximal phalanges at the MTP joints and flexing the middle phalanges at the PIP joints. (action 1)

Reverse Mover Action Notes

- The reverse action involves motion of the more proximal bone at each of the joints of the toes. In other words, the reverse action at the MTP joint is flexion of the metatarsal of the toe relative to a fixed proximal phalanx, and the reverse action at the proximal interphalangeal joint is flexion of the proximal phalanx relative to a fixed middle phalanx. These reverse actions are not likely to occur. (reverse action 1)

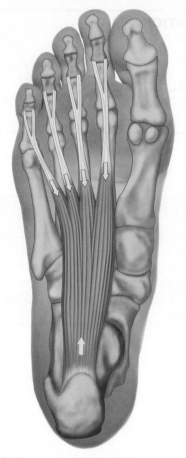

Figure 18-9 Plantar view of the right flexor digitorum brevis.

Eccentric Antagonist Functions

1. Restrains/slows extension of toes two through five at the MTP and PIP joints, and extension of metatarsals two through five at the MTP joints

Isometric Stabilization Functions

1. Stabilizes the MTP and PIP joints of toes two through five

INNERVATION
☐ The Medial Plantar Nerve
  ☐ S1, S2

ARTERIAL SUPPLY
☐ The Medial and Lateral Plantar Arteries (terminal branches of the Posterior Tibial Artery)

Flexor Digitorum Brevis—*cont'd*

 PALPATION

1. With the client prone or supine, place palpating fingers on the midline of the plantar side of the foot.
2. Have the client flex toes two through five and feel for the contraction of the flexor digitorum brevis deep to the plantar fascia. Resistance can be added.
3. Continue palpating proximally and distally toward its attachments.

■ RELATIONSHIP TO OTHER STRUCTURES

☐ The flexor digitorum brevis is located in the first plantar layer of intrinsic muscles of the foot along with the abductor hallucis and the abductor digiti minimi pedis (and the plantar fascia).

☐ The flexor digitorum brevis is lateral to the abductor hallucis, medial to the abductor digiti minimi pedis, and deep to the plantar fascia.

☐ Deep to the belly of the flexor digitorum brevis is the quadratus plantae.

☐ The tendons of the flexor digitorum brevis are superficial to the tendons of the flexor digitorum longus.

☐ The flexor digitorum brevis is located within the superficial back line myofascial meridian.

■ MISCELLANEOUS

1. All three muscles in the first plantar layer of intrinsic muscles of the foot attach proximally onto the tuberosity of the calcaneus and the plantar fascia, and attach distally onto the toes.

2. Each distal tendon of the flexor digitorum brevis splits to allow passage for the flexor digitorum longus' distal tendon to attach onto the distal phalanx (of toes two through five). (This arrangement is essentially identical to that of the splitting of each distal tendon of the flexor digitorum superficialis to allow passage for the flexor digitorum profundus' distal tendon onto the distal phalanx (of fingers two through five in the upper extremity).

18

PLANTER SURFACE: LAYER II
Quadratus Plantae

The name, quadratus plantae, *tells us that this muscle has a square shape and is located on the plantar side of the foot.*

Derivation	☐ quadratus: L. *squared.*
	plantae: L. *refers to the plantar surface of the foot.*
Pronunciation	☐ kwod-RAY-tus, PLAN-tee

■ ATTACHMENTS

☐ **The Calcaneus**
 ☐ the medial and lateral sides

to the

☐ **Distal Tendon of the Flexor Digitorum Longus Muscle**
 ☐ the lateral margin

■ FUNCTIONS

CONCENTRIC (SHORTENING) MOVER ACTIONS	
Standard Mover Actions	**Reverse Mover Actions**
☐ 1. Flexes toes two through five at the MTP, PIP, and DIP joints	☐ 1. Flexes metatarsals at the MTP joints and flexes the more proximal phalanges at the PIP and DIP joints

MTP joints = metatarsophalangeal joints; PIP joints = proximal interphalangeal joints; DIP joints = distal interphalangeal joints

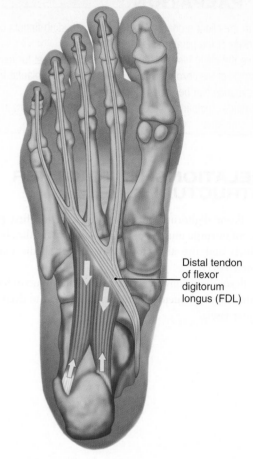

Figure 18-10 Plantar view of the right quadratus plantae.

Distal tendon of flexor digitorum longus (FDL)

Standard Mover Action Notes

- The quadratus plantae (with its fibers running horizontally in the sagittal plane) attaches into the distal tendon of the flexor digitorum longus (FDL) muscle. When the quadratus plantae contracts, it pulls on that tendon in the same way as if the belly of the FDL muscle itself had contracted. Therefore the quadratus plantae muscle has the same actions as the FDL muscle (in the foot), namely, flexion of toes two through five. Given that the attachments are onto the distal phalanx of these toes, the MTP, PIP, and DIP joints are all crossed and therefore are all flexed. (action 1)
- More specifically, flexing toes at the MTP, PIP, and DIP joints refers to flexing the proximal phalanges of the toes at the MTP joints, flexing the middle phalanges at the PIP joints, and flexing the distal phalanges at the DIP joints. (action 1)
- Similar to the FDL, the quadratus plantae has no individual control of flexion of toes two through five because all of its muscle fibers converge into the common distal tendon of the FDL before it splits to go to each of the toes. (action 1)

Reverse Mover Action Notes

- Reverse actions usually occur when the distal attachment is fixed and the proximal attachment moves instead. In other words, the reverse action of the quadratus plantae at the MTP joint is flexion of the metatarsal of the toe relative to a fixed proximal phalanx. The reverse action at the PIP joint is flexion of the proximal phalanx relative to a fixed middle phalanx. The reverse action at the DIP joint is flexion of the middle phalanx relative to a fixed distal phalanx. These reverse actions are not likely to occur. (reverse action 1)

Eccentric Antagonist Functions

1. Restrains/slows extension at the MTP, PIP, and DIP joints of toes two through five

Isometric Stabilization Functions

1. Stabilizes the MTP, PIP, and DIP joints of toes two through five

18

Quadratus Plantae—*cont'd*

Additional Notes on Functions

1. Given its assistance to the flexor digitorum longus, the quadratus plantae is also known as the *flexor accessorius* or the *flexor digitorum accessorius*. The quadratus plantae not only assists by adding further strength but also assists by modifying (straightening out) the line of pull of the flexor digitorum longus muscle. If not for the quadratus plantae's assistance, the contraction of the flexor digitorum longus would pull the toes slightly medially as it flexed them.

INNERVATION
- ☐ The Lateral Plantar Nerve
  - ☐ S2, S3

ARTERIAL SUPPLY
- ☐ The Medial and Lateral Plantar Arteries (terminal branches of the Posterior Tibial Artery)

🖐 PALPATION

1. With the client prone or supine, place palpating fingers on the midline of the proximal half of the plantar side of the foot and feel for the quadratus plantae deep to the plantar fascia and flexor digitorum brevis.
2. To further bring out the quadratus plantae, resist the client from actively flexing toes two through five.
3. Keep in mind that this will cause the more superficial flexor digitorum brevis to contract as well.

■ RELATIONSHIP TO OTHER STRUCTURES

- ☐ The quadratus plantae is in the second plantar layer of intrinsic muscles of the foot along with the lumbricals pedis (and the distal tendons of the flexor digitorum longus and the flexor hallucis longus).
- ☐ The quadratus plantae is deep to the flexor digitorum brevis.
- ☐ Deep to the quadratus plantae are the tarsal bones.
- ☐ The quadratus plantae is located within the superficial back line myofascial meridian.

■ MISCELLANEOUS

1. Proximally, the quadratus plantae has two heads. The medial head attaches onto the medial side of the calcaneus and the lateral head attaches onto the lateral side of the calcaneus.

18

Lumbricals Pedis

(There are four lumbrical pedis muscles, named one, two, three, and four.)

The name, lumbricals pedis, tells us that these muscles are shaped like earthworms and located in the foot.

Derivation	☐ lumbricals: L. *earthworms.*
	pedis: L. *refers to the foot.*
Pronunciation	☐ LUM-bri-kuls, PEED-us

■ ATTACHMENTS

☐ **The Distal Tendons of the Flexor Digitorum Longus Muscle**
  ☐ ONE: medial border of the tendon to toe two
  ☐ TWO: adjacent sides of the tendons to toes two and three
  ☐ THREE: adjacent sides of the tendons to toes three and four
  ☐ FOUR: adjacent sides of the tendons to toes four and five

  to the

☐ **Dorsal Digital Expansion**
  ☐ the medial sides of the extensor digitorum longus tendons merging into the dorsal digital expansion of toes two through five

■ FUNCTIONS

CONCENTRIC (SHORTENING) MOVER ACTIONS	
Standard Mover Actions	**Reverse Mover Actions**
☐ **1. Flex toes two through five at the MTP joints**	☐ 1. Flex the metatarsals at the MTP joints
☐ **2. Extend toes two through five at the PIP and DIP joints**	☐ 2. Extend the more proximal phalanges at the PIP and DIP joints

MTP joints = metatarsophalangeal joints; PIP joints = proximal interphalangeal joints; DIP joints = distal interphalangeal joints

Standard Mover Action Notes

• The lumbricals pedis cross the MTP joint of toes two through five on the plantar side (with their fibers running horizontally in the sagittal plane); therefore they flex toes two through five at the MTP joints. More specifically, flexing toes at the MTP joints refers to flexing the proximal phalanges of the toes at the MTP joints. (action 1)

• The lumbricals pedis, by attaching into the dorsal digital expansion of the tendons of the extensor digitorum longus (after the MTP joint but before the interphalangeal [IP] joints of the toes), in effect exert their pull (horizontally in the sagittal plane) at the attachments of the extensor digitorum longus, which are the middle and distal phalanges of toes two through five. The lumbricals pedis, in effect, cross

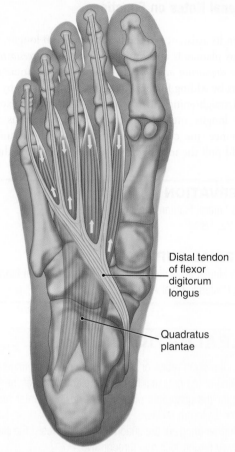

Figure 18-11 Plantar view of the right lumbricals pedis. The quadratus plantae has been ghosted in.

(labels on figure:)
Distal tendon of flexor digitorum longus
Quadratus plantae

the PIP and DIP joints on the dorsal side and therefore extend these joints of toes two through five. More specifically, extending toes at the IP joints refers to extending the middle phalanges of the toes at the proximal IP joints and extending the distal phalanges at the distal IP joints. (action 2)

Reverse Mover Action Notes

• Reverse actions usually occur when the distal attachment is fixed and the proximal attachment moves instead. In other words, the reverse action of the lumbricals pedis at the MTP joint is flexion of the metatarsal of the toe relative to a fixed proximal phalanx, the reverse action at the PIP joint is extension of the proximal phalanx relative to a fixed middle phalanx, and the reverse action at the DIP joint is extension of the middle phalanx relative to the fixed distal phalanx. The reverse action of flexion of the metatarsal at the MTP joint is not likely to occur. However, the reverse actions at the IP joints occur during toe-off in the gait cycle. (reverse actions 1, 2)

18

Lumbricals Pedis—cont'd

Eccentric Antagonist Functions

1. Restrains/slows flexion of the PIP and DIP joints of toes two through five
2. Restrains/slows extension of the MTP joints of toes two through five

Isometric Stabilization Functions

1. Stabilizes the MTP, PIP, and DIP joints of toes two through five

Additional Notes on Functions

1. The lumbricals pedis flex the MTP joints because they cross these joints on the plantar side. Because they attach into the dorsal digital expansion of the foot, their line of pull is transmitted across the dorsal side of the interphalangeal (IP) joints; therefore they extend the IP joints. All muscles that attach into the dorsal digital expansion of the foot flex the MTP joints and extend the IP joints.
2. The lumbricals manus of the hand have similar actions in that they flex the fingers at the metacarpophalangeal (MCP) joints and extend the fingers at the proximal and distal IP joints.

INNERVATION
- ☐ The Medial and Lateral Plantar Nerves
  - ☐ S1, S2, S3
  - ☐ medial plantar nerve to lumbrical pedis one
  - ☐ lateral plantar nerve to lumbricals pedis two through four

ARTERIAL SUPPLY
- ☐ The Medial and Lateral Plantar Arteries (terminal branches of the Posterior Tibial Artery)
  - ☐ branches of the Plantar Arch (an anastomosis between the Lateral Plantar Artery and the Dorsalis Pedis Artery)

🤚 PALPATION

1. With the client prone or supine, place palpating hand distally on the plantar surface of the foot and feel for the lumbricals pedis between the metatarsal bones.
2. To further bring out the lumbricals pedis, resist the client from actively flexing the metatarsophalangeal joint (with the interphalangeal joints extended) of toes two through five. Note: Many people are unable to isolate these actions.

■ RELATIONSHIP TO OTHER STRUCTURES

- ☐ The lumbricals pedis are in the second plantar layer of the intrinsic muscles of the foot along with the quadratus plantae (and the distal tendons of the flexor digitorum longus and flexor hallucis longus).
- ☐ The lumbricals pedis are located between the distal tendons of the flexor digitorum longus in the distal foot.
- ☐ The lumbricals pedis are deep to the plantar aponeurosis. No muscles are superficial to the lumbricals pedis except, perhaps, a small part of the flexor digitorum brevis.
- ☐ Deep to the lumbricals pedis are the metatarsals and the plantar interossei and dorsal interossei pedis muscles.
- ☐ The lumbricals pedis may be involved with the superficial back line and deep front line myofascial meridians.

■ MISCELLANEOUS

1. The lumbricals pedis are actually four small separate muscles named from the medial side: *one*, *two*, *three*, and *four*.
2. The lumbricals pedis are usually known as the *lumbricals*. However, this allows for confusion with the lumbricals manus of the hand.

18

PLANTAR SURFACE: LAYER III
Flexor Hallucis Brevis

The name, flexor hallucis brevis, *tells us that this muscle flexes the big toe and is short (shorter than the flexor hallucis longus).*

Derivation	☐ flexor:	L. *a muscle that flexes a body part.*
	hallucis:	L. *refers to the big toe.*
	brevis:	L. *shorter.*
Pronunciation	☐ FLEKS-or, hal-OO-sis, BRE-vis	

■ ATTACHMENTS

☐ **Cuboid and the third Cuneiform**

to the

☐ **Big Toe (Toe One)**
 ☐ the medial and lateral sides of the plantar surface of the base of the proximal phalanx

■ FUNCTIONS

CONCENTRIC (SHORTENING) MOVER ACTIONS	
Standard Mover Actions	**Reverse Mover Actions**
☐ **1. Flexes the big toe at the MTP joint**	☐ 1. Flexes the metatarsal of the big toe at the MTP joint

MTP joint = metatarsophalangeal joint

Standard Mover Action Notes

• The flexor hallucis brevis crosses the MTP joint of the big toe (toe number one) on the plantar side (with its fibers running horizontally in the sagittal plane) to attach onto the proximal phalanx of the big toe. Therefore the flexor hallucis brevis flexes the big toe at the MTP joint. (action 1)
• More specifically, flexing the big toe at the MTP joint refers to flexing the proximal phalanx of the big toe relative to a fixed first metatarsal at the MTP joint. (action 1)

Reverse Mover Action Note

• Reverse actions usually occur when the distal attachment is fixed and the proximal attachment moves instead. The reverse action of the flexor hallucis brevis is flexion of the metatarsal of the big toe relative to a fixed proximal phalanx at the MTP joint. This reverse action is not likely to occur. (reverse action 1)

Eccentric Antagonist Function

1. Restrains/slows extension of the MTP joint of the big toe

Isometric Stabilization Function

1. Stabilizes the MTP joint of the big toe

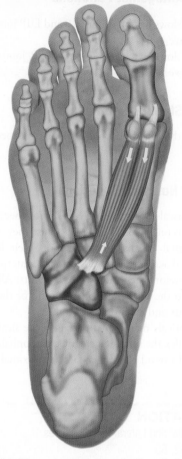

Figure 18-12 Plantar view of the right flexor hallucis brevis.

Additional Note on Functions

1. The flexor hallucis brevis splits distally to attach onto the medial and lateral sides of the proximal phalanx of the big toe. The medial head of the flexor hallucis brevis crosses the MTP joint medially to attach onto the proximal phalanx of the big toe, so it can pull the big toe medially away from the second toe (abduction). The lateral head of the flexor hallucis brevis crosses the MTP joint laterally to attach onto the proximal phalanx of the big toe, so it can pull the big toe laterally toward the second toe (adduction). Because the second toe is the axis for abduction/adduction of the toes, the flexor hallucis brevis can both abduct and adduct the big toe at the MTP joint.

INNERVATION
☐ The Medial Plantar Nerve
 ☐ S1, S2

ARTERIAL SUPPLY
☐ The Medial Plantar Artery (a branch of the Posterior Tibial Artery)

18

Flexor Hallucis Brevis—*cont'd*

 PALPATION

1. With the client prone or supine, place palpating hand distally on the medial side of the plantar surface of the foot and feel for the flexor hallucis brevis.
2. To further bring out the flexor hallucis brevis, resist the client from actively flexing the big toe at the metatarsophalangeal joint.
3. Continue palpating proximally and distally toward its attachments.

■ RELATIONSHIP TO OTHER STRUCTURES

☐ The flexor hallucis brevis is located in the third plantar layer of intrinsic muscles of the foot along with the flexor digiti minimi pedis and the adductor hallucis.

☐ The flexor hallucis brevis is medial to the oblique head of the adductor hallucis and lateral to the abductor hallucis.

☐ Even though the flexor hallucis brevis is in the third plantar layer, it is relatively superficial, because there is no belly of any other muscle directly superficial to it. Only the tendon of the flexor hallucis longus and the plantar fascia are superficial to it.

☐ Deep to the flexor hallucis brevis is the first metatarsal and the first dorsal interosseus pedis muscle.

☐ The flexor hallucis brevis is located within the superficial back line myofascial meridian.

■ MISCELLANEOUS

1. Distally, there is a sesamoid bone in each of the medial and lateral tendons of the flexor hallucis brevis.

18

Flexor Digiti Minimi Pedis

The name, flexor digiti minimi pedis, *tells us that this muscle flexes the little toe.*

Derivation	☐ flexor: L. *a muscle that flexes a body part.*
	digiti: L. *refers to a digit* (toe).
	minimi: L. *least.*
	pedis: L. *refers to the foot.*
Pronunciation	☐ FLEKS-or, DIJ-i-tee, MIN-i-mee, PEED-us

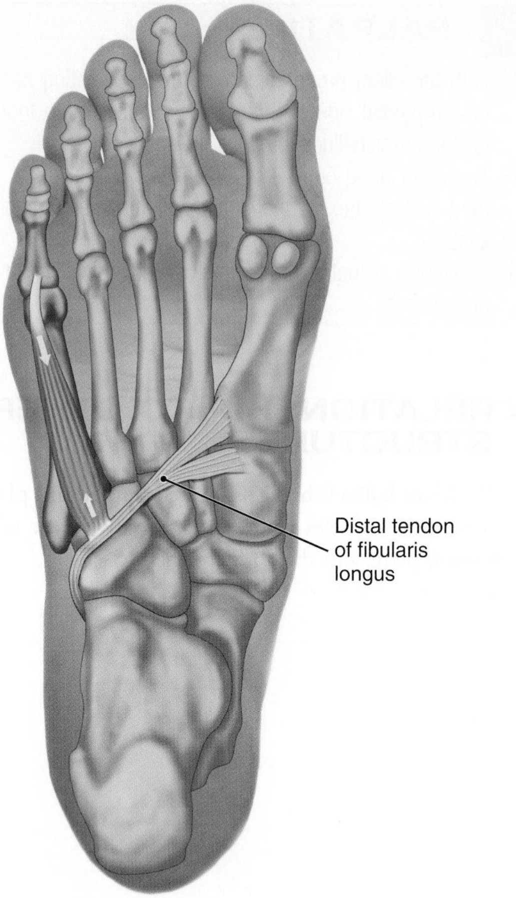

■ ATTACHMENTS

☐ **Fifth Metatarsal**
  ☐ the plantar surface of the base of the fifth metatarsal and the distal tendon of the fibularis longus

  to the

☐ **Little Toe (Toe Five)**
  ☐ the plantar surface of the proximal phalanx

■ FUNCTIONS

CONCENTRIC (SHORTENING) MOVER ACTIONS	
Standard Mover Actions	**Reverse Mover Actions**
☐ **1. Flexes the little toe at the MTP joint**	☐ 1. Flexes the metatarsal of the little toe at the MTP joint

MTP joint = metatarsophalangeal joint

Standard Mover Action Notes

- The flexor digiti minimi pedis crosses the MTP joint of the little toe (toe number five) on the plantar side (with its fibers running horizontally in the sagittal plane) to attach onto the proximal phalanx of the little toe. Therefore it flexes the little toe at the MTP joint. (action 1)
- More specifically, flexing the little toe at the MTP joint refers to flexing the proximal phalanx of the little toe relative to a fixed fifth metatarsal at the MTP joint. (action 1)

Reverse Mover Action Note

- The reverse action involves motion of the fifth metatarsal relative to the proximal phalanx of the little toe at the MTP joint, and would occur if the proximal phalanx is fixed and the fifth metatarsal is mobile. This reverse action is not very likely to occur.

Distal tendon of fibularis longus

Figure 18-13 Plantar view of the right flexor digiti minimi pedis.

Eccentric Antagonist Function

1. Restrains/slows extension of the MTP joint of the little toe

Isometric Stabilization Function

1. Stabilizes the MTP joint of the little toe

INNERVATION
☐ The Lateral Plantar Nerve
  ☐ S2, S3

ARTERIAL SUPPLY
☐ The Lateral Plantar Artery (a branch of the Posterior Tibial Artery)

18

Flexor Digiti Minimi Pedis—*cont'd*

 PALPATION

1. With the client prone or supine, place palpating hand distally on the lateral side of the plantar surface of the foot (just medial to the abductor digiti minimi pedis) and feel for the flexor digiti minimi pedis.
2. To further bring out the flexor digiti minimi pedis, resist the client from actively flexing the little toe at the metatarsophalangeal joint.
3. Continue palpating proximally and distally toward its attachments.

■ RELATIONSHIP TO OTHER STRUCTURES

☐ The flexor digiti minimi pedis is in the third plantar layer of intrinsic muscles of the foot along with the flexor hallucis brevis and the adductor hallucis.

☐ The flexor digiti minimi pedis lies directly medial to the abductor digiti minimi pedis and lateral to the fourth lumbrical pedis muscle.

☐ Even though the flexor digiti minimi pedis is in the third plantar layer, it is relatively superficial, because there is no belly of any other muscle directly superficial to it. It is deep only to the plantar fascia.

☐ Deep to the flexor digiti minimi pedis is the fifth metatarsal (and a small portion of the third plantar interosseus and the fourth dorsal interosseus pedis).

☐ The flexor digiti minimi pedis is located within the superficial back line myofascial meridian.

■ MISCELLANEOUS

1. The flexor digiti minimi pedis is also known as the *flexor digiti minimi.* However, this allows for confusion with the flexor digiti minimi manus of the hand, which flexes the little finger.
2. The flexor digiti minimi pedis is also known as the *flexor digiti minimi brevis,* although the addition of the word *brevis* at the end does not make sense in this case. Usually, the word *brevis* at the end of a muscle's name is added to distinguish the muscle from a longer muscle that does the same action. In this case, there is no flexor digiti minimi longus.
3. The flexor digiti minimi pedis occasionally has attachments that range from the tarsals proximally, onto the fifth metatarsal distally. When this occurs, this muscle has the ability to oppose the little toe toward the other toes; therefore it is named the *opponens digiti minimi pedis* (see Figure 18-4). This muscle is commonly found in apes, who have feet that are more *handy* than ours!

18

The name, adductor hallucis, *tells us that this muscle adducts the big toe.*

Derivation	☐ adductor: L. *a muscle that adducts a body part.*
	hallucis: L. *refers to the big toe.*
Pronunciation	☐ ad-DUK-tor, hal-OO-sis

■ ATTACHMENTS

☐ **Metatarsals**
  ☐ OBLIQUE HEAD: from the base of metatarsals two through four and the distal tendon of the fibularis longus
  ☐ TRANSVERSE HEAD: arises from the plantar metatarsophalangeal ligaments

to the

☐ **Big Toe (Toe One)**
  ☐ the lateral side of the base of the proximal phalanx

■ FUNCTIONS

CONCENTRIC (SHORTENING) MOVER ACTIONS	
Standard Mover Actions	**Reverse Mover Actions**
☐ **1. Adducts the big toe at the MTP joint**	☐ 1. Adducts the metatarsal of the big toe at the MTP joint
☐ 2. Flexes the big toe at the MTP joint	☐ 2. Flexes the metatarsal of the big toe at the MTP joint
MTP joint = metatarsophalangeal joint	

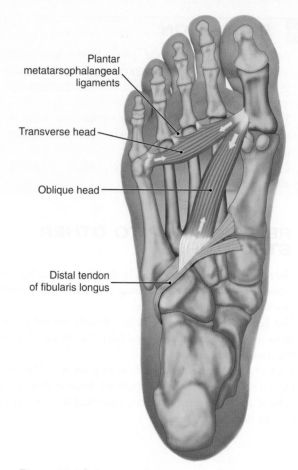

Figure 18-14 Plantar view of the right adductor hallucis.

Standard Mover Action Notes

• The adductor hallucis crosses the MTP joint to attach onto the proximal phalanx of the big toe on the lateral side (with its fibers running horizontally in the frontal plane). Therefore when the adductor hallucis contracts, it pulls the big toe laterally toward the second toe (which is the axis of abduction/adduction of the toes). Therefore the adductor hallucis adducts the big toe at the MTP joint. (action 1)

• The adductor hallucis crosses the MTP joint to attach onto the proximal phalanx of the big toe on the plantar side (with its fibers running horizontally in the sagittal plane). Therefore when the adductor hallucis pulls on the big toe, it flexes the big toe at the MTP joint. (action 2)

• More specifically, adduction and flexion of the big toe at the MTP joint refer to adduction and flexion of the proximal phalanx of the big toe relative to the first metatarsal at the MTP joint. (actions 1, 2)

Reverse Mover Action Note

• The reverse actions involve motion (adduction and flexion) of the metatarsal of the big toe relative to a fixed proximal phalanx at the MTP joint. These reverse actions are not likely to occur. (reverse actions 1, 2)

Eccentric Antagonist Functions

1. Restrains/slows abduction and extension of the MTP joint of the big toe

Isometric Stabilization Function

1. Stabilizes the MTP joint of the big toe

Isometric Stabilization Function Note

• The adductor hallucis (especially the transverse head) also stabilizes the transverse arch of the foot.

18

Adductor Hallucis—*cont'd*

INNERVATION

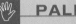

- ☐ The Lateral Plantar Nerve
  - ☐ S2, S3

ARTERIAL SUPPLY

- ☐ Branches of the Plantar Arch (an anastomosis between the Lateral Plantar Artery and the Dorsalis Pedis Artery)

🖐 PALPATION

1. With the client prone or supine, place palpating hand on the plantar surface of the foot over the second, third, and fourth metatarsals.
2. Have the client adduct the big toe and feel for the contraction of the adductor hallucis. Resistance can be added.

■ RELATIONSHIP TO OTHER STRUCTURES

- ☐ The adductor hallucis is located in the third plantar layer of intrinsic muscles of the foot along with the flexor hallucis brevis and the flexor digiti minimi pedis.
- ☐ The oblique head of the adductor hallucis is directly lateral to the flexor hallucis brevis.

- ☐ The oblique head of the adductor hallucis is deep to the lumbricals pedis and the quadratus plantae.
- ☐ The transverse head of the adductor hallucis is deep to the flexors digitorum longus and brevis tendons.
- ☐ Deep to the adductor hallucis are the interossei muscles and the metatarsals.
- ☐ The adductor hallucis is located within the superficial back line myofascial meridian.

■ MISCELLANEOUS

1. The adductor hallucis has two distinct heads: distally, there is the *transverse head*, with fibers that run transversely across the foot, and proximally, there is the *oblique head*, with fibers that run obliquely across the foot.
2. There is an adductor pollicis of the hand that also has two heads: an oblique head and a transverse head.
3. The adductor hallucis occasionally has attachments that attach distally onto the first metatarsal. When this occurs, this muscle has the ability to oppose the big toe toward the other toes and is named the *opponens hallucis* of the foot. This arrangement is common in apes, who have feet that are more *handy* than ours!
4. The oblique head of the adductor hallucis often blends with the flexor hallucis brevis.

18

PLANTAR SURFACE: LAYER IV

Plantar Interossei

(There are three plantar interossei, named one, two, and three.)

The name, plantar interossei, *tells us that these muscles are located between bones (metatarsals) on the plantar side.*

Derivation	☐ plantar: L. *refers to the plantar side of the foot.*
	interossei: L. *between bones.*
Pronunciation	☐ PLAN-tar, in-ter-OSS-ee-eye

■ ATTACHMENTS

☐ **Metatarsals**
  ☐ the medial side (*second-toe side*) of metatarsals three through five:
    ☐ ONE: attaches onto metatarsal three
    ☐ TWO: attaches onto metatarsal four
    ☐ THREE: attaches onto metatarsal five

to the

☐ ***Second-Toe Sides* of the Proximal Phalanges of Toes Three through Five, and the Dorsal Distal Expansion**
  ☐ the bases of the proximal phalanges,
    ☐ ONE: attaches to toe three
    ☐ TWO: attaches to toe four
    ☐ THREE: attaches to toe five

■ FUNCTIONS

CONCENTRIC (SHORTENING) MOVER ACTIONS	
Standard Mover Actions	**Reverse Mover Actions**
☐**1. Adduct toes three through five at the MTP joints**	☐ 1. Adduct the metatarsals of toes three through five at the MTP joints
☐ 2. Flex toes three through five at the MTP joints	☐ 2. Flex the metatarsals at the MTP joints
☐ 3. Extend toes three through five at the PIP and DIP joints	☐ 3. Extend the more proximal phalanges at the PIP and DIP joints

MTP joints = metatarsophalangeal joints; PIP joints = proximal interphalangeal joints; DIP joints = distal interphalangeal joints

Standard Mover Action Notes

• The plantar interossei cross the MTP joint of toes three through five medially (with their fibers running horizontally) and pull toes three through five medially toward the second toe (which is the axis for abduction/adduction of the toes). Therefore the plantar interossei adduct toes three through five at the MTP joints. (action 1)

• The plantar interossei cross the MTP joint of toes three through five on the plantar side (with their fibers running horizontally in the sagittal plane); therefore they flex toes three through five at the MTP joints. (action 2)

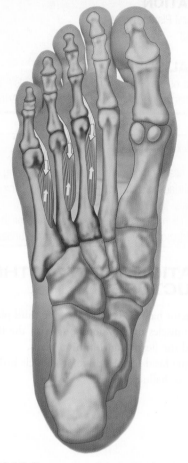

Figure 18-15 Plantar view of the right plantar interossei.

• More specifically, adducting and flexing toes at the MTP joints refers to adducting and flexing the proximal phalanges of the toes at the MTP joints. (actions 1, 2)

• The plantar interossei, by attaching into the dorsal digital expansion, in other words the tendons of the extensor digitorum longus muscle (after the MTP joint but before the interphalangeal [IP] joints of the toes), exert their pull at the attachments of the extensor digitorum longus, the distal phalanx of toes three through five. The plantar interossei, in effect, cross the PIP and DIP joints on the dorsal side (with their fibers running horizontally in the sagittal plane); therefore the plantar interossei extend both the PIP and DIP joints of toes three through five. (action 3)

• More specifically, extending toes at the IP joints refers to extending the middle phalanges of the toes at the PIP joints and extending the distal phalanges at the DIP joints. (action 3)

Plantar Interossei—*cont'd*

Reverse Mover Action Note

- The reverse actions involve motion of the more proximal bone at each of the joints of the toes. In other words, the reverse action at the MTP joint is adduction or flexion of the metatarsal of the toe relative to a fixed proximal phalanx, the reverse action at the PIP joint is extension of the proximal phalanx relative to a fixed middle phalanx, and the reverse action at the DIP joint is extension of the middle phalanx relative to the fixed distal phalanx. The reverse action at the MTP joint is not likely to occur. However, the reverse actions at the PIP and DIP joints occur during toe-off in the gait cycle. (reverse actions 1, 2, 3)

Eccentric Antagonist Functions

1. Restrains/slows abduction of the MTP joints of toes three through five
2. Restrains/slows extension of the MTP joints of toes three through five
3. Restrains/slows flexion of the IP joints of toes three through five

Isometric Stabilization Functions

1. Stabilizes of toes two through five of the MTP, PIP, and DIP joints

Additional Notes on Functions

1. The lumbricals pedis flex the MTP joints because they cross these joints on the plantar side. Because they attach into the dorsal digital expansion of the foot, their line of pull is transmitted across the dorsal side of the interphalangeal (IP) joints; therefore they extend the IP joints. All muscles that attach into the dorsal digital expansion of the foot flex the MTP joints and extend the IP joints.
2. The plantar interossei have the same actions as the lumbricals pedis of the foot, namely flexion of the MTP joints and extension of the IP joints. And the plantar interossei adduct toes three through five at the MTP joints.
3. There are also palmar interossei manus of the hand that have essentially identical actions (adduction and flexion of the fingers at the metacarpophalangeal [MCP] joints, and extension of the fingers at the PIP and DIP joints) to the plantar interossei of the foot.
4. A mnemonic for remembering the adduction and abduction actions of the plantar interossei and dorsal interossei pedis is *DAB PAD: **D**orsals **AB**duct, **P**lantars **AD**duct.*

INNERVATION
- [ ] The Lateral Plantar Nerve
  - [ ] S2, S3

ARTERIAL SUPPLY
- [ ] Branches of the Plantar Arch (an anastomosis between the Lateral Plantar Artery and the Dorsalis Pedis Artery)

PALPATION

- [ ] Given the thickness of the plantar fascia and the depth of the plantar interossei, it is difficult to distinguish them from other deep muscles of the foot on the plantar side. If attempted, resist the client from adducting toes three through five and feel for the contraction of the plantar interossei between the metatarsals on the plantar side of the foot.

■ RELATIONSHIP TO OTHER STRUCTURES

- [ ] The plantar interossei are in the fourth plantar layer of intrinsic muscles of the foot along with the dorsal interossei pedis (and the distal tendons of the fibularis longus and tibialis posterior).
- [ ] From the plantar perspective, the plantar interossei are deep to the lumbricals pedis.
- [ ] From the plantar perspective, the plantar interossei are somewhat superficial to (partially overlap) the metatarsals and the dorsal interossei pedis.
- [ ] The plantar interossei are involved with the superficial back line and deep front line myofascial meridians.

■ MISCELLANEOUS

1. There are three separate plantar interossei muscles. They are named, from the medial side, *one, two,* and *three.*
2. The first plantar interosseus attaches to the third digit of the foot and moves the third toe. Similarly, the second plantar interosseus attaches onto and moves the fourth toe, and the third plantar interosseus attaches onto and moves the fifth toe.
3. Knowing the number of plantar interossei muscles and knowing which toes have plantar interossei attached to them can be reasoned out; it does not need to be memorized. The big toe (toe number one) gets its own adductor (the adductor hallucis), and toe number two cannot adduct (its movement is described as being either tibial abduction or fibular abduction). That leaves three toes that can adduct: toes three, four, and five. The result is that there are three plantar interossei muscles attached to toes three, four, and five.

18

Dorsal Interossei Pedis

(There are four dorsal interossei pedis muscles, named one, two, three, and four.)

The name, dorsal interossei pedis, *tells us that these muscles are located between bones (metatarsals) on the dorsal side and located in the foot.*

Derivation	☐ dorsal: L. *refers to the dorsal side.*
	interossei: L. *between bones.*
	pedis: L. *refers to the foot.*
Pronunciation	☐ DOR-sul, in-ter-OSS-ee-eye, PEED-us

■ ATTACHMENTS

☐ **Metatarsals**
  ☐ each one arises from the adjacent sides of two metatarsals:
    ☐ ONE: attaches onto metatarsals one and two
    ☐ TWO: attaches onto metatarsals two and three
    ☐ THREE: attaches onto metatarsals three and four
    ☐ FOUR: attaches onto metatarsals four and five

  to the

☐ **Sides of the Phalanges and the Dorsal Digital Expansion**
  ☐ the bases of the proximal phalanges (on the sides away from the center of the second toe)
    ☐ ONE: attaches to the medial side of toe number two
    ☐ TWO: attaches to the lateral side of toe number two
    ☐ THREE: attaches to the lateral side of toe number three
    ☐ FOUR: attaches to the lateral side of toe number four

■ FUNCTIONS

CONCENTRIC (SHORTENING) MOVER ACTIONS	
Standard Mover Actions	**Reverse Mover Actions**
☐ **1. Abduct toes two through four at the MTP joints**	☐ 1. Abduct the metatarsals of toes two through four at the MTP joints
☐ 2. Flex toes two through four at the MTP joints	☐ 2. Flex the metatarsals at the MTP joints
☐ 3. Extend toes two through four at the PIP and DIP joints	☐ 3. Extend the more proximal phalanges at the PIP and DIP joints

MTP joints = metatarsophalangeal joints; IP joints = interphalangeal joints; PIP joints = proximal interphalangeal joints; DIP joints = distal interphalangeal joints

Standard Mover Action Notes

• All the dorsal interossei pedis cross the MTP joint to attach onto the proximal phalanx of toes two through four (with their fibers running horizontally). The first dorsal interosseus

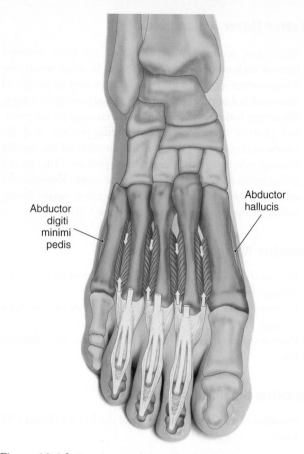

Figure 18-16 Dorsal view of the right dorsal interossei pedis. The abductor hallucis and abductor digiti minimi pedis have been ghosted in.

Abductor digiti minimi pedis

Abductor hallucis

pedis attaches onto the medial side of the second toe. When it contracts, it pulls the second toe medially away from the axis of abduction/adduction of the toes (which is an imaginary line drawn through the second toe when it is in anatomic position). Therefore the first dorsal interosseus pedis performs *tibial abduction* of the second toe at the MTP joint. The second dorsal interosseus pedis attaches onto the lateral side of the second toe. When it contracts, it pulls the second toe laterally away from the axis of abduction/adduction of the toes. Therefore the second dorsal interosseus pedis performs *fibular abduction* of the second toe at the MTP joint. The third and fourth dorsal interossei pedis attach onto the lateral sides of the third and fourth toes, respectively. When they contract, they pull the third and fourth toes laterally away from the second toe. Therefore the third and fourth dorsal interossei pedis abduct the third and fourth toes at the MTP joints. (action 1)

• The dorsal interossei pedis cross the MTP joints of toes two through four on the plantar side (with their fibers running horizontally in the sagittal plane); therefore they flex toes two through four at the MTP joints. (action 2)

18

Dorsal Interossei Pedis—*cont'd*

- More specifically, abduction and flexion of toes at the MTP joints refers to abduction and flexion of the proximal phalanges of the toes at the MTP joints. (actions 1, 2)
- The dorsal interossei pedis, by attaching into the dorsal digital expansion, in other words, tendons of the extensor digitorum longus muscle (after the MTP joint but before the interphalangeal [IP] joints of the toes), exert their pull at the attachment of the extensor digitorum longus (at the distal phalanx of toes two through four). The dorsal interossei pedis, in effect, cross the proximal and distal IP joints on the dorsal side (essentially exerting their pull horizontally in the sagittal plane); therefore the dorsal interossei pedis extend both the PIP and DIP joints of toes two through four. (action 3)
- More specifically, extending toes at the IP joints refers to extending the middle phalanges of the toes at the PIP joints and extending the distal phalanges at the DIP joints. (action 3)

Reverse Mover Action Note

- The reverse actions involve motion of the more proximal bone at each of the joints of the toes. In other words, the reverse action at the MTP joint is abduction or flexion of the metatarsal of the toe relative to a fixed proximal phalanx, the reverse action at the PIP joint is extension of the proximal phalanx relative to a fixed middle phalanx, and the reverse action at the DIP joint is extension of the middle phalanx relative to the fixed distal phalanx. The reverse action at the MTP joint is not likely to occur. However, the reverse actions at the PIP and DIP joints occur during toe-off in the gait cycle. (reverse actions 1, 2, 3)

Eccentric Antagonist Functions

1. Restrains/slows adduction of the MTP joints of toes two through four
2. Restrains/slows extension of the MTP joints of toes two through four
3. Restrains/slows flexion of the PIP and DIP joints of toes two through four

Isometric Stabilization Functions

1. Stabilizes the MTP, PIP, and DIP joints of toes two through four

Additional Notes on Functions

1. The dorsal interossei pedis flex the MTP joints because they cross these joints on the plantar side. Because they attach into the dorsal digital expansion of the foot, their line of pull is transmitted across the dorsal side of the IP joints; therefore they extend the IP joints. All muscles that attach into the dorsal digital expansion of the foot flex the MTP joints and extend the IP joints.
2. The dorsal interossei pedis have the same actions as the lumbricals pedis, namely flexion of the MTP joints and extension of the IP joints. And the dorsal interossei pedis abduct toes two through four at the MTP joints.
3. There are four dorsal interossei manus of the hand, which have essentially identical actions (abduction and flexion of the fingers at the metacarpophalangeal [MCP] joints, and extension of the fingers at the PIP and DIP joints) to the dorsal interossei pedis of the foot.
4. A mnemonic for remembering the adduction and abduction actions of the plantar interossei and dorsal interossei pedis is ***DAB PAD: D****orsals **AB**duct, **P**lantars **AD**duct.*

INNERVATION
- ☐ The Lateral Plantar Nerve
  - ☐ S2, S3

ARTERIAL SUPPLY
- ☐ Branches of the Plantar Arch (an anastomosis between the Lateral Plantar Artery and the Dorsalis Pedis Artery)

✋ PALPATION

1. With the client supine, place palpating fingers on the dorsal side of the foot between the first and second metatarsal bones.
2. Have the client abduct the second toe toward the big toe (tibial abduction) and feel for the contraction of the first dorsal interosseus pedis. Resistance can be added.
3. Repeat between the second and third metatarsal bones with fibular abduction of the second toe and feel for the contraction of the second dorsal interosseus pedis.
4. Repeat between metatarsals three-four and four-five with abduction of the third and fourth toes and feel for the contraction of the third and fourth dorsal interossei pedis, respectively.

■ RELATIONSHIP TO OTHER STRUCTURES

- ☐ The dorsal interossei pedis are in the fourth plantar layer of intrinsic muscles of the foot along with the plantar interossei (and the distal tendons of the fibularis longus and tibialis posterior).
- ☐ The dorsal interossei pedis are located between the metatarsals; hence they are bordered on either side by the metatarsal bones.
- ☐ From the dorsal perspective, the dorsal interossei pedis are deep to the tendons of the extensor digitorum longus and extensor digitorum brevis.

18

☐ From the plantar perspective, the dorsal interossei pedis are adjacent and deep to (partially overlapped by) the plantar interossei.

☐ The dorsal interossei pedis are involved with the superficial back line and deep front line myofascial meridians.

■ MISCELLANEOUS

1. There are four dorsal interossei pedis muscles named, from the medial side, *one*, *two*, *three*, and *four*.
2. Knowing the number of dorsal interossei pedis muscles and knowing which toes have dorsal interossei pedis attached to

them can be reasoned out; this information does not have to be memorized. The big toe and the little toe each get their own abductor muscle (the big toe has the abductor hallucis and the little toe has the abductor digiti minimi pedis). That leaves toes two, three, and four to have dorsal interossei pedis muscles attached. However, toe number two can abduct in the tibial (medial) direction and in the fibular (lateral) direction; therefore it gets two dorsal interossei pedis muscles attached to it (one on each side). The result is that there are four dorsal interossei pedis muscles: one attaching to toe number four, one attaching to toe number three, and two attaching to toe number two.

CHAPTER

19

Functional Groups of Muscles

This chapter contains functional groups of muscles.

The first part of the chapter (Figures 19-1 through 19-35) illustrates functional mover groups. All muscles of a functional mover group share the same concentric standard and reverse mover actions. They also share the same eccentric restraining/slowing and isometric stabilization functions as well. This part is divided into three sections: upper extremity, axial body, and lower extremity.

The second part of this chapter (Figures 19-36 through 19-38) illustrates muscles of the pelvic floor. The pelvic floor is just that, a floor to the pelvis upon which the contents of the abdominopelvic cavity sit. Medial, superior, and inferior views of the muscles of the pelvic floor are shown.

The third part of the chapter (Figures 19-39 through 19-43) illustrates myofascial meridians. A myofascial meridian is a line of myofascial tissues, in other words muscles embedded within a continuous line of fascial webbing that can serve to transmit tension (pulling) forces across the body. These pulling forces are important for creating mover actions as well as restraining/slowing and stabilization functions during posture and movement. (For more on myofascial meridians, see Myers T: *Anatomy trains: Myofascial meridians for manual and movement therapists*, ed 2, Edinburgh, 2009, Churchill Livingstone.)

FUNCTIONAL MOVER GROUPS: UPPER EXTREMITY

Scapulocostal Joint Elevators

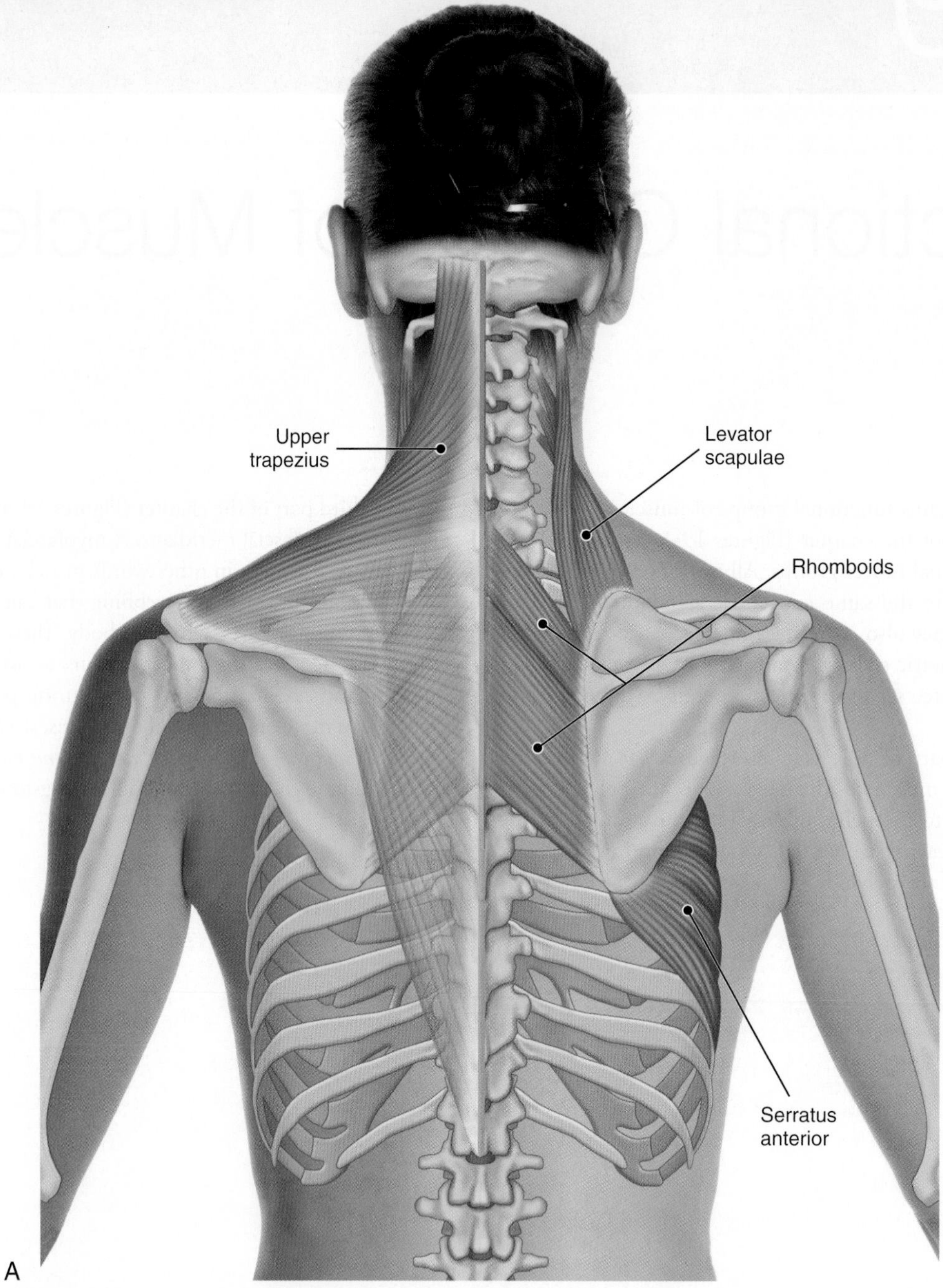

Figure 19-1 Scapulocostal joint elevators and depressors. **A,** Posterior view of the scapulocostal joint elevators. The middle and lower trapezius have been ghosted in on the left.

Scapulocostal Joint Elevators
Upper trapezius, levator scapulae, rhomboids, serratus anterior

Scapulocostal Joint Depressors

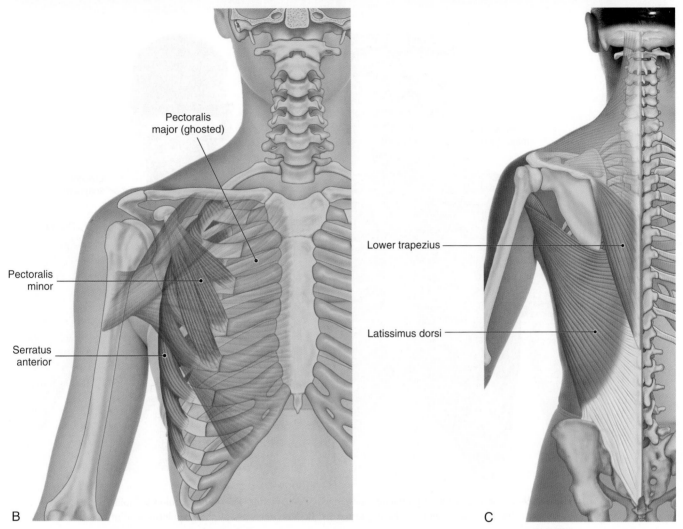

Figure 19-1, cont'd B, Anterior view of the scapulocostal joint depressors. **C,** Posterior view of the scapulocostal joint depressors. The upper and middle trapezius have been ghosted in on the left.

Scapulocostal Joint Depressors
Lower trapezius, pectoralis minor, pectoralis major, serratus anterior, latissimus dorsi

19

Scapulocostal Joint Protractors and Retractors

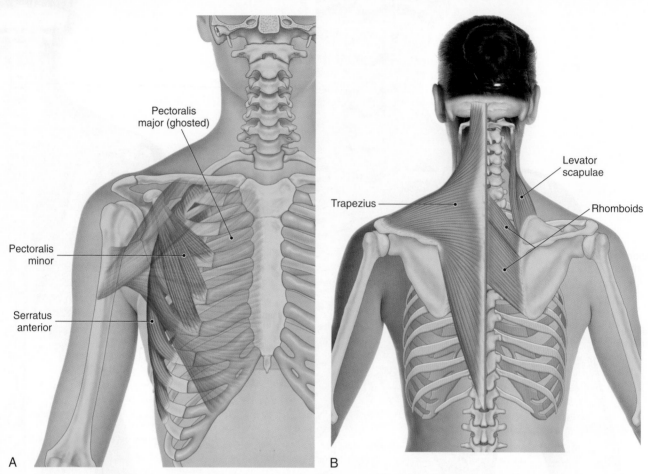

Figure 19-2 Scapulocostal joint protractors and retractors. **A,** Anterior view of the scapulocostal joint protractors. The pectoralis major has been ghosted in. **B,** Posterior view of the scapulocostal joint retractors.

Scapulocostal Joint Protractors
Serratus anterior, pectoralis minor, pectoralis major

Scapulocostal Joint Retractors
Rhomboids, trapezius, levator scapulae

19

Scapulocostal Joint Upward and Downward Rotators

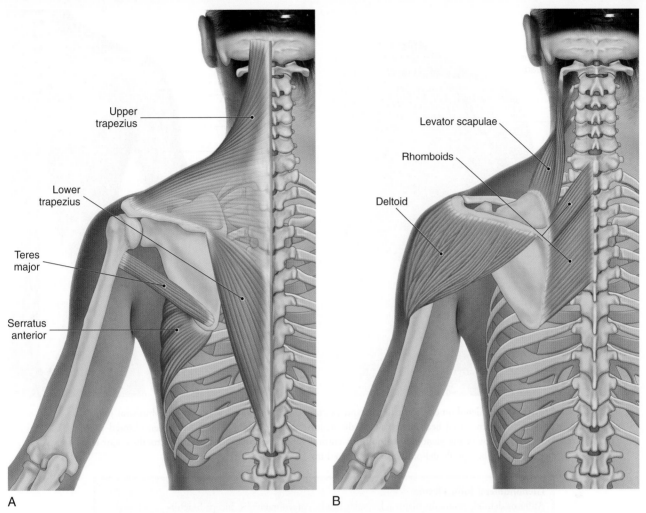

Figure 19-3 Scapulocostal joint upward rotators and downward rotators. **A,** Posterior view of the scapulocostal joint upward rotators. The middle trapezius has been ghosted in. **B,** Posterior view of the scapulocostal joint downward rotators. The pectoralis minor is not pictured.

Scapulocostal Joint Upward Rotators
Upper trapezius, lower trapezius, serratus anterior, teres major

Scapulocostal Joint Downward Rotators
Rhomboids, levator scapulae, deltoid, pectoralis minor (not seen)

19

Glenohumeral Joint Flexors and Extensors

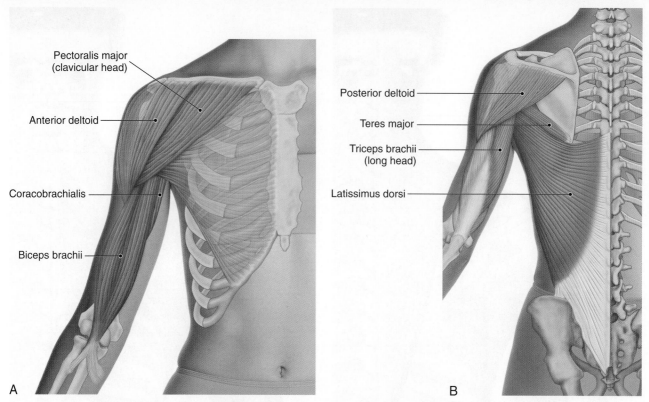

Pectoralis major (clavicular head)

Anterior deltoid

Coracobrachialis

Biceps brachii

A

Posterior deltoid

Teres major

Triceps brachii (long head)

Latissimus dorsi

B

Figure 19-4 Glenohumeral joint flexors and extensors. **A,** Anterior view of the glenohumeral joint flexors. The sternocostal head of the pectoralis major and the middle deltoid have been ghosted in. **B,** Posterior view of the glenohumeral joint extensors. The sternocostal head of the pectoralis major is not pictured. The middle deltoid has been ghosted in.

Glenohumeral Joint Flexors

Anterior deltoid, pectoralis major (clavicular head), coracobrachialis, biceps brachii

Glenohumeral Joint Extensors

Latissimus dorsi, teres major, posterior deltoid, pectoralis major (sternocostal head; not seen), triceps brachii (long head)

19

Glenohumeral Joint Abductors

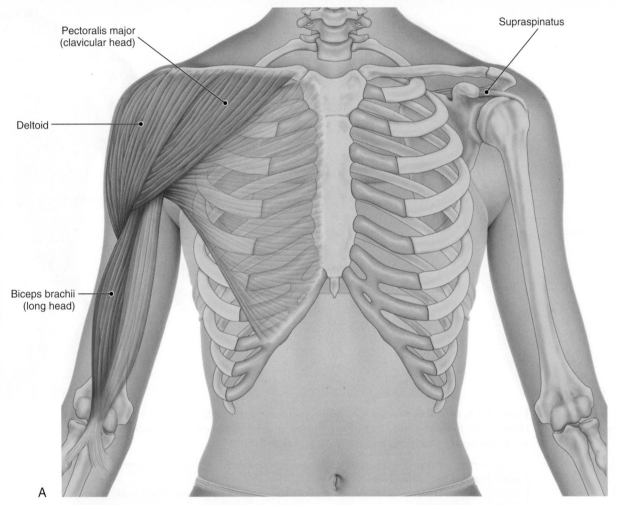

Pectoralis major
(clavicular head)

Supraspinatus

Deltoid

Biceps brachii
(long head)

A

Figure 19-5 Glenohumeral joint abductors and adductors. **A,** Anterior view of the glenohumeral joint abductors. The sternocostal head of the pectoralis major and the short head of the biceps brachii have been ghosted in.

Glenohumeral Joint Abductors
Deltoid, supraspinatus, biceps brachii (long head), pectoralis major (clavicular head)

19

Glenohumeral Joint Adductors

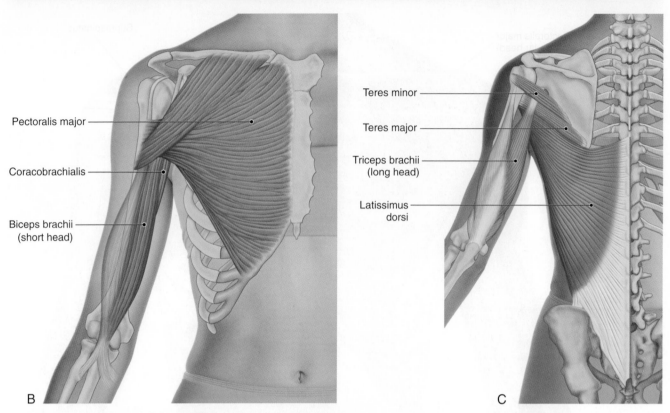

Pectoralis major

Coracobrachialis

Biceps brachii
(short head)

B

Teres minor

Teres major

Triceps brachii
(long head)

Latissimus
dorsi

C

Figure 19-5, cont'd B, Anterior view of the glenohumeral joint adductors. The long head of the biceps brachii has been ghosted in. **C,** Posterior view of the glenohumeral joint adductors. The lateral and medial heads of the triceps brachii have been ghosted in.

Glenohumeral Joint Adductors
Pectoralis major, latissimus dorsi, teres major, coracobrachialis, biceps brachii (short head), triceps brachii (long head), teres minor

Glenohumeral Joint Lateral and Medial Rotators

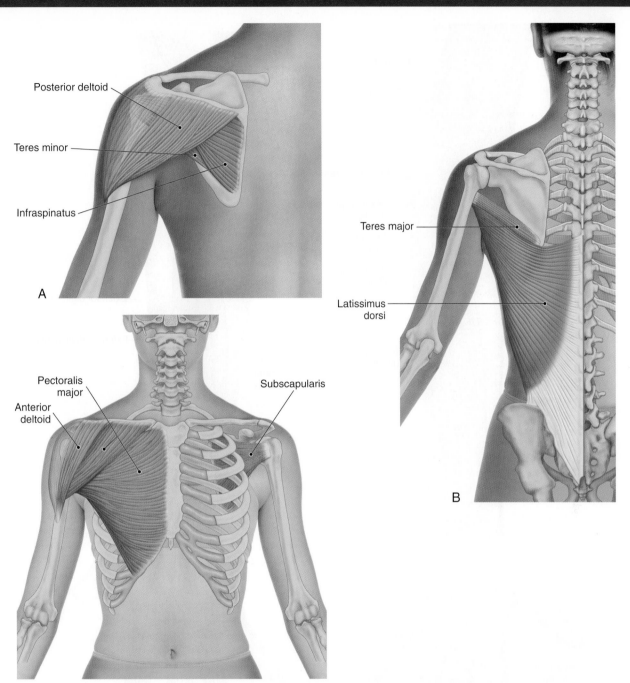

Posterior deltoid

Teres minor

Infraspinatus

A

Teres major

Latissimus dorsi

B

Pectoralis major

Anterior deltoid

Subscapularis

C

Figure 19-6 Glenohumeral joint lateral rotators and medial rotators. **A,** Posterior view of the glenohumeral joint lateral rotators. The middle deltoid has been ghosted in. **B,** Posterior view of the glenohumeral joint medial rotators. **C,** Anterior view of the glenohumeral joint medial rotators.

Glenohumeral Joint Lateral Rotators
Posterior deltoid, infraspinatus, teres minor

Glenohumeral Joint Medial Rotators
Pectoralis major, anterior deltoid, latissimus dorsi, teres major, subscapularis

19

Elbow Joint Flexors and Extensors

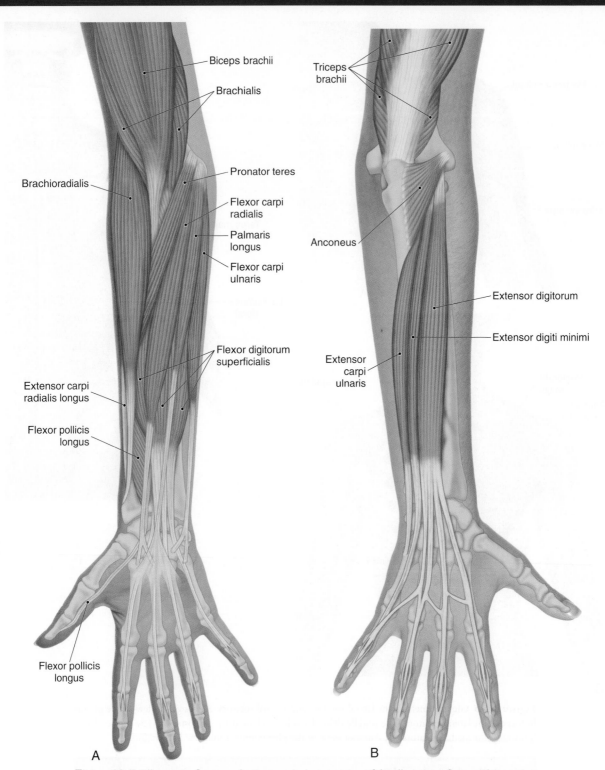

Figure 19-7 Elbow joint flexors and extensors. **A,** Anterior view of the elbow joint flexors. The extensor carpi radialis brevis is not pictured. **B,** Posterior view of the elbow joint extensors.

Elbow Joint Flexors

Brachialis, biceps brachii, brachioradialis, pronator teres, flexor carpi radialis, palmaris longus, flexor carpi ulnaris, flexor digitorum superficialis, flexor pollicis longus, extensor carpi radialis longus, extensor carpi radialis brevis (not seen)

Elbow Joint Extensors

Triceps brachii, anconeus, extensor digitorum, extensor digiti minimi, extensor carpi ulnaris

Radioulnar Joints Pronators and Supinators

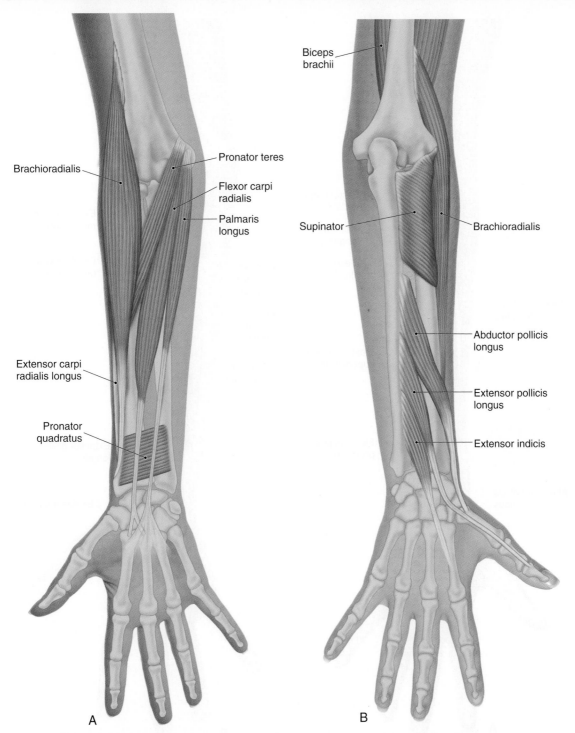

Figure 19-8 Radioulnar joints: pronators and supinators. **A,** Anterior view of the radioulnar joints pronators. The extensor carpi radialis brevis is not pictured. **B,** Posterior view of the radioulnar joints supinators. The extensors carpi radialis longus and brevis are not pictured.

Radioulnar Joints Pronation
Pronator teres, pronator quadratus, brachioradialis, flexor carpi radialis, palmaris longus, extensor carpi radialis longus, extensor carpi radialis brevis (not seen)

Radioulnar Joints Supination
Supinator, biceps brachii, brachioradialis, abductor pollicis longus, extensor pollicis longus, extensor indicis, extensor carpi radialis longus (not seen), extensor carpi radialis brevis (not seen)

Wrist Joint Flexors and Extensors

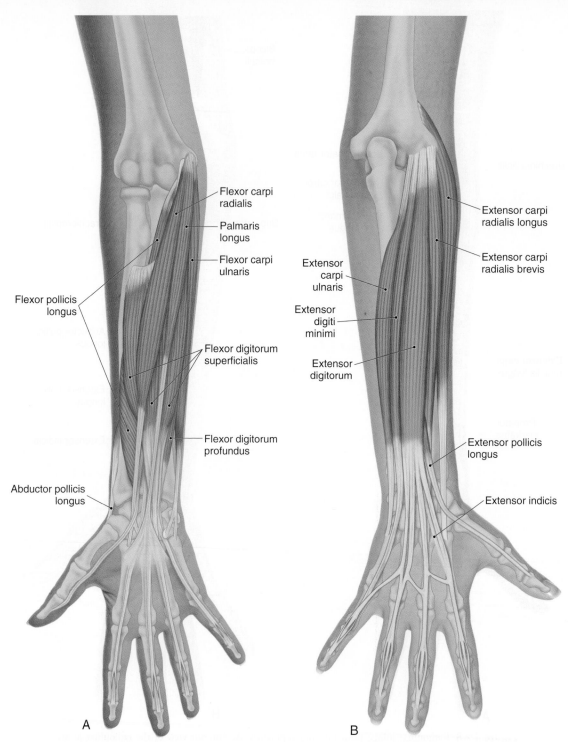

Flexor carpi radialis

Palmaris longus

Flexor carpi ulnaris

Flexor pollicis longus

Flexor digitorum superficialis

Flexor digitorum profundus

Abductor pollicis longus

Extensor carpi radialis longus

Extensor carpi radialis brevis

Extensor carpi ulnaris

Extensor digiti minimi

Extensor digitorum

Extensor pollicis longus

Extensor indicis

A

B

Figure 19-9 Wrist joint flexors and extensors. **A,** Anterior view of the wrist joint flexors. **B,** Posterior view of the wrist joint extensors.

Wrist Joint Flexors

Flexor carpi radialis, palmaris longus, flexor carpi ulnaris, flexor digitorum superficialis, flexor digitorum profundus, flexor pollicis longus, abductor pollicis longus

Wrist Joint Extensors

Extensor carpi radialis longus, extensor carpi radialis brevis, extensor digitorum, extensor digiti minimi, extensor carpi ulnaris, extensor pollicis longus, extensor indicis

Wrist Joint Radial Deviators

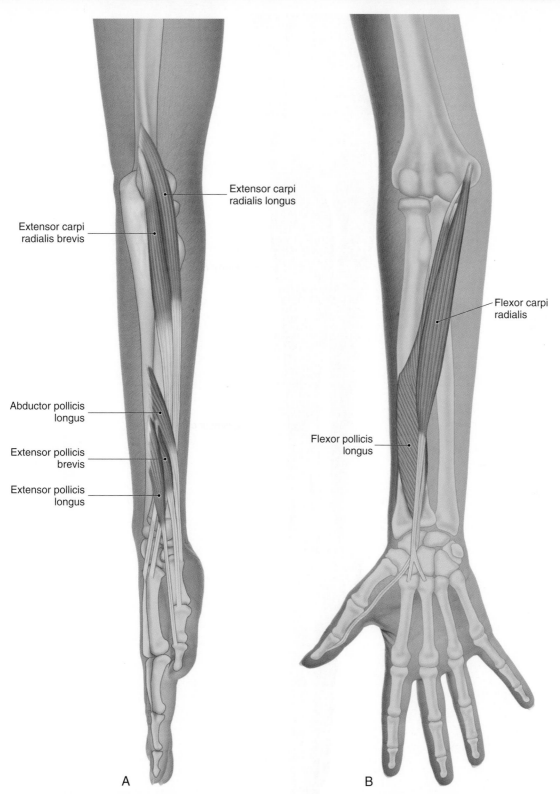

Figure 19-10 Wrist joint radial deviators and ulnar deviators. **A,** Radial (lateral) view of wrist joint radial deviators. **B,** Anterior view of wrist joint radial deviators.

Wrist Joint Radial Deviators
Flexor carpi radialis, extensor carpi radialis longus, extensor carpi radialis brevis, abductor pollicis longus, extensor pollicis brevis, extensor pollicis longus, flexor pollicis longus

Wrist Joint Ulnar Deviators

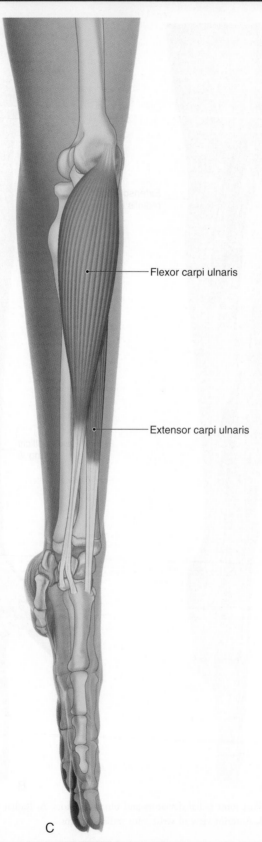

Flexor carpi ulnaris

Extensor carpi ulnaris

C

Figure 19-10, cont'd C, Ulnar (medial) view of wrist joint ulnar deviators.

Wrist Joint Ulnar Deviators
Flexor carpi ulnaris, extensor carpi ulnaris

Thumb Flexors and Extensors

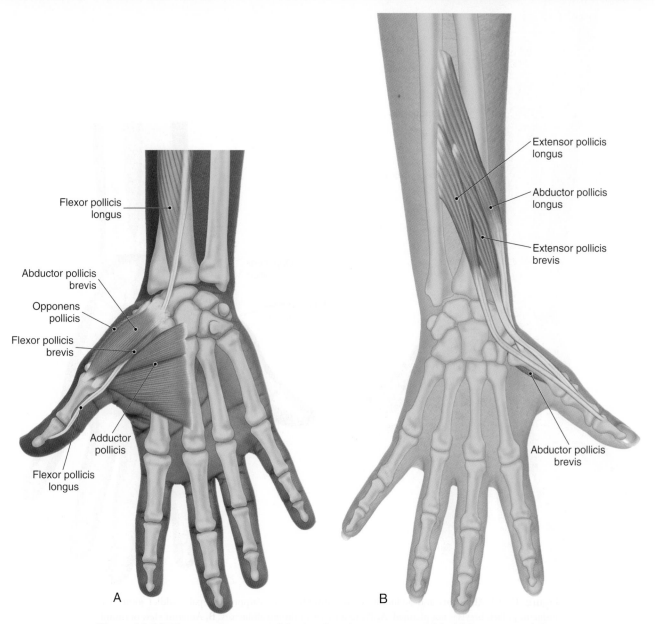

Figure 19-11 Flexors and extensors of the thumb at the carpometacarpal (saddle), metacarpophalangeal, and interphalangeal joints. **A,** Anterior view of thumb joint (CMC, MCP, IP) flexors. **B,** Posterior view of thumb joint (CMC, MCP, IP) extensors.

Thumb Joint (CMC, MCP, IP) Flexors
Flexor pollicis longus, flexor pollicis brevis, abductor pollicis brevis, opponens pollicis, adductor pollicis

Thumb Joint (CMC, MCP, IP) Extensors
Extensor pollicis longus, extensor pollicis brevis, abductor pollicis longus, abductor pollicis brevis

19

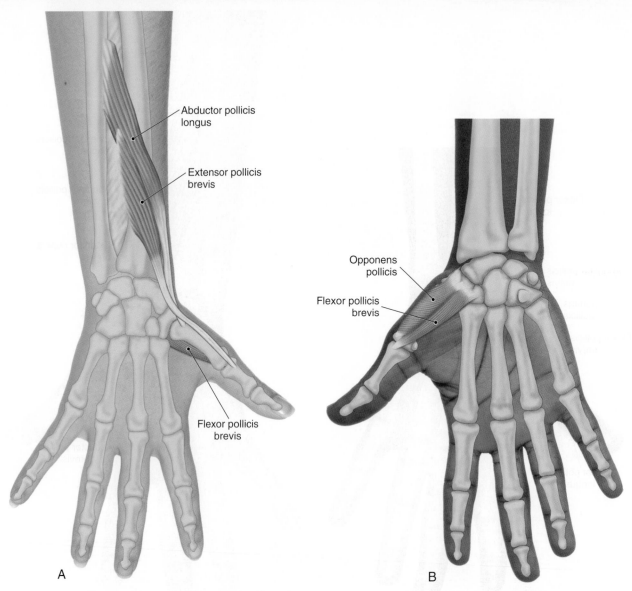

A

B

Figure 19-12 Abductors and adductors of the thumb at the carpometacarpal (saddle) joint. The abductor pollicis brevis is not pictured. **A,** Posterior view of thumb abductors. **B,** Anterior view of thumb abductors. Abductor pollicis brevis is not pictured.

Thumb Joint (CMC) Abductors
Abductor pollicis longus, abductor pollicis brevis (not seen), extensor pollicis brevis, flexor pollicis brevis, opponens pollicis

19

Thumb Adductors

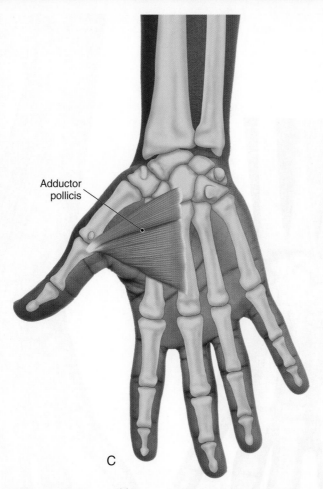

Adductor
pollicis

C

Figure 19-12, cont'd C, Anterior view of thumb adductor.

Thumb Joint (CMC) Adductors
Adductor pollicis

Thumb Medial and Lateral Rotators

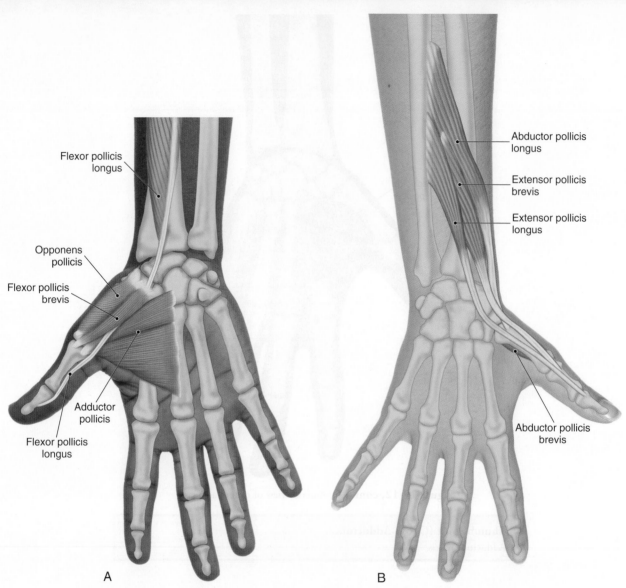

Figure 19-13 Medial rotators and lateral rotators of the thumb at the carpometacarpal (saddle) joint. **A,** Anterior view of the medial rotators. **B,** Posterior view of the lateral rotators.

Thumb Joint (CMC) Medial Rotators
Opponens pollicis, flexor pollicis brevis, flexor pollicis longus, adductor pollicis

Thumb Joint (CMC) Lateral Rotators
Extensor pollicis longus, extensor pollicis brevis, abductor pollicis longus, abductor pollicis brevis

Finger Flexors

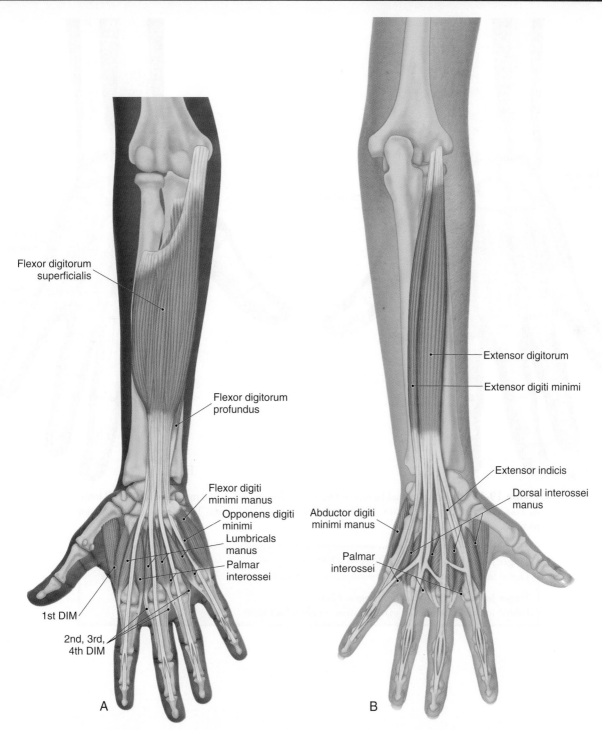

Figure 19-14 Flexors and extensors of fingers two through five at the metacarpophalangeal and proximal and distal interphalangeal joints. **A,** Anterior view of finger flexors. Dorsal interosseus/interossei manus, DIM. **B,** Posterior view of finger extensors. The lumbricals manus are not pictured.

Finger Joint (MCP, IP) Flexors (fingers #2-5)
Flexor digitorum superficialis, flexor digitorum profundus, flexor digiti minimi manus, opponens digiti minimi, palmar interossei, dorsal interossei manus, lumbricals manus

Finger Joint (MCP, IP) Extensors (fingers #2-5)
Extensor digitorum, extensor digiti minimi, extensor indicis, abductor digiti minimi manus, palmar interossei, dorsal interossei manus, lumbricals manus (not seen)

Finger Abductors and Adductors

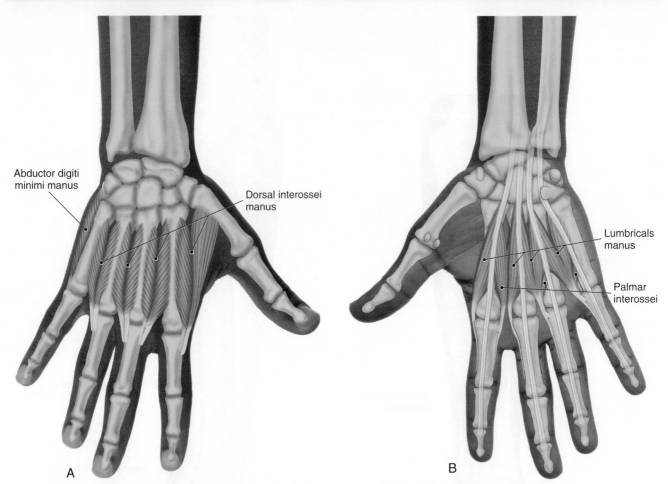

Abductor digiti
minimi manus

Dorsal interossei
manus

Lumbricals
manus

Palmar
interossei

A

B

Figure 19-15 Abductors and adductors of fingers two through five at the metacarpophalangeal joint. **A,** Posterior view of the abductors. **B,** Anterior view of the adductors. The extensor indicis is not pictured.

Finger Joint (MCP) Abductors (fingers #2-5)
Dorsal interossei manus, abductor digiti minimi manus

Finger Joint (MCP) Adductors (fingers #2-5)
Palmar interossei, lumbricals manus, extensor indicis (not seen)

19

FUNCTIONAL MOVER GROUPS: AXIAL BODY

Temporomandibular Joint (Mandible): Elevators and Depressors

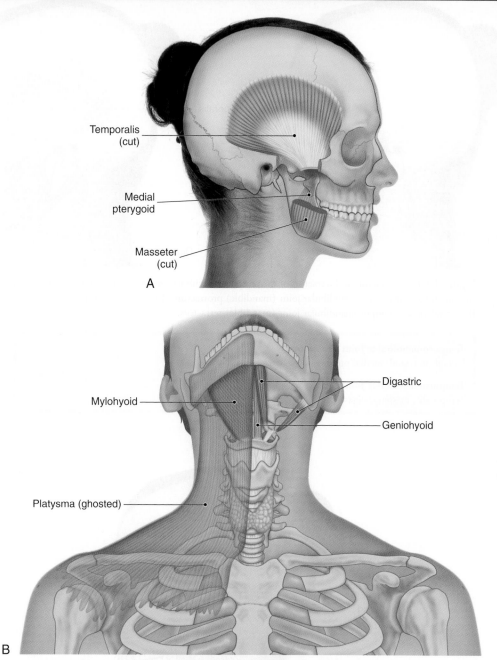

Figure 19-16 Elevators and depressors of the temporomandibular joints. **A,** Lateral view of temporomandibular joints (mandible) elevators. The zygomatic arch has been cut away. **B,** Anterior view of temporomandibular joints (mandible) depressors. The platysma has been ghosted in.

Temporomandibular Joint Elevators
Temporalis, masseter, medial pterygoid

Temporomandibular Joint Depressors
Digastric, mylohyoid, geniohyoid, platysma

19

Temporomandibular Joint (Mandible) Protractors, Retractors, and Contralateral Deviators

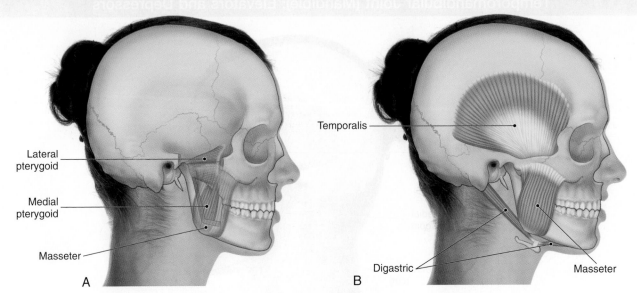

Figure 19-17 Protractors and retractors of the temporomandibular joints. The mandible has been cut. **A,** Lateral view of temporomandibular joint (mandible) protractors. The masseter has been ghosted in. **B,** Lateral view of temporomandibular joint (mandible) retractors.

Temporomandibular Joint Protractors
Lateral pterygoid, medial pterygoid, masseter

Temporomandibular Joint Retractors
Temporalis, masseter, digastric

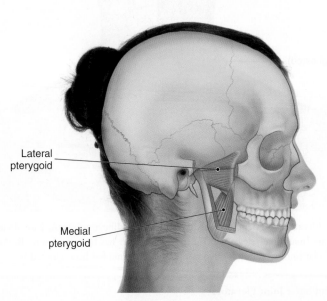

Figure 19-18 Lateral view of temporomandibular joint (mandible) contralateral deviators. The mandible has been cut.

Temporomandibular Joint Contralateral Deviators
Lateral pterygoid, medial pterygoid

Hyoid Bone Elevators and Depressors

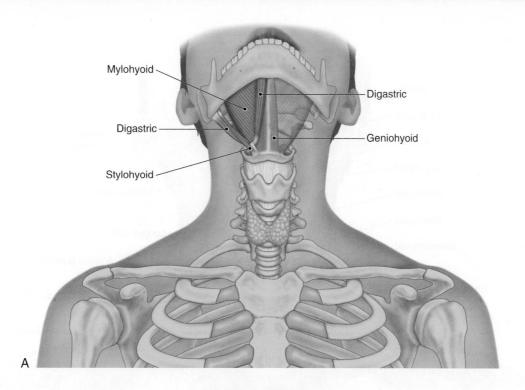

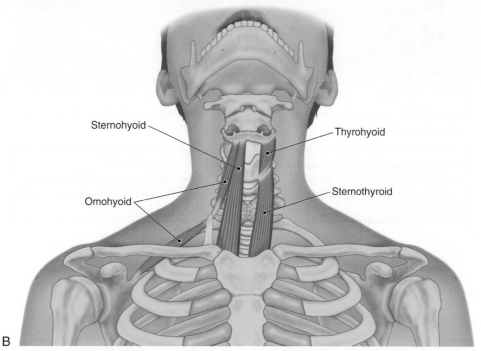

Figure 19-19 Elevators and depressors of the hyoid bone. **A,** Anterior view of hyoid bone elevators. The mylohyoid has been ghosted in on the left. **B,** Anterior view of hyoid bone depressors.

Hyoid Bone Elevators
Digastric, mylohyoid, geniohyoid, stylohyoid

Hyoid Bone Depressors
Sternohyoid, sternothyroid, thyrohyoid, omohyoid

19

Cervical Spinal Joint (Neck and Head) Flexors

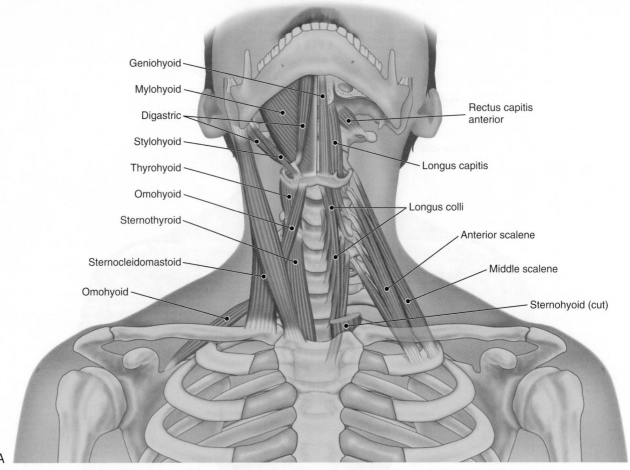

Geniohyoid

Mylohyoid

Digastric

Stylohyoid

Thyrohyoid

Omohyoid

Sternothyroid

Sternocleidomastoid

Omohyoid

Rectus capitis anterior

Longus capitis

Longus colli

Anterior scalene

Middle scalene

Sternohyoid (cut)

A

Figure 19-20 Flexors and extensors of the cervical spinal joints (neck and head). **A,** Anterior view of neck and head flexors.

Cervical Spinal (Head and Neck) Joint Flexors

Sternocleidomastoid, anterior scalene, middle scalene, longus colli, longus capitis, rectus capitis anterior, sternohyoid, sternothyroid, thyrohyoid, omohyoid, digastric, mylohyoid, geniohyoid, stylohyoid

19

Cervical Spinal Joint (Neck and Head) Extensors

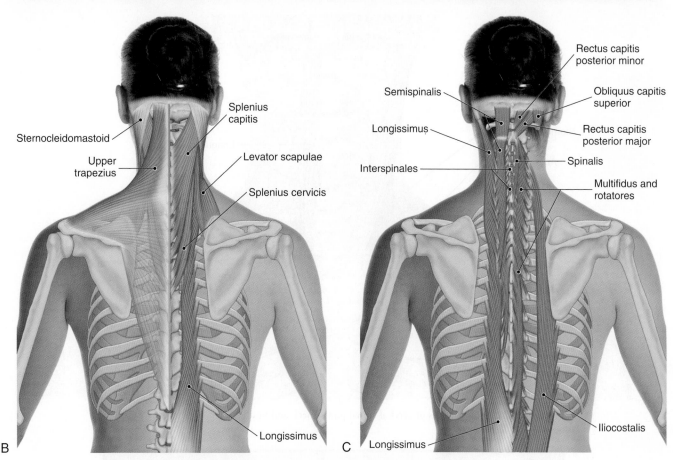

Figure 19-20, cont'd B, Posterior view of neck and head extensors (superficial). The middle and lower trapezius have been ghosted in. **C,** Posterior view of neck and head extensors (deep).

Cervical Spinal (Head and Neck) Joint Extensors

Semispinalis, upper trapezius, splenius capitis, splenius cervicis, levator scapulae, iliocostalis, longissimus, spinalis, sternocleidomastoid, multifidus, rotatores, interspinales, rectus capitis posterior major, rectus capitis posterior minor, obliquus capitis superior

19

Cervical Spinal Joint (Neck and Head) Lateral Flexors

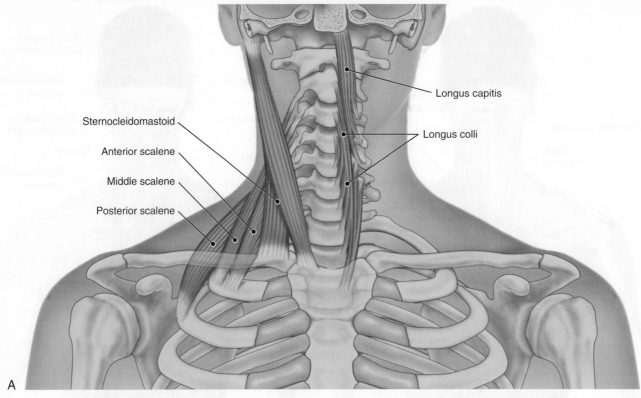

Figure 19-21 Lateral flexors of cervical spinal joints (neck and head). **A,** Anterior view of neck and head lateral flexors.

Cervical Spinal (Head and Neck) Joint Lateral Flexors
Upper trapezius, sternocleidomastoid, semispinalis, anterior scalene, middle scalene, posterior scalene, splenius capitis, splenius cervicis, levator scapulae, longus colli, longus capitis, iliocostalis, longissimus, spinalis, multifidus, rotatores, intertransversarii

Cervical Spinal Joint (Neck and Head) Lateral Flexors—*cont'd*

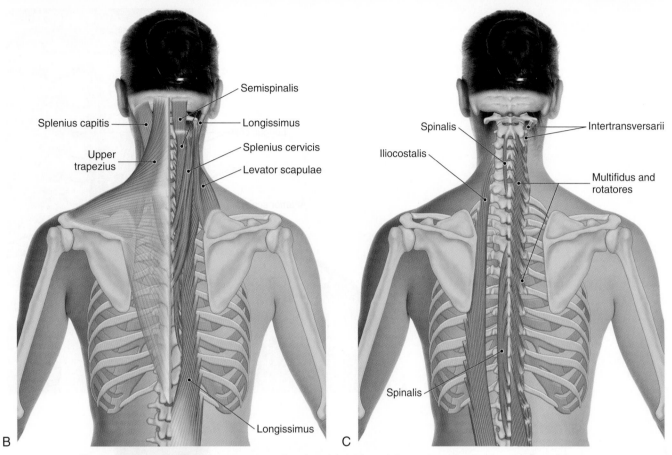

Figure 19-21, cont'd B, Posterior view of neck and head lateral flexors (superficial). The middle and lower trapezius have been ghosted in. **C,** Posterior view of neck and head lateral flexors (deep).

19

Cervical Spinal Joint (Neck and Head) Contralateral Rotators

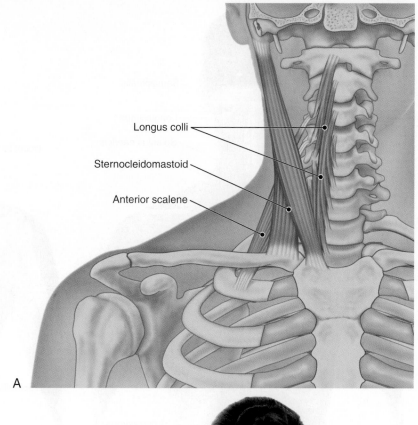

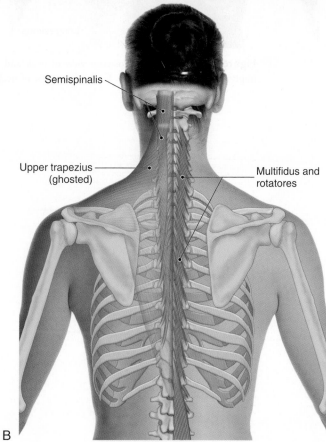

Figure 19-22 Contralateral rotators and ipsilateral rotators of the cervical spinal joints (neck and head). **A,** Anterior view of neck and head contralateral rotators. **B,** Posterior view of neck and head contralateral rotators. The trapezius has been ghosted in.

Cervical Spinal (Head and Neck) Joint Contralateral Rotators
Sternocleidomastoid, upper trapezius, rotatores, multifidus, semispinalis, anterior scalene, longus colli

19

Cervical Spinal Joint (Neck and Head) Ipsilateral Rotators

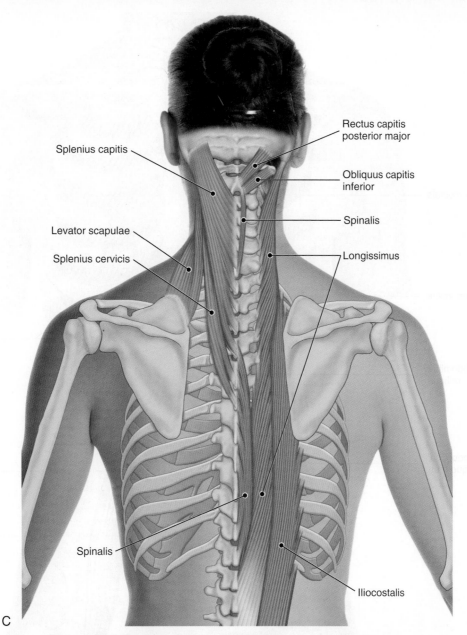

Splenius capitis

Levator scapulae

Splenius cervicis

Spinalis

Rectus capitis posterior major

Obliquus capitis inferior

Spinalis

Longissimus

Iliocostalis

C

Figure 19-22, cont'd C, Posterior view of neck and head ipsilateral rotators.

Cervical Spinal (Head and Neck) Joint Ipsilateral Rotators
Splenius capitis, splenius cervicis, obliquus capitis inferior, rectus capitis posterior major, levator scapulae, longissimus, iliocostalis, spinalis

19

Thoracolumbar Spinal Joint (Trunk) Flexors

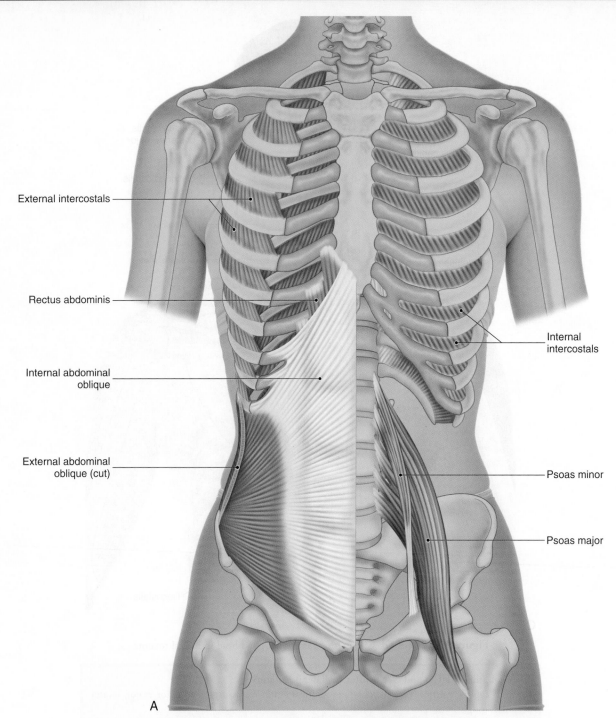

External intercostals

Rectus abdominis

Internal abdominal oblique

External abdominal oblique (cut)

Internal intercostals

Psoas minor

Psoas major

A

Figure 19-23 Flexors and extensors of the thoracolumbar spinal joints (trunk). **A,** Anterior view of trunk flexors.

Thoracolumbar Spinal Joint (Trunk) Flexors
Rectus abdominis, external abdominal oblique, internal abdominal oblique, external intercostals, internal intercostals, psoas major, psoas minor

19

Thoracolumbar Spinal Joint (Trunk) Extensors

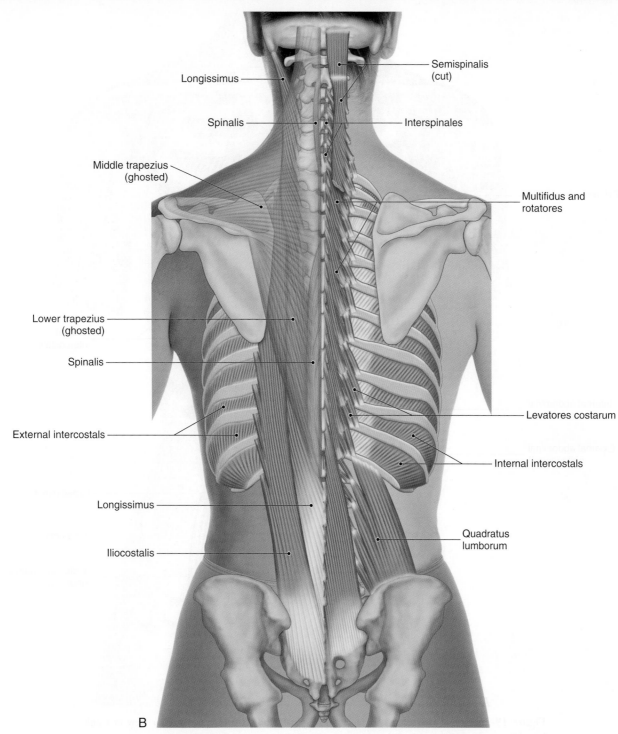

Longissimus

Semispinalis (cut)

Spinalis

Interspinales

Middle trapezius (ghosted)

Multifidus and rotatores

Lower trapezius (ghosted)

Spinalis

Levatores costarum

External intercostals

Internal intercostals

Longissimus

Quadratus lumborum

Iliocostalis

B

Figure 19-23, cont'd B, Posterior view of trunk extensors. The trapezius has been ghosted in. The latissimus dorsi is not pictured.

Thoracolumbar Spinal Joint (Trunk) Extensors
Iliocostalis, longissimus, spinalis, semispinalis, multifidus, rotatores, external intercostals, internal intercostals, quadratus lumborum, middle and lower trapezius, latissimus dorsi (not seen), interspinales, levatores costarum

Thoracolumbar Spinal Joint (Trunk) Lateral Flexors

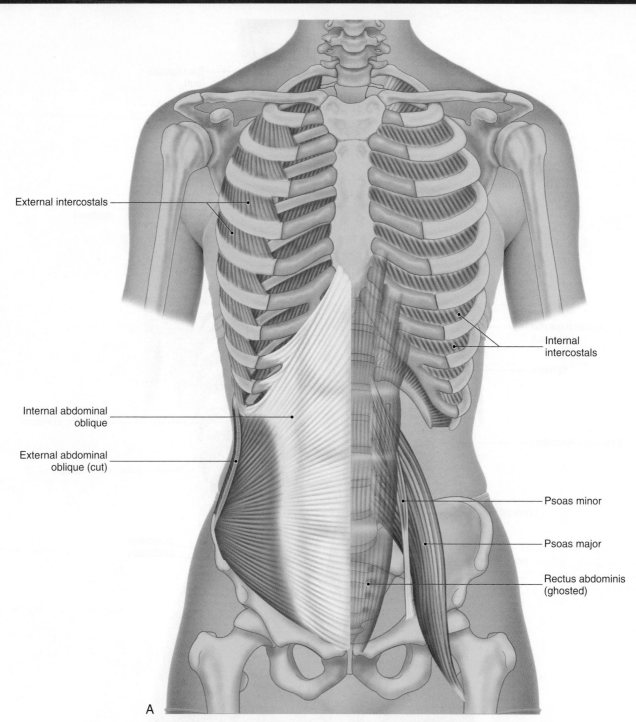

External intercostals

Internal intercostals

Internal abdominal oblique

External abdominal oblique (cut)

Psoas minor

Psoas major

Rectus abdominis (ghosted)

A

Figure 19-24 Lateral view of the thoracolumbar spinal flexors (trunk). **A,** Anterior view of trunk lateral flexors.

Thoracolumbar Spinal Joint (Trunk) Lateral Flexors
Iliocostalis, longissimus, spinalis, external abdominal oblique, internal abdominal oblique, rectus abdominis, external intercostals, internal intercostals, psoas major, psoas minor, quadratus lumborum, semispinalis, multifidus, rotatores, intertransversarii, levatores costarum

Thoracolumbar Spinal Joint (Trunk) Lateral Flexors—*cont'd*

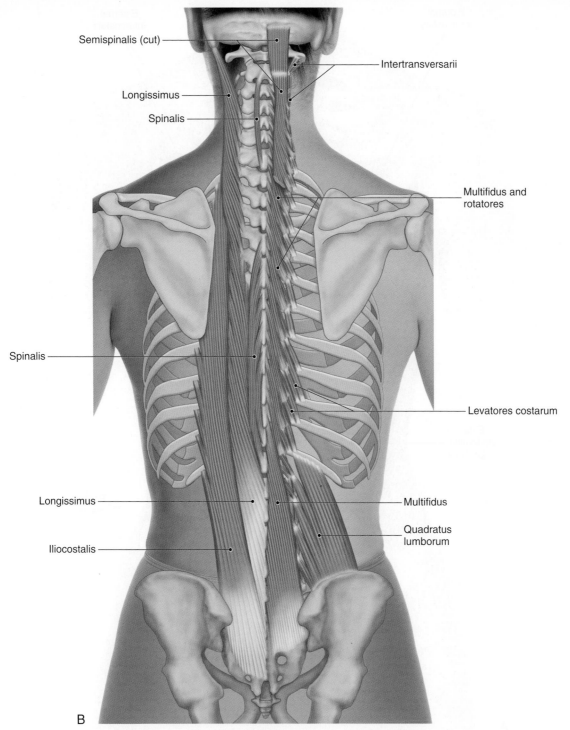

Figure 19-24, cont'd B, Posterior view of trunk lateral flexors.

Thoracolumbar Spinal Joint (Trunk) Contralateral Rotators

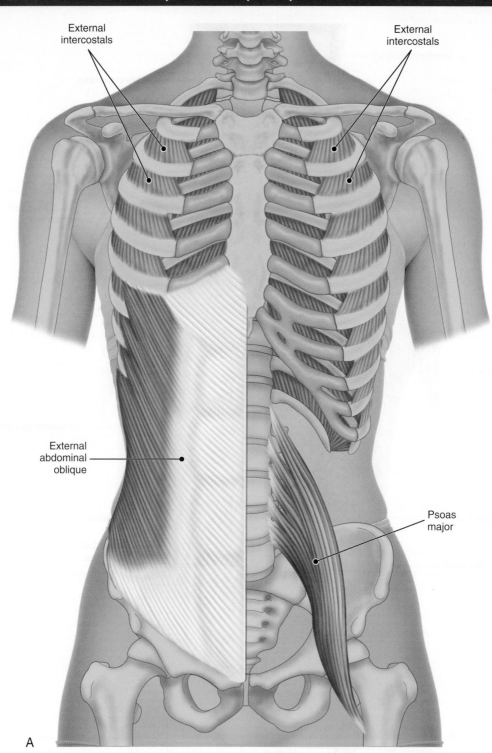

External
intercostals

External
intercostals

External
abdominal
oblique

Psoas
major

A

Figure 19-25 Contralateral rotators and ipsilateral rotators of the thoracolumbar spinal joints (trunk). **A,** Anterior view of trunk contralateral rotators.

> **Thoracolumbar Spinal Joint (Trunk) Contralateral Rotators**
> External abdominal oblique, external intercostals, rotatores, multifidus, semispinalis, psoas major, levatores costarum, rhomboids, serratus posterior superior, serratus posterior inferior

19

Thoracolumbar Spinal Joint (Trunk) Contralateral Rotators—*cont'd*

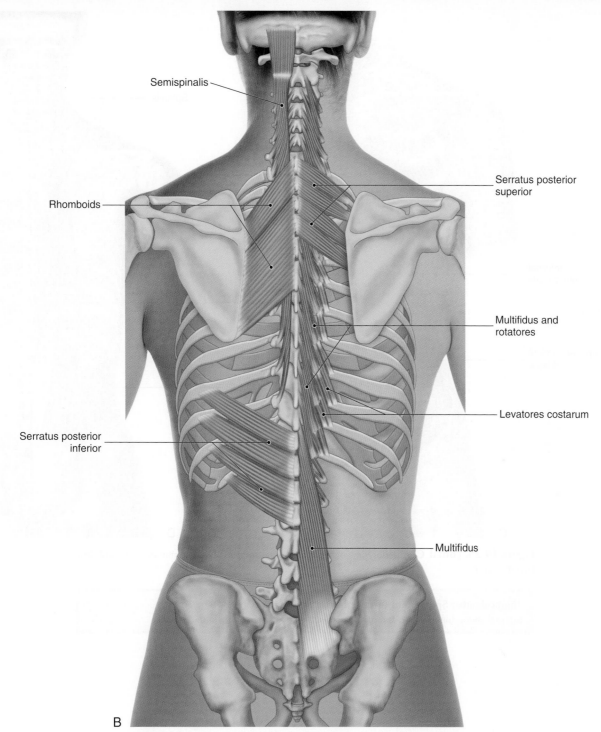

Semispinalis

Rhomboids

Serratus posterior superior

Multifidus and rotatores

Levatores costarum

Serratus posterior inferior

Multifidus

B

Figure 19-25, cont'd B, Posterior view of trunk contralateral rotators.

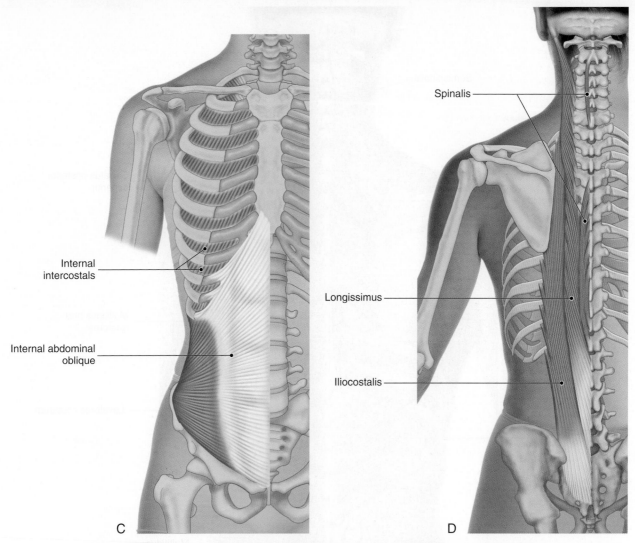

Internal intercostals

Internal abdominal oblique

Spinalis

Longissimus

Iliocostalis

C

D

Figure 19-25, cont'd C, Anterior view of trunk ipsilateral rotators. **D,** Posterior view of trunk ipsilateral rotators.

19

Thoracolumbar Spinal Joint (Trunk) Ipsilateral Rotators
Internal abdominal oblique, internal intercostals, iliocostalis, longissimus, spinalis

FUNCTIONAL MOVER GROUPS: LOWER EXTREMITY
Hip Joint Flexors and Extensors

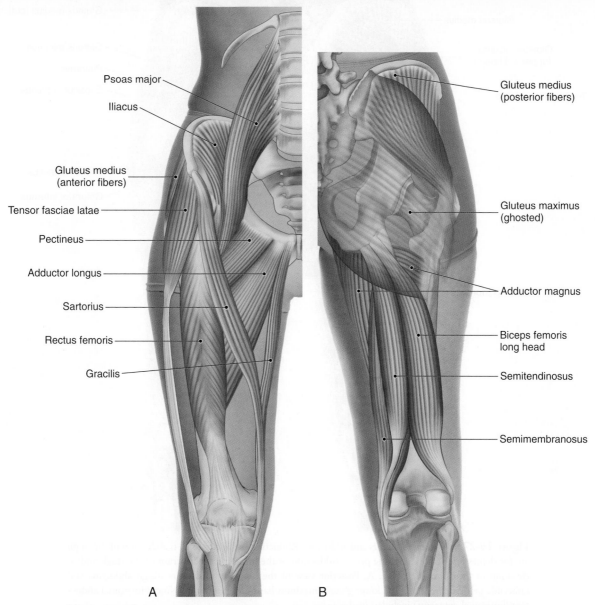

Figure 19-26 Hip joint flexors and extensors. Flexion of the hip joint is flexion of the thigh and/or anterior tilt of the pelvis at the hip joint. Extension of the hip joint is extension of the thigh and/or posterior tilt of the pelvis at the hip joint. **A,** Anterior view of the hip joint flexors (thigh flexors and pelvic anterior tilters). The adductor brevis and gluteus minimus are not pictured. **B,** Posterior view of the hip joint extensors (thigh extensors and pelvic posterior tilters). The gluteus maximus has been ghosted in. The gluteus minimus is not pictured.

Hip Joint Flexors (Thigh Flexors/Pelvis Anterior Tilters)
Psoas major, iliacus, tensor fasciae latae, rectus femoris, sartorius, pectineus, adductor longus, adductor brevis (not seen), gracilis, gluteus medius (anterior fibers), gluteus minimus (anterior fibers) (not seen)

Hip Joint Flexors (Thigh Extensors/Pelvis Posterior Tilters)
Gluteus maximus, semitendinosus, semimembranosus, biceps femoris (long head), adductor magnus, gluteus medius (posterior fibers), gluteus minimus (posterior fibers) (not seen)

19

Hip Joint Abductors (Pelvic Depressors)

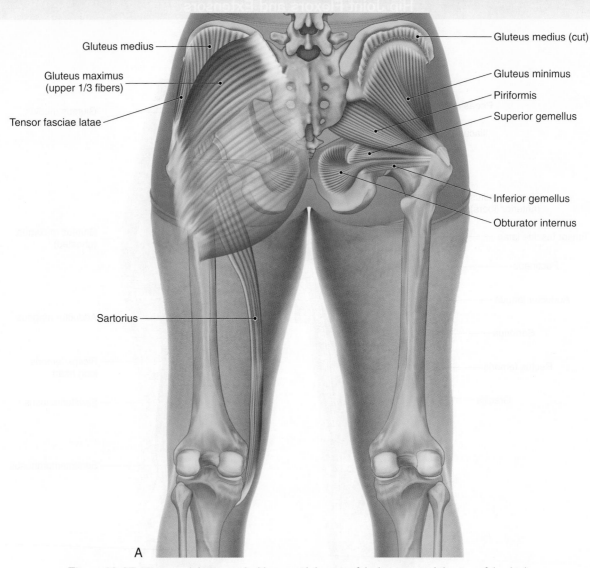

A

Figure 19-27 Hip joint abductors and adductors. Abduction of the hip joint is abduction of the thigh and/or depression of the same-side pelvis. Adduction of the hip joint is adduction of the thigh and/or elevation of the same-side pelvis. **A,** Posterior view of the hip joint abductors (thigh abductors and same-side pelvic depressors). The lower gluteus maximus has been ghosted in. Note: Horizontal abductors (horizontal extensors) included in this list.

Hip Joint Abductors (Thigh Abductors/Ipsilateral Pelvic Depressors)
Gluteus medius, gluteus minimus, gluteus maximus (upper 1/3), tensor fasciae latae, sartorius, piriformis, superior gemellus, obturator internus, inferior gemellus

19

Hip Joint Adductors (Pelvic Elevators)

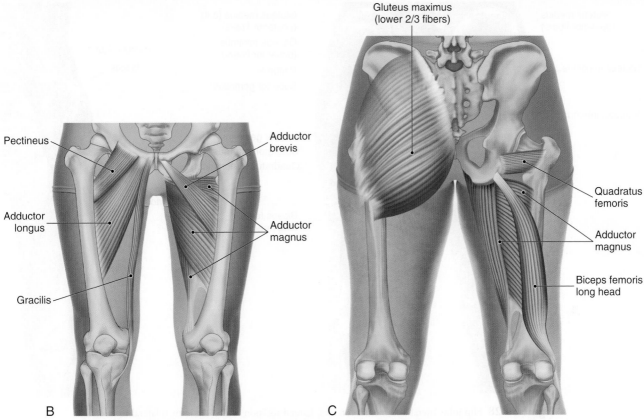

Figure 19-27, cont'd B, Anterior view of the hip joint adductors (thigh adductors and same-side pelvic elevators). **C,** Posterior view of the hip joint adductors (thigh adductors and same-side pelvic elevators). The upper gluteus maximus has been ghosted in.

Hip Joint Adductors (Thigh Adductors/Ipsilateral Pelvic Elevators)

Adductor magnus, adductor longus, adductor brevis, pectineus, gracilis, gluteus maximus (lower 2/3), quadratus femoris, biceps femoris (long head)

19

Hip Joint Lateral Rotators (Pelvic Contralateral Rotators)

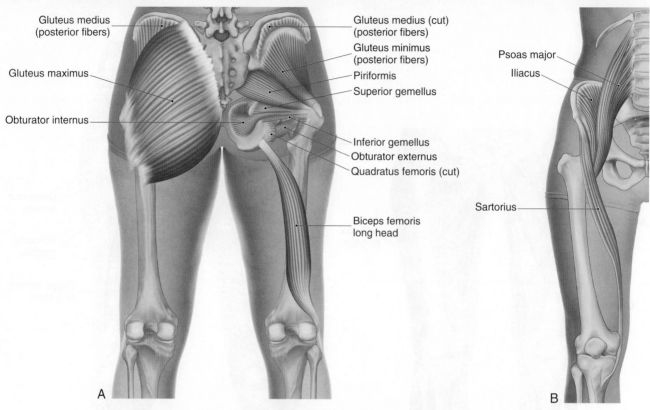

Gluteus medius (posterior fibers)

Gluteus maximus

Obturator internus

Gluteus medius (cut) (posterior fibers)

Gluteus minimus (posterior fibers)

Piriformis

Superior gemellus

Inferior gemellus

Obturator externus

Quadratus femoris (cut)

Biceps femoris long head

Psoas major

Iliacus

Sartorius

A

B

Figure 19-28 Hip joint lateral and medial rotators. Lateral rotation of the hip joint is lateral rotation of the thigh and/or contralateral rotation of the pelvis at the hip joint. Medial rotation of the hip joint is medial rotation of the thigh and/or ipsilateral rotation of the pelvis at the hip joint. **A,** Posterior view of the hip joint lateral rotators (thigh lateral rotators and pelvic contralateral rotators). **B,** Anterior view of the hip joint lateral rotators (thigh lateral rotators and pelvic contralateral rotators).

Hip Joint Lateral Rotators (Thigh Lateral Rotators/Pelvic Contralateral Rotators)
Gluteus maximus, gluteus medius (posterior fibers), gluteus minimus (posterior fibers), piriformis, quadratus femoris, superior gemellus, obturator internus, inferior gemellus, obturator externus, sartorius, psoas major, iliacus, biceps femoris (long head)

19

Hip Joint Medial Rotators (Pelvic Ipsilateral Rotators)

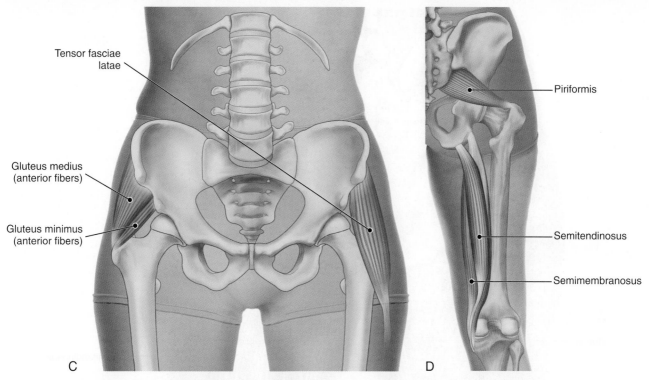

Figure 19-28, cont'd C, Anterior view of the hip joint medial rotators (thigh medial rotators and pelvic ipsilateral rotators). **D,** Posterior view of the hip joint medial rotators (thigh medial rotators and pelvic ipsilateral rotators).

Hip Joint Medial Rotators (Thigh Medial Rotators/Pelvic Ipsilateral Rotators)
Gluteus medius (anterior fibers), gluteus minimus (anterior fibers), tensor fasciae latae, piriformis, semitendinosus, semimembranosus

19

Knee Joint Flexors

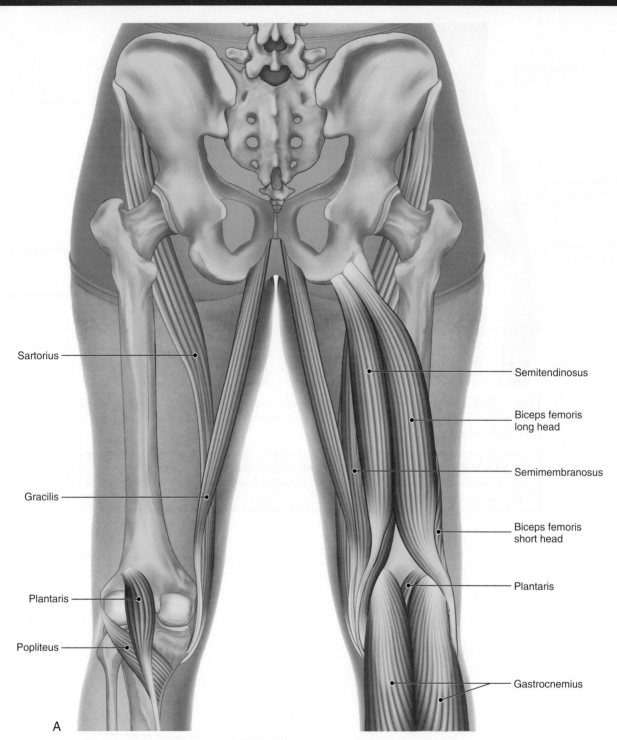

Sartorius

Semitendinosus

Biceps femoris
long head

Semimembranosus

Gracilis

Biceps femoris
short head

Plantaris

Plantaris

Popliteus

Gastrocnemius

A

Figure 19-29 Flexors and extensors of the knee joint. **A,** Posterior view of the knee joint flexors.

Knee Joint Flexors
Semitendinosus, semimembranosus, biceps femoris, sartorius, gracilis, popliteus, gastrocnemius, plantaris

19

Knee Joint Extensors

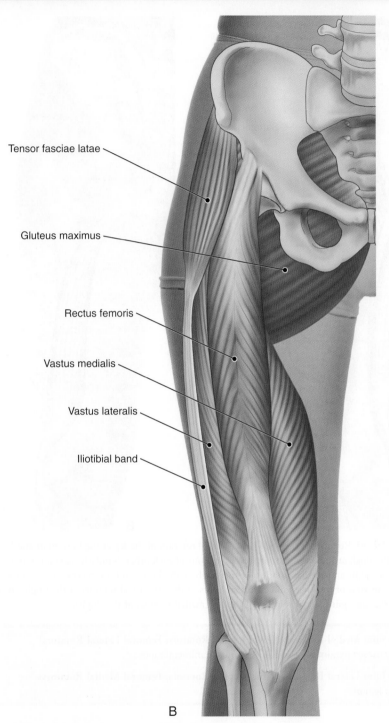

Tensor fasciae latae

Gluteus maximus

Rectus femoris

Vastus medialis

Vastus lateralis

Iliotibial band

B

Figure 19-29, cont'd B, Anterior view of the knee joint extensors. The vastus intermedius is not pictured.

Knee Joint Extensors
Rectus femoris, vastus lateralis, vastus medialis, vastus intermedius (not seen), tensor fasciae latae, gluteus maximus

19

Knee Joint Medial and Lateral Rotators

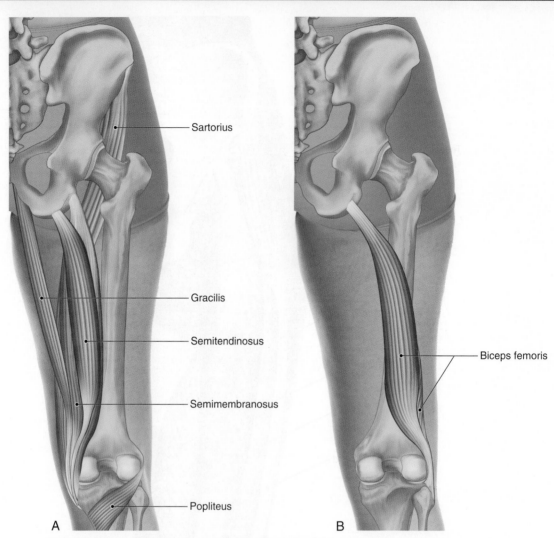

Sartorius

Gracilis

Semitendinosus

Semimembranosus

Biceps femoris

Popliteus

A

B

Figure 19-30 Rotators of the knee joint. Medial rotation of the leg at the knee joint and lateral rotation of the thigh at the knee joint are reverse actions of each other. Similarly, lateral rotation of the leg at the knee joint and medial rotation of the thigh at the knee joint are reverse actions of each other. **A,** Posterior view of the knee joint medial rotators of the leg (lateral rotators of the thigh). **B,** Posterior view of the knee joint lateral rotators of the leg (medial rotators of the thigh).

Knee Joint Medial Rotators (Tibial Medial Rotators; Femoral Lateral Rotators)
Popliteus, semitendinosus, gracilis, sartorius, semimembranosus

Knee Joint Lateral Rotators (Tibial Lateral Rotators; Femoral Medial Rotators)
Biceps femoris

19

Ankle Joint Dorsiflexors and Plantarflexors

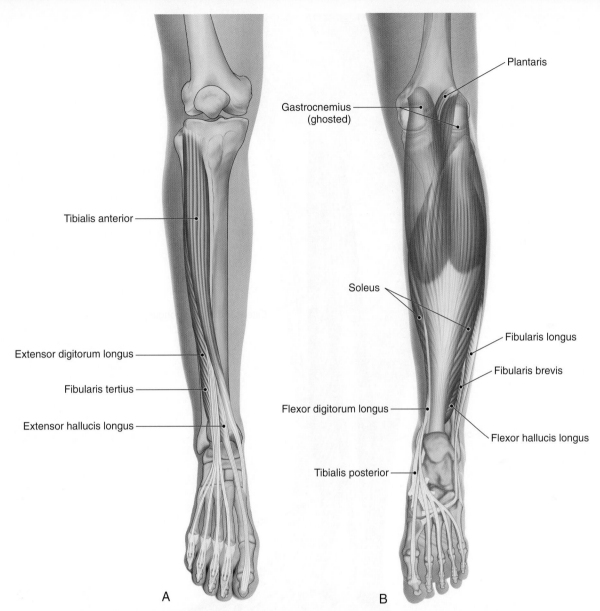

Figure 19-31 Dorsiflexors and plantarflexors of the ankle joint. **A,** Anterior view of the ankle joint dorsiflexors. **B,** Posterior view of the ankle joint plantarflexors. The gastrocnemius has been ghosted in.

Ankle Joint Dorsiflexors
Tibialis anterior, extensor digitorum longus, fibularis tertius, extensor hallucis longus

Ankle Joint Plantarflexors
Gastrocnemius, soleus, plantaris, tibialis posterior, flexor digitorum longus, flexor hallucis longus, fibularis longus, fibularis brevis

19

Subtalar Joint Pronators (Everters)

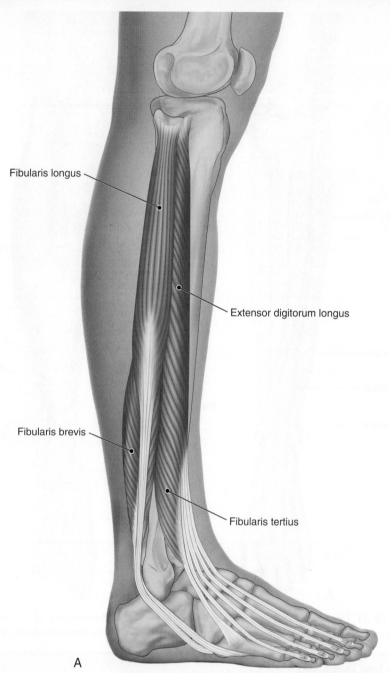

A

Figure 19-32 Pronators and supinators of the subtalar joint. Note: Eversion is the principle component of pronation; inversion is the principle component of supination. **A,** Lateral view of the subtalar joint pronators (everters).

Subtalar Joint Pronators (Everters)
Fibularis longus, fibularis brevis, fibularis tertius, extensor digitorum longus

19

Subtalar Joint Supinators (Inverters)

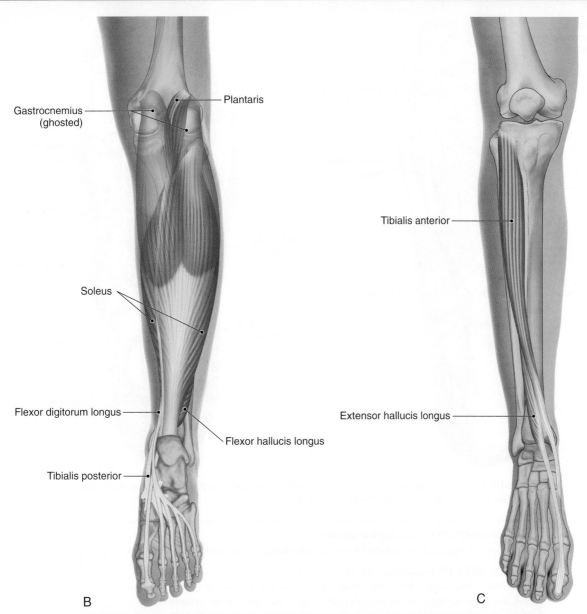

Gastrocnemius (ghosted)

Plantaris

Soleus

Flexor digitorum longus

Flexor hallucis longus

Tibialis posterior

Tibialis anterior

Extensor hallucis longus

B

C

19

Figure 19-32, cont'd B, Posterior view of the subtalar joint supinators (inverters). The gastrocnemius has been ghosted in. **C,** Anterior view of the subtalar joint supinators (inverters)

Subtalar Joint Supinators (Inverters)
Tibialis anterior, tibialis posterior, extensor hallucis longus, flexor digitorum longus, flexor hallucis longus, gastrocnemius, soleus, plantaris

Toe Flexors

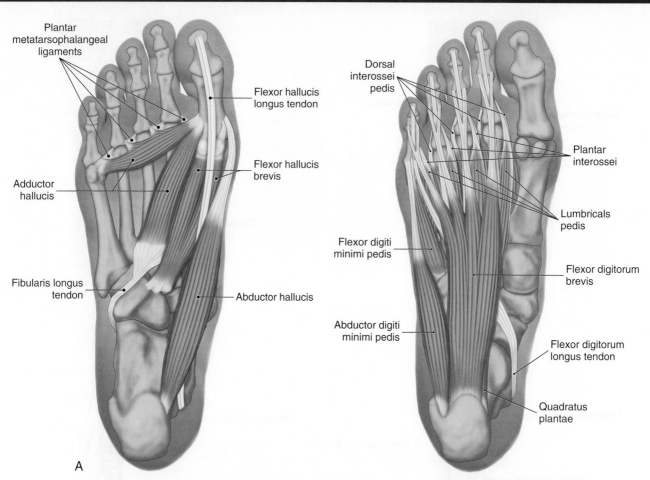

Figure 19-33 Flexors of the five toes at the metatarsophalangeal and interphalangeal joints. **A,** Plantar view of the flexors of the big toe. **B,** Plantar view of the flexors of toes two through five.

Toe Joint (MTP, IP) Flexors (big toe: toe #1)
Flexor hallucis longus, flexor hallucis brevis, adductor hallucis, abductor hallucis

Toe Joint (MTP, IP) Flexors (toes #2-5)
Flexor digitorum longus, flexor digitorum brevis, quadratus plantae, flexor digiti minimi pedis, abductor digiti minimi pedis, lumbricals pedis, plantar interossei, dorsal interossei pedis

Toe Extensors

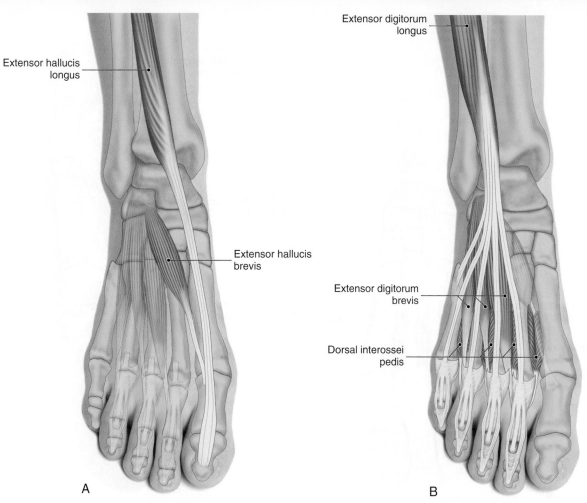

Extensor hallucis longus

Extensor digitorum longus

Extensor hallucis brevis

Extensor digitorum brevis

Dorsal interossei pedis

A

B

Figure 19-34 Extensors of the five toes at the metatarsophalangeal and interphalangeal joints. **A,** Plantar view of the extensors of the big toe. The extensor digitorum brevis has been ghosted in. **B,** Dorsal view of the extensors of toes two through five. The abductor hallucis brevis has been ghosted in. The lumbricals pedis and plantar interossei are not pictured.

Toe Joint (MTP, IP) Extensors (big toe: toe #1)
Extensor hallucis longus, extensor hallucis brevis

Toe Joint (MTP, IP) Extensors (toes #2-5)
Extensor digitorum longus, extensor digitorum brevis, dorsal interossei pedis, lumbricals pedis (not seen), plantar interossei (not seen)

19

Toe Abductors and Adductors

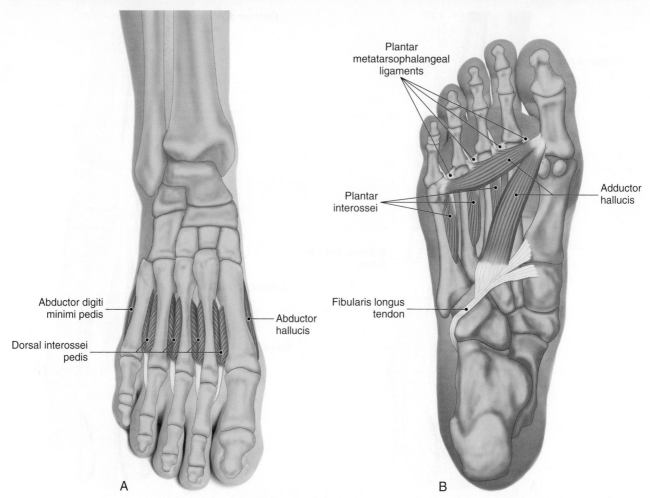

Figure 19-35 Abductors and adductors of the five toes at the metatarsophalangeal joints. **A,** Dorsal view of the toe abductors. **B,** Plantar view of the toe adductors.

Toe Joint (MTP) Abductors (toes #1-5)
Dorsal interossei pedis, abductor hallucis, abductor digiti minimi pedis

Toe Joint (MTP) Adductors (toes #1-5)
Plantar interossei, adductor hallucis

19

MUSCLES OF THE PELVIC FLOOR
Medial Views of the Pelvic Floor

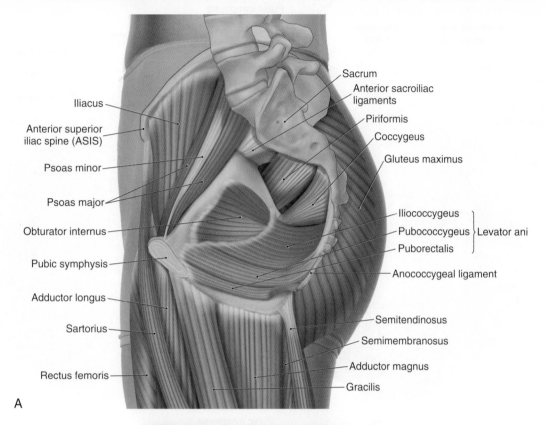

Iliacus
Anterior superior
iliac spine (ASIS)
Psoas minor
Psoas major
Obturator internus
Pubic symphysis
Adductor longus
Sartorius
Rectus femoris

Sacrum
Anterior sacroiliac
ligaments
Piriformis
Coccygeus
Gluteus maximus
Iliococcygeus
Pubococcygeus } Levator ani
Puborectalis
Anococcygeal ligament
Semitendinosus
Semimembranosus
Adductor magnus
Gracilis

A

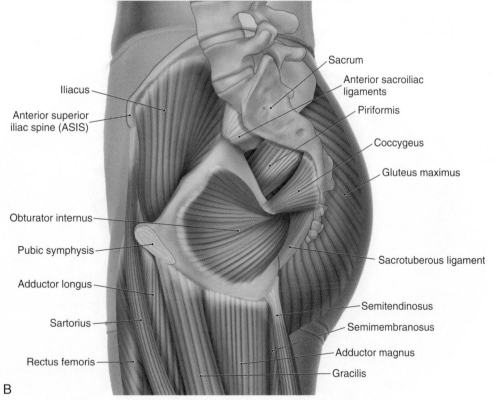

Iliacus
Anterior superior
iliac spine (ASIS)
Obturator internus
Pubic symphysis
Adductor longus
Sartorius
Rectus femoris

Sacrum
Anterior sacroiliac
ligaments
Piriformis
Coccygeus
Gluteus maximus
Sacrotuberous ligament
Semitendinosus
Semimembranosus
Adductor magnus
Gracilis

B

Figure 19-36 Medial views of the muscles of the right side of the pelvis. **A,** Superficial view. **B,** Deep view.

Superior Views of the Pelvic Floor

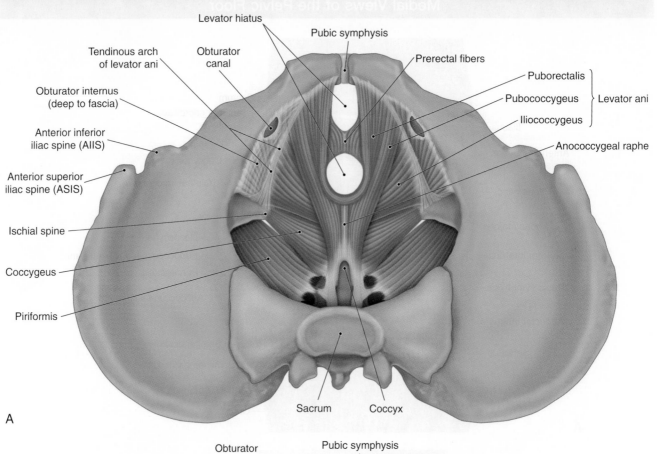

A

Levator hiatus
Pubic symphysis
Tendinous arch of levator ani
Obturator canal
Prerectal fibers
Obturator internus (deep to fascia)
Puborectalis
Pubococcygeus — Levator ani
Iliococcygeus
Anterior inferior iliac spine (AIIS)
Anterior superior iliac spine (ASIS)
Anococcygeal raphe
Ischial spine
Coccygeus
Piriformis
Sacrum
Coccyx

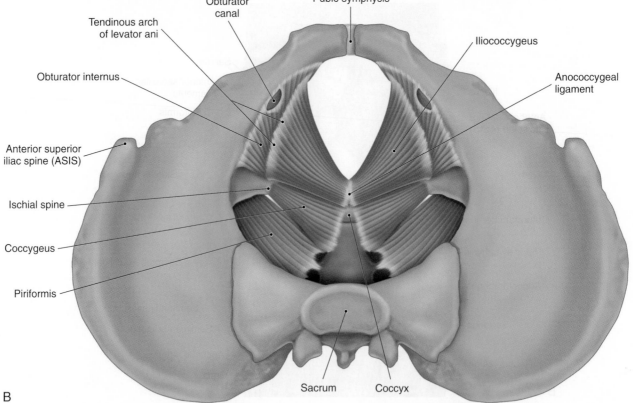

B

Obturator canal
Pubic symphysis
Tendinous arch of levator ani
Obturator internus
Iliococcygeus
Anococcygeal ligament
Anterior superior iliac spine (ASIS)
Ischial spine
Coccygeus
Piriformis
Sacrum
Coccyx

Figure 19-37 Superior views of the muscles of the female pelvic floor. **A,** Superficial view. **B,** Deep view.

19

Inferior Views of the Pelvic Floor

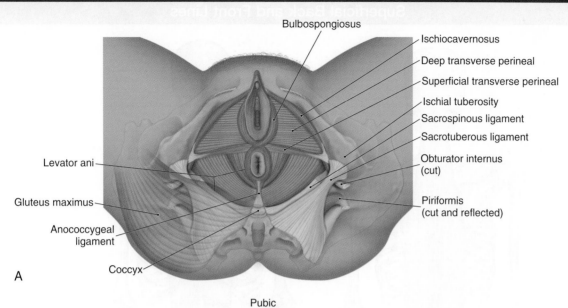

Bulbospongiosus
Ischiocavernosus
Deep transverse perineal
Superficial transverse perineal
Ischial tuberosity
Sacrospinous ligament
Sacrotuberous ligament
Obturator internus (cut)
Piriformis (cut and reflected)
Levator ani
Gluteus maximus
Anococcygeal ligament
Coccyx

A

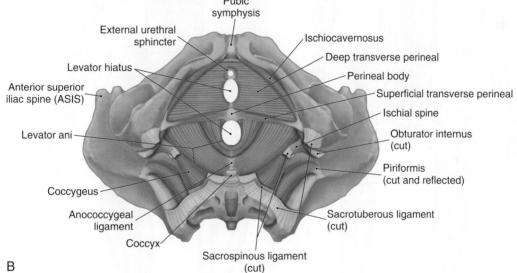

Pubic symphysis
External urethral sphincter
Ischiocavernosus
Levator hiatus
Deep transverse perineal
Perineal body
Anterior superior iliac spine (ASIS)
Superficial transverse perineal
Ischial spine
Levator ani
Obturator internus (cut)
Piriformis (cut and reflected)
Coccygeus
Anococcygeal ligament
Coccyx
Sacrotuberous ligament (cut)
Sacrospinous ligament (cut)

B

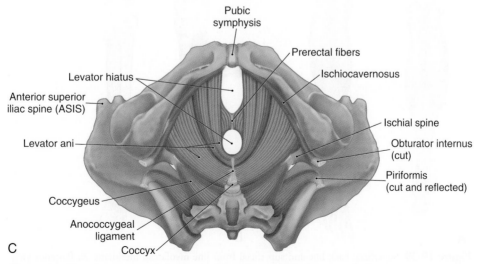

Pubic symphysis
Prerectal fibers
Levator hiatus
Ischiocavernosus
Anterior superior iliac spine (ASIS)
Ischial spine
Levator ani
Obturator internus (cut)
Piriformis (cut and reflected)
Coccygeus
Anococcygeal ligament
Coccyx

C

Figure 19-38 Inferior views of the muscles of the female pelvic floor. **A,** Superficial view. The gluteus maximus has been ghosted in on the right. **B,** Intermediate view. **C,** Deep view.

19

MYOFASCIAL MERIDIANS
Superficial Back and Front Lines

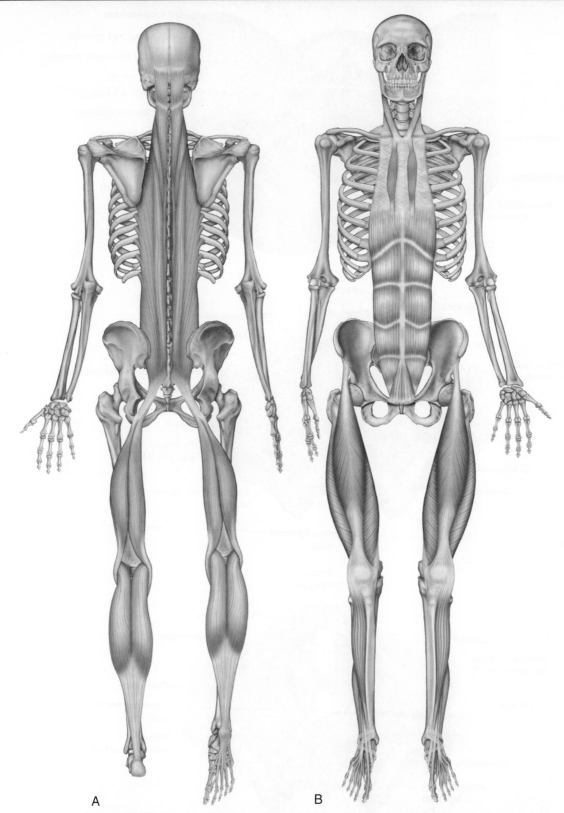

Figure 19-39 Superficial back line and superficial front line myofascial meridians. **A,** Posterior view of the superficial back line. **B,** Anterior view of the superficial front line. (From Myers TW: *Anatomy trains: myofascial meridians for manual and movement therapists,* ed. 2. Edinburgh, 2009, Churchill Livingstone.)

A

B

19

Lateral and Deep Front Lines

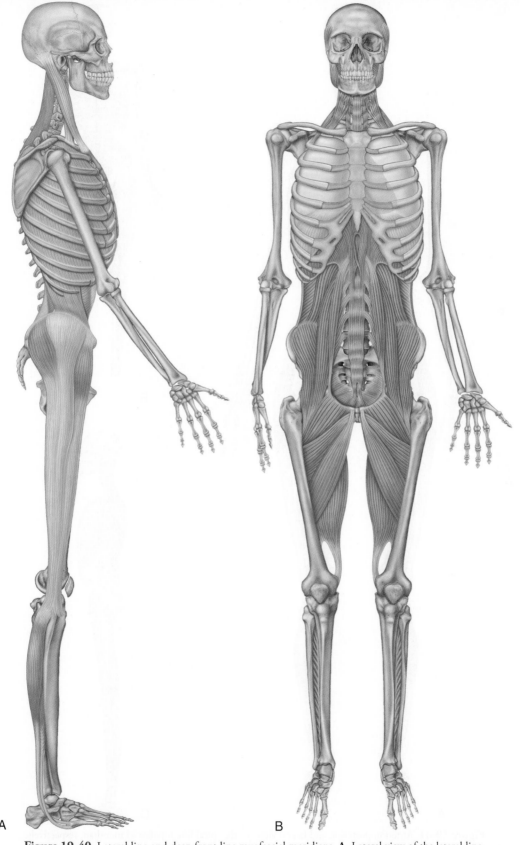

A   B

Figure 19-40 Lateral line and deep front line myofascial meridians. **A,** Lateral view of the lateral line. **B,** Anterior view of the deep front line. (From Myers TW: *Anatomy trains: myofascial meridians for manual and movement therapists*, ed. 2. Edinburgh, 2009, Churchill Livingstone.)

19

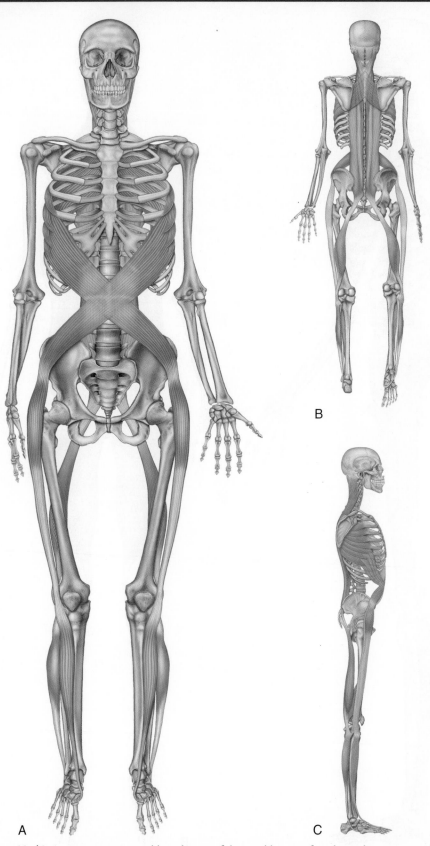

A

B

C

Figure 19-41 Anterior, posterior, and lateral views of the spiral line myofascial meridian, respectively. (From Myers TW: *Anatomy trains: myofascial meridians for manual and movement therapists*, ed. 2. Edinburgh, 2009, Churchill Livingstone.)

Arm Lines

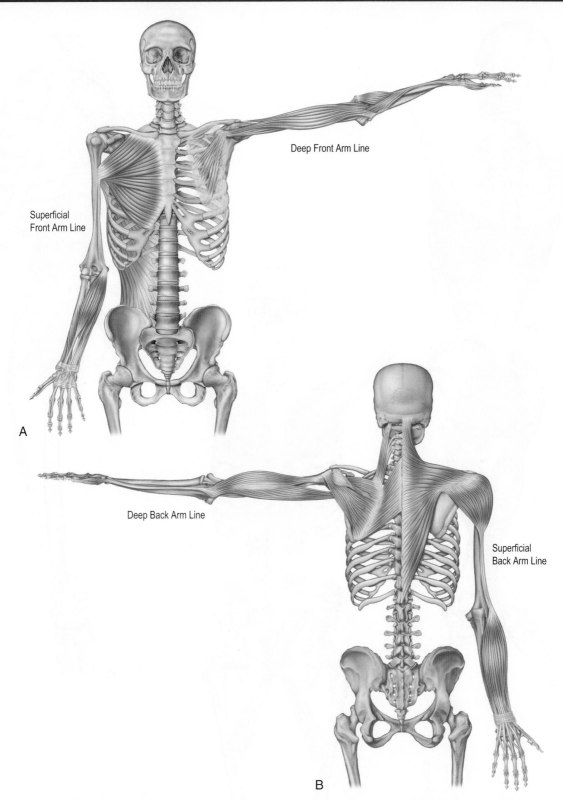

Deep Front Arm Line

Superficial
Front Arm Line

A

Deep Back Arm Line

Superficial
Back Arm Line

B

Figure 19-42 Arm line myofascial meridians. **A,** Anterior view of the superficial and deep front arm lines. **B,** Posterior view of the superficial and deep back arm lines. (From Myers TW: *Anatomy trains: myofascial meridians for manual and movement therapists*, ed. 2. Edinburgh, 2009, Churchill Livingstone.)

19

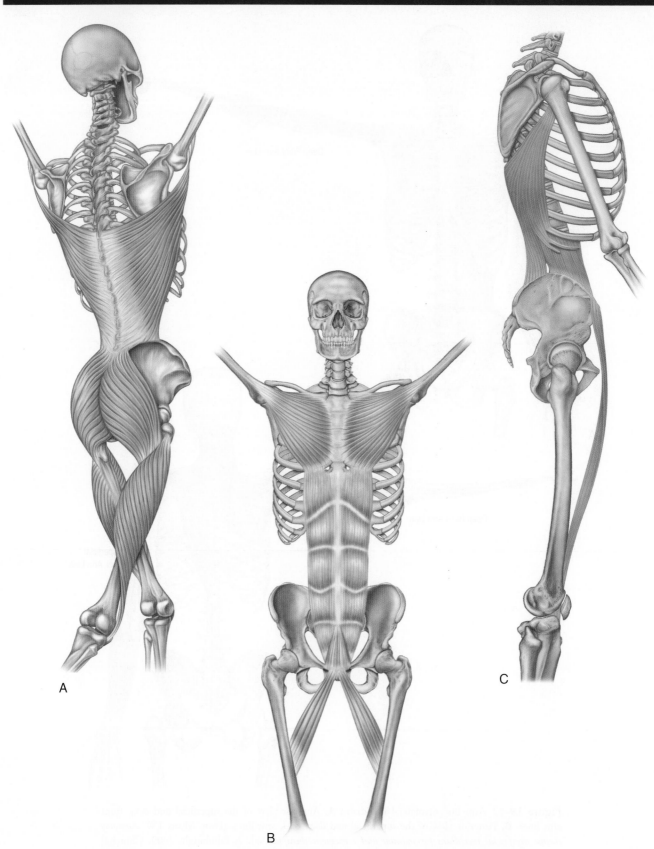

A

B

C

Figure 19-43 Functional line myofascial meridians. **A,** posterolateral view of the back functional line. **B,** Anterior view of the front functional line. **C,** Lateral view of the ipsilateral functional line. (From Myers TW: *Anatomy trains: myofascial meridians for manual and movement therapists*, ed. 2. Edinburgh, 2009, Churchill Livingstone.)

Aaberg E: *Muscle mechanics*, ed 2, Champaign, IL, 2006, Human Kinetics.

Abrahams PH, Marks Jr SC, Hutchings RT: *McMinn's color atlas of human anatomy*, ed 5, Edinburgh, 2003, Mosby.

Anderson JE: *Grant's atlas of anatomy*, ed 7, Baltimore, 1980, Williams & Wilkins.

Atlas of anatomy, Germany, 2005, Thieme.

Bandy WD, Reese NB: *Joint range of motion and muscle length testing*, Philadelphia, 2002, Saunders.

Basmajian JV, De Luca CJ: *Muscles alive: their functions revealed by electromyography*, ed 5, Baltimore, 1985, Williams & Wilkins.

Biel A: *Trail guide to the body*, ed 3, Boulder, CO, 2005, Books of Discovery.

Bisschop P, Ombregt L: *Atlas of orthopedic examination of the peripheral joints*, Edinburgh, 1999, Saunders.

Burkel WE, Woodburne RT: *Essentials of human anatomy*, ed 9, New York, 1994, Oxford University Press.

Cailliet R: *Neck and arm pain*, ed 2, Philadelphia, 2001, F.A. Davis Company.

Calais-Germain B: *Anatomy of movement*, Seattle, 1993, Eastland Press, Inc.

Chaitow L: *Palpation and assessment skills*, ed 2, Edinburgh, 2003, Churchill Livingstone.

Cipriano JJ: *Photographic manual of regional orthopaedic and neurological tests*, ed 4, Philadelphia, 2003, Williams & Wilkins.

Clay JH, Pounds DM: *Basic clinical massage therapy*, ed 2, Philadelphia, 2008, Williams & Wilkins.

Clemente CD: *Clemente anatomy*, ed 4, Philadelphia, 1997, Williams & Wilkins.

Cohen BJ: *Structure and function of the human body*, ed 8, Philadelphia, 2005, Williams & Wilkins.

Cramer GD, Darby SA: *Basic and clinical anatomy of the spine, spinal cord and ANS*, St. Louis, 1995, Mosby.

Deutsch H, Hamilton N, Luttgens K: *Kinesiology: scientific basis of human motion*, ed 8, Madison, WI, 1992, WCB.

Dixon M: *Joint play the right way: axial skeleton*, Port Moody, BC, 2006, Arthrokinetic Publishing.

Dixon M: *Joint play the right way: for the peripheral skeleton*, Port Moody, BC, 2003, Arthrokinetic Publishing.

Enoka RM: *Neuromechanics of human movement*, ed 3, Champaign, IL, 2002, Human Kinetics.

Field D, Palastanga N, Soames R: *Anatomy and human movement*, ed 4, Oxford, 2002, Butterworth Heinemann.

Findley TW, Schleip R: *Fascia research: basic science and implications for conventional and complementary health care*, Munich, Germany, 2007, Elsevier.

Frankel VH, Nordin M: *Basic biomechanics of the musculoskeletal system*, ed 3, Philadelphia, 2001, Williams & Wilkins.

Gardiner PF, MacIntosh BR, McComas AJ: *Skeletal muscle: form and function*, ed 2, Champaign, IL, 2006, Human Kinetics.

Gosling JA, Harris PF, Whitmore I, Willan PLT: *Human anatomy: color atlas and text*, ed 4, Edinburgh, 2002, Mosby.

Gray's anatomy for students, New York, 2005, Churchill Livingstone.

Gray's anatomy, ed 39, New York, 2005, Churchill Livingstone.

Greene DP, Roberts SL: *Kinesiology: movement in the context of activity*, ed 2, St. Louis, 2005, Elsevier.

Gunn C: *Bones & joints: a guide for students*, ed 4, Edinburgh, 2002, Churchill Livingstone.

Hamill J, Knutzen JM: *Biomechanical basis of human movement*, ed 2, Philadelphia, 2003, Williams & Wilkins.

Hoppenfeld S: *Physical examination of the spine and extremities*, New York, 1976, Appleton-Century-Crofts.

Jenkins DB: *Hollinshead's functional anatomy of the limbs and back*, ed 8, Philadelphia, 2002, Saunders.

Juhan D: *Job's body: a handbook for bodywork*, New York, 1987, Station Hill Press.

Kapandji IA: *The physiology of the joints*, vol 1, ed 5, Edinburgh, 2002, Churchill Livingstone.

Kapandji IA: *The physiology of the joints*, vol 3, ed 2, Edinburgh, 1980, Churchill Livingstone.

Kendall FP, McCreary EK, Provance PG: *Muscles: testing and function*, ed 4, Baltimore, 1993, Williams & Wilkins.

Lehmkuhl LD, Smith LK, Weiss EL: *Brunnstrom's clinical kinesiology*, ed 5, Philadelphia, 1996, F.A. Davis Company.

Levangie PK, Norkin CC: *Joint structure and function: a comprehensive analysis*, ed 3, Philadelphia, 2001, F.A. Davis Company.

Lieber RL: *Skeletal muscle, structure, function & plasticity*, ed 2, Baltimore, 2002, Lippincott Williams & Wilkins.

Lowe W: *Orthopedic assessment in massage therapy*, Sisters, OR, 2006, Daviau Scott Publishers.

Ludwig L, Rattray F: *Clinical massage therapy: understanding, assessing and treating over 70 conditions*, Toronto, 2000, Talus, Inc.

Lutjen-Drecoll E, Rohen JW, Yokochi C: *Color atlas of anatomy: a photographic study of the human body*, ed 5, Philadelphia, 2002, Williams & Wilkins.

Magee DJ: *Orthopedic physical assessment*, ed 4, Philadelphia, 2002, Saunders.

Mense S, Simons DG: *Muscle pain: understanding its nature, diagnosis, and treatment*, Baltimore, 2001, Williams & Wilkins.

Muscolino JE: *Kinesiology: the skeletal system and muscle function*, St. Louis, 2006, Mosby.

Muscolino JE: *The muscle and bone palpation manual*, St. Louis, MO, 2009, Mosby.

Myers TM: *Anatomy trains*, ed 2, New York, 2009, Churchill Livingstone.

Netter FH: *Atlas of human anatomy*, ed 3, Teterboro, NJ, 2003, ICON Learning Systems.

Neumann DA: *Kinesiology of the musculoskeletal system: foundations for physical rehabilitation*, St. Louis, 2002, Mosby.

Norkin CC, White DJ: *Measurement of join motion: a guide to goniometry*, ed 3, Philadelphia, 2003, F.A. Davis Company.

Oatis CA: *Kinesiology: the mechanics & pathomechanics of human movement*, Philadelphia, 2004, Williams & Wilkins.

Olson TR: *A.D.A.M. student atlas of anatomy*, Baltimore, 1996, Williams & Wilkins.

Patton KT, Thibodeau GA: *Anatomy & physiology*, ed 5, St. Louis, 2003, Mosby.

Simons DG, Travell JG: *Myofascial pain and dysfunction: the trigger point manual – the lower extremities*, vol 2, Baltimore, 1999, Williams & Wilkins.

Simons DG, Travell JG: *Myofascial pain and dysfunction: the trigger point manual – the upper half of the body*, vol 1, Baltimore, 1999, Williams & Wilkins.

Stone JA, Stone RJ: *Atlas of skeletal muscles*, ed 4, Boston, 2003, McGraw-Hill.

Tixa S: *Atlas of palpatory anatomy of limbs and trunk*, Teterboro, NJ, 2003, ICON Learning Systems.

Warfel JH: *The extremities*, ed 4, Philadelphia, 1981, Lea & Febiger.

Warfel JH: *The head, neck and trunk*, ed 4, Philadelphia, 1978, Lea & Febiger.

Watkins J: *Structure and function of the musculoskeletal system*, Champaign, IL, 1999, Human Kinetics.

White TD: *Human osteology*, ed 2, San Diego, 2000, Academic Press.

A

Page numbers followed by f indicate figures; t, tables; b, boxes.